Urothelial Malignan
Urinary Tract

Majid Eshghi
Editor

Urothelial Malignancies of the Upper Urinary Tract

A Textbook of Step by Step Management

Springer

Editor
Majid Eshghi, MD, FACS, MBA
Chief, Section of Endourology and
Minimally Invasive Urology
Westchester Medical Health Network
Valhalla, NY
USA

and

Professor, Department of Urology
New York Medical College
Valhalla, NY
USA

Additional material to this book can be downloaded from http://extras.springer.com.

ISBN 978-3-030-09597-0 ISBN 978-3-319-51263-1 (eBook)
https://doi.org/10.1007/978-3-319-51263-1

Printed on acid-free paper

This Springer imprint is published by the registered company Springer International Publishing AG part of Springer Nature
The registered company address is: Gewerbestrasse 11, 6330 Cham, Switzerland

To the memory of my parents,
They taught me first, they taught me best

To my wife Rosemary for her patience, advice, support and care through the hard years of training

To MY Fab Four: Maryam, Amanda, Cyrus, Blaise
They are the heart, soul, breath and light of my life

To my Mentor Arthur D. Smith
From him I learned the five p's of urology:
Passion, Perfection, Presence, Presentation, Publication
He led and we followed

To Moneer Hanna
Who taught me the principles of good surgery applies to all ages.

To the memory of my friends and colleagues from the pioneering days of Endourology
Joseph Segura, Ed Lyon, Steven Stream

My gratitude to all the patients who put their faith and trust in me to care for them

Special thanks to Carla McDonnell for all her help in preparing this book.

Prologue

The evolution in the treatment of upper tract urothelial carcinoma has for many years been overshadowed by the concentrated efforts toward diagnosis and treatment of urothelial carcinoma of the bladder. The upper tract was inadvertently regarded a subsidiary or an orphan child with mostly limited treatment options such as nephroureterectomy or segmental ureterectomy. Many distinguished periodicals, monthlies, e-pubs and *urozines* addressed the genetic studies, chemotherapy, and in more recent times, laparoscopic partial and total nephrectomy primarily for renal cell carcinoma and the *vital aqueduct* of the urinary tract remained to play a second fiddle.

After enduring many years of *inadequate* attention, with rapid development of endourology and minimally invasive techniques, urothelial carcinoma of the upper tract is being addressed with as much intensity as bladder carcinoma and at last this orphan child is coming of age.

Once the book's research process started many ideas, formats, and names flashed through my mind. I was convinced a systematic step-by-step approach would be the best route rather a mix bag of the usual journal article type of chapters. The basic principles to the most sophisticated management protocols would be described with the aim of being informative and with necessary details to allow readers to apply and incorporate them into their practice. At times parts of the texts take the form of a guide or manual to provide specifics to guide treating physicians who may want to consider such approaches. Considering that the upper tract may be virgin territory, in comparison to the bladder urothelial carcinoma, the number of definitive, evidence-based references are rather sparse and anecdotal at times due to paucity of such material in literature. In other areas such as imaging, basic science and laboratory research data are as strong as bladder urothelial carcinoma.

Conservative protocols of the upper tract urothelial carcinoma still remain controversial during the transitional phases and introduction of new modalities. The data in this book reflects partly existing literature as well as authors' choice and preferred approach. The text is a panorama of data, ideas, preference, techniques and individual choices by physician and at times desired by patients.

While formatting this text I initially struggled with two ideas: How to fill a whole book with just this one subject? Versus: With so much to say how can I limit myself to 35 sections. I quickly realized the latter being the harder of the two tasks. By reviewing the contents, the readers will realize that this text starts with the very basics of UTUC, covers specifics of prognostic factors, economics of preserving the kidneys, imaging, instruments, endoscopic, open and laparoscopic treatments. Conservative treatment is covered with several detailed section and followed by ancillary treatments. The section on case studies provides an actual review of variety of modalities discussed reflecting a timeline with a glimpse of the future at the end.

I consider myself unfortunate not to have every well-known or lesser-known expert to contribute to this book. That was not by choice rather due to circumstances such as their unavailability, other commitments, decline, or my unintentional negligence in not reaching out. I am indebted to more than 50 contributors from 25 outstanding academic departments and centers who unselfishly devoted hours of their valuable time to share their knowledge and expertise with no rewards and to only benefit their present and future colleagues, the field of urology and ultimately our patients who trust us with their most valuable asset: their health. I am humbled and grateful for their generosity.

Like most project as we neared the publication I felt the need to revise or update many sections which would leave us with a project that will never end. The future publications will carry that burden. Many magnificent texts have been written on the subject of urothelial carcinoma by divas and divos of urology. This tome, a genuine collective efforts of many physicians from different fields of medicine, is devoted specifically to the upper tract urothelial carcinoma with special chapters on conservative treatments to preserve the renal units. This text, which was designed to be comprehensive and instructive to cover all possible details, may not be the first, hoping it would not be the last but just a ***prologue***[1].

We should waste no nephron before its time: when and if it is necessary.

Valhalla, NY, USA
January 2018

Majid Eshghi

[1]William Shakespeare, The Tempest 1610: What is past is a prologue

Contents

Contributors

Ahmed A. Aboumohamed Urology Department, Montefiore Medical Center, Bronx, NY, USA

Nariman Ahmadi University of Southern California, Institute of Urology, Los Angeles, CA, USA

Arash Akhavein Glickman Urological and Kidney Institute, Cleveland Clinic, Cleveland, OH, USA; Cedar Sinai Medical Center, Los Angeles, CA, USA

Mitchell S. Anscher Department of Radiation Oncology, Virginia Commonwealth University School of Medicine, Richmond, VA, USA

Stuart Bentley-Hibbert Department of Radiology, Columbia University Medical Center, New York, NY, USA

Jonathan Bloom Urologic Oncology Branch, National Institute of Health, Bethesda, MD, USA; Department of Urology, Westchester Medical Health Network/New York Medical College, Valhalla, NY, USA

Muhammad S. Choudhury Department of Urology, Westchester Medical Health Network/New York Medical College, Valhalla, NY, USA

Jonathan A. Coleman Department of Surgery, Urology, Memorial Sloan Kettering Cancer Center, New York, NY, USA

Majid Eshghi Department of Urology, Westchester Medical Health Network/New York Medical College, Valhalla, NY, USA

Ali Fathollahi Department of Urology, New York Medical College, Valhalla, NY, USA

Mark Ferretti Department of Urology, Westchester Medical Health Network/New York Medical College, Valhalla, NY, USA

Cristina Fox Department of Urology, Westchester Medical Health Network/New York Medical College, Valhalla, NY, USA

Reza Ghavamian Department of Urology, Northwell Health, Northwell Hofstra School of Medicine, Hempsted, NY, USA

Anthony Gilet Department of Radiology, New York Medical College/Westchester Medical Health Network, Valhalla, NY, USA

Inderbir Gill University of Southern California, Institute of Urology, Los Angeles, CA, USA

David M. Golombos Department of Urology, New York Presbyterian Hospital—Weill Cornell Medical Center, New York, NY, USA

Sabina Hajiyeva Department of Pathology, Westchester Medical Health Network/New York Medical College, Valhalla, NY, USA

Jullet Han Department of Urology, Weill Cornell Medical College, New York, NY, USA

Harry Herr Department of Surgery, Urology, Memorial Sloan Kettering Cancer Center, New York, NY, USA

Joel Hillelsohn Department of Urology, Westchester Medical Health Network/New York Medical College, Valhalla, NY, USA

Scott G. Hubosky Department of Urology, Sidney Kimmel Medical College at Thomas Jefferson University, Philadelphia, PA, USA

Tobias Klatte Department of Urology, Vienna General Hospital, Comprehensive Cancer Center, Medical University of Vienna, Vienna, Austria

Patrick Lewicki Department of Urology, Weill Cornell Medical College, New York, NY, USA

Romain Mathieu Department of Urology, Vienna General Hospital, Comprehensive Cancer Center, Medical University of Vienna, Vienna, Austria; Department of Urology, Rennes University Hospital, Rennes, France

Surena F. Matin Department of Urology, University of Texas MD Anderson Cancer Center, Houston, TX, USA

Aurélie Mbeutcha Department of Urology, Vienna General Hospital, Comprehensive Cancer Center, Medical University of Vienna, Vienna, Austria; Department of Urology, University Hospital of Nice, University of Nice Sophia-Antipolis, Nice, France

Carla McDonnell Department of Urology, Westchester Medical Health Network, Valhalla, NY, USA

Reza Mehrazin Department of Urology and Oncological Science, Icahn School of Medicine at Mount Sinai, New York, NY, USA

Saman Moazami Department of Urology, Montefiore Medical Center/Albert Einstein College of Medicine, Bronx, NY, USA

Manoj Monga Glickman Urological and Kidney Institute, Cleveland Clinic, Cleveland, OH, USA

Eric J. Moskowitz Stamford Health Medical Group, Stamford, CT, USA

Jeffrey H. Newhouse Department of Radiology, Columbia University Medical Center, New York, NY, USA

Carl A. Olsson Department of Urology and Oncological Science, Icahn School of Medicine at Mount Sinai, New York, NY, USA; John K Lattimer Emeritus, Professor, Columbia University Medical Center, New York, NY, USA

Neel Patel Department of Urology, Westchester Medical Health Network/ New York Medical College, Valhalla, NY, USA

John L. Phillips Department of Urology, Westchester Medical Health Network/New York Medical College, Valhalla, NY, USA

Jay D. Raman Division of Urology, Penn State Milton S. Hershey Medical Center, Hershey, PA, USA

Grant P. Redrow Department of Surgery (Urology), University of Texas Houston, Houston, TX, USA

Barak Rosenzweig Department of Surgery, Urology, Memorial Sloan Kettering Cancer Center, New York, NY, USA

Douglas S. Scherr Department of Urology, New York Presbyterian Hospital —Weill Cornell Medical Center, New York, NY, USA

Mark P. Schoenberg Department of Urology, Montefiore Medical Center/Albert Einstein College of Medicine, Bronx, NY, USA

Ariel Schulman Division of Urology, Duke University School of Medicine, Durham, NC, USA; Department of Urology, New York Medical College, Valhalla, NY, USA

Shahrokh F. Shariat Department of Urology, Vienna General Hospital, Comprehensive Cancer Center, Medical University of Vienna, Vienna, Austria; Department of Urology, Weill Cornell Medical College, New York, NY, USA; Department of Urology, University of Texas Southwestern Medical Center, Dallas, TX, USA

Arthur D. Smith Department of Urology, Northwell Health and Hofstra University, Lake Success, NY, USA

Abhishek Srivastava Department of Urology, Montefiore Medical Center, Albert Einstein College of Medicine, Bronx, NY, USA

Joshua M. Stern Department of Urology, Montefiore Medical Center/Albert Einstein College of Medicine, Bronx, NY, USA

Angela Tong Department of Radiology, New York Medical College/Westchester Medical Health Network, Valhalla, NY, USA

Alfredo I. Urdaneta Department of Radiation Oncology, Virginia Commonwealth University School of Medicine, Richmond, VA, USA

Raghu Vikram Department of Diagnostic Radiology, University of Texas MD Anderson Cancer Center, Houston, TX, USA

Joshua L. Warrick Department of Pathology, Penn State Milton S. Hershey Medical Center, Hershey, PA, USA

Roger Yau Department of Urology, Westchester Medical Health Network/New York Medical College, Valhalla, NY, USA

Esther Chaewon Yoon Department of Pathology, Westchester Medical Health Network/New York Medical College, Valhalla, NY, USA

Minghao Zhong Department of Pathology, Westchester Medical Health Network/New York Medical College, Valhalla, NY, USA

Part I

Introduction

Epidemiology and Presentation

1

Muhammad S. Choudhury

Epidemiology

Incidence

The most common site of transitional cell cancer of the urinary tract is the bladder, accounting for 90–95% of all cases and the remaining 5–10% affect the upper urinary tract (UUT), specifically the renal pyelocalyceal system and the ureters [1]. The National Cancer Data Base (NCDB) collects data on approximately 75% of all newly diagnosed cancer cases annually in the U.S.' reported a total of 426,425 cases of urothelial malignancy between 1993 and 2005 and of these, 398,125 (93%) involved the urinary bladder and 28,300 (7%) affected the UUT [1]. The same report showed that 64% (18,172) of the UUT cancer involved the renal pelvis and 36% (10,128) were ureteral cancer.

The National Cancer Institute's Surveillance, Epidemiology and End Result (SEER) database from 1985 to 1996 revealed that the incidence of ureteral and renal pyelocalyceal tumors in the United States was 0.73 and 1.0 each per 100,000 person-years respectively [2]. The incidence of UUT cancer has been increasing in recent years, largely due to the identification of the in situ tumors: and an updated SEER data from 1973–2005 indicate that the incidence of UUT cancer (renal pelvis and ureter) has increased from 1.88 to 2.06 cases per 100,000 person-years [3].

Age

Typically, urothelial malignancy of the upper urinary tract (UUT) is a disease of the elderly. The mean age at presentation was 70.0 years, for a group of 5052 patients from the SEER database diagnosed between 1985 and 1996 [2]. In the same study, the mean age at diagnosis was 67.9 years for a group of 4020 patients who presented in the previous decade between 1973 and 1984. An international, multi-institutional study of 1363 patients, who underwent radical nephroureterectomy for UUT urothelial malignancy between 1992 and 2006, reported the median age of the patients as 69.7 ± 11.1 years [4]. A similar study involving 5918 patients who underwent nephroureterectomy between 1988 and 2006, identified through SEER data base, were randomly divided into two equal cohorts based on geographical location in the United States. The study reported mean age of 70.8 and 71.6 years in these two groups [5].

M. S. Choudhury (✉)
Department of Urology, Westchester Medical Health Network/New York Medical College,
40 Sunshine Cottage Road, 19 Skyline 1S-B46,
Valhalla, NY 10595, USA
e-mail: muhammad_choudhury@nymc.edu

M. Eshghi (ed.), *Urothelial Malignancies of the Upper Urinary Tract*,
https://doi.org/10.1007/978-3-319-51263-1_1

Sex

Urothelial malignancies of the upper urinary tract (UUT) is about twice as common in men than in women, approximately 60% of the patients are male and 30% are female [2, 4, 5]. The incidence of UUT urothelial malignancy in female appears to be increasing and review of the SEER data base over a two decade period by Munoz and Ellison [2], revealed that the incidence in men decreased from 64.1 (1973–1984) to 61.7% (1985–1996) but the incidence in female increased from 35.9 (1973–1984) to 38.3% (1985–1996).

Race

In the United States, approximately 90% of patients diagnosed with urothelial malignancy of the upper urinary tract (UUT) are Caucasian, 3–4% are African American and the remaining are of other races [2].

Presentation

Most patients with upper urinary tract urothelial cancer will manifest themselves during their life time with signs and symptoms and therefore, these tumors are a rare incidental autopsy finding [6]. Hematuria, gross or microscopic, is the presenting symptom in 56–98% of patients [7–9]. Flank pain is the second most common symptom and is reported by 10–40% of patients [10–12]. Typically, flank pain is dull in nature and is caused by gradual obstruction and progressive hydronephrosis due to ureteral tumor and acute exacerbation of flank pain is caused by blood clot from bleeding [13]. In about 15% of patients, UUT urothelial malignancy present as an incidental finding in radiologic examination, and symptoms of locally advanced and metastatic disease include flank pain, weight loss, anorexia, and bone pain [13]. In 1998, Hall et al. [14] reported their 30-year experience involving 252 patients with UUT urothelial malignancy and in this series, hematuria was the presenting symptom in 77.6% of their patients, followed by flank pain in 18.3%, dysuria in 6%, UTI in 4.8% and palpable mass in only 1.2% (Table 1.1).

Risk Factors: Upper Urinary Tract Urothelial Malignancy

The risk factors for the development of upper urinary tract urothelial cancer can be placed in four different categories. First, upper urinary tract urothelial cancer can be part of certain genetic syndrome. Second, certain risk factors are shared with bladder cancer such as smoking and occupation. Third, there are risk factors which are unique to UUT urothelial malignancy specifically phenacetin/analgesic abuse and exposure to Aristolochic Acid (AA) in Balkan Endemic Nephropathy (BEN), Chinese herb nephropathy (CHN), etc. Finally, patients treated for bladder cancer, especially non-muscle invasive bladder cancer (NMIBC) either with bladder in place or post-cystectomy are also at increased risk of UUT cancer.

Risk factors for Upper Urinary Tract Urothelial Cancer:

1. Genetic Factor: Hereditary Cancer Syndrome
2. Carcinogen Exposure: shared with bladder cancer
   Cigarette smoking
   Occupational exposure
3. Carcinogen Exposure: unique for UUT urothelial cancer
   Aristolochic Acid (AA):
   Balkan Endemic Nephropathy (BEN)
   Chinese Herb Nephropathy (CHN)
   Herbal Medicine use in Taiwan
   Phenacetin and Analgesic Nephropathy
4. Urothelial Cancer of the Bladder
   Patients with intact bladder
   Post cystectomy

Hereditary Upper Urinary Tract Urothelial Cancer: Genetic Risk Factors

Upper urinary tract urothelial malignancy can be part of certain genetic syndrome. The most common of which is Lynch Syndrome. Lynch Syndrome, also known as "Hereditary Non-polyposis Colon Cancer" (HNPCC)

Table 1.1 Presenting signs and symptoms of patients with urothelial malignancy of the upper urinary tract

Presentation	Incidence (%)
Gross or microscopic hematuria	56–98
Flank pain	10–40
Palpable mass	1–2
Incidental finding on radiologic study	~15

Syndrome, is the most common hereditary cancer syndrome associated with upper urinary tract urothelial cancer. It is an autosomal dominant genetic disease caused by germline mutation in four mismatch repair (MMR) genes, leading to accumulation of DNA errors in microsatellite region [15].

The most common cancer affecting families with Lynch Syndrome is colon cancer, but a spectrum of other cancers may affect these family members including endometrioid, ovarian, stomach, small bowel, hepatobiliary, sebaceous gland, central nervous system, and the upper urinary tract, which is considered a core cancer in Lynch Syndrome with a reported life time risk of 2.9% and the overall risk is 8–16-fold higher than the general population [16].

Clinically, compared to sporadic urothelial malignancy of the UUT, Lynch Syndrome patients affected with UUT urothelial malignancies are 8 years younger at presentation (62 vs. 70 years), has a higher proportion of ureteral cancer (51% vs. 28%), a greater female preponderance (male to female ratio 0.95 vs. 1.52) but the grade and stage of the tumor at presentation is not significantly different when compared to sporadic UUT urothelial cancer [17].

Pathological tissue based Microsatellite Instability—Polymerase Chain Reaction (MSI-PCR) and Immunohistochemistry (IHC) are the first means of evaluating clinically suspected Lynch Syndrome and high level of MSI, which is considered the hallmark of MMR deficiency, raises suspicion of Lynch Syndrome [15]. Immunohistochemistry stains a tumor for protein products of mismatch repair (MMR) genes and if one or more MMR proteins are absent, this indicates which gene should be targeted for germline genetic testing, which is the confirmatory test for Lynch Syndrome [15].

While treating patients with UUT urothelial malignancies in Lynch Syndrome patients, the potential for increased risk of bilateral disease should be considered, and a more conservative approach to treatment such as ureteroscopic management has been advocated when feasible rather than nephroureterectomy [18].

Carcinogen Exposure: Shared with Bladder Cancer

Smoking

Similar to bladder cancer, cigarette smoking is the most important of the modifiable risk factors for upper urinary tract cancer [13]. The aromatic amines present in cigarette smoke are metabolized by the body into N-hydroxylamine, which has carcinogenic activity [19]. McLaughlin et al. [20] found that this risk is dose dependent and increases with longer duration and heavier smoking. These authors reported that cigarette smoking is associated with 3.1-fold increased risk, with long-term (>45 years) smoker having a 7.2-fold increased risk, and subjects who smoke <20 cigarettes per day, the estimated risk is 2.4 (OR, odds ratio) but the risk doubles to 4.8 (OR, odds ratio) when they smoke >40 cigarettes per day. The same study revealed that, cessation of smoking decreases the risk and subjects who stop smoking for over 10 years, the risk decreases by 60–70% relative to current smoker.

Occupation

Occupational exposure to certain aromatic amines found in many industries including textile, rubber, chemicals, coals, petrochemical, etc., increases the risk of developing upper urinary tract urothelial cancer [19, 21]. The average duration of exposure needed to develop upper urinary tract urothelial malignancy is ~7 years with a latency period after the end of exposure of ~20 years [21].

Carcinogen Exposure: Unique to UUT Urothelial Malignancy

Exposure to Aristolochic Acid (AA), a chemical found it herbaceous plants of Aristolochia species has been identified as a unique risk factor for the development of UUT urothelial malignancy. The exposure can take place with dietary contamination or by the use of herbal medication containing Aristolochic Acid (AA).

Balkan Endemic Nephropathy (BEN)

The association of upper urinary tract urothelial malignancy and Balkan Endemic Nephropathy (BEN), a form of chronic kidney disease characterized by chronic tubulointerstitial fibrosis of the kidneys and invariable progression to renal failure, was first described in 1950s [22–25]. This disease complex is prevalent in Southern Europe along the tributaries of the Danube River especially in certain farming villages in Bosnia, Bulgaria, Croatia, Romania, and Serbia [23]. Epidemiologic studies conducted by Grollman et al. [25] revealed the chronic dietary poisoning with Aristolochic Acid (AA) as an etiologic factor in the development of BEN and its associated urothelial malignancy of the upper urinary tract. The researchers found that Aristolochic Acid (AA) is derived from the seeds of 'Aristolochic Clements', a plant native in the rural region of the Balkan countries, which grows in the field along with planted wheats and at the time of harvest, the seeds from 'Aristolochic clements' contaminate the wheat grain leading to the dietary exposure to Aristolochic acid through home-baked bread [19, 25].

Upper urinary tract urothelial malignancy develops in approximately half of all patients diagnosed with BEN and the incidence in some rural areas of Balkans was reported as 60–100 times higher than the rest of the world. [24]. However, the reported incidence in recent years has dramatically decreased and in 1998 it was considered only eleven times higher [26]. Upper urinary tract urothelial malignancy associated with BEN is usually low grade, multi-focal, and more frequently bilateral compared to sporadic upper tract urothelial cancer [27].

Chinese Herb Nephropathy (CHN)/ Aristolochic Acid Nephropathy (AAN)

In the early 1990s, a direct causal connection was established between Aristolochic Acid exposure, and the development of chronic kidney disease, in a cohort of Belgian women who used Chinese herbal medication for weight loss and were inadvertently exposed to Aristolochic Acid [28, 29]. The renal disease affecting the Belgian patients was originally named Chinese Herb Nephropathy (CHN) and later retitled Aristolochic Acid Nephropathy (AAN) to more accurately reflect the etiology of the disease [30]. The kidney disease affecting these patients are characterized by progressive, and irreversible tubulointerstitial disease, renal insufficiency, pronounced and early anemia, low molecular weight proteinuria, and variable glycosuria [31, 32]. Almost 40% of these patients were subsequently found to have upper tract urothelial cancer and subsequent investigation revealed an error in the manufacture of the herbal medication mix where "Stephania tetrandra" was replaced inadvertently by "Aristolochia Fangchi", which was the source of Aristolochic Acid in the herbal medication [33, 34]. Since the initial report less than 20 years ago implicating Aristolochic Acid exposure as a risk factor for upper tract urothelial cancer in human, Aristolochic Acid has been classified as a group 1 human carcinogen [35, 36].

Herbal Medicine Use in Taiwan

The incidence of upper urinary tract urothelial malignancy in certain regions of the island of Taiwan is reported to be one of the highest in the world and in some parts of Taiwan this represent 20–25% all urothelial cancer [37–39]. The characteristic of these UUT cancer include higher prevalence in female (male:female ratio 1:2), younger onset (55–60 years) and ureteric tumor being twice as common as the renal pelvic tumor [38, 39].

Exposure to arsenic from artesian well water has been investigated as a cause but never been formally proven [19, 38, 39]. Recent studies implicate the use of herbal medication in Taiwan containing Aristolochic acid as a likely cause of the high incidence of UUT urothelial malignancy [34, 40].

Analgesic Abuse

Phenacetin (p-ethoxyacetanilide), a pro-drug for acetaminophen, is a synthetic analgesic anti-pyretic agent that was first introduced into the pharmaceutical market in 1897 and habitual use of phenacetin containing analgesic compounds, have been known as a risk factor for urothelial malignancy of the upper urinary tract since the 1960s [34]. Phenacetin and compound analgesics containing phenacetin and other drugs such as caffeine, aspirin, and phenazone were widely used throughout the world for much of the twentieth century, because of its efficacy and easy availability.

Reports linking habitual use of phenacetin containing compound analgesics to renal insufficiency and tubulointerstitial kidney disease (Analgesic Nephropathy) was first reported in the 1950s [41]. Renal papillary necrosis is frequently associated with analgesic nephropathy.

The first report, linking abuse of phenacetin containing compound analgesic to epithelial tumors of the renal pelvis came from Sweden in 1965 [42] and this was soon followed by multiple reports from Australia, Switzerland, Belgium, and other countries confirming the relationship between phenacetin abuse, renal papillary necrosis, and the high incidence of upper tract urothelial cancer [43, 44]. An estimated 8–10% of patients diagnosed with phenacetin induced analgesic nephropathy eventually develop urothelial malignancy [34]. In the absence of other risk factors, habitual use of phenacetin containing analgesics alone increased the risk of upper tract urothelial cancer by 3½, renal papillary necrosis by itself increases the risk sevenfold but when phenacetin abuse and renal papillary necrosis were present in the same patient, the risk of upper tract urothelial cancer increased 20-fold compared to individuals who did not have either of the risk factors [45].

Based on the reports of high incidence of ESRD and upper tract urothelial cancer associated with phenacetin abuse, Phenacetin was banned starting in 1970s and since then the incidence of analgesic abuse-related urothelial malignancy of the upper tract has declined [46, 47]. Phenacetin is now listed as a group I carcinogen in human [48].

Urothelial Cancer of the Bladder

Upper Urinary Tract Urothelial Malignancy After Primary Bladder Cancer

Upper urinary tract urothelial malignancy develops in 0.7–25% of patients after primary bladder cancer [49, 50]. Most published series reports incidence of 2–4%. [51–54].

Wright et al. [55] reported on 99,938 patients with bladder cancer from the Surveillance, Epidemiology and End Result (SEER) database from 1988 to 2003, of that only 768 (0.8%) of these patients developed upper urinary tract urothelial cancer. The authors reported that the median time for the development of these metachronous upper urinary tract tumor, was 33 months and 71% of these tumors presented within 5 years, 20% presented between 5 and 10 years, and the remaining 9% were diagnosed after 10 years of the initial diagnosis of bladder cancer. These authors identified the following risk factors in patients who developed secondary

UUT tumor: high-grade bladder tumor (HR 2.16, 95% CI 1.71–2.74); non-muscle invasive bladder cancer (NMIBC) Ta and T1 disease (HR 1.16, 95% CI 0.97–1.39) and tumor location at trigone/ureteral orifice (HR 1.76, 95% CI1.48–2.09).

Another large population-based study reviewed 91,245 patients, also from the SEER database from 1973 to 1996, found secondary tumor involving the upper urinary tract in 657 (0.7%) patients at a median follow-up of 4.1 years [49]. Other studies have reported higher incidence of upper urinary tract urothelial tumor in patients with bladder cancer. Oldbring et al. [56] reported on 657 patients with primary bladder cancer followed for at least 10 years or death, 11 (1.7%) of them developed secondary UUT tumors. The authors identified multiple and recurrent bladder tumors, or tumor involving the ureteral orifice or patients who had prior cystectomy as risk factors and recommended upper tract study in this select group of patients. Solsona et al. [51] reported upper urinary tract tumor in 18 of 786 (2.2%) patients followed for a mean of 43.6 months for superficial bladder tumor without associated carcinoma in situ (CIS) of the bladder.

Millan-Rodriguez et al. [52] risk stratified non-muscle invasive bladder cancer into low risk (Ta or solitary T1, grade 2) and high risk (multiple T1 grade 2, Ta grade 3, T1 grade 3, or carcinoma in situ) groups. In their 40 low risk patients, only one (0.6%) patient developed upper tract tumor during a 10 year follow-up and in the high risk group the incidence of upper tract tumor during the same period was 4.1%, sevenfold higher compared to the low risk group. This finding led to the recommendation by the authors of every 1–2 year upper tract surveillance for the high-risk group and less rigorous or no surveillance for the low-risk group.

Canales et al. [53] risk stratified a group of 375 patients with Ta bladder tumors with a median follow-up of 6 years and reported that 13 patients (3.4%) developed an upper tract tumor at an average of 22 months after the initial diagnosis of bladder tumor. The authors found that among 280 patients with no recurrence or only one recurrence of bladder tumor, upper tract tumor developed in only 1.8% cases, and in patients with two or more recurrences with less than 12 month between recurrences developed upper tract tumor in 8.9% cases, a 4.5-fold higher risk. The authors concluded that this subgroup of Ta patients should be considered for more rigorous upper tract surveillance.

Upper Tract Urothelial Malignancy in Patients with Carcinoma in Situ of the Bladder

Several investigators have reported significantly higher incidence of upper tract urothelial malignancy in patient with carcinoma in situ of the bladder. Solsona et al. [51] reported on 132 patients with Tis of the bladder, 28 (21.2%) of whom developed upper tract tumor at a mean time of 38.1 months, and most of these patients had associated T1 grade 2 or T1 grade 3 disease in addition to Tis.

Herr et al. [57] followed 86 patients with Tis and accompanying Ta and T1 bladder cancer treated with intravesical BCG for 15 years or longer, and found 18 of these patients (21%) developed an upper tract urothelial malignancy at a median follow-up of 7.3 years (range 1–15 years or longer). The authors also reported that, six of these patients (30%) developed upper tract tumor in the first 5 years, seven (40%) between 5 and 10 years and the remaining five (27%) from 10 to 15 years or longer. The authors concluded that high-risk patients with non-muscle invasive bladder cancer require lifelong surveillance of the upper tract and recommended routine annual I.V.P. in this select group.

Risk Factors for Upper Urinary Tract Tumor in Patients with Bladder Cancer: [51–53, 55–57]

1. High-risk non-muscle invasive bladder cancer
2. Multifocal bladder tumor
3. Ta disease with more than one recurrence in 12 months
4. Tis of the bladder

5. Tumor involving bladder trigone or ureteral orifice
6. Patients treated with intravesical BCG.

Upper Urinary Tract Tumors After Radical Cystectomy (RC) for Transitional Cell Bladder Cancer

Similar to patients with history of bladder cancer with an intact bladder, subjects who undergo radical cystectomy for transitional cell cancer are also at increased risk of developing UUT urothelial malignancy. This topic has been discussed in detail in Chap. 25. In this section, only a brief discussion primarily of the epidemiology of UUT urothelial malignancy after radical cystectomy is included.

In a review of eight separate contemporary series (2007–2013) involving 7047 patients, who underwent radical cystectomy for transitional cell bladder cancer, the incidence of upper urinary tract tumor recurrence varied between 1.8 and 6%. The median follow-up in these eight series ranged between 38 and 172 months [58–64].

Risk Factors for UUT Tumor After RC

Volkmer et al. [62] reported on 1420 patients who underwent radical cystectomy for bladder cancer, and found that 25 of these patients (1.8%) developed UUT tumor recurrence at a median time of 39 months. The authors identified four risk factors for metachronous UUT tumor recurrence: carcinoma in situ in the bladder (RR 2.3), history of recurrent bladder cancer (RR 2.6), cystectomy for non-muscle invasive bladder cancer (RR 3.8), and tumor involvement of the distal ureter in the cystectomy specimen (RR 2.7). In this study, patients who had none of the above four risk factors, the UUT tumor recurrence rate was only 0.8% at 15 years, the risk increased to 8.4% in patients with 1–2 risk factors and 13.5% in those with 3–4 risk factors.

Another study by Sanderson et al. [58] involving 1069 patients who underwent radical cystectomy for transitional cell bladder cancer, reported that 27 patients (2.5%) developed upper tract tumor at a median follow-up of 3.3 years (range 0.4–9.3 years). The authors identified that involvement of the prostatic urethra in men by superficial transitional cell carcinoma with an increased risk of upper tract recurrence (p = <0.01) and at 10 years, these men were at fourfold cumulative increased risk compared to those without prostatic urethral involvement. Similarly, in women with urethral involvement in cystectomy specimen, 10 year estimated probability of recurrence in the upper tract was 6 times greater than in women without urethral involvement.

Interestingly, men with prostatic stromal invasion did not have higher risk of upper tract tumor likely because of advanced stage of the disease in these patients and early demise.

Tran et al. [59] reported on 1329 patients who had radical cystectomy for transitional cell bladder cancer, 80 (6%) patients developed upper tract tumor recurrence at a median recurrence time of 25.2 months (range 1–107). In this series, any ureteral involvement at radical cystectomy including carcinoma in situ portended a significantly higher risk of upper tract recurrence (Hazard ration 2.49 for ureteral involvement vs. noninvolvement; 95% CI 1.52, 4.05; $p <$ 0.0005).

Risk factors for UUT tumor recurrence after radical cystectomy: [58, 59, 62–64]

- Ureteral tumor involvement in cystectomy specimen
- Prostatic urethral involvement (superficial) in men
- Cystectomy done for non-muscle invasive bladder cancer
- Bladder carcinoma in situ
- Recurrent bladder cancer before cystectomy

- Urethral involvement in female
- Pathologically negative lymph node

Bladder Cancer After Treatment of Upper Urinary Tract Transitional Cell Cancer

The risk of developing bladder cancer within 5 years of being diagnosed with upper urinary tract urothelial malignancy varies between 15 and 75% and because of this high risk routine surveillance cystoscopy is recommended in patients with history of UUT urothelial cancer [13]. Multiple etiologies have been suggested for the high incidence of metachronous bladder cancer in patients with upper urinary tract cancer including: (i) downstream seeding of malignant cells (ii) longer exposure time of bladder mucosa to carcinogen and (iii) greater number of urothelial cells in the bladder that are subject to random carcinogenic events [13].

Risk Factors

Novara et al. [65] reported on 231 patients who underwent nephroureterectomy for UUT urothelial malignancy, and found 109 (47.2%) of these patients develop bladder cancer during a median follow-up of 38 months. In this study, a previous history of bladder transitional cell cancer was the only independent predictor of metachronous bladder cancer. Raman et al. [66] found risk of metachronous bladder cancer in 49.5% of 103 patients treated for UUT urothelial malignancy at a mean interval of 13.2 months. These authors also found previous history of bladder cancer as the only predictive risk factor. Matsui et al. [67] reported a metachronous incidence of bladder cancer of 41.6% in a group of 89 patients who underwent nephroureterectomy for UUT cancer during a median follow-up of 39.7 months. On multivariate analysis, the authors found tumor multiplicity ($p = 0.0075$), pathologic stage ($p = 0.0221$), tumor size ($p = 0.0377$), and surgical modality ($p = 0.0413$) had a statistically significant impact on the risk of intravesical tumor recurrence. Kang et al. [68] reported metachronous bladder tumor recurrence rate of 31.2% in a group of 189 patients treated for UUT urothelial malignancy with a median follow-up of 91 months. The authors identified multiplicity of UUT tumor as a significant and independent risk factor for the development of subsequent bladder tumor.

Risk Factors for Bladder Cancer in Patients Treated for UUT Cancer [65–68]

- History of prior bladder cancer
- Tumor multiplicity
- Tumor size
- Pathologic stage
- Surgical modality.

Conclusion

Urothelial malignancy of the upper urinary tract remains a relatively rare malignancy but the incidence seems to be increasing. The most significant modifiable risk factor is smoking. Patients with history of transitional cell bladder cancer are at increased risk of developing upper urinary tract urothelial malignancy and require careful long-term surveillance of the upper tract in high-risk group. The risk of metachronous bladder cancer in patients with history of upper tract cancer is significant and surveillance of the bladder is mandatory in these patients.

Summary Box

- Approximately 28,000 new cases of upper urinary tract (UUT) urothelial malignancy are diagnosed annually in the United States of America' and this represents about 7% of all urothelial cancer of the genitourinary tract.
- The mean age at presentation of UUT urothelial cancer is 70 years and it is twice as common in men as in women. Hematuria gross or microscopic is the most common presenting symptom.

- Certain risk factors such as smoking and occupational carcinogen exposure are shared between UUT and bladder cancer. On the other hand, analgesic abuse and exposure to Aristolochic Acid such as in Balkan and Chinese Herb Naphropathy are unique risk factors for UUT malignancy.
- UUT urothelial malignancy can also be part of certain genetic syndrome such as Lynch syndrome and patients treated for bladder cancer are also at increased risk.

Acknowledgements Author acknowledges the contribution of Michael Stern, MD, Westchester Medical Health Network, New York Medical College, Valhalla, NY and thanks him for his helpful comments and feedback.

References

1. David KA, Mallin K, Milowsky MI, et al. Surveillance of urothelial carcinoma: stage and grade migration, 1993–2005 and survival trends, 1993–2000. Cancer. 2009;115(7):1435–47.
2. Munoz JJ, Ellison LM. Upper tract urothelial neoplasms: incidence and survival during the last 2 decades. J Urol. 2000;164(5):1523–5.
3. Raman JD, Messer J, Sielatycki JA, et al. Incidence and survival of patients with carcinoma of the ureter and renal pelvis in the USA, 1973–2005. BJU Int. 2011;107(7):1059–64.
4. Margulis V, Shariat SF, Matin SF, Kamat AM, et al. Outcomes of radical nephroureterectomy: a series from the upper tract urothelial carcinoma collaboration. Cancer. 2009;115(6):1224–33.
5. Jeldres C, Sun M, Lughezzani G, et al. Highly predictive survival nomogram after upper urinary tract urothelial carcinoma. Cancer. 2010;116(16):3774–84.
6. Ressequie LT, Nobrega FT, Farrow GM, et al. Epidemiology of renal and ureteral cancer in Rochester, Minnesota, 1950–1974, with special reference to clinical and pathologic features. Mayo Clin Proc. 1978;53(8):503–10.
7. Murphy DM, Zincke H, Furlow WL. Management of high grade transitional cell cancer of the upper urinary tract. J Urol. 1981;125(1):25–9.
8. Guinan P, Vogelzang NJ, Randazzo R, et al. Renal pelvic cancer: a review of 611 patients treated in Illinois 1975–1985. Cancer incidence and end results committee. Urology. 1992;40(5):393–9.
9. Raabe NK, Fossa SD, Bjerkehagen B. Carcinoma of the renal pelvis. Scand J Urol Nephrol. 1992;26(4):357–61.
10. Babaian RJ, Johnson DE. Primary carcinoma of the ureter. J Urol. 1980;123(3):357–9.
11. Richie JP. Carcinoma of the renal pelvis and ureter. In: Skinner DG, Lieskovsky G, editors. Diagnosis and management of genitourinary cancer. Philadelphia: WB Saunders; 1988. p. 323–36.
12. Melamed MR, Reuter VE. Pathology and staging of urothelial tumors of the kidney and ureter. Urol Clin North Am. 1993;20(2):333–47.
13. Sagalowsky AI, Jarrett TW, Flanigan RC. Urothelial tumors of the upper urinary tract and ureter. In: Wein AJ, editor. Campbell-Walsh urology. 10th ed. Philadelphia, PA: Saunders Elsevier; 2011 (Chapter 53).
14. Hall MC, Womack S, Sagalowsky AI, et al. Prognostic factors, recurrence, and survival in transitional cell carcinoma of the upper urinary tract: a 30 year experience in 252 patients. Urology. 1998;52(4):594–601.
15. Mork M, Hubosky SG, Roupret M, et al. Lynch syndrome: a primer for urologists and panel recommendations. J Urol. 2015;194(1):21–9.
16. Barrow P, Khan M, Lalloo F, Evans DG, et al. Systematic review of the impact of registration and screening on colorectal cancer incidence and mortality in familial adenomatous polyposis and Lynch syndrome. Br J Surg. 2013;100(13):1719–31.
17. Crockett DG, Wagner DG, Holmang S, et al. Upper urinary tract carcinoma in Lynch syndrome cases. J Urol. 2011;185(5):1627–30.
18. Hubosky SG, Boman BM, Charles S, et al. Ureteroscopic management of upper tract urothelial carcinoma (UTUC) in patients with Lynch Syndrome (hereditary nonpolyposis colorectal cancer syndrome). BJU Int. 2013;112(6):813–9.
19. Colin P, Koenig P, Ouzzane A, et al. Environmental factors involved in carcinogenesis of urothelial cell carcinomas of the upper urinary tract. BJU Int. 2009;104(10):1436–40.
20. McLaughlin JK, Silverman DT, Hsing AW, et al. Cigarette smoking and cancers of the renal pelvis and ureter. Cancer Res. 1992;52(2):254–7.
21. Mazeman E. Tumors of the upper excretory urinary tract, calices, renal pelvis and ureter. J Urol Nephrol (Paris). 1972;78(Suppl. 9):1–219.
22. Bamias G, Boletis J. Balkan nephropathy: evolution of our knowledge. Am J Kidney Dis. 2008;52(3):606–16.
23. Tatu CA, Orem WH, Finkelman RB, et al. The etiology of Balkan endemic nephropathy: still more questions than answers. Environ Health Perspect. 1998;106(11):689–700.
24. Petkovic SD. Epidemiology and treatment of renal pelvic and ureteral tumor. J Urol. 1975;114(6):858–65.
25. Grollman AP, Shibutani S, Moriya M, et al. Aristolochic acid and the etiology of endemic (Balkan)

nephropathy. Proc Natl Acad Sci USA. 2007;104 (29):12129–34.
26. Markovic N, Ignjatovic I, Cukuranovic R, et al. Decreasing incidence of urothelial cancer in a Balkan endemic nephropathy region in Serbia. a surgery based study from 1969 to 1998. Pathol Biol (Paris). 1969;53(1):26–9.
27. Radovanovic Z, Krajinovic S, Jankovic S, et al. Family history of cancer among cases of upper urothelial tumours in the Balkan nephropathy area. J Cancer Res Clin Oncol. 1985;110(2):181–3.
28. Cosyns JP. Aristolochic acid and 'Chinese herbs nephropathy': a review of the evidence to date. Drug Saf. 2003;26(1):33–48.
29. Nortier JL, Vanherwegham JL. Renal interstitial fibrosis and urothelial carcinoma associated with the use of Chinese herb (Aristolochia fangchi). Toxicology. 2002;27(181–182):577–80.
30. Gillerot G, Jadoul M, Arlt VM, et al. Aristolochic acid nephropathy in a Chinese patient: time to abandon the term "Chinese herbs nephropathy"? Am J Kidney Dis. 2001;38(5):E26.
31. Cosyns JP, Jadoul M, Squifflet JP, et al. Chinese herbs nephropathy: a clue to Balkan endemic nephropathy? Kidney Int. 1994;45(6):1680–8.
32. Reginster F, Jadoul M, van Ypersele de Strihou C. Chinese herbs nephropathy presentation, natural history and fate after transplantation. Nephrol Dial Transplant. 1997;12(1):81–6.
33. Nortier JL, Martinez MC, Schmeiser HH, et al. Urothelial carcinoma associated with the use of a Chinese herb (Aristolochia fangchi). N Engl J Med. 2000;342(23):1686–92.
34. Dickman KG, Fritsche HM, Grollman AP, et al. Epidemiology and risk factors for upper urinary urothelial cancers. In: Shariat SF, Xylinas E, editors. Upper tract urothelial carcinoma. New York: Springer Science & Business Media; 2015. p. 1–30 (Chapter 1).
35. National Toxicology Program. Aristolochic acids. Rep Carcinog. 2011;12:45–9.
36. IARC. Plants containing aristolochic acid. IARC Monogr Eval Carcinog Risk Chem Hum. 2012;100A:347–61.
37. Lai MN, Wang SM, Chen PC, et al. Population-based case-control study of Chinese herbal products containing aristolochic acid and urinary tract cancer risk. J Natl Cancer Inst. 2010;102(3):179–86.
38. Tan LB, Chen KT, Guo HR. Clinical and epidemiological features of patients with genitourinary tract tumour in a blackfoot disease endemic area of Taiwan. BJU Int. 2008;102(1):48–54.
39. Yang MH, Chen KK, Yen CC, et al. Unusually high incidence of upper urinary tract urothelial carcinoma in Taiwan. Urology. 2002;59(5):681–7.
40. Chen CH, Dickman KG, Huang CY, et al. Aristolochic acid-induced upper tract urothelial carcinoma in Taiwan: clinical characteristics and outcome. Int J Cancer. 2013;133(1):14–20.
41. Spuhler O, Zollinger HU. Chronic interstitial nephritis. Z Klin Med. 1953;151(1):1–50.
42. Hultengren N, Lagergren C, Ljungqvist A. Carcinoma of the renal pelvic in renal papillary necrosis. Acta Chir Scand. 1965;130(4):314–20.
43. Nanra RS. Renal effects of antipyretic analgesics. Am J Med. 1983;75(5A):70–81.
44. Prescott LF. Analgesic nephropathy: a reassessment of the role of phenacetin and other analgesics. Drugs. 1982;23(1–2):75–149.
45. McCredie M, Stewart JH, Carter JJ, et al. Phenacetin and papillary necrosis: independent risk factors for renal pelvic cancer. Kidney Int. 1986;30(1):81–4.
46. McCredie M, Stewart J, Smith D, et al. Observations on the effect abolishing analgesic abuse and reducing smoking on cancers of the kidney and bladder in New South Wales, Australia, 1972–1995. Cancer Causes Control. 1999;10(4):303–11.
47. McCredie M, Stewart JH, Mathew TH, et al. The effect of withdrawal of phenacetin-containing analgesics on the incidence of kidney and urothelial cancer and renal failure. Clin Nephrol. 1989;31 (1):35–9.
48. IARC. Phenacetin. IARC Monogr Eval Carcinog Risk Chem Hum. 2012;100A:377–98.
49. Rabbani F, Perrotti M, Russo P, et al. Upper-tract tumors after an initial diagnosis of bladder cancer: argument for long-term surveillance. J Clin Oncol. 2001;19(1):94–100.
50. Herr HW. Extravesical tumor relapse in patients with superficial bladder tumors. J Clin Oncol. 1998;16 (3):1099–102.
51. Solsona E, Iborra I, Ricos JV, et al. Upper urinary tract involvement in patients with bladder carcinoma in situ (Tis): its impact on management. Urology. 1997;49(3):347–52.
52. Millan-Rodriguez F, Chechile-Toniolo G, Salvador-Bayarri J, et al. Upper urinary tract tumors after primary superficial bladder tumors: prognostic factors and risk groups. J Urol. 2000;164(4):1183–7.
53. Canales BK, Anderson JK, Premoli J, et al. Risk factors for upper tract recurrence in patients undergoing long-term surveillance for stage Ta bladder cancer. J Urol. 2006;175(1):74–7.
54. Hurle R, Losa A, Manzetti A, et al. Upper urinary tract tumors developing after treatment of superficial bladder cancer: 7-year follow-up of 591 consecutive patients. Urology. 1999;53(6):1144–8.
55. Wright JL, Hotaling J, Porter MP. Predictors of upper tract urothelial carcinoma after primary bladder cancer: a population based analysis. J Urol. 2009;181(3):1035–9.
56. Oldbring J, Glifberg I, Mikulowski P, et al. Carcinoma of the renal pelvis and ureter following bladder carcinoma: frequency, risk factors and clinicopathological findings. J Urol. 1989;141(6):1311–3.
57. Herr HW, Cookson MS, Soloway SM. Upper tract tumors in patients with primary bladder cancer followed for 15 years. J Urol. 1996;156(4):1286–7.

58. Sanderson KM, Cai J, Miranda G, et al. Upper tract urothelial recurrence following radical cystectomy for transitional cell carcinoma of the bladder: an analysis of 1069 patients with 10-year follow up. J Urol. 2007;177(6):2088–94.
59. Tran W, Serio AM, Raj GV, et al. Longitudinal risk of upper tract recurrence following radical cystectomy for urothelial cancer and the potential implications for long-term surveillance. J Urol. 2008;179(1):96–100.
60. Furukawa J, Miyake H, Hara I, et al. Upper urinary tract recurrence following radical cystectomy for bladder cancer. Int J Urol Off Jpn Urol Assoc. 2007;14(6):496–9.
61. Meissner C, Giannarini G, Schumacher MC, et al. The efficiency of excretory urography to detect upper urinary tract tumors after cystectomy for urothelial cancer. J Urol. 2007;178(6):2287–90.
62. Volkmer BG, Schnoeller T, Kuefer R, et al. Upper urinary tract recurrence after radical cystectomy for bladder cancer—who is at risk? J Urol. 2009;182 (6):2632–7.
63. Umbreit EC, Crispen PL, Shimko MS, et al. Multifactorial, site-specific recurrence model after radical cystectomy for urothelial carcinoma. Cancer. 2010;116(14):3399–407.
64. Takayanagi A, Masumori N, Takahashi A, et al. Upper urinary tract recurrence after radical cystectomy for bladder cancer: incidence and risk factors. Int J Urol Off Jpn Urol Assoc. 2012;19(3):229–33.
65. Novara G, De Marco V, Dalpiaz O, et al. Independent predictors of metachronous bladder transitional cell carcinoma (TCC) after nephroureterectomy for TCC of the upper urinary tract. BJU Int. 2008;101 (11):1368–74.
66. Raman JD, Ng CK, Boorjian SA, et al. Bladder cancer after managing upper urinary tract transitional cell carcinoma: predictive factors and pathology. BJU Int. 2005;96(7):1031–5.
67. Matsui Y, Utsunomiya N, Ichioka K, et al. Risk factors for subsequent development of bladder cancer after primary transitional cell carcinoma of the upper urinary tract. Urology. 2005;65(2):279–83.
68. Kang GH, Yu TJ, Hsieh HH, et al. The development of bladder tumors and contralateral upper urinary tract tumors after primary transitional cell carcinoma of the upper urinary tract. Cancer. 2003;98(8):1620–6.

2 Prognostic Factors and Predictive Tools in Upper Tract Urothelial Carcinoma

Aurélie Mbeutcha, Tobias Klatte, Romain Mathieu and Shahrokh F. Shariat

Introduction

Upper tract urothelial carcinoma (UTUC) is a rare and biologically heterogeneous disease that accounts for less than 5% of all urothelial tumors [1]. The standard treatment for patients with non-metastatic UTUC who have a normal contralateral kidney remains open radical nephro-ureterectomy (RNU) with bladder cuff excision (BCE) [2]. Less invasive approaches, such as laparoscopic RNU, endoscopic ablation and segmental resection are adequate alternatives with regard to functional and oncologic outcomes in well-selected candidates [3, 4].

Oncologic outcomes after RNU are excellent for patients with low-stage UTUC with a survival rate reaching 90%, but drop to less than 30% for patients with advanced stages and/or lymph node metastasis [5]. These poor survival rates call for a better understanding of the biological and clinical markers that would improve the selection of high-risk patients who could benefit from multimodal therapy or from a close monitoring.

Beside well-established prognostic factors such as tumor stage, grade, lymph node metastasis, and lympho-vascular invasion (LVI), several preoperative and postoperative factors have been recently identified [6]. Such studies were hampered by the low incidence of UTUC, and retrospective single-center design. Lately, several multi-center and international studies have been performed and the combination of their outcomes have led to the development of predictive tools such as nomograms and risk stratification models helping clinical decision-making in pursuit of tailored, individual patient care. This review provides an overview of existing prognostic factors and predictive tools for the management of patients with UTUC.

A. Mbeutcha · T. Klatte · R. Mathieu · S. F. Shariat
Department of Urology, Vienna General Hospital, Comprehensive Cancer Center, Medical University of Vienna, Vienna, Austria
e-mail: ambeutcha@hotmail.com

T. Klatte
e-mail: tobias.klatte@meduniwien.ac.at

A. Mbeutcha
Department of Urology, University Hospital of Nice, University of Nice Sophia-Antipolis, Nice, France

R. Mathieu
Department of Urology, Rennes University Hospital, Rennes, France
e-mail: romain.mathieu@chu-rennes.fr

S. F. Shariat
Department of Urology, Weill Cornell Medical College, New York, NY, USA

S. F. Shariat (✉)
Department of Urology, University of Texas Southwestern Medical Center, Dallas, TX, USA
e-mail: sfshariat@gmail.com

M. Eshghi (ed.), *Urothelial Malignancies of the Upper Urinary Tract*,
https://doi.org/10.1007/978-3-319-51263-1_2

Evidence Acquisition

A literature search was performed using PubMed/Medline on articles published in English between January 2000 and July 2015 using combinations of the following keywords: upper tract urothelial carcinoma, urothelial carcinoma, prognosis, prognostic factors, predictive tools, nomogram, risk grouping, risk table, markers, and survival. A preselection of relevant papers was made among the 900 retrieved articles by using the following criteria: highlight of large cohorts by using a threshold of 300 patients included for clinical studies and 100 patients for biomarkers studies. In case of redundancy, we privileged multi-institutional and/or international and/or prospective studies over retrospective and/or single-center cohorts. After qualitative review of full articles, we retained 108 articles with the consensus of all authors (Fig. 2.1).

Evidence Synthesis

Prognostic Factors and Predictive Tools of Advanced-Stage and Non-Organ-Confined Disease

Patient-Related Factors

Epidemiologic data showed that at the time of diagnosis, up to 45% of the patients present with non-organ-confined (NOC) UTUC (i.e., T3+ or N+ or M+) [7]. Therefore, accurate preoperative prediction of advanced stage would help the

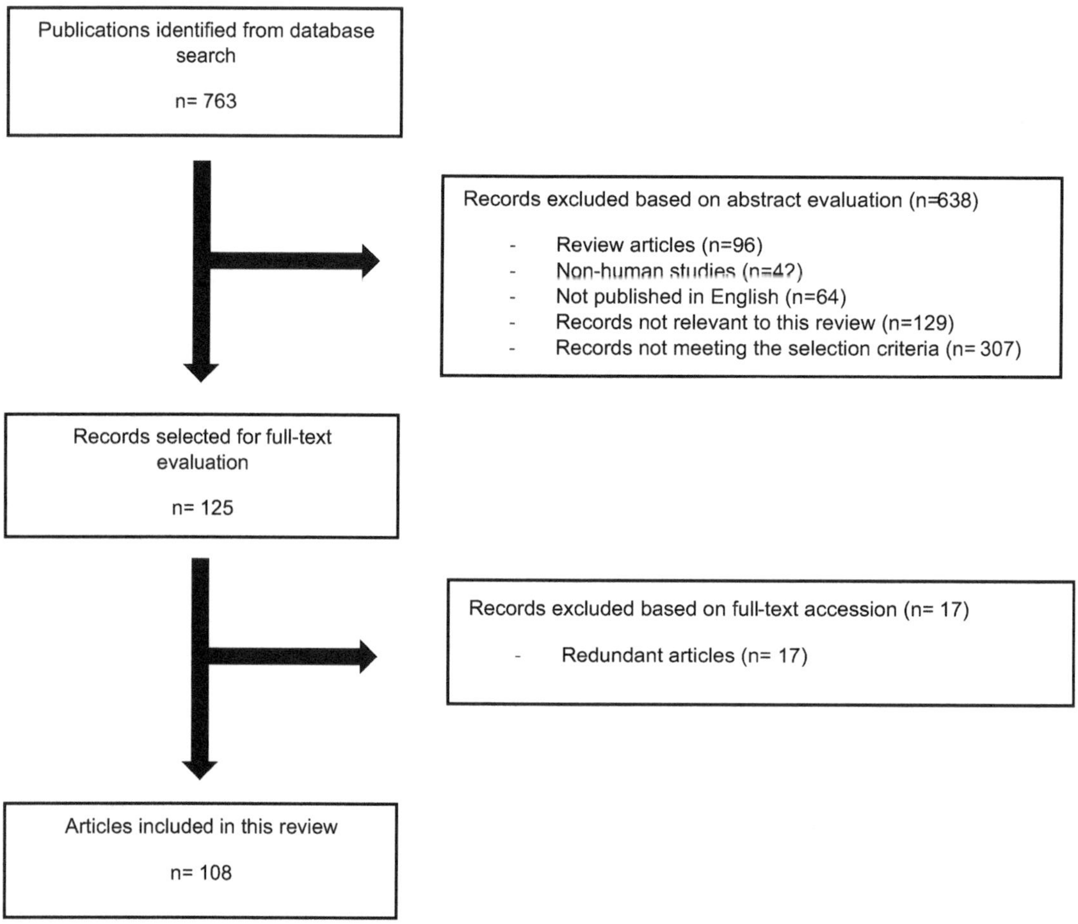

Fig. 2.1 Flow-chart of evidence acquisition in a systematic review on prognostic factors and prediction models for UTUC

identification of those high-risk patients who could benefit from more aggressive management, such as neoadjuvant chemotherapy, RNU, and extended lymph node dissection.

Despite improvement in imaging and ureteroscopy, preoperative assessment of tumor aggressiveness remains difficult, if not close to impossible. Many retrospective studies have been able to identify independent prognostic factors (Table 2.1), which have been eventually integrated in tools predicting muscle-invasiveness and/or NOC disease (Table 2.2).

Among the patient-related predictive factors associated with advanced-stage disease and/or NOC, smoking status is the only well-established variable. Former and current smokers are more likely to develop high grade and stage tumors associated with lymph node metastasis and LVI [8, 9].

Systemic symptoms [10] such as anorexia, weight loss and night sweat, and imaging features such as local invasion [11] and hydronephrosis [12, 13] have also been associated with advanced disease. Indeed, the combination of imaging and established clinical features such as cytology and biopsy grading can achieve an excellent negative predictive value for T2 and higher stage UTUC [11].

Compared with other urologic malignancies, the mean age of patients with UTUC at the time of diagnosis is rather advanced. Advanced-age has been identified as a factor for more aggressive tumors in several studies, including nationwide epidemiologic-based studies [14]. Yet, in large multi-institutional studies, chronical age was not an independent predictor of worse survival when the effect of performance status was adjusted for [15, 16].

Gender is another controversial prognostic factor for advanced-stage and/or NOC disease. Female gender has been associated with higher stage and grade at the time of diagnosis in nationwide epidemiologic databases [17] but these findings have not been confirmed in cohort studies. In contrast to bladder cancer, it seems that gender does not affect outcomes independently [18, 19].

Finally, obese patients (body mass index ≥30) are more likely features of biologically and clinically aggressive UTUC such as LVI and sessile architecture; in addition, obese patients seems to have worse prognosis compared to non-obese patients [20].

Tumor Pathology Features and Biomarkers

A few pathologic elements associated with muscle-invasive and/or NOC UTUC are identifiable preoperatively. Ureteroscopy is accurate and could help in the preoperative risk stratification of patients [21]. Ureteroscopy can help identify tumor architecture [22, 23] and tumor multifocality [24]. When combined with biopsies, ureteroscopy may help identify pathologic features associated with worse prognosis, such as concomitant carcinoma in situ (CIS) [25, 26], variant histology [27–29], LVI [30–32] or tumor necrosis [33, 34].

The association between tumor location and aggressive tumors is still unclear. Contradictory findings have been reported [13, 35–38] and a recent meta-analysis including more than 12,000 patients did not find any statistical difference between both locations in patients presenting with NOC disease [39]. Nevertheless, these results were limited by a significant heterogeneity among the studies.

Beyond patient and tumor pathologic characteristics, several tissue-based biomarkers involved in different steps of UTUC carcinogenesis have been identified lately (Table 2.1). These biomarkers are implicated in diverse mechanisms of tumorigenesis, such as cell proliferation (Ki-67 [40, 41], CDCA5 [42], PAK1 [43], INHBA [44], PTP4A3 [45], COX2 [46] and EPR4R [46]), cell cycle regulation (mTOR pathway [47], PAK1 [43]), apoptosis (Bcl-xL [48]), cell differentiation (ALDH1 [49]), and immunity (CD204+ macrophages [50]). The identification of these markers on ureteroscopic diagnostic biopsy might help risk not only to better understand UTUC carcinogenesis, but also to stratify patients according to their risk group. For the moment, most of these biomarkers have been evaluated in small single-center retrospective cohorts. Further

Table 2.1 Prognostic factors of advanced-stage and non-organ-confined disease

Factors	High tumor stage	High tumor grade	Lymph node metastasis	Other associations	Ref.
Preoperative factors					
Advanced age	✓	✓			[14]
Female gender	✓	✓			[17]
Obesity (BMI ≥ 30)				Sessile architecture and LVI	[20]
Smoking	✓	✓	✓	LVI	[8, 9]
History of bladder CIS		✓		Sessile architecture	[62]
Hydronephrosis	✓	✓	✓		[12, 13]
Symptoms	✓	✓	✓	Necrosis, LVI	[10]
Local invasion on imaging	✓		✓		[11]
Postoperative/pathologic factors					
Concomitant CIS	✓	✓	✓	LVI	[25, 26]
LVI	✓	✓	✓	Positive surgical margins	[30]
Tumor multifocality	✓	✓	✓	LVI	[13, 24, 94]
Sessile tumor	✓	✓	✓	LVI, concomitant CIS	[13, 22]
Tumor necrosis	✓	✓	✓	LVI, sessile architecture, concomitant CIS	[33, 34]
Concomitant histology variant	✓	✓	✓	LVI, tumor diameter, positive surgical margins, sessile architecture	[27, 28]
Molecular markers					
Tissue-based					
Ki-67	✓		✓	LVI, necrosis, sessile architecture, concomitant CIS	[40, 41]
mTOR pathway	✓	✓	✓	LVI, concomitant CIS	[47]
IMP3	✓	✓	✓	LVI, sessile tumors, concomitant CIS, necrosis	[95]
BCAT 1	✓	✓	✓	LVI	[76]
INHBA	✓	✓	✓	LVI	[44]
ALDH1	✓	✓		LVI	[49]
CDCA5	✓	✓	✓	LVI	[42]
GPX2	✓	✓	✓	LVI	[77]
PTP4A3	✓		✓	LVI	[45]
High cd204 + cell density	✓	✓	✓	LVI, sessile architecture, concomitant CIS	[50]
mi-149	✓				[96]
KPNA2	✓	✓			[97]
PAK1	✓	✓		LVI	[43]

(continued)

Table 2.1 (continued)

Factors	High tumor stage	High tumor grade	Lymph node metastasis	Other associations	Ref.
COX2 and EP4R co-expression	✓	✓			[46]
IGFBP5	✓	✓	✓	LVI	[98]
Bcl-xl	✓	✓		LVI	[48]
Blood-based					
NLR	✓	✓	✓	LVI, concomitant CIS	[52]
Fibrinogen	✓	✓			[53]

Notes LVI lymphovascular invasion; *CIS* carcinoma in situ; *BMI* body mass index

Table 2.2 Predictive tools of advanced-stage and non-organ-confined disease

Reference	Prediction form	Outcome	N° of patients	Variables	Accuracy	Validation
Chen et al. 2013 [13]	Preoperative nomogram	Muscle-invasive disease	693	Gender, architecture, multifocality, location, grade, hydronephrosis	79%	Internal
Chen et al. 2013 [13]	Preoperative nomogram	Non-organ confined disease	693	Gender, architecture, multifocality, location, grade	79%	Internal
Favaretto et al. 2012 [11]	Preoperative risk stratification	Muscle-invasive disease	274	Ureteroscopic grade, location, invasion and hydronephrosis on imaging	71%	None
Favaretto et al. 2012 [11]	Preoperative risk group stratification	Non-organ-confined disease	274	Ureteroscopic grade, location, invasion and hydronephrosis on imaging	70%	None
Margulis et al. 2010 [38]	Preoperative nomogram	Non-organ-confined disease	659	Grade, architecture, location	77%	Internal
Brien et al. 2010 [21]	Preoperative risk group stratification	Muscle-invasive disease	172	Hydronephrosis, ureteroscopic grade and urinary cytology	PPV 89% NPV 100%	–
Brien et al. 2010 [21]	Preoperative risk group stratification	Non-organ-confined disease	172	Hydronephrosis, ureteroscopic grade and urinary cytology	PPV 73% NPV 100%	–

validations of their clinical utility by conducting large multi-center and prospective studies are, therefore, still necessary before their introduction in the clinical use [51].

High preoperative neutrophil-to-lymphocyte ration (NLR) [52] and high fibrinogen [53] are the only two preoperative blood-based biomarkers that have been associated with advanced-stage disease. Both these biomarkers reflect systemic inflammation which has a known role in carcinogenesis and tumor progression. Nevertheless, here also validation is necessary.

Predictive Tools

The available predictive tools are shown in Table 2.2. In a study of 683 patients, Chen et al. [13] developed a preoperative nomogram predicting muscle-invasive disease and another one predicting NOC disease with an accuracy of 79% each. Together with gender, these nomograms include features based on the ureteroscopy and imaging, such as tumor architecture, multifocality, tumor location, and hydronephrosis.

The risk group stratification proposed by Favaretto et al. [11] reached an accuracy of 70% for muscle-invasive disease prediction and 71% for NOC disease by combining ureteroscopic grade, tumor location, hydronephrosis, and invasion on imaging.

By combining tumor grade, architecture, and tumor location, Margulis et al. [38] managed to develop a nomogram predicting NOC disease with an accuracy of 77%.

Unfortunately, none of these tools were assessed in external validation cohorts, thereby limiting their generalizability, reliability, and validity in the clinical setting. Nevertheless, since staging based on today's tools is difficult, risk stratification based on tissue and fluid biomarkers will likely allow accurate risk stratification to guide therapy.

By identifying tissue-based biomarkers and pathological features associated with advanced-stage and/or NOC disease, in the near future, ureteroscopy combined with biopsies will provide an accurate preoperative prediction of those high-risk patients who would benefit from a more aggressive management.

Prognostic Factors and Predictive Tools Associated with Intravesical, Loco-Regional and Distant Metastatic Recurrence

Patient-Related Factors

In order to be able to propose adjuvant chemotherapy and risk-based surveillance to patients at high-risk for disease recurrence and ultimately death from UTUC, several studies have focused on the identification of postoperative prognostic factors (Table 2.3). Indeed, several relatively accurate tools predicting UTUC recurrence have been recently developed (Table 2.4).

Table 2.3 Prognostic factors associated with intravesical, loco-regional and distant metastatic recurrence

Factors	Intravesical recurrence	Loco-regional recurrence	Metastatic recurrence	Ref.
Preoperative factors				
Advanced-age	✓	✓		[16, 54]
Male gender	✓			[19, 54]
Obesity (BMI ≥ 30)		✓		[20]
Smoking	✓	✓		[8, 9, 63]
DM with poor glycemic control	✓	✓		[64–66]
Previous/concomitant BC	✓			[54, 61, 62, 87]
Hydronephrosis			✓	[69]
Absence of RAS inhibitor administration			✓	[70]
Postoperative/pathologic factors				
High tumor stage	✓	✓	✓	[54–58, 82]
High tumor grade		✓		[57, 58]

(continued)

Table 2.3 (continued)

Factors	Intravesical recurrence	Loco-regional recurrence	Metastatic recurrence	Ref.
Lymph node metastasis	✓	✓		[54, 56, 58]
Ureteral location	✓	✓	✓	[24, 39, 54, 82]
Multifocal tumors		✓	✓	[24, 71]
Tumor size > 3 cm	✓			[73]
LVI		✓	✓	[30, 56, 58–60]
Concomitant CIS	✓	✓		[25, 26, 54]
Sessile architecture		✓		[22, 23, 56]
Concomitant variant histology		✓	✓	[28]
Laparoscopic RNU	✓			[67]
Endoscopic BCE	✓	✓		[54, 74]
Extravesical BCE	✓	✓		[54, 67, 74]
Positive surgical margin	✓		✓	[67, 99, 100]
Molecular markers				
Tissue-based				
Ki-67		✓		[40, 41]
IMP3		✓		[95]
KPNA2	✓	✓		[97]
ALDH1		✓		[49]
PAK1		✓		[43]
FAS	✓	✓		[101]
HER2	✓			[102]
BCAT1			✓	[76]
INHBA			✓	[44]
CDCA5			✓	[42
GPX2			✓	[77]
PTP4A3			✓	[45]
High CD204+ cell density			✓	[50]
IGFBP5			✓	[98]
mTOR pathway		✓		[47]
p53		✓		[103]
HIF1-alpha		✓		[104]
Blood-based				
Anemia		✓	✓	[78]
High CRP		✓		[79]
High NLR		✓	✓	[52]
Urine-based				
Cytology	✓			[80]

Beside well-established pathologic factors, such as tumor stage [54–58], lymph node metastasis [54, 56, 58] and LVI [30, 32, 56, 58–60], many patient- and surgery-related factors have been tested.

Unfortunately, the retrospective setting of most of the studies rarely allows a precise definition of disease recurrence specifically when it comes to the site (bladder, loco-regional, contralateral or visceral metastasis). Nevertheless, some factors seem to be associated with specific recurrence patterns and localizations. Whether it is due to the biological aspect of the tumor or if it just a bias due to lack of precise data in a retrospective analysis remains unclear.

Advanced-age is one of the well-documented prognostic factors associated with intravesical and loco-regional recurrence [16, 54].

Despite being different diseases, bladder cancer (BC) is also a consequence of a pan-urothelial

Table 2.4 Predictive tools associated with intravesical, loco-regional and distant metastatic recurrence

Reference	Prediction form	Patient population	Outcome	N° of patients	Variables	Accuracy (%)	Validation
Kim et al. [105]	Postoperative nomogram	All RNU	2- and 5-year RFS	277	Stage, LVI, BCE, dNLR	78	External
Xylinas et al. [54]	Risk group stratification and nomogram	All RNU	3, 6, 9, 12, 18, 24 and 36 months IVR	1839	age, gender, previous BC, location, stage, CIS, lymph node metastasis, ureteral management, surgical approach	69	External
Ehdaie et al. [81]	Postoperative nomogram	RNU without neoadjuvant chemotherapy	5-year RFS	253	preoperative GFR, tumor grade, stage, lymph node metastasis	82	None
Ishioka et al. [55]	Risk group stratification and nomogram	All RNU	1- and 5-year IVR	754	Papillary architecture, stage, LVI, gender	62	None
Colin et al. [82]	Risk group stratification	pT2–3 pNx	2- and 5-year MFS	151	Tumor location, stage, LVI, surgical margin	–	None
Cha et al. [56]	Postoperative nomogram	RNU without perioperative chemotherapy	2- and 5-year RFS	2244	Age, stage, grade, lymph node metastasis, LVI, architecture, CIS	77	External
Bolenz et al. [106]	Risk group stratification	RNU with lymphadenectomy	5-year RFS	432	Stage, grade, LVI, lymph node density	70	Internal

IVR intravesical recurrence; *RNU* radical nephro-ureterectomy; *dNLR* derived neutrophil to lymphocyte ratio; *BC* bladder cancer; *CIS* carcinoma in situ; *GFR* glomerular filtration rate; *LVI* lymphovascular invasion disease. Therefore, it is not surprising that previous/concomitant BC is associated with intravesical UTUC recurrence [54, 61, 62].

Others well-established factors associated with intravesical and loco-regional recurrence are smoking status [8, 9, 63] and diabetes mellitus with poor glycemic control [64–66].

Male gender and preoperative chronic kidney disease have also been identified as independent predictors of intravesical recurrence in meta-analyses [67, 68].

Hydronephrosis [69] and absence of renin-angiotensin system (RAS) inhibitor treatment for patient with hypertension [70] have been established as specific predictors of metastatic recurrence. Both of these results have been obtained in relatively small single-center studies and need, therefore, to be confirmed in multi-institutional and/or prospective analysis.

Tumor- and Surgery-Related Factors

Beside the pathological features associated with intravesical and loco-regional recurrence previously discussed, concomitant CIS [25, 26, 54] and multifocal tumors [24, 71] have also been identified as independent predictors. Therefore, the presence of either of these features should be emphasized in order to propose a more intense follow-up to patients with these features.

Once again, the prognostic impact of tumor location is debated. Several large-scale studies found contradictory results according to tumor location focusing on loco-regional recurrences [36, 37, 71, 72] or intravesical recurrences [19]. Meta-analyses have, however, shown that ureteral location is associated with shorter recurrence-free survival (RFS) for both loco-regional [39] and intravesical locations [67, 68].

Other pathological features that would benefit from more research are tumor size and tumor necrosis. To our knowledge, the influence of tumor size on RFS has been studied in a few studies including only one large cohort. The authors of this study showed that large tumors were associated with shorter time to intravesical recurrence [73]. A meta-analysis including the previous study and 6 others (of which the majority had less than 100 patients) confirmed these data [68]. Studies on tumor necrosis and RFS showed variable results [33, 34].

Interestingly, tumor architecture is associated with different recurrence sites. Papillary architecture has been established as a predictor of intravesical recurrence [55] whereas sessile architecture is associated with loco-regional recurrence [22, 23, 56]. This supports the idea that recurrence sites are related to the underlying biological potential of the primary tumor.

Although open RNU with BCE remains the standard making it mandatory for patients with high-risk noninvasive UTUC or invasive disease [2], better understanding of UTUC prognostic factors has allowed the development of less invasive surgical techniques, such as laparoscopic RNU, endoscopic BCE, and segmental resection. Current data have shown that the choice of the surgical technique may have an impact on recurrence rates, albeit modest. A meta-analysis found that laparoscopic RNU was associated with lower urinary recurrence and distant metastasis [3], but more recent and well-conducted retrospective studies and meta-analysis established that laparoscopic RNU, endoscopic BCE, and extravesical BCE were associated with higher intravesical and loco-regional recurrence rates [54, 67, 74]. International guidelines insist on the indications for laparoscopic RNU and kidney-sparing treatment. Concerning the BCE technique, it remains at the discretion of the surgeon according to its personal experience, although stripping and stapling leads to higher intravesical recurrence rates [75].

Biomarkers

The identification of molecular markers predictors associated with disease recurrence is a major challenge and hope. Tissue-based biomarkers implicated in each step of tumorigenesis have been identified (Table 2.3). Interestingly, some of them seem to be associated with specific recurrence patterns. For example, cell proliferation markers, such as BCAT1 [76], INHBA [44], CDCA5 [42], and PTP43A [45], or markers implicated in oxidative stress such as GPX2 [77] seem to be specifically associated with visceral metastatic patterns. These findings are anyway limited by the retrospective design of the studies. A validation in a prospective setting would implement their accuracy and potentially enable their use in a clinical setting.

Anemia [78], high CRP [79] and high NLR [52] are all known systemic inflammation blood-based biomarkers correlated with shorter RFS (Table 2.3). The volume of studies and their level of evidence is still low but the role of inflammation in cancer is well established. Therefore, more studies exploring this subject should be performed in order to allow evidence-based care of UTUC patients.

Urinary cytology is the only noninvasive biomarker that has been associated with intravesical recurrence so far. For low grade tumors, selective ureteral cytology in UTUC has a rate of false-negative of up to 50% which is a major limitation. Further investigations need to be performed to confirm these findings as only one large cohort study has established it up to date [80].

Predictive Tools

Based on these different findings, tools predicting intravesical RFS, loco-regional RFS and metastasis-free survival have been developed (Table 2.4).

Based on the data from the UTUC Collaboration group, Xylinas et al. developed a risk group stratification and a nomogram predicting intravesical recurrence at 3, 6, 9, 12, 18, and 36 months [54]. By combining information on age, gender, previous BC, tumor location, stage, concomitant CIS, lymph node metastasis, BCE management, and surgical approach, they created a nomogram reaching an accuracy of 69%.

Edhaie et al. constructed a postoperative nomogram based on the preoperative glomerular filtration rate (GFR), tumor grade, stage, and lymph node metastasis [81]. Their model had an accuracy of 82% but lacked external or internal validation.

Finally, data from the French national database on UTUC, Colin et al. proposed a risk stratification model predicting 2- and 5-year metastasis-free survival by using tumor location, stage, LVI, and surgical margin [82].

All these nomograms and predictive tools are promising for the management of UTUC. However, external validation and integration of the most promising biomarkers may be the next step to improve their clinical use and accuracy.

Data seem to indicate that some factors (both clinical and pathological) are associated with different specific recurrence patterns and localizations. Taking this issue into account would improve the accuracy of the upcoming predictive tools for disease recurrence.

Prognostic Factors and Predictive Tools for Cancer-Specific and Overall Survival

Patient-Related Factors

In the last two decades, UTUC-related mortality has not decreased [83]. Though, in the latest years, the increase of research has permitted to identify factors of biologically and clinically aggressive disease (Table 2.5) and therefore help the establishment of tools predicting UTUC related mortality (Table 2.6).

Advanced-age has been associated with a shorter cancer-specific survival (CSS) [14–16, 58]. Beside the hypothesis on the biological potential of tumors in elderlies explained earlier, this could also be explained by the reluctance of physicians to propose a radical therapy to these patients. International guidelines insist on the fact that old age should not be an exclusion criterion in treatment decision-making for potentially curable UTUC [2]. In contrast, performance status may be one.

Smoking status is also an independent predictor of shorter CSS, but interestingly, patients who have quitted smoking for more than 10 years have similar oncologic outcomes than those who never smoked [8, 63]. This information should invigorate physicians to perform smoking cessation counseling.

The other well-documented patient-related factors associated with CSS are obesity [20], diabetes mellitus with poor glycemic control [64]

Table 2.5 Prognostic factors for cancer-specific and overall survival

Factors	Cancer-specific survival	Overall survival	Ref.
Preoperative factors			
Advanced-age	✓	✓	[14–16, 58]
ECOG-PS	✓	✓	[4, 84]
Obesity (BMI ≥ 30)	✓	✓	[20]
Smoking	✓		[8, 63]
DM with poor glycemic control	✓		[64]
Hydronephrosis		✓	[69]
Postoperative/pathologic factors			
High tumor stage	✓	✓	[20, 26, 56–58]
High tumor grade	✓		[22, 36, 58]
Lymph node metastasis	✓	✓	[20, 56, 58]
Ureteral location	✓		[39]
Multifocal tumor	✓	✓	[24, 39, 71]
LVI	✓	✓	[60]
Concomitant CIS	✓		[25, 26]
Sessile architecture	✓		[22, 23, 56, 58]
Concomitant variant histology	✓	✓	[28]
Lack of BCE	✓		[88]
Molecular markers			
Tissue-based			
Ki-67	✓		[41, 107]
IMP3	✓	✓	[95]
KPNA2		✓	[97]
ALDH1	✓	✓	[49]
COX2 and EP4R co-expression	✓		[46]
BCAT1	✓		[76]
INHBA	✓		[44]
PTP4A3	✓		[45]
IGFBP5	✓		[98]
mi-149	✓		[96]
mTOR pathway	✓		[47]
CDCA5	✓		[42]
Bcl-xL	✓		[48]
p53	✓	✓	[103]
Nuclear p-AKT	✓		[108]
FGFR3 mutation	✓		[109]
Osteopontin	✓		[110]
HIF-1alpha		✓	[104]
PAK1	✓	✓	[43, 111]
GPX2 (under-expressed)	✓		[77]
Blood-based			
Anemia	✓		[78]
High CRP	✓		[79]
High NLR	✓		[52]
Fibrinogen	✓	✓	[53]
Low sodium	✓		[78]

Table 2.6 Predictive tools for cancer-specific and overall survival

Reference	Prediction form	Patient population	Outcome	N° of patients	Variables	Accuracy (%)	Validation
Kim et al. [105]	Postoperative nomogram	All RNU	2- and 5-year CSS	277	Stage, LVI, BCE, dNLR	80	External
Fujita et al. [78]	Preoperative risk group stratification	All RNU	5-year CSS	357	Preoperative sodium and hemoglobin level	–	External
Ehdaie et al. [81]	Postoperative nomogram	RNU without neoadjuvant chemotherapy	5-year CSS	253	Stage, grade, lymph node metastasis, preoperative GFR	83	None
Seisen et al. [92]	Postoperative nomogram	pT1–3/N0-x M0 without preoperative chemotherapy	5-year CSS	1563	Age, stage, grade, location, architecture, LVI	81	External
Sakano et al. [112]	Risk group stratification	All RNU	5-year CSS	536	Stage, cytology, white blood cell counts	–	None
Rouprêt et al. [93]	Postoperative nomogram	All RNU	5-year CSS	2371	Age, stage, lymph node metastasis, architecture and LVI	80	External
Ku et al. [113]	Online nomogram of Yates	RNU without neoadjuvant chemotherapy	3- and 5-years CSS	328	Age, stage, grade, lymph node metastasis, location	72	External
Cha et al. [56]	Postoperative nomogram	RNU without perioperative chemotherapy	2- and 5-year CSS	2244	Age, stage, grade, lymph node metastasis, LVI, architecture, concomitant CIS	82	External
Yates et al. [114]	Postoperative nomogram	All RNU	3- and 5-year CSS	667	Age, stage, grade, lymph node metastasis, location	78	External
Jeldres et al. [91]	Postoperative nomogram	All RNU	5-year CSS	2959	Age, stage, grade, lymph node metastasis	75	External
Bolenz et al. [106]	Risk group stratification	RNU with lymphadenectomy	5-year CSS	432	Stage, grade, LVI, lymph node density	68	Internal

RNU radical nephro-ureterectomy; *CSS* cancer-specific survival; *LVI* lymphovascular invasion; *BCE* bladder cuff excision; *dNLR* derived neutrophil to lymphocyte ration; *GFR* glomerular filtration rate and Eastern Cooperative group Performance Status (ECOG-PS) [4, 84].

Male gender has been identified as an independent prognostic factor for shorter CSS in population-based epidemiologic studies [7], but large single- and multicenter studies failed to confirm this finding [17, 18, 85]. Therefore, according to guidelines, gender is no longer considered an independent prognostic factor influencing UTUC mortality [2].

Few studies explored the influence of ethnical background on UTUC-related outcomes. A multi-institutional international study comparing Caucasian and Japanese patient's outcomes did not find any difference in CSS between these two groups [86], but an epidemiologic nationwide study found that African-American patients with UTUC had shorter survival than other ethnic groups [7]. Yet, these findings could be biased by socioeconomical features.

Tumor-and Surgery-Related Factors

Surprisingly, BC is an independent predictor of CSS according its stage: concomitant non-muscle invasive BC is not associated with CSS in UTUC [87], whereas bladder CIS is [62]. These findings need to be confirmed in further studies.

Widely studied and validated postoperative features associated with CSS and/or overall survival (OS) are tumor stage [20, 26, 56–58], grade [22, 36, 58], lymph node metastasis [20, 56, 58], multifocality [24, 39, 71], LVI [60], concomitant CIS [25, 26] and sessile architecture [22, 23, 56, 58].

Non-pure urothelial carcinoma with the presence of concomitant histologic variant seems also to be associated with worse survival. In a retrospective study including 1648 patients, the 5-year CSS was superior to 60% for patients with pure UTUC whereas it dropped to less than 50% for patients with variant histology ($p = 0.003$) [29].

Finally, the lack of BCE is associated with worse CSS [88, 89], confirming the necessity to pay special care during this procedure in accordance with guidelines [2].

Contradictory outcomes on tumor location need to be assessed. Some studies supported the idea that ureteral location was associated with worse CSS [24, 90] whereas some supported the contrary [35, 36, 71, 72]. A recent meta-analysis found that ureteral location was associated with worse CSS, but this study suffered from significant heterogeneity [39].

In the same way, tumor necrosis also suffers from contradictory findings [33, 34, 86] and its role in CSS needs to be further evaluated.

Biomarkers

Promising biomarkers associated with CSS are listed in Table 2.5.

Amongst the tissue-based biomarkers some, such as Bcl-xL are implicated in apoptosis and are potential therapy targets [48]. But all these biomarkers have been evaluated only in small cohorts; therefore further studies are needed to validate or reject these findings.

Systemic inflammation-associated blood-based biomarkers, such as anemia [78], high CRP [79], high NLR [52] and high fibrinogen [53] are associated with CSS.

Hyponatremia is a phenomenon associated with CSS in different types of cancers, including UTUC [78], but its mechanism remains unclear to date.

Predictive Tools

The first postoperative nomogram assessing CSS was proposed by Jeldres et al. [91]. In a study including a cohort of 2959 patients, the authors managed to construct a postoperative nomogram integrating age, tumor stage, grade, and lymph node metastasis. This model predicting the 5-year CSS had an accuracy of 75%.

Since then, many tools have been developed to predict CSS (Table 2.6).

Edhaie et al. developed a nomogram integrating tumor stage, grade, lymph node metastasis, and preoperative GFR [81]. To our knowledge, this model reached the highest accuracy rate (83%), but these results are limited by the small size of the cohort ($n = 253$) and the absence of external validation.

Three other nomograms, each of them developed from retrospective cohorts including more than 2000 patients and beneficiating from an external validation cohort, reached an accuracy rate above 80% [56, 92, 93].

Widely studied clinical and pathological features, such as age, stage, grade and lymph node metastasis have permitted to elaborate highly accurate predictive tools for CSS. Nevertheless, the integration of promising biomarkers in the conception of these tools would very probably increase their accuracy.

Conclusion

Until recently, the studies on UTUC were limited by small sample sizes and selection biases due to their retrospective nature. Efforts provided by international collaboration groups have permitted to identify new prognostic factors (LVI, necrosis, architecture) aside of the established pathologic clinical factors (stage, grade, and lymph node metastasis).

As the current staging system is not optimal, new prognostic factors and tools are needed to help decision-making process and help identifying high-risk patients who could benefit from intensified therapy and those who could be spared from the side effects of an unnecessary therapeutic intervention and/or follow-up. In order to select these patients and include them in clinical trials on multimodal therapy schemes, highly accurate tools estimating individual prognosis are needed.

Therefore, a prospective validation of the existing predictive models and further investigations to discover new biomarkers is necessary.

Summary Box

- Amongst the patient-related predictive factors associated with advanced-stage disease and/or NOC, smoking status is the only well-established variable.
- Ureteroscopy is accurate and could help in the preoperative risk stratification of patients. When combined with biopsies, ureteroscopy may help identifying architectural and pathological patterns associated with adverse outcomes, such as sessile architecture, multifocal tumors, concomitant CIS, or tumor necrosis.
- In the near future, identification of tissue-based biomarkers on ureteroscopically obtained biopsies will provide an accurate preoperative prediction of those high-risk patients who would benefit from a more aggressive management.
- Data seem to indicate that some factors (both clinical and pathological) are associated with different specific recurrence patterns and localizations. Taking this issue into account would improve the accuracy of the upcoming predictive tools for disease recurrence.
- Widely studied clinical and pathological features, such as age, stage, grade, and lymph node metastasis have permitted to elaborate highly accurate predictive tools for CSS. Nevertheless, the integration of promising biomarkers in the conception of these tools would very probably increase their accuracy.

References

1. Siegel RL, Miller KD, Jemal A. Cancer statistics, 2015. CA Cancer J Clin. 2015;65:5–29.
2. Rouprêt, M. et al. European association of urology guidelines on upper urinary tract urothelial cell carcinoma: 2015 update. Eur Urol 2015;68:1–12. doi:10.1016/j.eururo.2015.06.044.
3. Rai BP, Shelley M, Coles B, Somani B, Nabi G. Surgical management for upper urinary tract transitional cell carcinoma (UUT-TCC): a systematic review. BJU Int. 2012;110:1426–35.
4. Bagrodia A, et al. Comparative analysis of oncologic outcomes of partial ureterectomy vs radical nephroureterectomy in upper tract urothelial carcinoma. Urology. 2013;81:972–7.
5. Rink M, et al. Stage-specific impact of tumor location on oncologic outcomes in patients with upper and lower tract urothelial carcinoma following radical surgery. Eur Urol. 2012;62:677–84.
6. Lughezzani G, et al. Prognostic factors in upper urinary tract urothelial carcinomas: a comprehensive

review of the current literature. Eur Urol. 2012;62:100–14.
7. Raman JD, Messer J, Sielatycki JA, Hollenbeak CS. Incidence and survival of patients with carcinoma of the ureter and renal pelvis in the USA, 1973–2005. BJU Int. 2011;107:1059–64.
8. Rink M, et al. Impact of smoking on oncologic outcomes of upper tract urothelial carcinoma after radical nephroureterectomy. BJU Int. 2012;63:1082–90.
9. Xylinas E, et al. Impact of smoking status and cumulative exposure on intravesical recurrence of upper tract urothelial carcinoma after radical nephroureterectomy. BJU Int. 2014;114:56–61.
10. Raman JD, et al. Does preoperative symptom classification impact prognosis in patients with clinically localized upper-tract urothelial carcinoma managed by radical nephroureterectomy? Urol Oncol. 2011;29:716–23.
11. Favaretto RL, et al. Combining imaging and ureteroscopy variables in a preoperative multivariable model for prediction of muscle-invasive and non-organ confined disease in patients with upper tract urothelial carcinoma. BJU Int. 2012;109:77–82.
12. Messer JC, et al. Multi-institutional validation of the ability of preoperative hydronephrosis to predict advanced pathologic tumor stage in upper-tract urothelial carcinoma. Urol Oncol. 2013;31:904–8.
13. Chen X-P, et al. Predictive factors for worse pathological outcomes of upper tract urothelial carcinoma: experience from a nationwide high-volume centre in China. BJU Int. 2013;112:917–24.
14. Yap SA, Schupp CW, Chamie K, Evans CP, Koppie TM. Effect of age on transitional cell carcinoma of the upper urinary tract: presentation, treatment, and outcomes. Urology. 2011;78:87–92.
15. Shariat SF, et al. Advanced patient age is associated with inferior cancer-specific survival after radical nephroureterectomy. BJU Int. 2010;105:1672–7.
16. Chromecki TF, et al. Chronological age is not an independent predictor of clinical outcomes after radical nephroureterectomy. World J Urol. 2011;29:473–80.
17. Lughezzani G, et al. Gender-related differences in patients with stage I to III upper tract urothelial carcinoma: results from the surveillance, epidemiology, and end results database. Urology. 2010;75:321–7.
18. Shariat SF, et al. Gender differences in radical nephroureterectomy for upper tract urothelial carcinoma. World J Urol. 2011;29:481–6.
19. Kusuda Y, et al. Gender as a significant predictor of intravesical recurrence in patients with urothelial carcinoma of the upper urinary tract following nephroureterectomy. Urol Oncol. 2013;31:899–903.
20. Ehdaie B, et al. Obesity adversely impacts disease specific outcomes in patients with upper tract urothelial carcinoma. J Urol. 2011;186:66–72.
21. Brien JC, et al. Preoperative hydronephrosis, ureteroscopic biopsy grade and urinary cytology can improve prediction of advanced upper tract urothelial carcinoma. J Urol. 2010;184:69–73.
22. Remzi M, et al. Tumour architecture is an independent predictor of outcomes after nephroureterectomy: a multi-institutional analysis of 1363 patients. BJU Int. 2009;103:307–11.
23. Fritsche H-M, et al. Macroscopic sessile tumor architecture is a pathologic feature of biologically aggressive upper tract urothelial carcinoma. Urol Oncol. 2012;30:666–72.
24. Ouzzane A, et al. Ureteral and multifocal tumours have worse prognosis than renal pelvic tumours in urothelial carcinoma of the upper urinary tract treated by nephroureterectomy. Eur Urol. 2011;60:1258–65.
25. Otto W, et al. Concomitant carcinoma in situ as an independent prognostic parameter for recurrence and survival in upper tract urothelial carcinoma: a multicenter analysis of 772 patients. World J Urol. 2011;29:487–94.
26. Wheat JC, et al. Concomitant carcinoma in situ is a feature of aggressive disease in patients with organ confined urothelial carcinoma following radical nephroureterectomy. Urol Oncol. 2012;30:252–8.
27. Masson-Lecomte A, et al. Impact of micropapillary histological variant on survival after radical nephroureterectomy for upper tract urothelial carcinoma. World J Urol. 2014;32:531–7.
28. Shibing Y, et al. Effect of concomitant variant histology on the prognosis of patients with upper urinary tract urothelial carcinoma after radical nephroureterectomy. Urol Oncol. 2015;33(204):e9–16.
29. Rink M, et al. Impact of histological variants on clinical outcomes of patients with upper urinary tract urothelial carcinoma. J Urol. 2012;188:398–404.
30. Hurel S, et al. Impact of lymphovascular invasion on oncological outcomes in patients with upper tract urothelial carcinoma after radical nephroureterectomy. BJU Int. 2013;111:1199–207.
31. Novara G, et al. Prognostic role of lymphovascular invasion in patients with urothelial carcinoma of the upper urinary tract: an international validation study. Eur Urol. 2010;57:1064–71.
32. Kikuchi E, et al. Lymphovascular invasion predicts clinical outcomes in patients with node-negative upper tract urothelial carcinoma. J Clin Oncol. 2009;27:612–8.
33. Zigeuner R, et al. Tumour necrosis is an indicator of aggressive biology in patients with urothelial carcinoma of the upper urinary tract. Eur Urol. 2010;57:575–81.
34. Seitz C, et al. Association of tumor necrosis with pathological features and clinical outcome in 754 patients undergoing radical nephroureterectomy for

upper tract urothelial carcinoma: an international validation study. J Urol. 2010;184:1895–900.
35. Isbarn H, et al. Location of the primary tumor is not an independent predictor of cancer specific mortality in patients with upper urinary tract urothelial carcinoma. J Urol. 2009;182:2177–81.
36. Raman JD, et al. Impact of tumor location on prognosis for patients with upper tract urothelial carcinoma managed by radical nephroureterectomy. Eur Urol. 2010;57:1072–9.
37. Favaretto RL, et al. The effect of tumor location on prognosis in patients treated with radical nephroureterectomy at Memorial Sloan-Kettering Cancer Center. Eur Urol. 2010;58:574–80.
38. Margulis V, et al. Preoperative multivariable prognostic model for prediction of nonorgan confined urothelial carcinoma of the upper urinary tract. J Urol. 2010;184:453–8.
39. Wu Y, Dong Q, Liu L, Han P, Wei Q. The impact of tumor location and multifocality on prognosis for patients with upper tract urothelial carcinoma: a meta-analysis. Sci Rep. 2014;4:6361.
40. Krabbe L-M, et al. Prospective analysis of Ki-67 as an independent predictor of oncologic outcomes in patients with high grade upper tract urothelial carcinoma. J Urol. 2014;191:28–34.
41. Krabbe L.-M, et al. Multi-institutional validation of the predictive value of ki-67 in patients with high-grade urothelial carcinoma of the upper urinary tract. J Urol. 2014. At <http://www.ncbi.nlm.nih.gov/pubmed/25451830>.
42. Chang I-W, et al. CDCA5 overexpression is an indicator of poor prognosis in patients with urothelial carcinomas of the upper urinary tract and urinary bladder. Am J Transl Res. 2015;7:710–22.
43. Kuroda K, et al. Clinical significance of p21-activated kinase 1 expression level in patients with upper urinary tract urothelial carcinoma. Jpn J Clin Oncol. 2015;45:103–10.
44. Lee H-Y, et al. INHBA overexpression indicates poor prognosis in urothelial carcinoma of urinary bladder and upper tract. J Surg Oncol. 2015;111:414–22.
45. Yeh H-C, et al. PTP4A3 independently predicts metastasis and survival in upper tract urothelial carcinoma treated with radical nephroureterectomy. J Urol. 2015;. doi:10.1016/j.juro.2015.05.101.
46. Miyata Y, Kanda S, Nomata K, Eguchi J, Kanetake H. Expression of cyclooxygenase-2 and EP4 receptor in transitional cell carcinoma of the upper urinary tract. J Urol. 2005;173:56–60.
47. Bagrodia A, et al. Evaluation of the prognostic significance of altered mammalian target of rapamycin pathway biomarkers in upper tract urothelial carcinoma. Urology. 2014;84:1134–40.
48. Yoshimine S, et al. Prognostic significance of Bcl-xL expression and efficacy of Bcl-xL targeting therapy in urothelial carcinoma. Br J Cancer. 2013;108:2312–20.
49. Liu J, et al. Prognostic impact of ALDH1 expression in transitional cell carcinoma of the renal pelvis. Anticancer Res. 2015;35:4829–36.
50. Ichimura T, et al. Prognostic significance of CD204-positive macrophages in upper urinary tract cancer. Ann Surg Oncol. 2014;21:2105–12.
51. Bensalah K, Montorsi F, Shariat SF. Challenges of cancer biomarker profiling. Eur Urol. 2007;52:1601–9.
52. Tanaka N, et al. A multi-institutional validation of the prognostic value of the neutrophil-to-lymphocyte ratio for upper tract urothelial carcinoma treated with radical nephroureterectomy. Ann Surg Oncol. 2014;21:4041–8.
53. Pichler M, et al. Validation of the preoperative plasma fibrinogen level as a prognostic factor in a European cohort of patients with localized upper tract urothelial carcinoma. J Urol. 2014;191:920–5.
54. Xylinas E, et al. Prediction of intravesical recurrence after radical nephroureterectomy: development of a clinical decision-making tool. Eur Urol. 2014;65:650–8.
55. Ishioka J, et al. Risk stratification for bladder recurrence of upper urinary tract urothelial carcinoma after radical nephroureterectomy. BJU Int. 2015;115:705–12.
56. Cha EK, et al. Predicting clinical outcomes after radical nephroureterectomy for upper tract urothelial carcinoma. Eur Urol. 2012;61:818–25.
57. Shariat SF, et al. Subclassification of pT3 urothelial carcinoma of the renal pelvicalyceal system is associated with recurrence-free and cancer-specific survival: proposal for a revision of the current TNM classification. Eur Urol. 2012;62:224–31.
58. Margulis V, et al. Outcomes of radical nephroureterectomy: a series from the upper tract urothelial carcinoma collaboration. Cancer. 2009;115:1224–33.
59. Novara G, et al. Prognostic role of lymphovascular invasion in patients with urothelial carcinoma of the upper urinary tract: an international validation study. Eur Urol. 2010;57:1064–71.
60. Ku JH, et al. Lymphovascular invasion as a prognostic factor in the upper urinary tract urothelial carcinoma: a systematic review and meta-analysis. Eur J Cancer. 2013;49:2665–80.
61. Pignot G, et al. Influence of previous or synchronous bladder cancer on oncologic outcomes after radical nephroureterectomy for upper urinary tract urothelial carcinoma. Urol Oncol. 2014;32 (23):e1–8.
62. Youssef RF, et al. Prognostic effect of urinary bladder carcinoma in situ on clinical outcome of subsequent upper tract urothelial carcinoma. Urology. 2011;77:861–6.
63. Rink M, et al. Gender-specific effect of smoking on upper tract urothelial carcinoma outcomes. BJU Int. 2013;112:623–37.

64. Rieken M, et al. Diabetes mellitus without metformin intake is associated with worse oncologic outcomes after radical nephroureterectomy for upper tract urothelial carcinoma. Eur J Surg Oncol. 2014;40:113–20.
65. Hu C-Y, et al. Ureteral involvement and diabetes increase the risk of subsequent bladder recurrence after nephroureterectomy for upper urinary tract urothelial carcinoma. Biomed Res Int. 2015;2015:1–8.
66. Tai Y-S, et al. Quality assessment and improvement in diabetes care-an issue now and for the future. Diabetes Metab Res Rev. 2015;31:307–14.
67. Seisen T, et al. A systematic review and meta-analysis of clinicopathologic factors linked to intravesical recurrence after radical nephroureterectomy to treat upper tract urothelial carcinoma. Eur Urol. 2015;67:1122–33.
68. Yuan H, et al. Risk factors for intravesical recurrence after radical nephroureterectomy for upper tract urothelial carcinoma: a meta-analysis. Urol Oncol Semin Orig Investig. 2014;32:989–1002.
69. Bozzini G, et al. Influence of preoperative hydronephrosis on the outcome of urothelial carcinoma of the upper urinary tract after nephroureterectomy: the results from a multi-institutional French cohort. World J Urol. 2013;31:83–91.
70. Tanaka N, et al. Prognonstic impact of renin-angiotensin system blockade in localised upper-tract urothelial carcinoma. Br J Cancer. 2012;106:290–6.
71. Williams AK, et al. Multifocality rather than tumor location is a prognostic factor in upper tract urothelial carcinoma. Urol Oncol. 2013;31:1161–5.
72. Catto JWF, et al. Behavior of urothelial carcinoma with respect to anatomical location. J Urol. 2007;177:1715–20.
73. Kates M, Badalato GM, Gupta M, McKiernan JM. Secondary bladder cancer after upper tract urothelial carcinoma in the US population. BJU Int. 2012;110:1325–9.
74. Kapoor A, et al. The impact of method of distal ureter management during radical nephroureterectomy on tumour recurrence. Can Urol Assoc J. 2014;8:845–52.
75. Rouprêt M, et al. European association of urology guidelines on upper urinary tract urothelial cell carcinoma: 2015 update. Eur Urol. 2015;. doi:10.1016/j.eururo.2015.06.044.
76. Chang I-W, et al. BCAT1 overexpression is an indicator of poor prognosis in patients with urothelial carcinomas of the upper urinary tract and urinary bladder. Histopathology. 2015;. doi:10.1111/his.12778.
77. Chang I-W, et al. GPX2 underexpression indicates poor prognosis in patients with urothelial carcinomas of the upper urinary tract and urinary bladder. World J Urol. 2015;. doi:10.1007/s00345-015-1522-7.
78. Fujita K, et al. Preoperative risk stratification for cancer-specific survival of patients with upper urinary tract urothelial carcinoma treated by nephroureterectomy. Int J Clin Oncol. 2015;20:156–63.
79. Luo Y, Fu SJ, She DL, Xiong HU, Yang LI. Preoperative C-reactive protein as a prognostic predictor for upper tract urothelial carcinoma: a systematic review and meta-analysis. Mol Clin Oncol. 2015;3:924–8.
80. Tanaka N, et al. The predictive value of positive urine cytology for outcomes following radical nephroureterectomy in patients with primary upper tract urothelial carcinoma: a multi-institutional study. Urol Oncol. 2014;32(48):e19–26.
81. Ehdaie B, Shariat SF, Savage C, Coleman J, Dalbagni G. Postoperative nomogram for disease tee on cancer staging classification. Urol J. 2014;11:1435–41.
82. Colin P, et al. Risk stratification of metastatic recurrence in invasive upper urinary tract carcinoma after radical nephroureterectomy without lymphadenectomy. World J Urol. 2014;32:507–12.
83. Brown GA, et al. Nephroureterectomy for treating upper urinary tract transitional cell carcinoma: time to change the treatment paradigm? BJU Int. 2006;98:1176–180.
84. Martinez-Salamanca JI, et al. Prognostic role of ECOG performance status in patients with urothelial carcinoma of the upper urinary tract: an international study. BJU Int. 2012;109:1155–61.
85. Choo MS, Jeong CW, Kwak C, Kim HH, Ku JH. Effect of sex on prognosis of urothelial carcinoma: propensity score matching analysis. Clin Genitourin Cancer. 2015;13:e113–21.
86. Matsumoto K, et al. Racial differences in the outcome of patients with urothelial carcinoma of the upper urinary tract: an international study. BJU Int. 2011;108:304–9.
87. Fang D, et al. Presence of concomitant non-muscle-invasive bladder cancer in chinese patients with upper tract urothelial carcinoma: risk factors, characteristics, and predictive value. Ann Surg Oncol. 2015;22:2789–98.
88. Lughezzani G, et al. Should bladder cuff excision remain the standard of care at nephroureterectomy in patients with urothelial carcinoma of the renal pelvis? A population-based study. Eur Urol. 2010;57:956–62.
89. Xylinas E, et al. Impact of distal ureter management on oncologic outcomes following radical nephroureterectomy for upper tract urothelial carcinoma. Eur Urol. 2014;65:210–7.
90. Yafi FA, et al. Impact of tumour location versus multifocality in patients with upper tract urothelial carcinoma treated with nephroureterectomy and bladder cuff excision: a homogeneous series without perioperative chemotherapy. BJU Int. 2012;110: E7–13.

91. Jeldres C, et al. Highly predictive survival nomogram after upper urinary tract urothelial carcinoma. Cancer. 2010;116:3774–84.
92. Seisen T, et al. Postoperative nomogram to predict cancer-specific survival after radical nephroureterectomy in patients with localised and/or locally advanced upper tract urothelial carcinoma without metastasis. BJU Int. 2014;114:733–40.
93. Rouprêt M, et al. Prediction of cancer specific survival after radical nephroureterectomy for upper tract urothelial carcinoma: development of an optimized postoperative nomogram using decision curve analysis. J Urol. 2013;189:1662–9.
94. Chromecki TF, et al. The impact of tumor multifocality on outcomes in patients treated with radical nephroureterectomy. Eur Urol. 2012;61:245–53.
95. Lee DJ, et al. Insulin-like growth factor messenger RNA-binding protein 3 expression helps prognostication in patients with upper tract urothelial carcinoma. Eur Urol. 2014;66:379–85.
96. Izquierdo L, et al. Prognostic value of microRNA expression pattern in upper tract urothelial carcinoma. BJU Int. 2014;113:813–21.
97. Shi B, et al. High expression of KPNA2 defines poor prognosis in patients with upper tract urothelial carcinoma treated with radical nephroureterectomy. BMC Cancer. 2015;15:380.
98. Liang P-I, et al. IGFBP-5 overexpression as a poor prognostic factor in patients with urothelial carcinomas of upper urinary tracts and urinary bladder. J Clin Pathol. 2013;66:573–82.
99. Ouzzane A, et al. The impact of lymph node status and features on oncological outcomes in urothelial carcinoma of the upper urinary tract (UTUC) treated by nephroureterectomy. World J Urol. 2013;31:189–97.
100. Colin P, et al. Influence of positive surgical margin status after radical nephroureterectomy on upper urinary tract urothelial carcinoma survival. Ann Surg Oncol. 2012;19:3613–20.
101. Hamada S, et al. Prognostic impact of fatty acid synthase expression in upper urinary tract urothelial carcinoma. Jpn J Clin Oncol. 2014;44:486–92.
102. Sasaki Y, et al. HER2 protein overexpression and gene amplification in upper urinary tract urothelial carcinoma-an analysis of 171 patients. Int J Clin Exp Pathol. 2014;7:699–708.
103. Ku JH, et al. The role of p53 on survival of upper urinary tract urothelial carcinoma: a systematic review and meta-analysis. Clin Genitourin Cancer. 2013;11:221–8.
104. Nakanishi K, et al. Expression of hypoxia-inducible factor-1alpha protein predicts survival in patients with transitional cell carcinoma of the upper urinary tract. Clin Cancer Res. 2005;11:2583–90.
105. Kim M, et al. Prognostic value of systemic inflammatory responses in patients with upper urinary tract urothelial carcinoma. World J Urol. 2015;. doi:10.1007/s00345-015-1484-9.
106. Bolenz C, et al. Risk stratification of patients with nodal involvement in upper tract urothelial carcinoma: value of lymph-node density. BJU Int. 2009;103:302–6.
107. Jeon HG, et al. Expression of Ki-67 and COX-2 in patients with upper urinary tract urothelial carcinoma. Urology 2010;76:513.e7–12.
108. Izquierdo L, Truan D, Mengual L, Mallofre C, Alcaraz A. HER-2/AKT expression in upper urinary tract urothelial carcinoma: prognostic implications. Anticancer Res. 2010;30:2439–45.
109. Van Oers JMM, et al. FGFR3 mutations indicate better survival in invasive upper urinary tract and bladder tumours. Eur Urol. 2009;55:650–7.
110. Ke H-L, et al. Osteopontin overexpression predicts poor prognosis of upper urinary tract urothelial carcinoma. Urol Oncol. 2011;29:703–9.
111. Kamai T, et al. Increased Rac1 activity and Pak1 overexpression are associated with lymphovascular invasion and lymph node metastasis of upper urinary tract cancer. BMC Cancer. 2010;10:164.
112. Sakano S, et al. Risk group stratification based on preoperative factors to predict survival after nephroureterectomy in patients with upper urinary tract urothelial carcinoma. Ann Surg Oncol. 2013;20:4389–96.
113. Ku JH, et al. External validation of an online nomogram in patients undergoing radical nephroureterectomy for upper urinary tract urothelial carcinoma. Br J Cancer. 2013;109:1130–6.
114. Yates DR, et al. Cancer-specific survival after radical nephroureterectomy for upper urinary tract urothelial carcinoma: proposal and multi-institutional validation of a post-operative nomogram. Br J Cancer. 2012;106:1083–8.

What is a Kidney Worth?

3

Eric J. Moskowitz

Introduction

Traditionally, UTUC has been managed with radical nephroureterectomy with excision of the bladder cuff [1]. Conservative management of UTUC with kidney-sparing surgery had typically been limited to patients with imperative indications, such as bilateral disease, renal insufficiency, or a solitary kidney. However, current recommendations suggest selected patients with low risk disease and normal, functioning contralateral kidneys should also be considered for such an approach due to its similar oncological efficacy [2].

Presently, in our current era of cost-effective management, it now also becomes imperative to understand the overall costs of preserving a kidney with UTUC [3]. These costs specifically refer to the direct, financial expenses of kidney-sparing conservative measures versus radical nephroureterectomy and subsequent CKD or ESRD. Alternatively, a kidney's "worth" in the setting of UTUC can also be evaluated via an analysis of the subsequent development and progression of CKD and ESRD after nephroureterectomy. Naturally, CKD and ESRD also impose their own set of "costs" on a patient's quality of life. In this chapter, we will review the financial implications of sparing a kidney with UTUC along with its value in preventing the development and progression of CKD and ESRD and their associated negative impact on a patient's quality of life.

E. J. Moskowitz (✉)
Stamford Health Medical Group, Stamford, CT, USA
e-mail: eric.moskowitz@gmail.com

Financial Costs of Nephron-Sparing Surgery in UTUC

From a financial cost perspective, renal-sparing management of UTUC has been shown to be effective in reducing ESRD health care-related expenses [3]. A retrospective review of 57 patients with UTUC with a minimum follow-up of 2 years calculated the direct costs of ureteroscopic ablation versus traditional nephroureterectomy and potentially hemodialysis in patients with a solitary kidney. The annual cost to maintain a kidney was calculated and projected over a period of 5 years against other treatment options. These annual costs were based upon a standardized surveillance protocol that included retrograde pyelography and ureteroscopy at three month intervals from last recurrence and extended to six months for negative surveillance. In this series of patients, renal preservation approached 81%, with cancer-specific survival at 94.7%.

In those patients with absolute indications for renal-sparing surgery, Pak et al. [3] found that the cost savings over a 5-year period ranged from three fold to almost tenfold when compared with the ESRD and hemodialysis cohort. Assuming a worst-case scenario of a solitary kidney with

M. Eshghi (ed.), *Urothelial Malignancies of the Upper Urinary Tract*,
https://doi.org/10.1007/978-3-319-51263-1_3

recurrences at each follow-up for 5 years versus nephroureterectomy and dialysis for the same period, an estimated $252,272 US dollars would have been saved, which would cover the expenses of five cadaveric renal transplantations.

The Value of Renal Preservation in Delaying CKD and ESRD

Renal-sparing surgery for UTUC in the setting of low risk disease not only achieves similar oncological efficacy as traditional radical nephroureterectomy but also offers value in delaying progression to CKD and ESRD and their associated cardiovascular morbidity and mortality, and providing savings in avoiding the expenses associated with chronic renal insufficiency. This value of renal preservation in preventing CKD can be extrapolated from research in renal cortical masses, where partial nephrectomy of small renal masses has been shown to produce adequate outcomes in cancer-specific survival. As Russo highlights [4], serum creatinine determination and more accurate formulas to estimate glomerular filtration rate (GFR) both demonstrate that partial nephrectomy preserves renal function compared with radical nephrectomy.

Initial studies assessing the difference between partial and radical nephrectomy typically relied upon serum creatinine. In 2000, a retrospective review of 164 patients with renal tumors less than or equal to 4 cm treated by partial or radical nephrectomy found that those patients treated with partial nephrectomy had a decreased cumulative incidence of chronic renal insufficiency, as defined by a serum creatinine of greater than 2 mg/dl (11.6 vs. 22.4%, respectively, at 10 years), and a decreased risk of proteinuria (34.5% in the partial vs. 55.2% in the radical) when compared with the patients undergoing radical nephrectomy [5]. These findings were confirmed in a retrospective review of 290 patients, 117 of whom underwent partial and 173 radical nephrectomy, all for tumors that were 4 cm or less. After a median follow-up of 25 months, the mean postoperative serum creatinine in the radical nephrectomy group was 1.5 (0.8–3.8) versus 1.0 mg/dl for the partial nephrectomy group (0.5–1.9; $p < 0.001$) [6].

Subsequent studies utilized formulas to estimate GFR, as opposed to simply the changes in serum creatinine, in order to analyze the effects of partial and radical nephrectomy on kidney function. In a retrospective cohort study of 662 patients with a normal serum creatinine and healthy native kidneys who underwent either elective partial or radical nephrectomy for a renal cortical mass of 4 cm or less, GFR was approximated using the MDRD equation. Postoperatively, the 3-year probability of freedom from new onset of a GFR of less than 60 was 80% after partial nephrectomy but only 35% after radical nephrectomy. Corresponding values for 3-year probability of freedom from new onset of a GFR of less than 45 was 95% for partial nephrectomy and 64% for radical nephrectomy. Multivariable analysis ultimately indicated that radical nephrectomy remained an independent risk factor for the development of new onset CKD [7]. The concerns regarding the long-term effects of radical nephrectomy in a population of patients with small renal masses with minimal risk of metastatic disease development and a long anticipated survival [4] can therefore be transposed to those effects of radical nephroureterectomy in a population of patients with low-volume, low-grade UTUC with likewise minimal risk of metastatic disease and a long anticipated survival.

Despite the above findings, Li et al.'s review reveals that prospective data on the incidence of *de novo* and accelerated CKD after cancer nephrectomy is lacking [8]. Furthermore, the only randomized clinical trial of partial versus radical nephrectomy conducted to date [9] was closed prematurely because of poor accrual and was limited by high crossover between the treatment groups. However, in order to negate the effect of malignancy on overall survival and chronic renal insufficiency, Kaushik et al. sought to assess for differences in overall survival and the development of stage IV CKD for patients undergoing partial or radical nephrectomy for benign renal masses. Their retrospective review of 442 patients with unilateral sporadic benign renal masses treated surgically with partial or radical nephrectomy found that estimated overall survival (95% confidence interval [CI]) rates at 10 and 15 years were 69% (62–76%) and 53% (45–62%) for radical nephrectomy compared with 80% (73–87%) and 74% (65–83%) following partial nephrectomy ($p = 0.023$). In addition, adjusting for covariates of interest demonstrated that patients treated with radical nephrectomy were significantly more likely to die from any cause (hazard ratio [HR]: 1.75; 95% CI, 1.08–2.83; $p = 0.23$) or develop stage IV CKD (HR: 4.23; 95% CI, 1.80–9.93; $p < 0.001$) compared with patients who underwent partial nephrectomy [10].

Financial Costs of CKD and ESRD

Kidney-sparing surgery for UTUC also eliminates the financial expenses associated with CKD and/or ESRD that are more likely to be associated with radical extirpative surgery. The magnitude of these CKD-related costs only continues to increase. A recent review by the National Kidney Foundation indicated that in 2007, CKD contributed 27.6% of costs, and CKD subjects constituted 9.8% of the population. Between 1993 and 2007, not only did overall Medicare costs nearly double but CKD-associated costs increased approximately fivefold. The Medicare cost of ESRD had risen from $12.2 in 2000 to $20.8 billion in 2007 [11].

The main contributors to these costs, particularly in those patients with moderate-to-severe CKD, are renal replacement therapy and major vascular events. These findings were produced by the Study of Heart and Renal Protection (SHARP), a randomized trial that prospectively collected information on kidney disease progression, serious adverse events, and hospital care use in a cohort of patients with moderate-to-severe CKD. In this study, over 7200 SHARP patients from Europe, North America, and Australasia contributed over 28,000 years of data. CKD patients without diabetes or vascular disease incurred annual hospital care costs ranging from £403 (95% CI: 345–462) in CKD stages 1–3B to £525 (449–602) in CKD stage 5 (not on dialysis). However, patients undergoing routine dialysis incurred annual hospital costs of £18,986 (18,620–19,352) in the year of initiation and £23,326 (23,321–23,421) annually thereafter. Furthermore, nonfatal major vascular events increased annual costs in the year of the event by £6133 (5608–6658) for patients on dialysis and by £4350 (3819–4880) for patients not on dialysis [12].

Wyld et al.'s examination of data from the Australian Diabetes, Obesity and Lifestyle study (AusDiab), a national longitudinal population-based study of non-institutionalized Australian adults aged ≥25 years, closely matches recent US data and reaffirms the conclusion that CKD imparts a large economic "cost" on high-income countries. Among 6138 study participants, there was a significant difference in the per-person annual direct healthcare costs by CKD status, increasing from $1829 (95% CI: $1740–1943) for those without CKD to $14,545 (95% CI: $5680–44,842) for those with stage 4 or 5 CKD ($p < 0.01$). Similarly, there was a significant difference in the per-person annual direct non-healthcare costs by CKD status from $524 (95% CI: $413–641) for those without CKD to $2349 (95% CI: $386–5156) for those with stage 4 or 5 CKD ($p < 0.01$) [13]. The above analyses [11–13] all suggest that prevention and slowing progression of CKD is cost-effective, reaffirming the value of kidney-sparing management of UTUC in delaying CKD and ESRD.

A Kidney's "Worth" in Terms of Quality of Life

The Effect of Nephron-Sparing Management of UTUC

The cost of conservative management of UTUC in terms of its effect on quality of life has never been examined [3]. Many studies have reported on the health-related quality of life of patients with cancer of the urinary bladder [14–25], but the majority has sought to assess the relationship between the types of urinary diversion and health-related quality of life after radical cystectomy for muscle invasive cancer of the bladder. However, the surgical management of non-muscle invasive urothelial carcinoma of the bladder requires a strict surveillance schedule similar to that required for conservative endoscopic management of UTUC. As a result, the impact of the management of non-muscle invasive urothelial carcinoma of the bladder on a patient's quality of life offers our best assessment of the cost of conservative management of UTUC in terms of its effect on quality of life.

Yoshimura et al. performed such an assessment a total of 178 times for 133 patients with non-muscle invasive bladder cancer before multiple transurethral resections (TURs) [26]. General health-related quality of life was examined using the Medical Outcome Study Short-Form 36-item survey. Compared to age-matched and sex-matched Japanese controls, the general health perception in those patients with non-muscle invasive bladder cancer was severely impaired. However, after demonstrating a nadir at the second or third TUR, the scores of all other domains subsequently increased if TUR was repeated a minimum of four times. These domains included physical functioning, social functioning, and role limitations because of emotional problems.

The Effect of CKD and ESRD

As discussed previously, renal-sparing surgery for UTUC in the setting of low risk disease not only achieves similar oncological efficacy as traditional radical nephroureterectomy but also offers value in delaying progression to CKD and ESRD and their associated cardiovascular morbidity and mortality. From a financial standpoint, if the rate of decline in GFR decreased by 10% and 30% in every patient with GFR of 60 mL/min/1.73 m^2 or less, the gross direct cumulative healthcare savings over the next 10 years would amount to $18.6 and $60.6 billion, respectively [11]. Further emphasizing the cost-effectiveness of the prevention and slowing progression of CKD though are the additional benefits that would accrue as a result of diminishing disability and gain in productivity.

If a patient ultimately progresses to CKD or ESRD, the effect of these on his/her quality of life is devastating and much poorer than initially reported. Evaluations of quality of life in ESRD hemodialysis patients have revealed that patients would give up to half of their remaining life expectancy in current health if the sacrifice would provide them with perfect health for a shorter time [27]. In addition, cost-utility analysis of nephron-sparing surgery in the management of small renal masses while adjusting for the burden of ensuing CKD demonstrates that partial nephrectomy, either open or laparoscopic, is considerably less costly and yields more quality-adjusted life years (QALYs) than laparoscopic radical nephrectomy [28]. Laparoscopic partial nephrectomy yielded 0.098 additional QALYs at an additional cost of $888 for an incremental cost-effectiveness ratio of $9057 per QALY, far below a commonly cited willingness-to-pay ratio of $50,000 per QALY. Alternatively, laparoscopic radical nephrectomy was more costly and yielded fewer QALYs than both open and laparoscopic partial nephrectomy.

Conclusion

Renal-sparing surgery for UTUC in the setting of low risk disease demonstrates its "worth" in not only achieving similar oncological efficacy as traditional radical nephroureterectomy but also offering value in delaying progression to CKD and ESRD and their associated cardiovascular morbidity and mortality. From a financial cost perspective, renal-sparing management of UTUC has been shown to be effective in reducing ESRD health care-related expenses [3] and preventing ESRD's "costly," negative impact on a patient's quality of life [27, 28].

Summary Box

- The conservative management of UTUC with kidney-sparing endoscopic surgery is an oncologically effective treatment modality in appropriate patients that has several significant cost implications.
- Despite the financial cost of its strict surveillance schedule, the conservative endoscopic management of UTUC effectively reduces ESRD expenditures by delaying the progression to CKD and ESRD that can occur after radical extirpative surgery.
- Although this strict surveillance schedule may initially impose an emotional cost on a patient's quality of life, the progression to CKD and/or ESRD after radical extirpative surgery imparts a more devastating and longer-lasting impact on a patient's quality of life.

References

1. Rai BP, Shelley M, Coles B, Somani B, Nabi G. Surgical management for upper urinary tract transitional cell carcinoma (UUT-TCC): a systematic review. BJU Int. 2012;110(10):1426–35.
2. Seisen T, Colin P, Roupret M. Risk-adapted strategy for the kidney-sparing management of upper tract tumours. Nat Rev Urol. 2015;12(3):155–66.
3. Pak RW, Moskowitz EJ, Bagley DH. What is the cost of maintaining a kidney in upper-tract transitional-cell carcinoma? An objective analysis of cost and survival. J Endourol. 2009;23(3):341–6.
4. Russo P. Partial nephrectomy achieves local tumor control and prevents chronic kidney disease. Expert Rev Anticancer Ther. 2006;6(12):1745–51.
5. Lau WK, Blute ML, Weaver AL, Torres VE, Zincke H. Matched comparison of radical nephrectomy vs nephron-sparing surgery in patients with unilateral renal cell carcinoma and a normal contralateral kidney. Mayo Clin Proc. 2000;75(12):1236–42.
6. McKiernan J, Simmons R, Katz J, Russo P. Natural history of chronic renal insufficiency after partial and radical nephrectomy. Urology. 2002;59(6):816–20.
7. Huang WC, Levey AS, Serio AM, Snyder M, Vickers AJ, Raj GV, et al. Chronic kidney disease after nephrectomy in patients with renal cortical tumours: a retrospective cohort study. Lancet Oncol. 2006;7(9):735–40.
8. Li L, Lau WL, Rhee CM, Harley K, Kovesdy CP, Sim JJ, et al. Risk of chronic kidney disease after cancer nephrectomy. Nat Rev Nephrol. 2014;10(3):135–45.
9. Van Poppel H, Da Pozzo L, Albrecht W, Matveev V, Bono A, Borkowski A, et al. A prospective, randomised EORTC intergroup phase 3 study comparing the oncologic outcome of elective nephron-sparing surgery and radical nephrectomy for low-stage renal cell carcinoma. Eur Urol. 2011;59(4):543–52.
10. Kaushik D, Kim SP, Childs MA, Lohse CM, Costello BA, Cheville JC, et al. Overall survival and development of stage IV chronic kidney disease in patients undergoing partial and radical nephrectomy for benign renal tumors. Eur Urol. 2013;64(4):600–6.
11. Trivedi H. Cost implications of caring for chronic kidney disease: are interventions cost-effective? Adv Chronic Kidney Dis. 2010;17(3):265–70.
12. Kent S, Schlackow I, Lozano-Kuhne J, Reith C, Emberson J, Haynes R, et al. What is the impact of chronic kidney disease stage and cardiovascular disease on the annual cost of hospital care in moderate-to-severe kidney disease? BMC Nephrol. 2015;16:65.
13. Wyld ML, Lee CM, Zhuo X, White S, Shaw JE, Morton RL, et al. Cost to government and society of chronic kidney disease stage 1–5: a national cohort study. Intern Med J. 2015;45(7):741–7.
14. Miyakawa M, Yoshida O. [The quality of life in patients with bladder cancer after radical cystectomy with ileal conduit: II. Results of questionnaire surveys to compare the impact of treatments]. Nihon Gan Chiryo Gakkai shi. 1987;22(7):1296–303.
15. Mack D, Frick J. Quality of life in patients undergoing bacille calmette-guerin therapy for superficial bladder cancer. Br J Urol. 1996;78(3):369–71.
16. Hart S, Skinner EC, Meyerowitz BE, Boyd S, Lieskovsky G, Skinner DG. Quality of life after radical cystectomy for bladder cancer in patients with an ileal conduit, cutaneous or urethral kock pouch. J Urol. 1999;162(1):77–81.
17. Kitamura H, Miyao N, Yanase M, Masumori N, Matsukawa M, Takahashi A, et al. Quality of life in patients having an ileal conduit, continent reservoir or orthotopic neobladder after cystectomy for bladder carcinoma. Int J Urol. 1999;6(8):393–9.
18. Fujisawa M, Isotani S, Gotoh A, Okada H, Arakawa S, Kamidono S. Health-related quality of life with orthotopic neobladder versus ileal conduit according to the SF-36 survey. Urology. 2000;55(6):862–5.
19. Hardt J, Filipas D, Hohenfellner R, Egle UT. Quality of life in patients with bladder carcinoma after cystectomy: first results of a prospective study. Qual Life Res Int J Qual Life Aspects Treat Care Rehabil. 2000;9(1):1–12.

20. McGuire MS, Grimaldi G, Grotas J, Russo P. The type of urinary diversion after radical cystectomy significantly impacts on the patient's quality of life. Ann Surg Oncol. 2000;7(1):4–8.
21. Dutta SC, Chang SC, Coffey CS, Smith JA Jr, Jack G, Cookson MS. Health related quality of life assessment after radical cystectomy: comparison of ileal conduit with continent orthotopic neobladder. J Urol. 2002;168(1):164–7.
22. Hara I, Miyake H, Hara S, Gotoh A, Nakamura I, Okada H, et al. Health-related quality of life after radical cystectomy for bladder cancer: a comparison of ileal conduit and orthotopic bladder replacement. BJU Int. 2002;89(1):10–3.
23. Mansson A, Davidsson T, Hunt S, Mansson W. The quality of life in men after radical cystectomy with a continent cutaneous diversion or orthotopic bladder substitution: is there a difference? BJU Int. 2002;90 (4):386–90.
24. Matsuda T, Aptel I, Exbrayat C, Grosclaude P. Determinants of quality of life of bladder cancer survivors five years after treatment in France. Int J Urol Official J Japanese Urol Assoc. 2003;10(8):423–9.
25. Yoneda T, Igawa M, Shiina H, Shigeno K, Urakami S. Postoperative morbidity, functional results and quality of life of patients following orthotopic neobladder reconstruction. Int J Urol. 2003;10(3):119–25.
26. Yoshimura K, Utsunomiya N, Ichioka K, Matsui Y, Terai A, Arai Y. Impact of superficial bladder cancer and transurethral resection on general health-related quality of life: an SF-36 survey. Urology. 2005;65 (2):290–4.
27. Churchill DN, Torrance GW, Taylor DW, Barnes CC, Ludwin D, Shimizu A, et al. Measurement of quality of life in end-stage renal disease: the time trade-off approach. Clin Invest Med. 1987;10(1):14–20.
28. Klinghoffer Z, Tarride JE, Novara G, Ficarra V, Kapoor A, Shayegan B, et al. Cost-utility analysis of radical nephrectomy versus partial nephrectomy in the management of small renal masses: adjusting for the burden of ensuing chronic kidney disease. Can Urol Assoc J (Journal de l'Association des urologues du Canada). 2013;7(3–4):108–13.

Part II

Diagnostic Workup

The Radiology of Upper Tract Collecting System Neoplasms

4

Stuart Bentley-Hibbert and Jeffrey H. Newhouse

Tumor Identification and Screening

Which imaging technique to choose when searching for an upper tract urothelial tumor depends upon the clinical presentation creating the concern. If the evaluation is prompted by persistent hematuria, a host of conditions other than urothelial tumors, such as renal parenchymal tumors, stones, vascular abnormalities, polycystic syndromes, and so forth must be sought [1], therefore techniques which demonstrate the renal parenchyma and vascular structures, as well as the urothelial surfaces must be employed. Sometimes the search may be limited to the urothelium. This is often the case when searching for synchronous tumors in patients with recently diagnosed urothelial malignancy or for metachronous tumors in patients undergoing surveillance after treatment of a first urothelial malignancy [2].

In either case, since a CT urogram can evaluate the parenchyma, vessels, and urothelial surfaces, it is the best test to employ [3]. This test has virtually replaced excretory pyelography wherever modern CT scanners are available [4]. In CT urography, the urinary system is first scanned without intravenous contrast and then rescanned at a later phase—or at several later phases—during which contrast administered intravenously has opacified the renal parenchyma and the intrarenal collecting systems, ureters, and urinary bladder [5–7]. Specific protocols for CT urography have been proposed; they differ primarily with regard to the number of post-contrast scans which are obtained [5, 8–11]. The most elaborate ones involve repeated scans, but these entail a large radiation dose and repeated imaging to fully opacify the ureters. Repeated imaging to fully opacify the peristalsing ureters in the absence of an identifiable mass has been shown to be of no added value [12]. At our institution we use a "split contrast bolus" technique which produces simultaneous opacification of the cortical and medullary tissue and of the pyelocalyceal system and ureter and permits a single post-contrast scan to visualize all pertinent structures [11]. It should be noted that in CT examinations without a pyelography phase urothelial cancers may still be detected, appearing as enhancing lesions situated within or upon the walls of the pyelocalyceal system or ureter (Fig. 4.1). Pyelography makes them easier to see, however, so CT urography remains the best technique to use. Regardless of how intravenous contrast is administered and how much post-contrast imaging is performed, enteric contrast generally is not needed although it is unclear if it truly limits evaluations.

S. Bentley-Hibbert (✉) · J. H. Newhouse
Department of Radiology, Columbia University Medical Center, 185 Fort Washington Avenue, New York, NY 10032, USA
e-mail: sb2390@cumc.columbia.edu

J. H. Newhouse
e-mail: jhn2@cumc.columbia.edu

M. Eshghi (ed.), *Urothelial Malignancies of the Upper Urinary Tract*,
https://doi.org/10.1007/978-3-319-51263-1_4

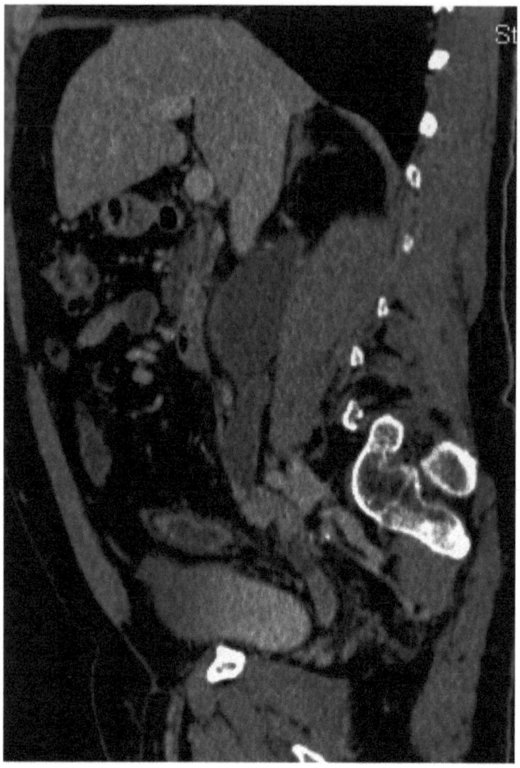

Fig. 4.1 Sagittal reconstruction of a contrast enhanced single phase CT. The *white* point towards 2 intraluminal mass lesions. Note the upstream dilated collecting system and the small amount of excreted contrast within the urinary bladder

If upper tract urothelial tumors are being sought, and a complete hematuria workup is not necessary, pyelography is crucial, and there are a number of ways this can be achieved in addition to CT urography. As mentioned above, excretory pyelography has been largely abandoned in communities with easy access to modern CT, but it is probably true that for upper tract urothelial malignancies excretory pyelography is as accurate as the pyelographic phase of CT. Properly performed retrograde pyeloureterography is also satisfactory, and may be performed simultaneously with cystoscopic evaluation for bladder tumors. MR urography can produce pyeloureterograms, but MR urography is more likely to be technically suboptimal than CT and retrograde pyelography [13] and extensive evidence to show that its accuracy matches that of CT urography is lacking (Fig. 4.2).

Ultrasound of the urinary tract is not sufficiently sensitive to be reliable in searching for urothelial tumors, although the development of contrast enhanced ultrasounds shows promising results [14]. It can detect large intrarenal tumors, but not small ones, and although it is relatively accurate in assessing hydronephrosis, it often fails to differentiate between tumors and other conditions which may produce obstruction. It is also relatively insensitive for detecting many of the wide array of conditions which can produce hematuria, and should not be the sole modality used in hematuria evaluation. Color Doppler does allow for the assessment of internal vascularity of a lesion as well as dynamic assessment of its mobility as the patient moves, allowing on to differentiate a mass from entities such as blood clots and fungus balls (Fig. 4.3). The American College of Radiology Appropriateness Criteria can provide online guidance when one is trying to determine the best imaging test for a large variety of conditions involving the upper tract (http://www.acr.org/quality-safety/appropriateness-criteria).

PET scanning, with or without fusion with CT images, has little role in diagnosing primary urothelial cancer, since activity found normally in the collecting system may obscure any abnormal activity which the tumor might display. It does however play a role in monitoring response to treatment as assessing for recurrent and metastatic disease (Fig. 4.4).

Retrograde ureteropyeloscopy may be used instead of ureteropyelography, of course, and has the advantage of permitting biopsy. It is, however, more expensive than most imaging techniques, and its complications are more frequent and serious [15].

Radiologic Appearance of Upper Tract Tumors

Urothelial tumors may be detected because they are directly visible or because of the secondary urinary tract abnormalities which they produce, or both.

Small tumors appear as filling defects within the lumina of the collecting system or ureter. These have a variety of appearances, including

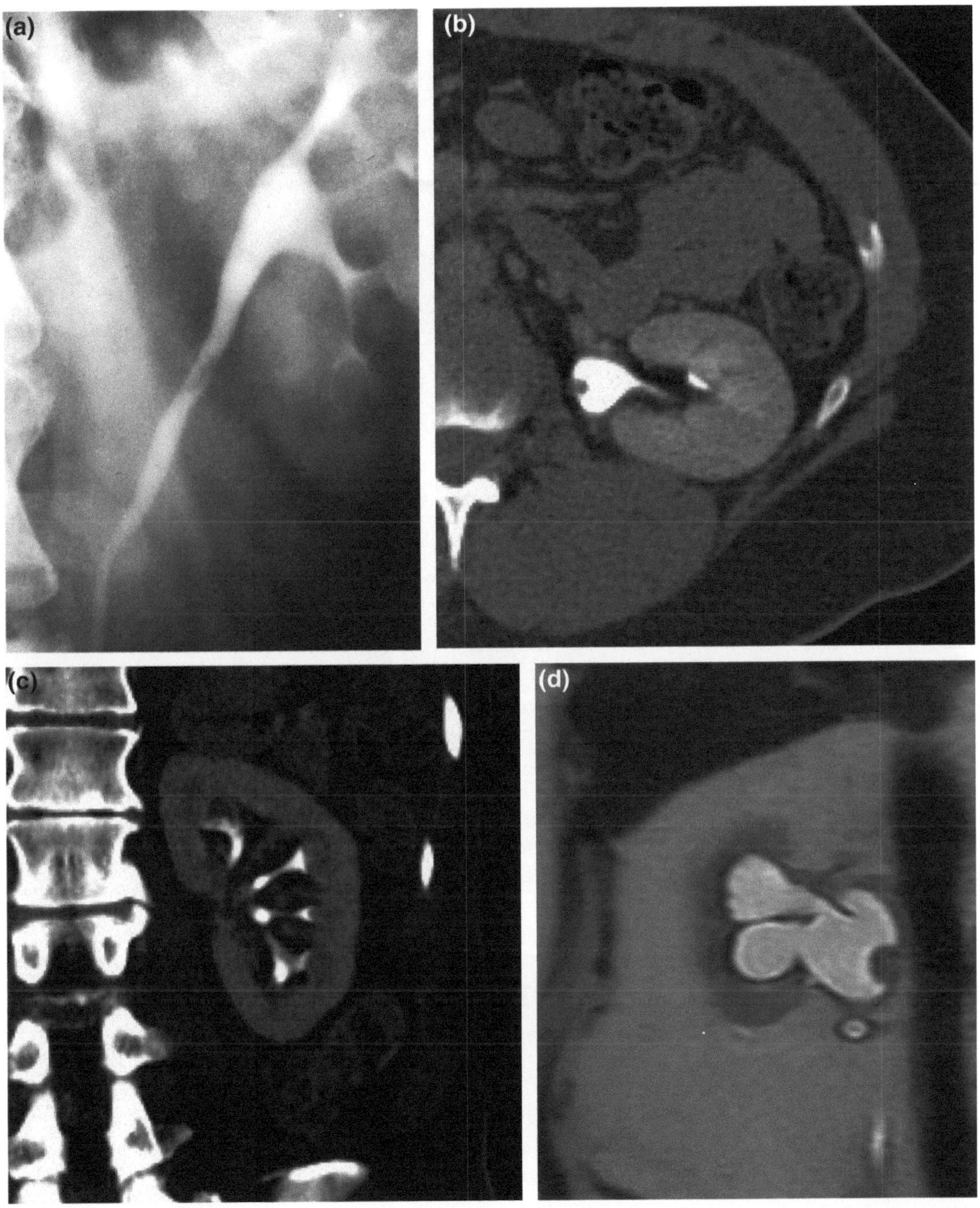

Fig. 4.2 Four images including excretory pyelogram (**a**), CT pyelogram (**b**, **c**) and coronal T2-weighted MRI images (**d**) demonstrates small sites of transitional cell carcinoma appearing as filling defects. Unlike fluoroscopy and CT, the intrinsic high T2 signal of urine allows one to look for filling defects without intravenous contrast

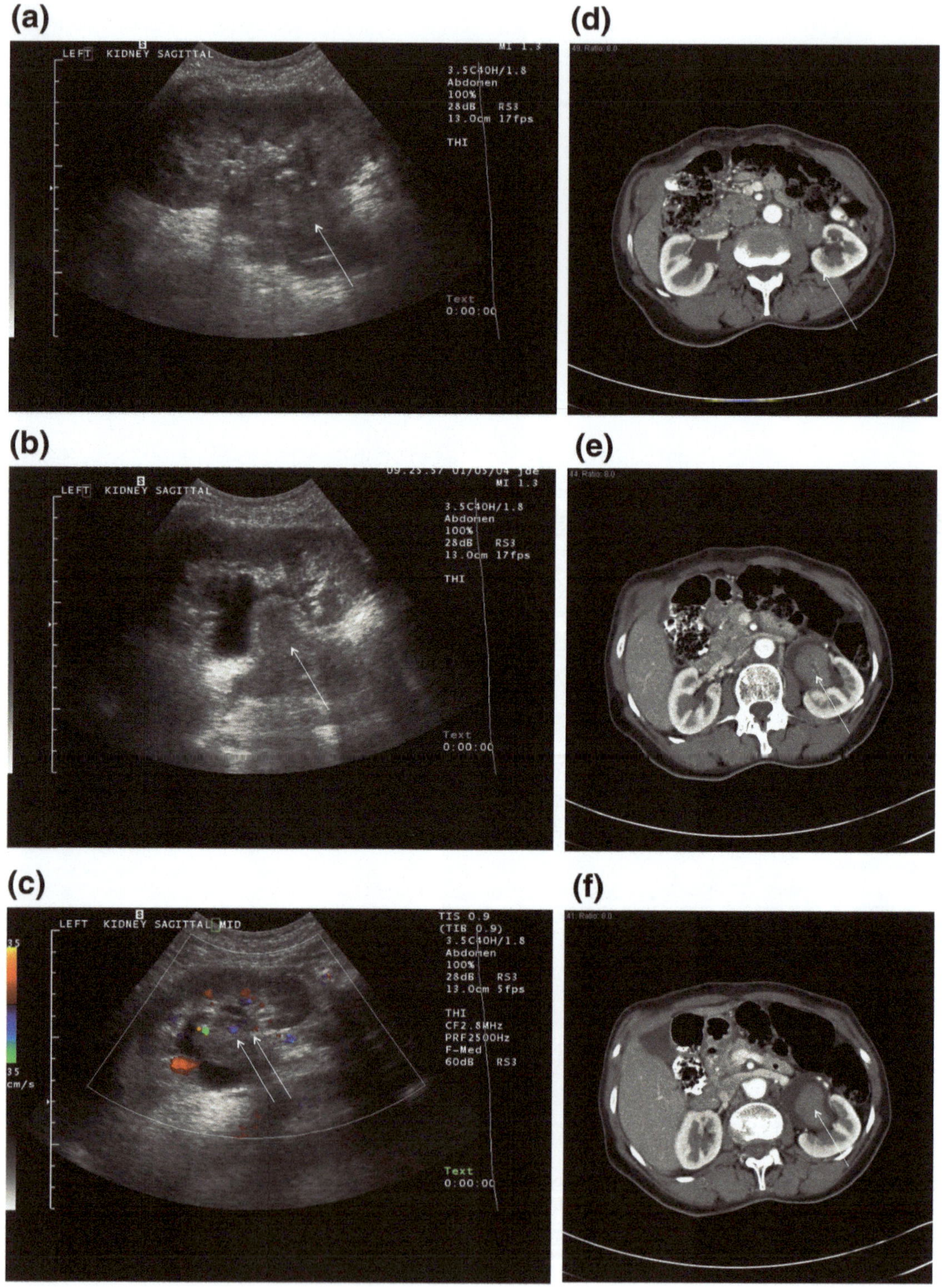

Fig. 4.3 Three ultrasound images (**a–c**) and 3 axial contrast CT images (**d–f**) demonstrate a large mass lesion within the collecting system with associated hydronephrosis. Grayscale images show the isoechoic mass along with a dilated anechoic collecting system. Color Doppler (**c**) demonstrates internal flow indicating the mass is vascularised. 3 CT images from the patient CT demonstrate the same findings, although it allows for a more complete evaluation of other findings including metastasis, smaller lesions and lymphadenopathy

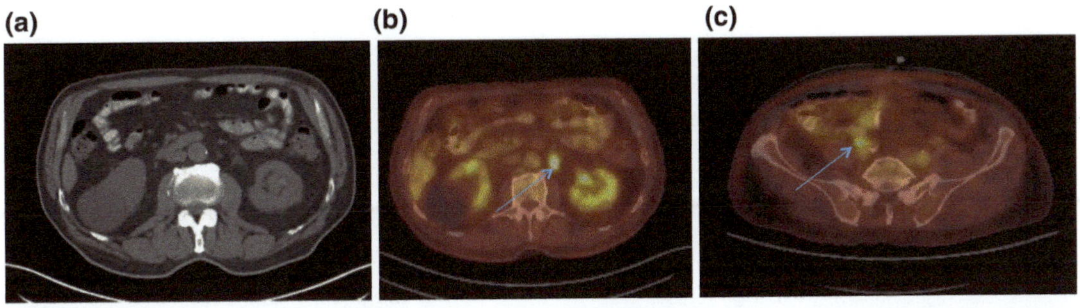

Fig. 4.4 PET L renal pelvis TCC and adjacent nodes and PET TCC recurrence p nephrectomy. Non-contrast CT (**a**) and FDG-PET reveals a hypermetabolic mass lesion within the collecting system, compatible with the primary mass (**b**). It also reveals a hypermetabolic lymph node, that although not pathologically enlarged by CT criteria is clearly concerning for a metastatic deposit. Follow up surveillance 1 year later (**c**) imaging post nephrectomy demonstrated recurrence in a right pelvis (*arrow*)

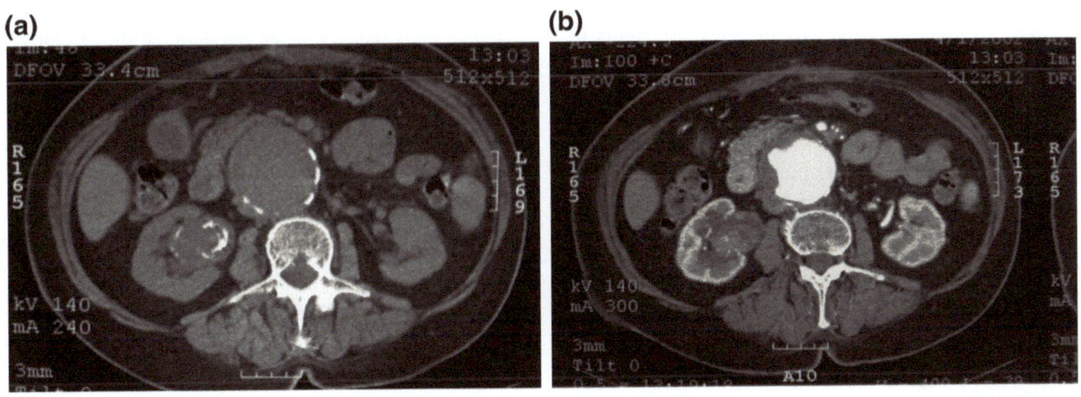

Fig. 4.5 Axial CT Images without (**a**) and with (**b**) intravenous contrast demonstrate large enhancing partially calcified mass within the right renal pelvis. The high density material on the pre-contrast (**a**) images is calcium. Non-contrast imaging in the work up of hematuria permits detection of stones and calcified portions of masses

those of polypoid masses or flatter sessile mural lesions which focally thicken the wall of the pyelocalyceal system and protrude into the lumen. The surfaces of these tumors are often irregular or shaggy, but may be smooth. The tumors may be only a few millimeters in diameter, large enough to fill the entirety of a dilated renal pelvis, or anywhere in between. If they are large enough, imaging may reveal internal blood flow, manifested as an increase in density on CT examinations, enhancement on MRI or Doppler flow on ultrasound (Fig. 4.3). Rarely, the tumors may calcify (Fig. 4.5).

A filling defect may also be produced by a variety of non-neoplastic lesions, but the short differential of tumor, blood clot, and stone almost always contains the correct diagnosis, and the specific diagnosis is usually easy to reach (Fig. 4.6). Only tumors demonstrate internal blood flow, and only tumors, by expanding, enlarge the specific lumen (usually ureteral) they occupy (Fig. 4.7). Clots have specific CT and MRI characteristics, are only seen in patients with gross hematuria and, since they usually lyse spontaneously, often resolve within a few days or weeks (Fig. 4.8). Stones—even relatively lucent

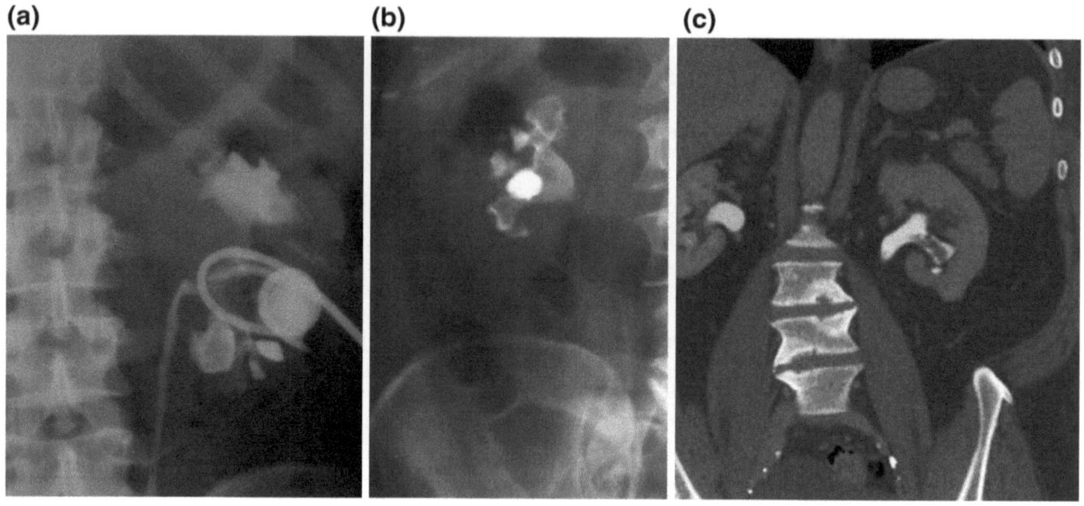

Fig. 4.6 Excretory pyelography of sloughed papilla (**a**) and fungus balls (**b**). CT of an intraluminal blood clot (**c**). Although imaging appearance may overlap, the clinical history allows for accurate diagnosis

ones like uric acid calculi are much denser than tumors or clots on CT, appear black on MRI and cast acoustic shadows in ultrasound examinations.

There are a number of other conditions which may produce upper tract filling defects, but their infrequent occurrence and specific appearances make serious differential diagnosis problems rare. Papillary necrosis which may occasionally cause a complete papilla to separate from the medullary tissue and appear as a filling defect, can be suspected if no normal papilla is found in the calyx, and can be confirmed by finding small amounts of papillary tissue in the urine [16, 17]. Fungal infections may produce mycetomas ("fungus balls"); in these cases, patients are often severely ill with fungal pyelonephritis and excrete detectable hyphae in their urine [18] (Fig. 4.6). Intramural hemorrhage (Antopol-Goldman syndrome) may cause local thickening of pyelocalyceal or ureteral walls; unlike tumors, these lesions spontaneously resolve and can sometimes be identified by demonstrating the characteristic features of hemorrhage with CT or MRI examination [19–21]. Pyeloureteritis cystica may produce filling defects, but these lesions are usually too smooth, round, uniform in size, and numerous to be confused with tumors [22]. Malacoplakia may produce focal mural thickening, but the thickening is often too diffuse to be likely to be due to tumors [23]. Leukoplakia is often morphologically very similar to tumors and usually requires pathologic examination for diagnosis. Fortunately, when these unusual lesions appear, ureteropyeloscopy and biopsy permit correct diagnosis.

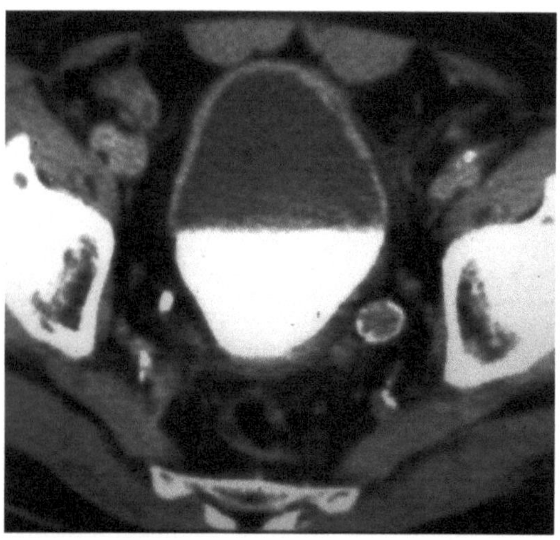

Fig. 4.7 Axial CT pyelogram image taken through the pelvis demonstrates a soft tissue filling defect within an expanded *left* distal ureter. Hyperdense ring is excreted contrast surrounding the mass, not calcium (pre-contrast imaging not shown)

Urothelial tumors often obstruct the upper tract at the infundibular, pelvic and ureteral

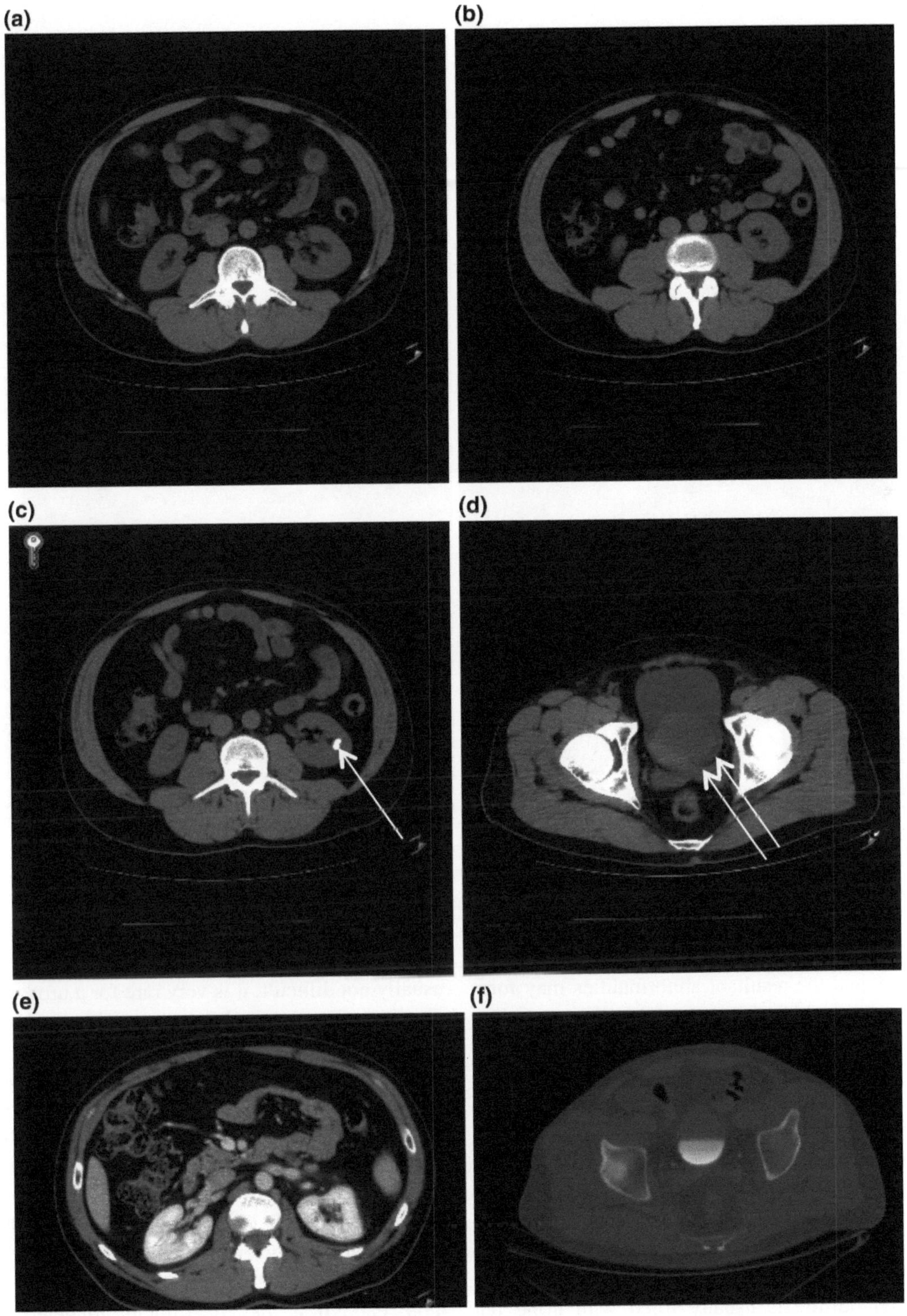

Fig. 4.8 Non-contrast CT (**a–d**) of patient who presented to the emergency department with left upper quadrant pain and hematuria. The scans revealed non-hydronephrotic kidneys without surrounding fat stranding, a non-obstructing stone within the *left* kidney (*white arrow*) and a large mass within the urinary bladder (*double arrow*). Repeat imaging (**e–f**) performed the next day to evaluate the mass and upper collecting system showed no mass. Additional history, not provided at time of imaging, revealed patient just passed blood clot

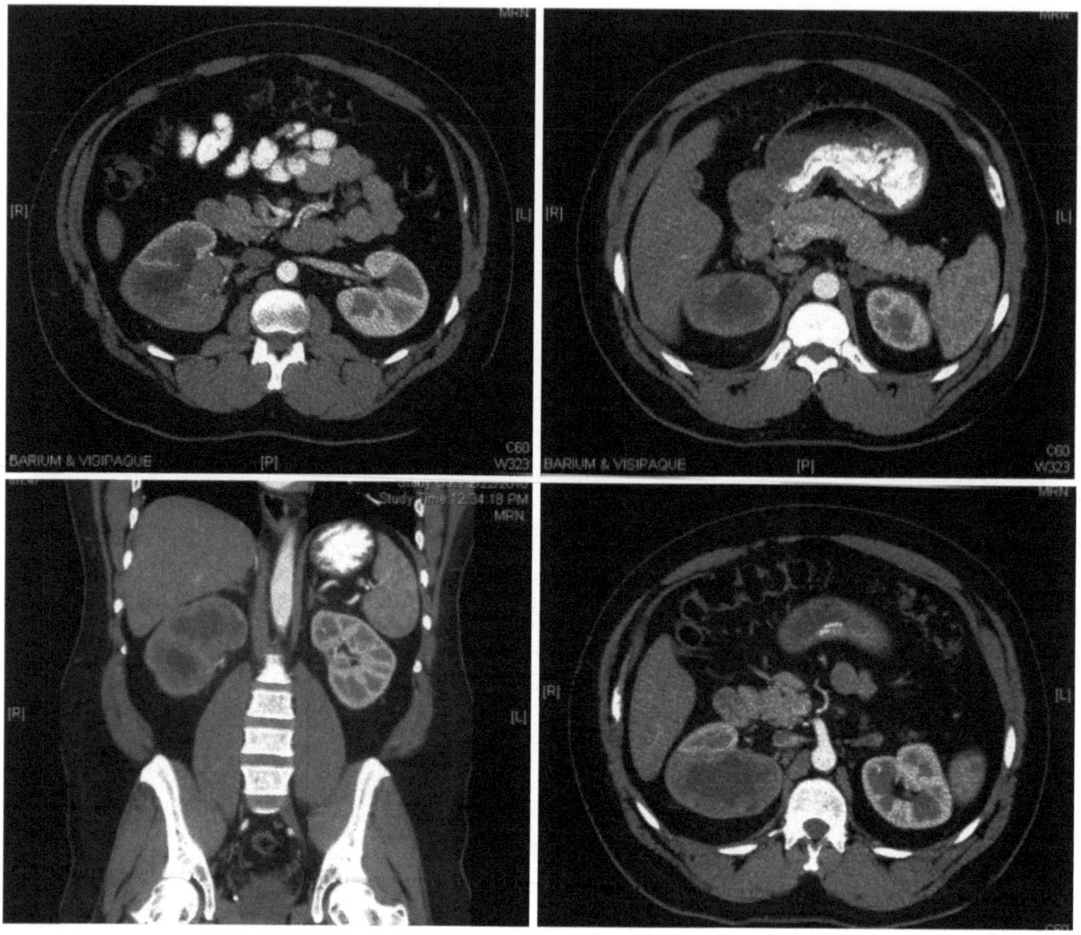

Fig. 4.9 Contrast enhanced CT demonstrates large transitional cell carcinoma in the right renal pelvis. The mass cases moderate hydropnephrosis of the *right* kidney. Comparison of the kidney's enhancement shows decreased and slowed enhancement of the *right* kidney relative to the *left*, a phenomenon known as a delayed nephrogram

levels, and the resultant abnormalities may form the most striking features of imaging examinations. The obstructed kidney, or portion of kidney, can be identified in the same way as obstruction from any other cause. The obstructed parenchyma usually displays diminished contrast enhancement relative to the non-obstructed kidney, often referred to as a "delayed nephrogram" (Fig. 4.9) in CT and MRI, and eventually becomes thinned. The obstructed ureter and collecting system (or part) becomes dilated; the dilated portion is usually filled with urine but may be occupied by the tumor itself. The differential diagnosis of the cause of obstruction is usually not difficult: it is very rare for a urothelial tumor to produce obstruction without being directly visible.

As urothelial tumors grow, they may become larger than what are usually thought of as filling defects, and become structures which, when visualized, are usually called masses. They may invade through the wall of the collecting system and ureter (Fig. 4.10). In the kidney, as they become larger they tend to occupy the renal sinus and then invade the parenchyma, and if they are large enough it may be difficult to determine whether they have originated in the collecting system or the solid parts of the kidney, and

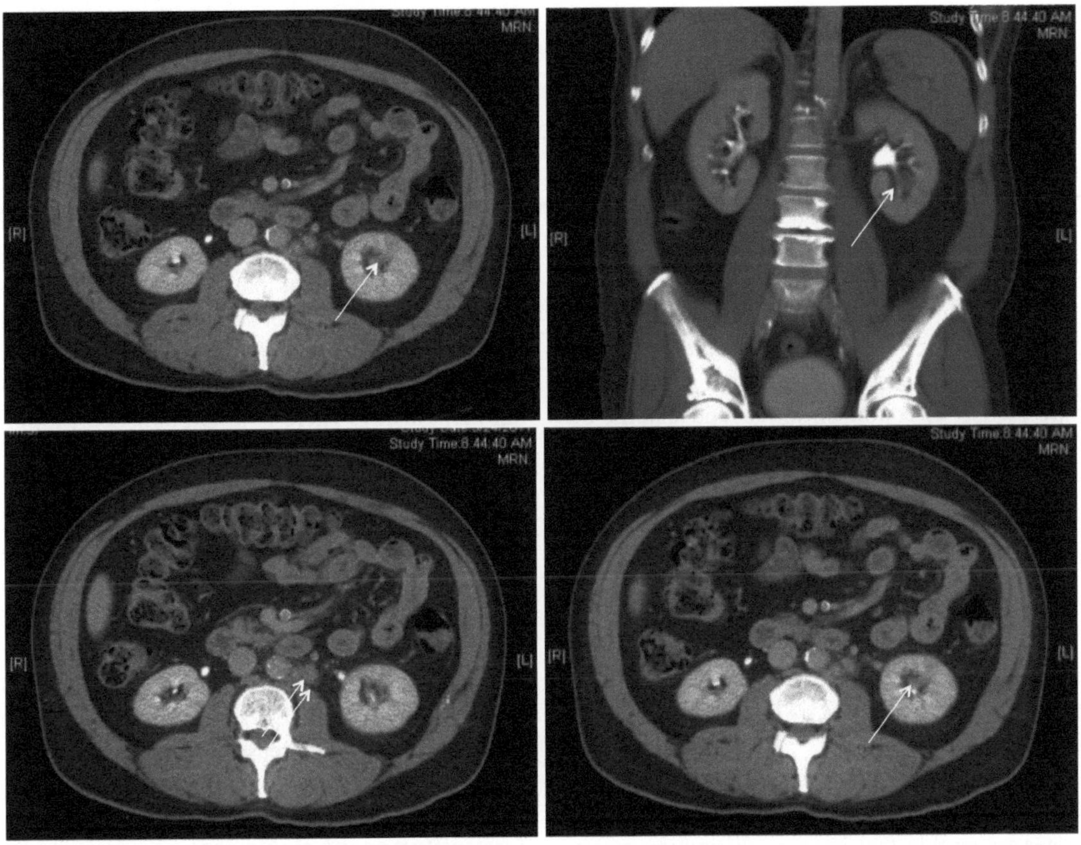

Fig. 4.10 Filling defect within the lower pole of the *left* kidney collecting system with haziness and thickening of the calyceal wall indicating invasion (*white arrow*). Un additional there is retroperitoneal lymphadenopathy with enlarged hazy lymph node (*double arrow*) indicating metastatic involvement

therefore become difficult to distinguish from renal cell carcinoma (Fig. 4.11). In this case, biopsy is often necessary to plan appropriate management. Tumors growing within the ureter may remain primarily in the lumen and thus cause local luminal enlargement with or without

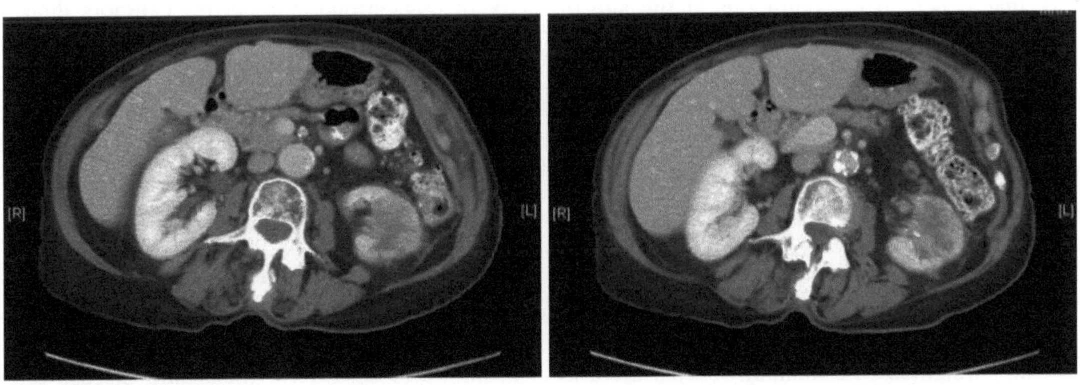

Fig. 4.11 Contrast enhanced CT through the kidneys demonstrate a large infiltrative mass lesion in the *left* kidney. Although this is pathological proven transitional cell carcinoma, none of the features are classic, and renal cell carcinoma would have a similar appearance

obstruction. As they invade the ureteral wall and adjacent structures it may become difficult to distinguish them from extraureteral tumors, which in turn may be metastases or direct ureteral invasion by adjacent malignancies. Having complete oncologic information about each patient becomes important, since of all malignancies involving the ureter, more begin in other organs, than the ureter itself.

Ultrasound can, of course, visualize most cases of obstruction caused by urothelial tumors. As mentioned above, small tumors anywhere may escape detection on ultrasound exams, but larger tumors in the kidney and in the uretero-pelvic and ureterovesicle junctions may be demonstrated. Tumors usually appear solid but relatively hypoechoic on ultrasound images, and they may be shown to be perfused by Doppler flow imaging (Fig. 4.3).

Staging Upper Tract Urothelial Carcinoma

The walls of the intrarenal collecting system and ureter are so thin that imaging distinction among tumors which do not invade, or only partially invade, the muscularis—that is, stages Ta, Tis, T1, and T2—is not accurately performed by imaging. Many stage T3 lesions invade the renal sinus or periureteral fat sufficiently deeply that their stage can be established with reasonable confidence, though, either by CT or MRI. MRI sometimes demonstrates the muscularis as a thin dark line which, if discontinuous at the site of tumor, permits diagnosis of T3 tumors even when they are relatively small.

Nodal metastases are usually detected by identifying nodal enlargement; 5 mm measured as the shortest diameter is a commonly used threshold, although there is obviously no size threshold which is simultaneously perfectly sensitive and specific. Node size can be established both by CT and MRI; normal or marginally enlarged nodes can be assumed to be more likely to harbor tumor is diffusion-weighted MR imaging reveals them to have abnormally low diffusion constants. FDG-PET/CT scanning may identify non-enlarged nodes which harbor metastatic tumor. PET/CT will however have limited sensitivity for nodes less than 5 mm in short axis diameter (Fig. 4.4).

Metastatic disease in non-nodal sites can usually be evaluated by the images of the entire abdomen and pelvis which are included in CT urography or MR urography. Chest radiography is usually obtained both for staging purposes and for the pre-anesthesia evaluation which is necessary for most patients with recently diagnosed urothelial malignancy. There is little published support for employing chest CT routinely, although it may be useful when chest radiography suggests metastases or when widespread abdominal metastases are found (Fig. 4.12). Radionuclide bone scans and brain imaging are not routinely necessary, although they can be requested if symptoms suggesting metastases in the brain or bones appear. PET/CT scans may be employed if less expensive techniques are ambiguous with regard to metastatic disease (Fig. 4.4).

Surveillance of Patients with Urothelial Cancer

Most patients with urothelial cancer have their tumors found in the bladder, and those who develop subsequent primary tumors usually have them in the bladder as well. Most patients with bladder cancer do not develop subsequent upper tract urothelial cancer, but they still have a higher risk of metachronous upper tract tumors than is seen in the general population. The chances of metachronous upper tract tumor can be stratified; patients with high-grade bladder cancer, or CIS, or who have failed intravesical chemotherapy are felt to have a high risk, and should probably have periodic upper tract imaging. Imaging intervals and duration of imaging surveillance are not firmly agreed upon; yearly imaging is probably the lowest test frequency likely to be effective. A common strategy is to use CT urography as the technique to screen for metastatic disease after

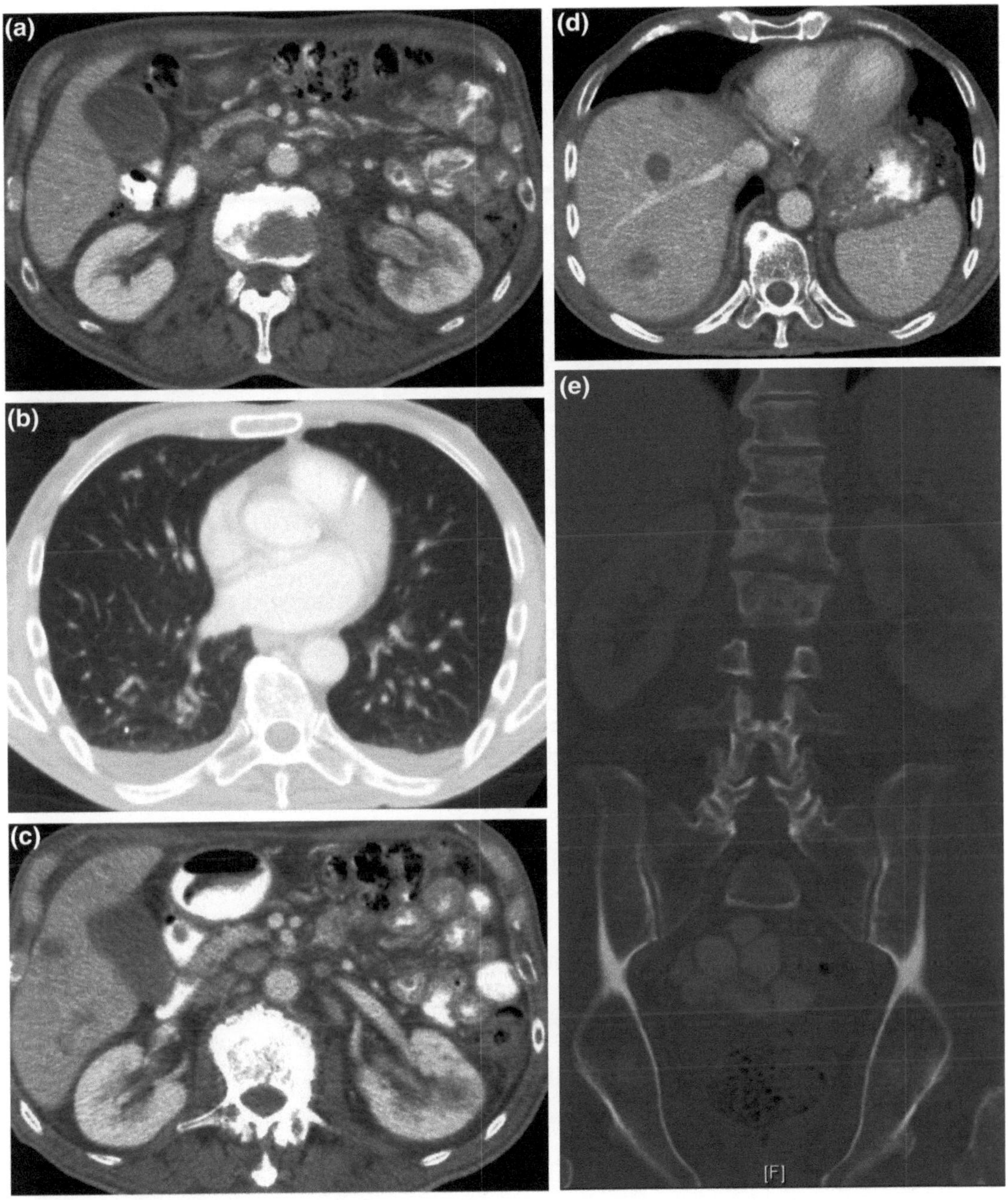

Fig. 4.12 Contrast enhanced CT of patient with metastatic transitional cell carcinoma demonstrates wide spread metastatic disease with retroperitoneal lympadenopathy (**a**), pulmonary metastasis (**b**), Renal lesions (**c**), Liver metastasis (**d**) and bone lesions (**e**)

treatment for bladder cancer, so that the upper tract urothelium can be investigated at intervals and for durations felt to be appropriate for surveillance for metastases.

There is some evidence that a condition called ureteral diverticulosis may be associated with upper tract urothelial malignancy. It is not clear whether patients with it require surveillance.

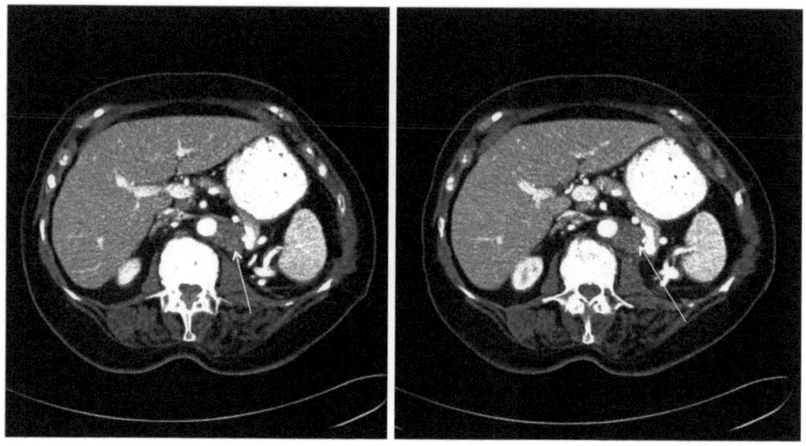

Fig. 4.13 Contrast enhanced CT of patient, post left nephrectomy for transitional cell carcinoma, undergoing routine surveillance. There is new conglomerate retroperitoneal lymphadenopathy (*arrow*) indicative of recurrent disease

Most metastases which appear first after treatment of urothelial cancer appear in locations included in a standard CT of the abdomen and pelvis (Fig. 4.13). Recurrent masses often appear at resection sites, in local draining lymph nodes or in bones. Initial metastases can, of course, appear in sites outside the anatomy usually included in a CT of the abdomen and pelvis, but most surveillance programs only include chest radiographs routinely, leaving additional imaging to be employed only if there are localizing symptoms.

Other Ureteral and Pyelocalyceal Tumors

Of all primary tumors in these sites, those of urothelial origin are by far the most common. They are usually transitional cell carcinomas,

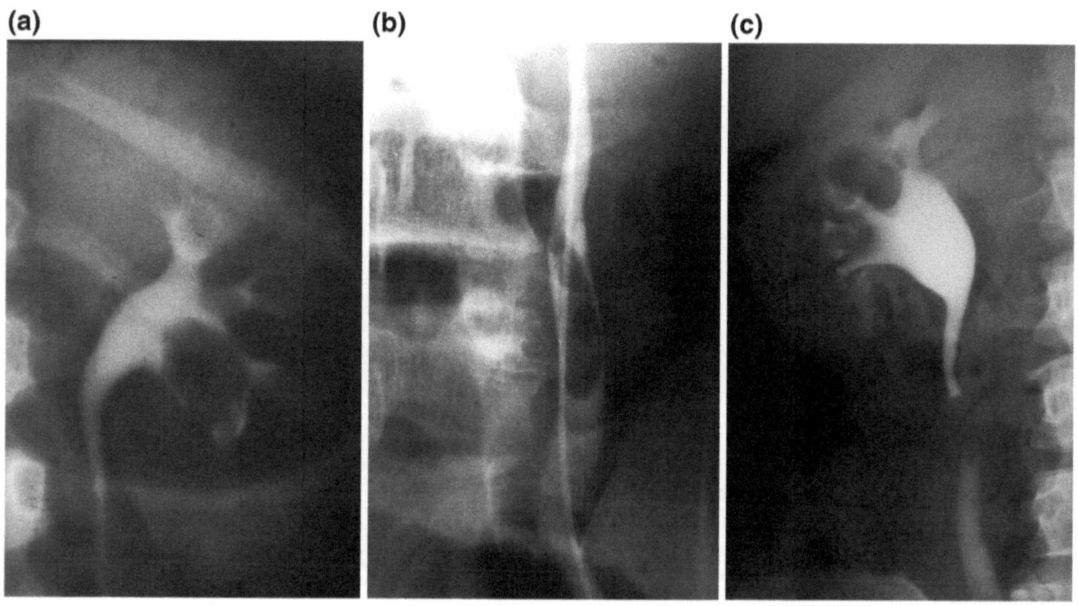

Fig. 4.14 Three excretory pyelograms demonstrating fibroepithelial polyps which appear as well circumscribed rounded filling defect within the lower pole calyx (**a**), midureter (**b**) and proximal ureter (**c**). This clearly intraluminal mass has smooth borders and does extend though the wall

although squamous cell carcinomas may appear. Squamous cell carcinomas are difficult to distinguish from transitional cell tumors on imaging, but may be suspected if they appear at sites which have been subjected to long-term inflammation. Rarely, non-epithelial tissues may also generate neoplasms, such as leiomyomas, leiomyosarcomas, lymphangiomas, hemangiomas, fibromas, and tumors of neural origin [24]. Imaging usually does not permit definitive diagnoses of these, but they can be suspected if their surfaces are smooth and if they have extramural components without irregular intraluminal surfaces.

As mentioned above, direct invasion or compression of the ureter by malignant lesions arising in adjacent organs, or by more remote malignancies which metastasize to the retroperitoneum, are common. Rarely, extraureteral malignancies may metastasize directly to the ureteral wall; melanomas and lymphomas have been documented. These are difficult to distinguish from primary urothelial tumors.

A specific benign tumor, known as a fibroepithelial polyp, occasionally appears in the ureter or collecting system. Its central portion consists of fibrovascular tissue and its surface is relatively normal transitional epithelium. It occurs in children and young adults, and is more likely to appear in the collecting system or proximal ureter than in the distal ureter (Fig. 4.14). These tumors grow entirely intraluminally and tend to have smoother surfaces than urothelial malignancies. They are relatively soft, and tend to adopt their shapes to the configuration of the space in which they grow, so they often appear lobular in the renal pelvis and cylindrical when in the ureter [25].

Summary Box

- The imaging evaluation of suspected urothelial carcinoma of the upper urinary tract includes CT, ultrasound and MRI, with CT being the preferred modality
- Pre- and post-contrast imaging should be performed in the evaluation of hematuria.
- Correct clinical history is critical in the evaluation of filling defects within the collecting system.
- CT urography is well suited to screen for upper tract recurrence in patients with bladder cancer.
- PET-CT is suitable for monitoring response to treatment and assessment of metastatic disease
- Cold Cup Biopsy is essential in the renal pelvic calyceal area for accurate staging.

References

1. Moloney F, et al. Haematuria: an imaging guide. Adv Urol. 2014;2014:414125.
2. Shinagare AB, Sadow CA, Silverman SG. Surveillance of patients with bladder cancer following cystectomy: yield of CT urography. Abdom Imaging. 2013;38(6):1415–21.
3. Pabon-Ramos W, et al. Excretory urography: trends in clinical use and diagnostic yield. Abdom Imaging. 2010;35(5):607–11.
4. Sallami S, et al. Imaging findings of urinary tuberculosis on computerized tomography versus excretory urography: through 46 confirmed cases. Tunis Med. 2014;92(12):743–7.
5. Helenius M, et al. Comparison of post contrast CT urography phases in bladder cancer detection. Eur Radiol. 2016;26(2):585–91.
6. Lin N, et al. Computed tomography urography for diagnosis of calyceal diverticulum complicated by urolithiasis: the accuracy and the effect of abdominal compression and prolongation of acquisition delay. Urology. 2013;82(4):786–90.
7. Takeuchi M, et al. CT urography for diagnosis of upper urinary tract urothelial carcinoma: are both nephrographic and excretory phases necessary? AJR Am J Roentgenol. 2015;205(3):W320–7.
8. Al-Amin M, et al. Cutting down the radiation dose on CT urography: how it is done and what results are received? Radiat Prot Dosimetry. 2015;165(1–4):172–4.
9. Sahni VA, Shinagare AB, Silverman SG. Virtual unenhanced CT images acquired from dual-energy CT urography: accuracy of attenuation values and variation with contrast material phase. Clin Radiol. 2013;68(3):264–71.
10. Sun H, et al. Application of single-bolus dual-source dual-energy CT urography in upper tract opacification and diagnostic performance for painless

hematuria. Zhongguo Yi Xue Ke Xue Yuan Xue Bao. 2014;36(3):283–90.
11. Takeuchi M, et al. Split-bolus CT-urography using dual-energy CT: feasibility, image quality and dose reduction. Eur J Radiol. 2012;81(11):3160–5.
12. Hack K, Pinto PA, Gollub MJ. Targeted delayed scanning at CT urography: a worthwhile use of radiation? Radiology. 2012;265(1):143–50.
13. Childs DD, et al. Contrast-enhanced magnetic resonance urography at 3T: clinical feasibility. J Comput Assist Tomogr. 2013;37(1):29–36.
14. Drudi FM, et al. Contrast-enhanced ultrasonography in the diagnosis of upper urinary tract urothelial cell carcinoma: a preliminary study. Ultraschall Med. 2013;34(1):30–7.
15. Kirkali Z, Tuzel E. Transitional cell carcinoma of the ureter and renal pelvis. Crit Rev Oncol Hematol. 2003;47(2):155–69.
16. Braden GL, et al. Ultrasound diagnosis of early renal papillary necrosis. J Ultrasound Med. 1991;10(7):401–3.
17. Jung DC, et al. Renal papillary necrosis: review and comparison of findings at multi-detector row CT and intravenous urography. Radiographics. 2006;26(6):1827–36.
18. Kauffman CA. Diagnosis and management of fungal urinary tract infection. Infect Dis Clin North Am. 2014;28(1):61–74.
19. Branchereau J, et al. Goldman Antopol syndrome associated with bilateral congenital severe factor V deficiency. Prog Urol. 2010;20(8):604–7.
20. Antopol W, Goldman L. Urol Cutaneous Rev. 1948;52:189.
21. Gayer G, et al. Spontaneous suburothelial hemorrhage in coagulopathic patients: CT diagnosis. Am J Roentgenol. 2011;197(5):W887–90.
22. Heo SH, et al. Pyeloureteritis cystica. Kidney Int. 2014;85(4):983–4.
23. Wang J, et al. Transitional cell carcinoma of upper urinary tract vs. benign lesions: distinctive MSCT features. Abdom Imaging. 2009;34(1):94–106.
24. Kenney PJ, Stanley RJ. Computed tomography of ureteral tumors. J Comput Assist Tomogr. 1987;11(1):102–7.
25. Hughes FA, Davis CS. Multiple benign ureteral fibrous polyps. AJR Am J Roentgenol. 1976;126(4):723–7.

5 Virtual Ureteroscopy of Upper Tract Urothelial Tumors

Angela Tong and Anthony Gilet

Introduction

Hematuria is the presence of red blood cells in urine. It often signifies renal or urinary tract pathology. It is important to elucidate the etiology of the hematuria as the differential is wide including renal stones versus pyelonephritis versus various malignant etiologies. Treatment of each disease entity is varied and thus accurate and efficient diagnosis is imperative [1]. Imaging can assist in the process of diagnosis [2].

One of the more harrowing etiologies of hematuria is urothelial cell carcinoma. It is the fourth most common cancer worldwide after breast/prostate, lung, and colorectal cancer. Most urothelial cancers occur in the bladder, however, upper tract urothelial carcinomas (UTUC) are less common and account for only 5–10% of the urothelial cancers [3] and 15% of renal pelvis cancers. Most of these renal pelvis cancers are transitional cell carcinomas (90%), however 10% are squamous cell carcinomas, and 1% is adenocarcinomas [4]. These cancers are usually silent during the first stages, limiting the opportunity for early diagnosis. 60% of UTUCs are invasive at diagnosis [5].

Visualization of the upper urinary tract system including the ureters and renal pelvises is important for diagnosis and localization of such cancers. Traditional ureteroscopy, performed by urologists, is often employed to do so, and has the advantages of direct visualization with possible immediate biopsy or treatment opportunities [6], however it is an invasive procedure that requires sedation [5, 7]. Dedicated imaging of the upper urinary tract with noninvasive techniques can be performed preliminarily or in conjunction with ureteroscopy [6–9]. These exams have an added benefit of visualization of the entire abdomen and pelvis, which allows for the detection of disease spread in addition to the visualization of the primary cancer; thus, it is important to cancer staging. Imaging of the upper urinary tract can also be used in posttreatment follow up to evaluate for recurrence of disease [7].

Imaging of the upper urinary tract system began with intravenous urography utilizing fluoroscopy, which was developed in the 1920s. It continued to be the mainstay of the upper tract imaging until computed tomography (CT) was

Electronic supplementary material The online version of this chapter (doi:10.1007/978-3-319-51263-1_5) contains supplementary material, which is available to authorized users.

A. Tong · A. Gilet (✉)
Department of Radiology, New York Medical College/Westchester Medical Health Network, Valhalla, NY 10595, USA
e-mail: anthony.gilet@wmchealth.org

A. Tong
e-mail: angela.tong@wmchealth.org

M. Eshghi (ed.), *Urothelial Malignancies of the Upper Urinary Tract*,
https://doi.org/10.1007/978-3-319-51263-1_5

invented in the 1970s. With the advent of CT came increased spatial resolution allowing for better visualization of anatomy and pathology. However, CT urogram (CTU) was not feasible until multidetector CT (MDCT) scanners were developed in the 1990s. This advancement in technology allowed for the imaging of the urinary tract in less than 1 mm slices with one breath hold, which was necessary to minimize motion artifact from breathing as well as to visualize the subtle details in the small ureters. The isotropic voxels, volume elements, also allowed for reconstructions of the images in different planes, helpful for diagnosis of disease entities, and evaluation of disease extent [10]. As new software is developed, 3D reconstructions of the acquired data can be made to simulate the more invasive ureteroscopy [11]. With these new advances, CT urography has become the first line of imaging UTUC [12].

CT Urography

Technique

The sensitivity of CT urography in detecting UTUCs ranges from 67 to 100% and the specificity ranges from 93 to 99%, depending on technique [13]. There are no standardized techniques, and many variations exist. They can be loosely divided into single bolus, split-bolus, and triple-bolus techniques. All require the administration of intravenous contrast and exploits the renal excretion of the contrast. The goal of CTU is to fill and distend the renal pelvis and ureters with contrast so that any potential neoplasm will manifest as a filling defect or stricture [14]. The use of CT allows for simultaneous evaluation of all the surrounding structures including the renal parenchyma as well as vasculature for surgery planning. Optimizing the scan is often difficult due to the peristalsis of the ureters and the variability of renal function in patients. Another limitation is the inherent nephrotoxicity of the contrast agents. As a result, only a limited quantity of contrast can be administered at one exam [15]. In addition to contrast enhanced scans, a non-contrast scan should be performed prior to the administration of contrast to exclude less ominous causes for hematuria such as renal stones [10, 16–18].

Single Bolus

Single bolus technique is one of the most commonly used techniques. It utilizes a non-diluted full dose of intravenous contrast in one bolus. Separate acquisitions are obtained, first prior to contrast administration then following the contrast through the corticomedullary phase (25–70 s post contrast), nephrographic phase (100 s post contrast), and a delayed renal excretory phase (10 min post contrast) [4, 19, 20]. Because this method dedicates the entire dose of contrast to the excretory phase, the contrast fully opacifies and distends the renal pelvis and ureters. Since multiple phases are obtained, this also allows for better evaluation of the renal parenchyma for renal cell carcinomas, which is another major cause of hematuria [21, 22].

The non-diluted contrast in the ureters appears very dense. This is helpful for post-processing of images, however the exaggerated difference of density between the ureter lumen and the surrounding soft tissue may obscure subtle details of the ureter. In addition, because three or four full acquisitions are performed, the radiation dose is high, which may be a consideration if the patient is to be monitored frequently [14, 23–25].

Split-Bolus

The split-bolus technique divides the contrast bolus into two. After the first portion of the contrast bolus is administered, the second portion of the bolus is administered approximately 5 min later. Images are acquired approximately 7 min after the initial bolus was administered. This allows for simultaneous acquisition of nephrographic and excretory phase, decreasing the number of total acquisitions [12, 21, 22, 26, 27].

Triple-Bolus

The triple-bolus technique is similar to the split-bolus technique, however the contrast bolus is split into three portions. The portions are administered such that the corticomedullary, nephrographic, and excretory phases may be acquired in one acquisition [28].

The advantage of the split-bolus and triple-bolus techniques is the decreased number of acquisitions, thus decreasing the radiation dose. However, the smaller contrast bolus in the excretory phase decreases contrast opacification of the ureters, especially the distal ureters. In addition, the lack of separate corticomedullary and nephrographic phases limits the ability to detect small renal cell carcinomas, which may be a confounding cause of painless hematuria [19].

Ancillary Techniques

Several ancillary techniques may also be implemented to improve some of the deficiencies in these techniques. To promote distention of the ureters, IV saline and oral water can be administered prior to the scan. IV furosemide during the scan can also be administered to help distend the ureters [25]. However, the evidence of the efficacy of these techniques is equivocal and the addition of medication such as furosemide can create additional complications as the patient's allergies, medications, blood pressure, and renal function need to be considered [27].

Another frequently used supplemental technique is abdominal compression, usually with an inflatable device. The lower abdomen is compressed to fully distend the proximal ureters. Separate acquisitions are needed without compression to visualize the distal ureters. The method is not consistent as compression may be less effective on a patient with a larger body habitus. In addition, care must be taken to ensure there are no contraindications to abdominal compression such as abdominal aortic aneurysm [26].

Contraindications

There are few contraindications to performing CTU. The most significant is decreased renal function. CTU utilizes iodine-based contrast, which is excreted through the kidneys. If renal function is not adequate, contrast will not be excreted in a timely manner to produce quality images of the excretory phase. In addition, the iodinated contrast material is nephrotoxic. Davenport et al. showed that, there is a decrease in glomerular filtration rate (GFR) after use of low-osmolality iodinated contrast, the least nephrotoxic iodinated contrast, in patients who have GFR of less than 30 mL/min/1.73 mm [2, 15, 29].

Another relative contraindication is a history of anaphylactoid reactions. In the general population, the risk of a severe adverse allergic reaction is 0.04% [30, 31]. These severe reactions are defined as one or the combination of the following symptoms that required treatment: dyspnea, sudden hypotension, cardiac arrest, and loss of consciousness. However, those who have experienced severe reactions to iodinated intravenous contrast reaction have a five to sixfold increased risk of having a subsequent reaction [30]. However, in the United States, it is the standard of care to administer prophylactic steroids with or without diphenhydramine prior to contrast administration to decrease the risk of allergic reaction. This was proven to be effective with the use of high-osmolality iodinated contrast agents, however, has not been proven to prevent severe reactions to iso or low-osmolality iodinated intravenous contrast agents, which are commonly used today [29].

3D Reconstruction

Source images are acquired in the axial plane and must be acquired at a thickness of less than 1 mm to gain the anatomic resolution necessary to make subtle findings. Standard coronal and sagittal reconstructions are then performed. There are several other reconstruction techniques that add value to interpretation. These include the maximum intensity projection (MIP), volume formation (VF), and volume rendering (VR).

MIP utilizes an algorithm that selects the highest attenuation voxels (a volume element similar to a 3D pixel) along lines projected through a volumetric data set. The selected voxels are then incorporated into a 2D image which highlights the hyperdense objects on the images [27, 32, 33]. This technique is often used for CT angiography, however it is also advantageous for evaluating well-distended collecting systems and ureters in the excretory phase of a CT urogram. The disadvantage is that other high-density tissue, such as calcifications and calcified or enhanced vasculature may obscure the ureters. In addition, the two-dimensionality may obscure 3D relationships that exist between some structures [34].

VF is a more primitive method, however, and allows for better awareness of 3D relationships between structures when compared to MIP. In the VF technique, each voxel is designated a tissue type based on thresholding of Hounsfield units. The system is binary and can only assign one tissue type to each Hounsfield unit. This limits the evaluation of tissue interfaces where more than one tissue type can occupy one voxel producing a Hounsfield unit that averages between the two (volume averaging). For example, VF would have difficulties in identifying the exact interface of a contrast filled ureter and the ureter itself [34].

VR is a complex calculation intensive technique, which identifies the percentage of designated tissue types (e.g., fat, water, soft tissue, bone) in a voxel according to Hounsfield units. This contrasts the VF technique, which assumes each voxel only has one tissue type within it. Each of the formed tissue category is then assigned a color and transparency. A 3D image is then rendered from casting simulated rays of light onto the voxels which modulate the color of the rays [34]. With the data from a CTU, the virtual light rays can be cast onto the designated ureteral tissue, which creates a rendering of the urinary tract system, and produces images for virtual ureteroscopy [4].

Virtual ureteroscopy is a 3D rendering of the ureters in an endoluminal view utilizing either source data or volume reconstructed data. These renderings allow visualization of endoluminal contents as they would appear during traditional ureteroscopy. Similar to traditional ureteroscopy, the renderings allow readers to "drive" and view endoluminal structures in any orientation. Lesions and strictures can be evaluated in their entirety rather than in a single plane as in planar reformatted images [19, 35].

Imaging Interpretation

Understanding the appearance of urothelial tumors on CT urography is important to diagnosis as well as identifying tumor recurrence. All images including source images, coronal, sagittal reconstructions, and 3D reconstructions add value to interpretation. On a CTU, urothelial tumors can present with ureteral thickening, filling defects, ureteral stricture, periureteral fat stranding, urothelial enhancement, ureteral calcification, and hydronephrosis/hydroureter [6, 25, 35]. Ureteral thickening and filling defects in the ureters are the most sensitive and specific findings for diagnosing urothelial tumors [5, 21, 36].

Ureteral wall thickening is helpful in determining the presence of urothelial cancer in the upper urinary tract [37]. Caoili et al. showed that of 24 urothelial tumors, 14 had circumferential wall thickening [12]. In another study, Xu et al. demonstrated that 14 of 38 lesions found on CT urography had ureteral wall thickening. Only nine were proven to have urothelial tumor (PPV, 64%). Further investigation showed that there was 87% positive predictive value (7/8 pelvicalyceal wall thickening) for diagnosing urothelial tumors in the renal pelvicalyceal region as opposed to in the ureters, which had a positive predictive value of 33.3% (2/6 lesions). This indicates that wall thickening has better correlation with urothelial carcinoma in the renal pelvicalyceal region [21].

Ureteral wall thickening may be a subtle finding and is best visualized on the nephrographic phase as the ureters are enhanced the most during this phase [5, 12, 32]. Evaluation on excretory phase may also be helpful as the contrast between the ureteral lumen and the ureter itself is heightened because of the contrast in the ureters. Care must be taken to review all phases. False negatives are possible on the excretory phase [6]. With administration of fluids and furosemide, the ureters may distend, thus altering the apparent thickness of the ureteral wall giving the impression that the wall is thinner than in actuality [21].

Filling defects or masses in the upper urinary tract are also indicative of urothelial cancers. These are best evaluated on the excretory phase. In addition to the standard axial, coronal, and sagittal images, 3D reconstructions are also beneficial in detecting filling defects as the contour of the upper urinary tract is readily

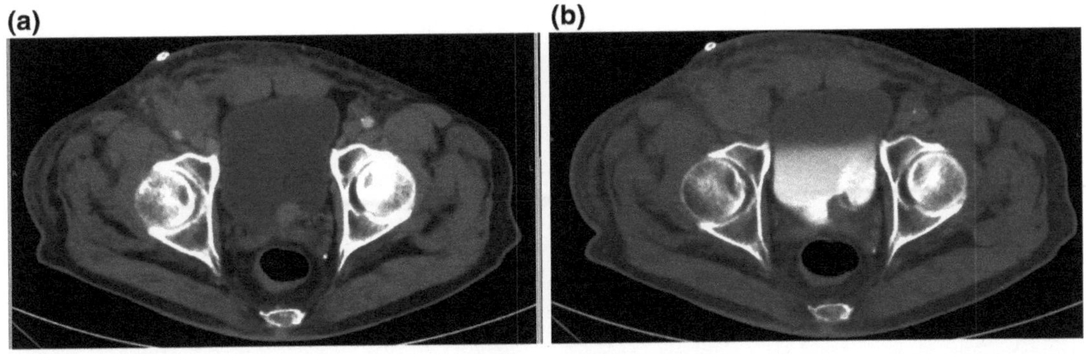

Fig. 5.1 Transitional Cell Carcinoma of the *left* bladder trigone. **a** Post contrast axial image through the bladder shows a 1.1 cm enhancing soft tissue lesion at the *left* ureterovesicular junction that is slightly hyperdense to the intraluminal urine [mass was completely inconspicuous on the non-contrast image (not shown), as it was isodense to the bladder contents]. **b** Axial excretory phase image more clearly delineates the borders of the 1.1 cm mass, which demonstrates greater conspicuity when outlined by the hyperdense intraluminal excreted contrast within the bladder. A contrast 'jet' can be seen ejected into the bladder lumen, as the ureterovesicular junction remains patent and contrast opacified as it traverses the mass. The mass is now less dense (measures a lower Hounsfield Unit attenuation) than on the arterial phase scan, indicating tumor washout. This is a helpful feature to discriminate the lesion from a pseudotumor such as a blood clot, which could have a similar appearance and mimic tumor if only a single CT phase was obtained

visualized if the ureters are well distended with contrast. Caoili et al. found that small masses (≤5 mm in maximum diameter) (n = 5 of 24) and large masses (>5 mm in maximum diameter) (n = 5 of 24) correlated with urothelial carcinomas [12]. In the study performed by Xu et al., 24/38 lesions had filling defects in the collecting systems or ureters. 15 of 24 lesions that showed filling defects were proven to be urothelial tumors (PPV 62.5%). There was a higher PPV (87.5%) for filling defects in the ureters than in the pelvicalyceal region (PPV 50%) [21].

Large filling defects or masses are readily visible and also cause secondary effects such as hydronephrosis and hydroureter, thus are easily diagnosed. Smaller filling defects and masses are subtler and can be difficult to identify (Fig. 5.1). This is especially true because of beam hardening artifacts from the dense contrast in the collecting system and ureters on excretory phase. Widening the window settings can allow for improved visualization. Subtle small filling defects may also be obscured on excretory phase MIP reconstructions as well because the algorithm utilizes only the highest attenuation voxel and may obscure the lower attenuated urothelial tumor mass.

Although urothelial neoplasms manifest as ureteral thickening and filling defects, there are additional secondary findings that may help diagnosis. Urothelial neoplasms may exhibit arterial enhancement from neovascularity [14, 38]. There may also be periureteral fat stranding from extraluminal extension of tumor mass. Hydronephrosis and hydroureter can result from obstruction due to stenosis from ureteral wall thickening and filling defects. Although these findings are nonspecific and are associated with many other pathologic processes, when found in conjunction with ureteral wall thickening and masses, these findings increase the likelihood of an urothelial mass diagnosis.

Benefits of 3D Imaging

Although 3D images require additional time to process and analyze, they add value to the final interpretation of the study. Caoli et al. showed that utilizing VR and MIP reconstructions of images collected from 4 and 8 detector MDCT allowed the group to diagnose six more lesions than they were able to with only the standard axial, coronal, and sagittal imaging. Current MDCTs have up to 256 detectors allowing for CT acquisitions with even thinner slices, which

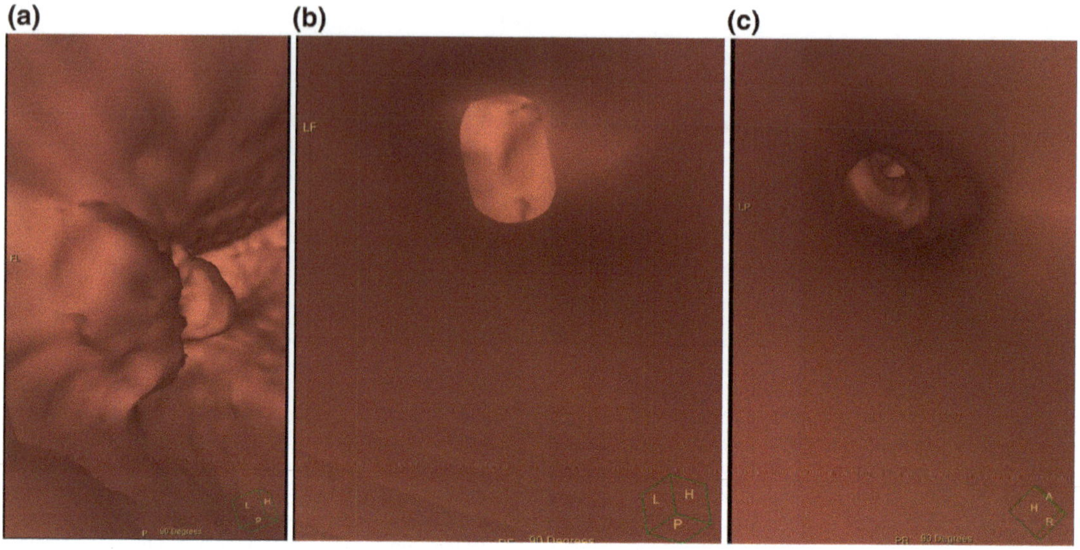

Fig. 5.2 **a** A single frame from a volume rendered CT Virtual Ureteroscopy, providing an endoluminal view of a 0.5 mm lesion transitional cell carcinoma. A polypoid lesion is demonstrated along the *right* anterolateral wall of the distal ureter. The green 3-D orientation box in the lower *left* hand of the screen as well as a cross-referenced line with the axial acquired imaged (not shown) provides a roadmap for the clinician. **b** and **c** demonstrate the normal intraluminal appearance of the ureter pre- and post-lesion respectively

can be obtained at a faster rate resulting in higher resolution images and reconstructions thus facilitating the use of 3D reconstructions.

3D reconstructions excel in several specific instances. VR and MIP can assist in the detection of subtle differences in ureteral caliber. Unlike axial source images and planar reformats, VR and MIP allow for the visualization of the entire ureter such that subtle dilatation or narrowing are more apparent. Areas of interest may be compared to source axial images to correlate for subtle wall thickening or enhancement. Cross-referencing with all series is imperative as the subtle differences in caliber may be due to normal peristalsis. The ability to visualize the entire ureter also increases the ease of detecting abrupt caliber changes or irregularity of the ureteral caliber, ominous signs for malignancy (Fig. 5.2) (Video 5.1).

In additional to VR and MIP, endoluminal views in virtual ureteroscopy also add to the value of source images in the diagnosis of upper urothelial tract tumors. The luminal contour is presented in its entirety and may be viewed in any orientation. In addition, cine movies can be made of traversing through the ureter, emphasizing the subtle differences in contour. This allows for the improved detection of small masses and irregularities in the ureteral wall. Again, suspicious regions should be correlated with contrast enhanced source images to confirm the presence of a tumor.

The advancement of CT technology has improved the quality and the ease at which 3D reconstructions and renderings are made. Although they are not sufficient in standalone evaluation of the upper urothelial tract, they present the source data in multiple different ways and can assist in the detection of subtle findings in the ureters [39]. With the correlation of findings on the source images to the reconstructions, accurate diagnosis of upper tract urothelial tumors is possible.

Summary Box

- Imaging is a critical component in the workup and management of a patient with known or suspected mass of the urinary collecting system.

- State of the art and emerging techniques in CT and MRI have revolutionized the role radiology plays in urothelial carcinoma.
- Novel post-processing techniques in CT and MR, including 3D and volume rendered imaging and 'Virtual Ureteroscopy' have increased the sensitivity of these examinations, allowing detection of increasingly smaller lesions.
- In addition to diagnosis, these techniques can act as a roadmap for interventions and treatments.
- Optimized technique is critical to the performance of these examinations. This entails adequate patient hydration, diuretic administration, tailored contrast administration to the clinical question, advanced scanners and cutting-edge post processing.

References

1. Cauberg ECC, Nio CY, de la Rosette JM, Laguna MP, de Reijke TM. Computed tomography-urography for upper urinary tract imaging: is it required for all patients who present with hematuria? J Endourol. 2011;25(11):1733–40.
2. Cowan N. CT Urography for hematuria. Nat Rev Urol. 2012;9:218–26.
3. Chandarana H, Taouli B. Diffusion and perfusion imaging of the liver. Eur J Radiol. 2010;76(3):348–58.
4. Raman SP, Horton KM, Fishman EK. MDCT Evaluation of ureteral tumors: advantages of 3D reconstruction and volume visualization. Am J Roentgenol. 2013;201(6):1239–47. doi:10.2214/AJR.13.10880.
5. Rouprêt M, Babjuk M, Compérat E, et al. European guidelines on upper tract urothelial carcinomas: 2013 update. Eur Urol. 2013;63(6):1059–71. doi:10.1016/j.eururo.2013.03.032.
6. Lee KS, Zeikus E, DeWolf WC, Rofsky NM, Pedrosa I. MR urography versus retrograde pyelography/ureteroscopy for the exclusion of upper urinary tract malignancy. Clin Radiol. 2010;65(3):185–92. doi:10.1016/j.crad.2009.11.003.
7. Lucca I, Leow JJ, Shariat SF, Chang SL. Diagnosis and management of upper tract urothelial carcinoma. Hematol Oncol Clin North Am. 2015;29(2):271–88. doi:10.1016/j.hoc.2014.10.003.
8. Latchamsetty KC, Porter CR. Treatment of upper tract urothelial carcinoma: a review of surgical and adjuvant therapy. Rev Urol. 2006. 8(2):61–70. http://www.pubmedcentral.nih.gov/articlerender.fcgi?artid=1578534&tool=pmcentrez&rendertype=abstract.
9. Razavi SA, Sadigh G, Kelly AM, Cronin P. comparative effectiveness of imaging modalities for the diagnosis of upper and lower urinary tract malignancy: a critically appraised topic. Acad Radiol. 2012;19(9):1134–40. doi:10.1016/j.acra.2012.05.004.
10. Silverman SG, Leyendecker JR, Amis ES. What is the current role of CT urography and MR urography in the evaluation of the urinary tract? Radiology. 2009;250(2):309–23. doi:10.1148/radiol.2502080534.
11. Mullen KM, Sahni VA, Sadow CA, Silverman SG. Yield of urinary tract cancer diagnosis with repeat CT urography in patients with hematuria. Am J Roentgenol. 2015;204(2):318–23. doi:10.2214/AJR.14.12825.
12. O'Connor OJ, McSweeney SE, Maher MM. Imaging of hematuria. Radiol Clin North Am. 2008;46(1):113–32. doi:10.1016/j.rcl.2008.01.007.
13. Anderson EM, Murphy R, Rennie TM, Cowan NC. Multidetector computed tomography urography (MDCTU) for diagnosing urothelial malignancy. Clin Radiol. 2007;62(4):324–32. doi:10.1016/j.crad.2006.10.008.
14. Takeuchi M, Konrad AJ, Kawashima A, Boorjian SA, Takahashi N. CT urography for diagnosis of upper urinary tract urothelial carcinoma: are both nephrographic and excretory phases necessary? Am J Roentgenol. 2015;205(3):W320–7. doi:10.2214/AJR.14.14075.
15. Davenport MS, Khalatbari S, Cohan RH, Dillman JR, Myles JD, Ellis JH. Contrast material-induced nephrotoxicity and intravenous low-osmolality iodinated contrast material: risk stratification by using estimated glomerular filtration rate. Radiology. 2013;268(3):719–28. doi:10.1148/radiol.13122276.
16. Chlapoutakis K, Theocharopoulos N, Yarmenitis S, Damilakis J. Performance of computed tomographic urography in diagnosis of upper urinary tract urothelial carcinoma, in patients presenting with hematuria: systematic review and meta-analysis. Eur J Radiol. 2010;73(2):334–8. doi:10.1016/j.ejrad.2008.10.026.
17. Chow LC, Kwan SW, Olcott EW, Sommer G. Split-bolus MDCT urography with synchronous nephrographic and excretory phase enhancement. Am J Roentgenol. 2007;189(2):314–22. doi:10.2214/AJR.07.2288.
18. Browne RFJ, Meehan CP, Colville J, Power R, Torreggiani WC. Transitional cell carcinoma of the upper urinary tract: spectrum of imaging findings. Radiographics. 2005;25(6):1609–27. doi:10.1148/rg.256045517.
19. Raman SP, Horton KM, Fishman EK. Transitional cell carcinoma of the upper urinary tract: optimizing image interpretation with 3D reconstructions. Abdom Imaging. 2012;37(6):1129–40. doi:10.1007/s00261-011-9838-2.

20. Yuh BI, Cohan RH. Different phases of renal enhancement: role in detecting and characterizing renal masses during helical CT. 1999;(Sept):747–55.
21. Xu AD, Ng CS, Kamat A, Grossman HB, Dinney C, Sandler CM. Significance of upper urinary tract urothelial thickening and filling defect seen on MDCT urography in patients with a history of urothelial neoplasms. Am J Roentgenol. 2010;195 (4):959–65. doi:10.2214/AJR.09.4177.
22. Dillman JR, Caoili EM, Cohan RH, et al. Comparison of urinary tract distension and opacification using single-bolus 3-phase vs split-bolus 2-phase multidetector row CT urography. J Comput Assist Tomogr. 2007;31(5):750–7. doi:10.1097/RCT.0b013e318033df36.
23. Hwang I, Cho JY, Kim SY, et al. Low tube voltage computed tomography urography using low-concentration contrast media: comparison of image quality in conventional computed tomography urography. Eur J Radiol. 2015;. doi:10.1016/j.ejrad.2015.09.010.
24. O'Connor OJ, McLaughlin P, Maher MM. MR urography. Am J Roentgenol. 2010;195(3):W201–6. doi:10.2214/AJR.09.4176.
25. Ergen FB, Hussain HK, Carlos RC, et al. 3D excretory MR urography: improved image quality with intravenous saline and diuretic administration. J Magn Reson Imaging. 2007;25(4):783–9. doi:10.1002/jmri.20875.
26. Maheshwari E, O'Malley ME, Ghai S, Staunton M, Massey C. Split-bolus MDCT urography: upper tract opacification and performance for upper tract tumors in patients with hematuria. Am J Roentgenol. 2010;194(2):453–8. doi:10.2214/AJR.09.3228.
27. Van Der Molen AJ, Cowan NC, Mueller-Lisse UG, Nolte-Ernsting CCA, Takahashi S, Cohan RH. CT urography: definition, indications and techniques. A guideline for clinical practice. Eur Radiol. 2008;18 (1):4–17. doi:10.1007/s00330-007-0792-x.
28. Kekelidze M, Dwarkasing RS, Dijkshoorn ML, Sikorska K, Verhagen PCMS, Krestin GP. Kidney and urinary tract imaging: triple-bolus multidetector CT urography as a one-stop shop-protocol design, opacification, and image quality analysis. Radiology. 2010;255 (2):508–16. doi:10.1590/S1677-55382010000400019.
29. Davenport MS, Cohan RH, Ellis JH. Contrast media controversies in 2015: imaging patients with renal impairment or risk of contrast reaction. Am J Roentgenol. 2015;(June):1–8. doi:10.2214/AJR.14.14259.
30. Beckett KR, Moriarity AK, Langer JM. Safe use of contrast media: what the radiologist needs to know. RadioGraphics. 2015;35(3):1738–50.
31. Katayama H, Yamaguchi K, Kozuka T, Takahima T, Seez P, Matsuura K. adverse nonionic reactions contrast to ionic media the japanese on the safety of contrast. Radiology. 1990;1775:621–8.
32. Ramamurthy NK, Moosavi B, McInnes MDF, Flood TA, Schieda N. Multiparametric MRI of solid renal masses: pearls and pitfalls. Clin Radiol. 2015;70(3):304–16. doi:10.1016/j.crad.2014.10.006.
33. Dickerson EC, Dillman JR, Smith EA, DiPietro MA, Lebowitz RL, Darge K. Pediatric MR urography: indications, techniques, and approach to review. RadioGraphics. 2015;35(4):1208–30. doi:10.1148/rg.2015140223.
34. Fishman EK, Ney DR, Heath DG, Corl FM, Horton KM, Johnson PT. Volume rendering versus maximum intensity projection in CT angiography: what works best, when, and why. Radiographics. 2006;26(3):905–22. doi:10.1148/rg.263055186.
35. Neri E, Boraschi P, Caramella D, et al. MR virtual endoscopy of the upper urinary tract. Am J Roentgenol. 2000;175(6):1697–702. http://www.scopus.com/inward/record.url?eid=2-s2.0-0033654115&partnerID=40&md5=4d77f6f06410ff7c0c330b19b3dfd232.
36. Mueller-Lisse UG, Mueller-Lisse UL, Hinterberger J, Schneede P, Meindl T, Reiser MF. Multidetector-row computed tomography (MDCT) in patients with a history of previous urothelial cancer or painless macroscopic haematuria. Eur Radiol. 2007;17 (11):2794–803. doi:10.1007/s00330-007-0609-y.
37. Bokacheva L, Rusinek H, Zhang J, Lee V. Assessment of renal function with dynamic contrast-enhanced mr imaging. Magn Reson Imaging Clin N Am. 2008;16(4):597–611.
38. Takeuchi M, Matsuzaki K, Kubo H, Nishitani H. High- *b* -value diffusion-weighted magnetic resonance imaging of pancreatic cancer and mass-forming chronic pancreatitis: preliminary results. Acta Radiol. 2008;49(4):383–6. doi:10.1080/02841850801895381.
39. Chahal R, Taylor K, Eardley I, Lloyd SN, Spencer JA. Patients at high risk for upper tract urothelial cancer: evaluation of hydronephrosis using high resolution magnetic resonance urography. J Urol. 2005;174(2):478–82. doi:10.1097/01.ju.0000165169.94286.3d.

Endoluminal Ultrasound for Upper Tract Urothelial Carcinoma

6

Scott G. Hubosky, Raghu Vikram and Surena F. Matin

Endoluminal Ultrasound for Upper Tract Urothelial Carcinoma

The pathologic stage of upper tract urothelial carcinoma (UTUC) has reliably and reproducibly been shown to be the best predictor of patient outcome after extirpative surgical treatment [1, 2]. In high-risk UTUC patients, neoadjuvant chemotherapy has been retrospectively shown to downstage nephroureterectomy (NU) specimens, result in occasional remissions [3] and increase survival versus those high-risk patients who are treated immediately with NU alone [4]. Additionally, given the potential nephrotoxic side effects of cisplatin-based chemotherapy, a window of opportunity to offer it may close after immediate radical NU since patient eligibility based on glomerular filtration rate (GFR) drops from 49 to 19% in the postoperative setting [5]. Nevertheless, chemotherapy use still needs to be justified and ideally only those patients standing to benefit, namely those with at least locally advanced disease (≥pT2) would be selected for treatment. Conversely, it is equally important to offer nephron-sparing options to patients with low-risk superficial disease given the benefit of endoscopic treatment to preserve renal function and provide long-term effective oncological control in this carefully selected population [6, 7]. Therefore, proper patient selection is critical to direct treatment for UTUC and relies heavily on the ability of the clinician to predict tumor stage.

Highly accurate clinical staging of UTUC remains elusive and the topic of much focused research. Almost twenty years ago, Keeley et al. [8] described the correlation of ureteroscopically derived UTUC biopsy grade to tumor grade and stage on final NU specimen. Out of this work grew the concept that ureteroscopic biopsy grade could serve as a surrogate for pathologic stage. Their results were confirmed by Brown et al. [9] ten years later in a larger cohort of patients. Findings from both groups demonstrated that low-grade disease on ureteroscopic biopsy correlated with noninvasive stage (≤pT1) in 73–86% and that high-grade disease resulted in more invasive cases (≥pT2) in 66%. Although correlation was shown to exist by both groups, it was not always reproducible by others and room for improvement existed. Historically, cross-sectional imaging with computerized tomography (CT) has been useful

S. G. Hubosky
Department of Urology, Sidney Kimmel Medical College at Thomas Jefferson University, Philadelphia, PA 19107, USA
e-mail: scott.hubosky@jefferson.edu

R. Vikram
Department of Diagnostic Radiology, University of Texas MD Anderson Cancer Center, Houston, TX 77030, USA
e-mail: rvikram@mdanderson.org

S. F. Matin (✉)
Department of Urology, University of Texas MD Anderson Cancer Center, Houston, TX 77030, USA
e-mail: surmatin@mdanderson.org

M. Eshghi (ed.), *Urothelial Malignancies of the Upper Urinary Tract*,
https://doi.org/10.1007/978-3-319-51263-1_6

for ruling out overt metastatic disease but has not performed well for predicting pathological stage and frequently results in understaging [10, 11]. Favaretto et al. [12] combined ureteroscopic biopsy findings with cross-sectional imaging in a preoperative predictive model and found that the combination performed better than ureteroscopic biopsy information alone but still only predicted ≥pT2 stage with 71% accuracy.

Endoluminal ultrasound (ELUS) has been used in vascular and nonvascular applications dating back almost 40 years with its use in upper gastrointestinal (GI) endoscopes [13]. It is a technique that provides anatomic detail of structures such as blood vessels or neoplasms, which may lie beyond the lumen of a hollow viscus, not visualized by endoscopy alone. In 1991 Goldberg, Bagley and associates were among the first to apply ELUS to the upper urinary tract when they described their experience with a commercially available 95 cm long, 6Fr probe which contained a 20 MHz transducer capable of achieving axial resolution of 0.1 mm (100 μm) with scanning penetration of about 2 cm. It was not possible to delineate the multiple histological layers of the ureter but a plane was usually discernable between the relatively hypoechoic muscularis and the hyperechoic periureteral fat [14]. Urologic application of ELUS in the upper urinary tract allows for detection of crossing vessels in cases of ureteropelvic junction (UPJ) obstructions, as well as characterization of submucosal calculi and upper tract neoplasms.

Equipment and Preparation

ELUS is performed in the same setting as retrograde pyelogram (RGP) and ureteroscopy (URS) for the evaluation of suspected UTUC. Preoperative imaging should be carefully studied to determine the level of the ureter or intrarenal collecting system affected. Sterile, disposable or limited reusable ELUS probes (Fig. 6.1) contain small high-frequency transducers (12.5–30 MHz), capable of mechanical radial scanning, contained within catheters, which can range between 3 and 9Fr. These probes are designed to be placed over a guidewire and both blunt-tipped and side-saddle designs are available and cost approximately $350–500(US) each. Sonographic systems for ELUS are available from multiple companies including Olympus (Center Valley, PA) and Boston Scientific Corporation (Marlborough, MA) and are shown in Fig. 6.1.

Technique

After thorough cystoscopy and documentation of any bladder tumors, a careful retrograde ureteropyelogram (RGP) is performed with an 8 or 10Fr cone-tipped catheter and approximately 5–8 mL of 30% contrast diluted with saline at a 1:2 ratio. This is slowly injected and fluoroscopy is performed to create the image. Careful attention is paid to the location, possible multifocality, size, shape, and origin of any filling defects.

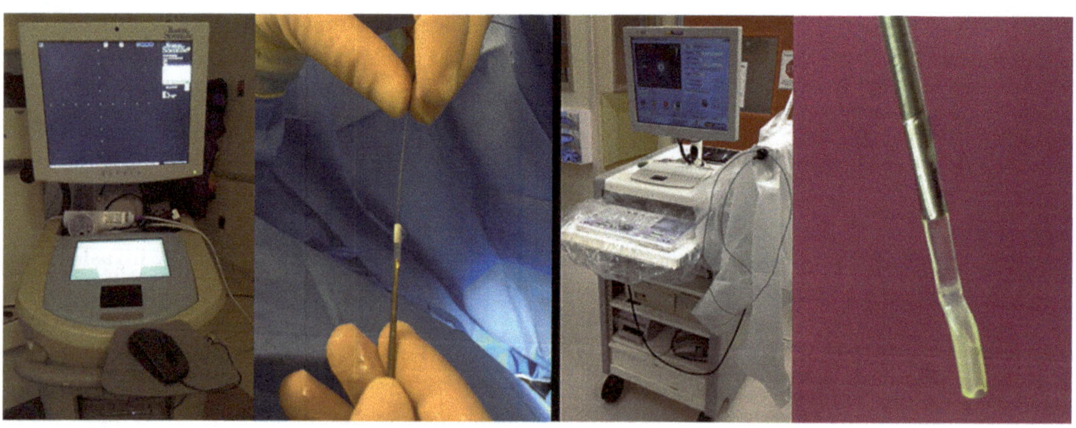

Fig. 6.1 The two different probes and machines used by the authors are shown. On *left* is the unit and device by Boston Scientific, on the *right* Olympus. Copyright SF Matin 2015

Ureteroscopic evaluation is then performed with either a semi-rigid or flexible ureteroscope using "no-touch" technique and avoiding initial blind guidewire placement whenever possible [15]. Once complete upper tract surveillance is achieved, all viable appearing lesions including size and location are documented. A 0.035-in. stainless steel, floppy tip, fixed core wire is then inserted under direct ureteroscopic visualization in an atraumatic fashion. ELUS is then performed prior to any biopsy or laser resection. The ELUS probe is placed over the guide wire and directed to the area of interest guided by fluoroscopy (Fig. 6.2). Bony landmarks serve as useful guides in this step in order to correlate with RGP findings. Fluoroscopy is utilized to orient the ELUS probe with the guidewire and the image on the ultrasound monitor is adjusted accordingly. Video or still pictures can be obtained during the evaluation.

Normal Ureteral Appearance on ELUS

ELUS provides 360°, real-time cross-sectional high-frequency (20–30 MHz) imaging of the ureteral lumen with penetration to several centimeters beyond the lumen. Due to the nature of such high frequencies however, there is less penetration and thus most optimal images are gained within a couple of centimeters. Images of the normal ureter are best when the lumen is well dilated and a column of fluid surrounds the probe. The appearance of fluid within the ureteral lumen will be very dark, typically black—as is the case with any notable blood vessels. The fluid can be used as a standard when adjusting the gain and contrast. A normal ureteral wall is typically symmetric but may be difficult to distend, especially the mid- and distal intramural ureter backed by the detrusor. The normal inner mucosal layer is rarely discernable but may appear as a very thin hyperechoic rim when contrasted against the muscularis layer of the ureter, which is usually readily seen as a hypoechoic, typically symmetric rim. Just beyond the muscularis, lays the periureteral fat, which is visualized as a very bright hyperechoic layer, which is normally quite symmetric (Fig. 6.3). Within the renal pelvis, the same hypoechoic muscularis layer is appreciated with slightly more hyperechoic normal renal parenchyma lying just beyond. Safety guidewires will appear as a hyperechoic focus with acoustic shadowing extending outwards, which can sometimes appear as a disruption of the

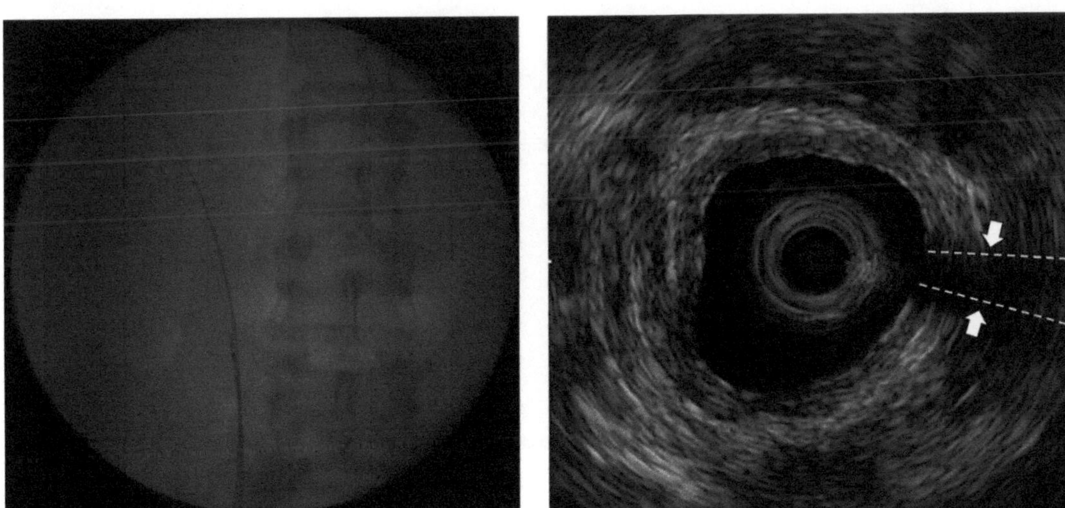

Fig. 6.2 Fluoroscopic image showing ELUS probe over a guide wire in the proximal ureter (*left panel*), and corresponding ELUS image (*right panel*); *arrows* and *dotted lines* indicate acoustic shadow from the guide wire. Copyright SF Matin 2015

periureteral fat layer (Fig. 6.3). Rotation of the probe will identify the wire shadow.

Abnormal Findings on ELUS/Typical UTUC Appearance

RGP and direct ureteroscopic evaluation will direct the surgeon to areas of interest to be studied by ELUS. It is helpful to scan from normal ureter to abnormal areas in order to pick up any subtle findings. Intraluminal (noninvasive) tumors usually will be hypoechoic relative to the hyperechoic periureteral fat layer and tend to distort the lumen as an asymmetric bulge (Figs. 6.4 and 6.5). Lesions however may also be symmetric and this usually will correlate with concentric appearing intraluminal tumor on ureteroscopy. Given the limitations of resolution with ELUS, the exact histological layers of the ureteral wall are not clearly depicted. However, invasive disease is suspected when an irregular hypoechoic mass extends into or beyond the muscularis layer and appears to disrupt the normally concentric, contiguous hyperechoic layer of periureteral fat (Fig. 6.6).

Validation Studies of ELUS for UTUC

A paucity of the literature exists regarding the staging accuracy of ELUS for UTUC and most reports are retrospective, single center experiences with small numbers of patients. The most recent validation study to date, described a series of 15 consecutive patients of which seven underwent NU without neoadjuvant chemotherapy [16]. Eight patients were excluded from analysis due to four not having UTUC and four others getting neoadjuvant chemotherapy prior to NU. Of the seven patients in the analysis, six were correctly categorized while one was overstaged by ELUS to have invasive disease while surgical pathology was noninvasive. The negative predictive value for invasive disease in this study was 100% (four patients) while positive predictive value was 66%. The authors mentioned one patient who had neoadjuvant chemotherapy that was classified by ELUS to be noninvasive but still had muscle invasive disease on final pathology thus indicating at least one likely case of understaging in this series.

In an earlier study, Liu et al. [17] described ELUS findings and attempted staging in 26

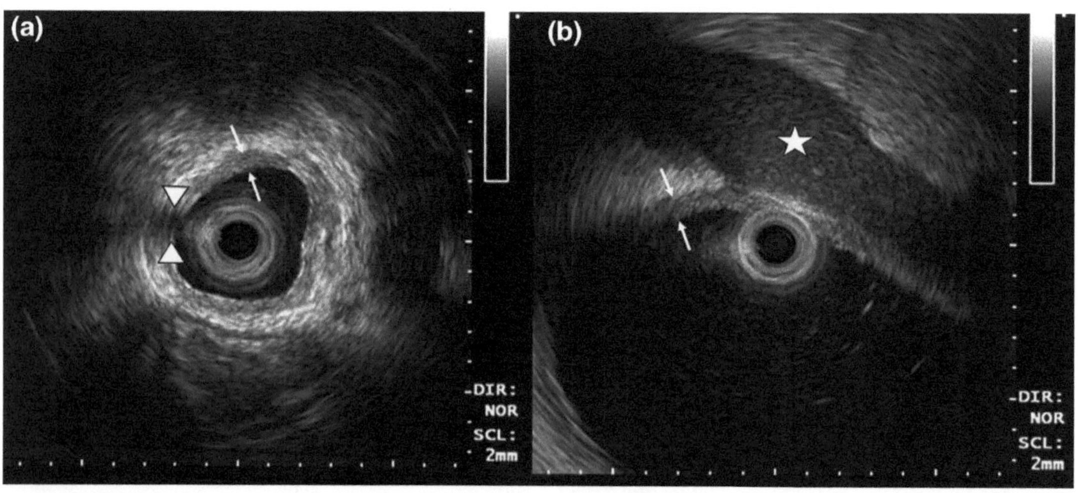

Fig. 6.3 Ultrasound images showing normal findings in varying parts of the upper urinary tract. **a** Mid and proximal ureter; **b** renal pelvis, with renal vein (*star*). An acoustic shadow is seen from the guide wire (*arrowheads*). The urothelial layer is not seen well except for occasional very thin hyperechoic edge due to refraction. The muscularis is primarily what is seen, appearing as a hypoechoic layer (*arrows*) surrounded by the hyperechoic fat (ureter) or renal parenchyma (renal pelvis). Copyright SF Matin 2015

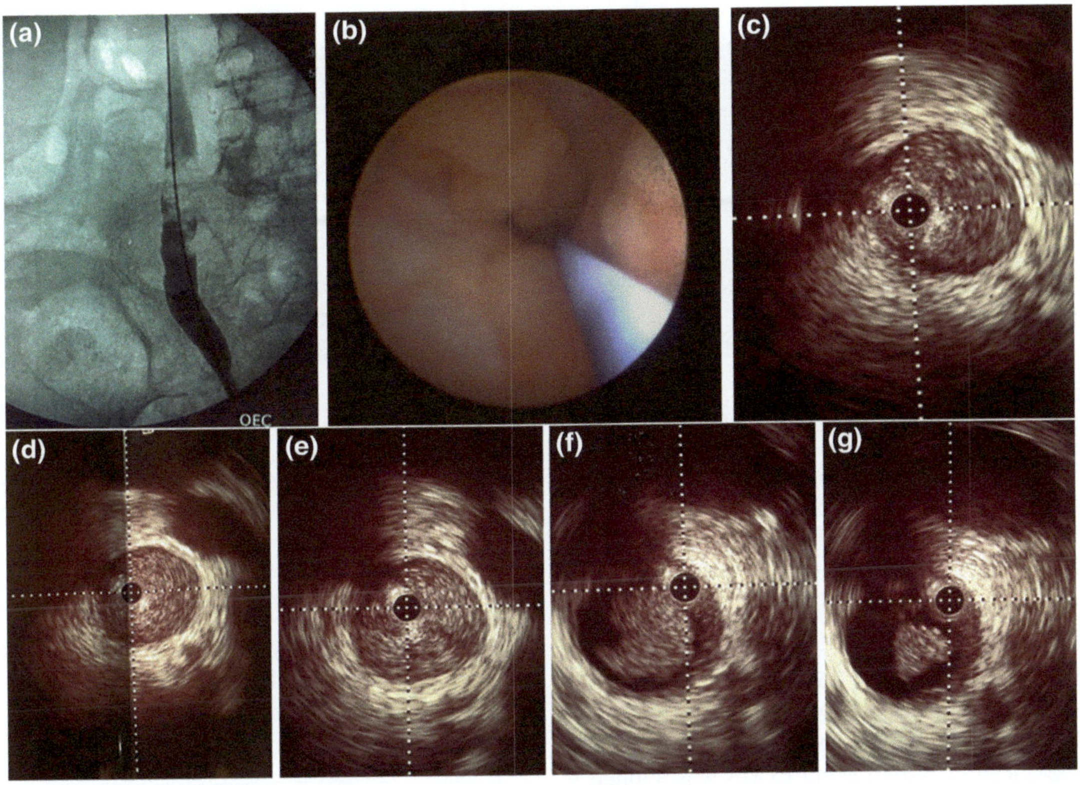

Fig. 6.4 2.5 cm papillary multifocal right lower proximal ureteral tumor on **a** retrograde pyelogram and **b** ureteroscopy (photo courtesy of Kelly A. Healy, MD); **c–e** endoluminal ultrasound shows eccentric hypoechoic tumor well contained within hyperechoic periureteral fat layer in all images obtained at multiple levels of the tumor. **f–g** Image of tumor tip dangling in the ureteral lumen consistent with papillary and noninvasive morphology. This patient was noted to have low-grade UTUC on ureteroscopic biopsy and was clear on second look ureteroscopic surveillance six weeks after initial laser resection. Surgical pathological validation is unavailable due to patient undergoing endoscopic treatment. Copyright SF Matin 2015

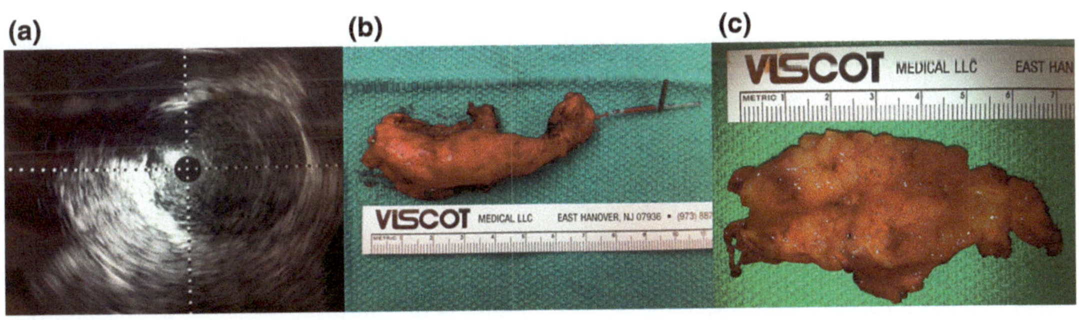

Fig. 6.5 73 year-old with solitary kidney and 7 cm distal UTUC which appeared low grade, papillary and multifocal on ureteroscopy. **a** Endoluminal ultrasound shows asymmetric hypoechoic mass extending towards the 3 o'clock position without overt infiltration of the hyperechoic periureteral fat layer. Safety wire is located at 10 o'clock with acoustic shadow; **b–c** distal ureterectomy demonstrated high volume but low-grade UTUC pTaN0. Copyright SF Matin 2015

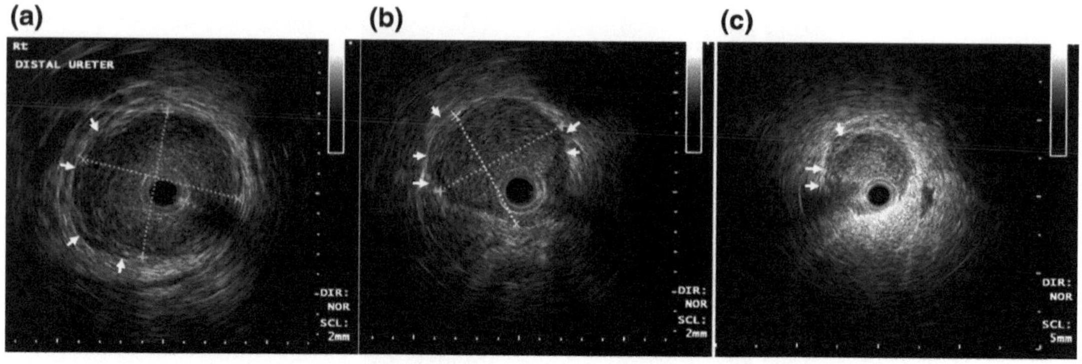

Fig. 6.6 Three examples of invasive disease as seen on endoluminal ultrasound and confirmed pathologically to represent T3 disease. *Arrows* indicate areas of asymmetric or irregular tumor bulging suggesting extraureteral extension. **a** Although there is symmetrical widening of the ureter due to tumor mass, an area of asymmetrical bulging with irregular borders is evident; **b** this figure shows both areas of irregular borders bulging into the periureteral fat, as well as a voluminous tumor asymmetrically protruding into the soft tissue; **c** *arrows* show areas of irregular tumor protruding into the periureteral fat. Copyright SF Matin 2015

patients with ureteroscopically proven UTUC. Unfortunately, only eight patients underwent extirpative surgery in that series as the majority were treated conservatively with ureteroscopic laser ablation for low-risk disease. A three-step classification system using ELUS was applied in which level A lesions were confined to the mucosal layer or lamina propria, level B lesions had presumed muscularis involvement and level C lesions were thought to extend beyond the ureteral or renal pelvic wall into surrounding fat or renal parenchyma. Of the eight patients with surgical validation, two in level A were both found to be pTa or pT1, all four in level B were noted to be $\leq$pT2, and two in level C were both found to be pT3. Thus, although only small numbers were reported, ELUS tended to not understage UTUC in this small series.

Taking these two small studies together, it appears that even though ELUS may not be able to differentiate tumor stage as specifically as histopathology, it still may give reasonable insight into those patients with $\geq$pT3 disease. As noted above, those patients with pT2 disease may not be detected by ELUS and this would seem to be the population which would most likely make up those patients comprising the false negative groups for UTUC staging by ELUS. There may be benefit however for those patients with $\geq$pT3 disease since detection by ELUS would be more likely and given that this population probably has the most to gain by receiving neoadjuvant chemotherapy given only an approximate 50% or less five year survival after NU alone [1, 2, 18].

Challenges and Limitations

The ability of ELUS to display even the normal layers of the ureter relies on how well the ureter can be distended. Anecdotally, more proximal portions of the ureter are easier to distend compared to the intramural distal ureter secondary to the potential compression of the detrusor muscle in that location. A small open-ended ureteral catheter can be placed below the ELUS probe in order to maintain some consistent distention but leakage at the level of the ureteral orifice limits the effectiveness of this maneuver.

As mentioned in previous reports, another limitation to ELUS is that it can be placed only wherever the guidewire can take it. The ELUS probe is unable to be steered into specific locations. The intrarenal collecting system morphology can pose difficulties in this regard, especially in dependent lower pole positions. Specific guidewire placement can sometimes be well directed with either direct ureteroscopic visualization or with an angled-tip ureteral catheter. Mention has been made of combining ELUS capability directly within a flexible ureteroscope [16], either with a probe small enough to be placed through a working channel or as a built-in compound endoscope, similar to those used in GI and pulmonary applications. Unfortunately, the importance of endoscope miniaturization is greatest in ureteral applications and the rate limiting step of creating a compound ELUS ureteroscope would clearly be the diameter of the ureteroscope tip and proximal shaft as both of these affect not only rate of successful retrograde access but also the ability to reach within narrow parts of the intrarenal collecting system [19].

A potential confounding situation occurs when patients come for ELUS evaluation with a previously placed stent that is sometimes necessary to prevent obstruction in the case of an intraluminal ureteral lesion. Previously placed stents have been reported as a source of false positive findings on ELUS evaluating for UTUC [17]. Mucosal thickening and wall edema may obscure the different layers of the ureter thereby posing additional challenges in interpreting the study. Direct visualization with ureteroscopy can help in some situations but still differentiating mucosal swelling from viable tumor is not always clear, even with conventional ureteroscopy. Narrow band Imaging (NBI) used during digital flexible ureteroscopy has anecdotally been shown to help differentiate surface mucosal swelling from viable intraluminal UTUC since the latter is usually more vascularized compared to the former.

The fact that ELUS has been available for UTUC evaluation for more than 20 years and that only a small number of reports exist describing its use and validation speaks volumes about its widespread application in this setting. In addition to the aforementioned technical constraints, ELUS is a relatively expensive technology and UTUC is a relatively uncommon malignancy. That combination does not make for a tremendous amount of interest from hospitals or medical device manufacturers. The emergence of neoadjuvant chemotherapy for UTUC, has however, raised the stakes for those patients with the disease and those clinicians who treat them. Given the relatively dismal and stagnant cancer specific survival rates for those with advanced UTUC [18], any modality that may help justify the use of neoadjuvant chemotherapy when appropriate in these patients, deserves attention and support. Only directed multi-institutional efforts will drive the data and experience needed to further characterize the benefits of ELUS in UTUC staging.

Summary Box

- Current clinical staging of UTUC is still not completely accurate and ELUS has the potential for providing high-resolution visualization of ureter and renal pelvis tumors.
- With ELUS the primary visualization is the hypoechoic muscularis and the hyperechoic periureteral fat. Tumors are seen as hypoechoic lesions in comparison to muscularis and periureteral fat.
- Invasive disease is suspected when an irregular hypoechoic mass extends into or beyond the muscularis layer and appears to disrupt the normally concentric, contiguous hyperechoic layer of periureteral fat.
- Limitations of ELUS currently include limited ability to assess invasion of the muscularis, poor visualization in a non-distended system, and inability to steer the probe into mid- or lower pole calyces.

References

1. Hall MC, Womack S, Sagalowsky AI, et al. Prognostic factors, recurrence, and survival in transitional cell carcinoma of the upper urinary tract: a 30-year experience in 252 patients. Urology. 1998;52:594–601.
2. Margulis V, Shariat SF, Matin SF, et al. Outcomes of radical nephroureterectomy: a series from the upper tract urothelial carcinoma collaboration. Cancer. 2009;115:1224–33.

3. Matin SF, Margulis V, Kamat A, et al. Incidence of downstaging and complete remission after neoadjuvant chemotherapy for high-risk upper tract transitional cell carcinoma. Cancer. 2010;116:3127–34.
4. Porten S, Siefker-Radtke MD, Xiao L, et al. Neoadjuvant chemotherapy improves survival of patients with upper tract urothelial carcinoma. Cancer. 2014;120:1794–9.
5. Kaag MG, O'Malley RL, O'Malley P, et al. Changes in renal function following nephroureterectomy may affect the use of perioperative chemotherapy. Euro Urol. 2010;58:581–7.
6. Grasso M, Fishman AI, Cohen J, et al. Ureteroscopic and extirpative treatment of upper urinary tract urothelial carcinoma: a 15-year comprehensive review of 160 consecutive patients. BJUI. 2012;110:1618–26.
7. Cutress ML, Stewart GD, Wells Cole S, et al. Long-term endoscopic management of upper tract urothelial carcinoma: 20-year single-centre experience. BJUI. 2012;110:1608–17.
8. Keeley FX, Kulp DA, Bibbo M, McCue PA, Bagley DH. Diagnostic accuracy of ureteroscopic biopsy in upper tract transitional cell carcinoma. J Urol. 1997;157:33–7.
9. Brown GA, Matin SF, Busby JE, et al. Ability of clinical grade to predict final pathologic stage in upper urinary tract transitional cell carcinoma: implications for therapy. Urology. 2007;70(2):252–6.
10. Scolieri MJ, Paik ML, Brown SL, et al. Limitations of computed tomography in the preoperative staging of upper tract urothelial carcinoma. Urology. 2000;56:930–4
11. Planz B, George R, Adam G, et al. Computed tomography for detection and staging of transitional cell carcinoma of the upper urinary tract. Euro Urol. 1995;27:146–50.
12. Favaretto RL, Shariat SF, Savage C, et al. Combining imaging and ureteroscopy variables in a preoperative multivariable model for prediction of muscle-invasive and non-organ confined disease in patients with upper tract urothelial carcinoma. BJUI. 2011;109:77–82.
13. Fukuda M, Hirata K, Saito K, et al. On the diagnostic use of echoendoscope in abdominal diseases: diagnostic experiences with a new type of echoendoscope in abdominal diseases. Proc Jpn J Med Ultrasound. 1980;37:409–10.
14. Goldberg BB, Bagley DH, Liu JB, et al. Endoluminal sonography of the urinary tract: preliminary observations. AJR. 1991;156:99–103.
15. Johnson GB, Portela D, Grasso M. Advanced ureteroscopy: wireless and sheathless. J Endourol. 2006;20:552–5.
16. Matin SF, Kamat AM, Grossman HB. High-frequency endoluminal ultrasonography as an aid to the staging of upper tract urothelial carcinoma. J Ultrasound Med. 2010;29:1277–84.
17. Liu JB, Bagley DH, Conlin MJ, et al. Endoluminal sonographic evaluation of ureteral and renal pelvic neoplasms. J Ultrasound Med. 1997;16:515–21.
18. Brown GA, Busby JE, Wood CG, et al. Nephroureterectomy for treating upper urinary tract transitional cell carcinoma: time to change the treatment paradigm? BJUI. 2006;98:1176–80.
19. Hubosky SG, Healy KA, Grasso M, et al. Accessing the difficult ureter and the importance of ureteroscope miniaturization: history is repeating itself. Urology. 2014;84(4):740–2.

Genetics Factors and Tumor Markers in Upper Urinary Tract-Urothelial Carcinoma

7

Mark Ferretti and John L. Phillips

Introduction

Urothelial carcinoma of the upper urinary tract (UUT) urothelial carcinoma (UC) shares many genetic features with bladder UC since the two neoplasms arise from the urothelium, an environment said to have a 'field defect' [1]. UUT and bladder UC are both strongly related to tobacco use and acquire somatic mutations that lead toward the development of invasive or noninvasive tumors via different pathways [2, 3]. Both UUT and bladder UC are potentially lethal when metastatic and patients who develop either tumor when advanced (i.e., >T3) disease have poor 1- and 3-year survival rates [4–6]. Unlike bladder UC, however, less is in known in the upper urinary tract about the genetic events of tumor development and progression, inheritable disease and somatic genetics, and how clinical tumor markers of bladder UC may or may not be applicable to UUT-UC [7–9]. Presumably, the knowledge gap regarding UUT-UC is potentially due to the relative infrequency of the tumor. Bladder UC occurred at a rate of 15.2–19.4/100,000 in UK males compared to 1.7–2.0/100,000 for renal pelvis UC (National Cancer Intelligence Network, 2013). Many genetic studies of bladder UC have been derived from biopsies of low-grade tumors in which recurrences in a patient's bladder have not only provided more specimen but prognostic information [10, 11]. Most studies of UUT-UC are derived from the nephroureterectomy specimen and there is little data concerning the natural history of treated low- versus high-grade tumors in subjects when tumors are small and would otherwise allow organ-preserving therapies [12]. The upper urinary tract is difficult to access, clinical stage, and isolate all of which make genetic and tumor marker studies of UUT-UC much more challenging [13–15]. This chapter will focus on the genetics of UUT-UC and specifically what urinary genetic markers can be used for diagnostic or prognostic purposes.

Genetics

Any discussion of the genetics of UUT-UC must first come within the context of cancer genetics in general and then what is specifically known about the genetics of bladder UC. Classically, tumors are thought to arise from 'somatic' mutations—DNA breaks which have occurred, either by chance or environmental influence, only in the tissue giving rise to a tumor. Somatic

M. Ferretti · J. L. Phillips (✉)
Department of Urology, Westchester Medical Health Network/New York Medical College, Valhalla, NY, USA
e-mail: john_phillips@nymc.edu

M. Ferretti
e-mail: mark.ferretti@gmail.com

M. Eshghi (ed.), *Urothelial Malignancies of the Upper Urinary Tract*,
https://doi.org/10.1007/978-3-319-51263-1_7

mutations are thought to arise at some point after the formation of the zygote and would include the very early intrauterine events which occur in the development of testis cancer or very late events in which years of genetic mutations must occur and accumulate before a 'sporadic 'tumor phenotype is established in the adult (e.g., lung cancer). Germline mutations, in contrast, are DNA changes that are inherited and therefore present in all tissues. It is now known that there are some mutations which occur after the zygotic stage and in adult life which are inheritable such as the histone acetylation mutations that fall within the field of 'epigenetics'. The human genome contains about 30,000 genes arranged on 22 somatic chromosomes. It appears that a low threshold of mutations are required to induce the phenotype of cancer, probably on the order of 15–20 'driver' mutations, although the expression of 100 s of other genes can be upregulated by mutation events elsewhere in the genome [16]. Bladder UC appears to occur as a result of mutations in either p53 or in FGFR3 [17]. TP53, the protein derived from p53, regulates the cell cycle, controlling the expression of p21 and cyclin D1. TP53 mutation-positive bladder UC is highly malignant, often presents with muscle-invasive bladder cancer (MIBC), and leads to other genetic features (i.e., expression of Ki67, RAS, VEGF, p63) that predict high rates of recurrence, lymphatic invasion, and perineural involvement [18, 19]. FGFR3, in contrast, is more associated with lower grade and stage bladder cancers, often nonmuscle-invasive bladder cancer (NMIBC), express wild-type p53, normal levels of p21 and cyclins, and expresses few dysregulated enzymes associated with invasion [20, 21]. FGFR-3 positive tumors are slow growing and rarely become MIBC, often because they have acquired p53 mutations late. Upper Urinary Tract UC is, in theory, similar, in that germline mutations or long-term exposure to urinary tract mutagens that induce somatic mutations, will induce p53-positive or FGFR-3 positive tumors [22]. In whole organ studies of nephroureterectomy specimens, the proportion of p53 and FGFR3 positive tumors in renal pelvis cancer is similar to that found in bladder cancer [20]. There have been few [7, 12] studies, however, that have conclusively analyzed the genetics of UUT-UC at the smallest tumor size presumably because endoscopically acquired biopsies yield insufficient tissue for traditional genomic analysis. Molecular profiling, however, requires mere picograms of tissue and may prove to be an ideal method to comprehensively analyze endoscopically derived biopsies in low-volume UUT-UC. Affymetrix gene array analysis by one group has revealed that expression of FXDY3 appears prevalent in both UUT- and bladder UC and suggests a potentially prognostic role [23]. Another study of 10 bladder carcinomas and 14 unrelated UUT-UCs demonstrated 21 genes could be used to differentiate BC from UUT including increased expression of CLCA2 and GABRA [24]. Such an approach could be used to determine the origin of cells found in a positive cytology based solely on their genetic fingerprint.

Germline mutations can cause cancers, most prevalently in family members who inherited germline mutations of tumor suppressor genes or other negative oncogenes that lead to tumors in specific end organs. Mutations in the Von Hippel Lindau protein are associated with tumors of the retina, cerebellum, pancreas, adrenal, and kidney but VHL-associated kidney cancers are, as a rule, clear cell, or 'conventional' carcinomas derived from the cells of the renal cortex and proximal tubule [25]. Families with inherited tumors of the renal collecting system, i.e., the urothelium, are far rarer. Still, such families and subjects who live in endemic regions of UUT-UC reveal other molecular insights into the disease that could potentially explain patients with sporadic or noninheritable forms. Balkan endemic nephropathy (BEN) has been long shown to increase the rate of UUT-UC nearly 100-fold in endemic areas and potentially through a p53 mutation pathway associated with proteinuria, renal failure, and mutations of the oncogene c-myb [26]. BEN patients with end-stage renal failure have undergone preventative bilateral nephroureterectomy. Certainly, any patient with multifocal and/or bilateral UUT-UC who is of Balkan descent may be a carrier of a predisposing germline mutation [27]. However, other familial conditions with genetic predispositions toward UUT-UC include Lynch Syndrome or Hereditary Non-polyposis Colorectal Cancer (HNPCC). Patients with HNPCC have germline mutations in the DNA mismatch repair (MMR) genes which may play a major role in UUT-UC that is distinct from bladder UC. MMR genes are most commonly comprised of mutations in MSH2 (also known as HNPCC 1) and MLH1 (or HNPCC 2), and are at nearly a 22-fold risk of UUT-UC, occur at an earlier age, and have a higher rate of bilaterality [28]. MMR mutations are thought to lead to inability to repair DNA copy errors during replication causing microsatellite instability (MSI) and chromosomal breakage, the hallmark of carcinogenesis. MSI mutations pathways may be important in nonfamilial cases of UUT-UC as well and thus point to a pathway in sporadic cancers of the upper urinary tract that is different than for bladder UC [29]. MSI mutations, in turn, are thought to be the driver of other mutations, such as p53 or FGFR3. Mismatch repair mutations were found in nearly 15% of potentially sporadic UUT tumors compared to only 1% of bladder cancers in a study of surgical specimens in sporadic cases.

In summary, the genetic features of UUT-UC are similar to those of bladder UC underlying the shared, 'field defect' hypothesis of urothelial carcinoma and point to mutations in FGFR3 for low-grade, noninvasive disease, mutations in p53 and p21 cyclin dysregulation in high-grade invasive disease, and mutations in DNA mismatch repair which may be a distinctive feature of UUT UC. It follows, then, that these features may be exploited in the use of urinary markers in the clinical management and prognosis of UUT-UC.

Molecular Markers

Cytology is the standard care method to assess for the presence or absence of urothelial carcinoma cells in the voided urine. The sensitivity of cytology, or the number of patients with cancer that are detectable by cytology, depends on the presence of sloughed or shed urothelial cells in the urine. Carcinoma in situ (CIS), which classically is shown to shed superficial layers of malignant cells from the involved mucosa, is readily detected by cytology leading to sensitivities of greater 90% [30, 31]. However, noninvasive, low-grade disease, such as FGFR3-positive urothelial cancers, may have relatively stable cytoarchitecture around its central fibrovascular scaffold, and have a low rate of urothelial shedding. Cytology for Ta disease can, therefore, be as low as 25% [32, 33]. In general, the sensitivity of cytology ranges from 40–85%. Specificity, or the number of patients who do not have cancer that is confirmed by cytology, is high, typically reaching 90–95% [30, 34, 35]. Cytology may be limited by the copious presence of blood, debris, bacterial breakdown products, or mucus such as seen in a urinary diversion. Cytology also requires the input of a trained cytopathologist, sufficiently viable cells, and the time and cost required for processing and interpretation. Alternatives to cytology, which may be specific for UUT-UC, have been sought and are typically derived from the clinical experience with markers of UC in bladder cancer.

DNA-Based Markers

Chromosomal Enumeration

The most common DNA-based marker for urothelial carcinoma remains fluorescent in situ hybridization (FISH) [36, 37]. DNA probes, covalently linked to fluorescently labeled congeners, are developed to bind to the highly repetitive but chromosome specific regions of the centromere of chromosomes 3, 7, and 17, and the 9p21 band. Aneuploidy of chromosomes 3, 7, and 17 are the hallmark of bladder cancers but homozygous and hemizygous deletions of 9p21 are also seen early in pathogenesis [38]. It is thought that two important cell cycle regulators, CDKN2 and CDKN2B, reside in the 9p21 region and their loss may be one of the earliest and most common genetic alterations in bladder cancer [39]. FISH is derived from the same technology used in amniocentesis for chromosomal enumeration and Y sex-chromosome identification, but is also used on tumor samples where individual cells can be readily identified as in a voided urine sample. FISH is not ideal, however, on tumor blocks as cell layers can be of irregular thickness and make it difficult to distinguish one cell nucleus from another. FISH requires the cytolysis of the cell membrane and fixation of the nucleus onto glass slides. The preparation for FISH, therefore, is ideal when a gross hematuria sample must be processed. All red blood cells will be removed during fixation leaving only the nuclei of urothelial cells behind for chromosomal staining. After FISH probe binding, fluorescent microscopy through a CCD camera is required to count each probe signal. Two signals from each 3, 7, and 17 chromosome, and two 9p21 locus signals, represent the diploid status of normal cells. However, up to 4% of normal cells may be tetraploid or captured during mitosis when the chromosomes have duplicated but the nuclei have not [38]. Deletions of 9p21 may be quite common in poorly preserved specimens and therefore must be found consistently in a large number of cells, by convention, 25 or more cells per test. Therefore, a FISH test is positive when at least 4% of cells have uneven gains of chromosomes 3, 7, or 17, or there are at least 12 or more of 25 total cells counted with deletions of 9p21. FISH tests have a specificity equivalent to cytology, in the >90% range but a superior sensitivity, of 65, 100, and 95% for pTa, pTis, and pT1–pT4 cases, respectively [40]. FISH is particularly useful to help resolve 'atypical' cytologies, patients who have completed BCG therapy, or patients with urinary diversions where the interpretation of cytology can be challenging [35, 36]. In urinary diversion patients who must be assessed for the risk of upper tract disease, however, cytology and FISH have similar and poor sensitivity [and positive predictive values (PPV)] of just 80% (and 10.7%) and 85.7% (and 23.1%), respectively. The poor PPV of both assays may suggest that the urinary diversion environment (e.g., inflammation, sloughed endothelial cells, infection) can induce morphologic and chromosomal changes that are often indistinguishable from a more malignant phenotype. Alternatively, a positive cytology or FISH may require intense investigation of small recurrent upper tract tumors that are notoriously difficult to find and may elude timely diagnosis [15, 41–43]. FISH is, however, expensive, requires a time-consuming process typically in centralized laboratories, and still requires a cytopathologist to 'enumerate' or count the FISH signals.

The use of FISH in the upper urinary tract is far less common than for bladder cancer but may ultimately prove far more useful (Fig. 7.1). FISH, for example, has been shown to have higher detectability for upper urinary tract UC than CT urography in patients with CIS or sessile nonobstructive masses. When derived from renal pelvis washings via a ureteral catheter, FISH performed better than cytology and had a higher predictive value [35, 36]. One study found that in no case did a positive FISH test from a renal unit yield to a negative ureteroscopic finding

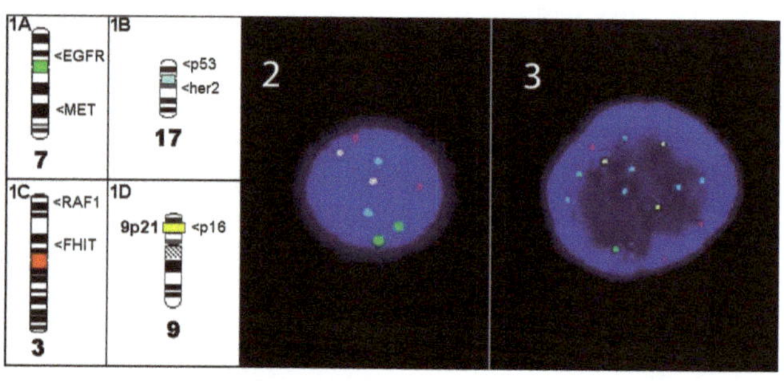

Fig. 7.1 Urinary fluorescent in situ hybridization (FISH) in upper urinary tract-urothelial carcinoma (UUT-UC). FISH probes bind to the centromere of chromosomes 7, 17, 3, and the 9p21 band of chromosome 9, respectively (Fig. 1A, 1B, 1C, 1D, respectively). 2. A normal cell from a renal pelvis showing two signals from each probe, i.e., diploid. 3. An abnormal cell from a ureteral washing showing gains of chromosomes 7 and 3 (multiple *green* and *red* signals). The patient had a pT2aNxMx renal UUT-UC

(whereas a negative FISH test did not rule out a ureteroscopically identified tumor [44]). A positive FISH test derived from a lateralized side, especially with a suspicious renal medullary mass, would be highly suspicious of UUT-UC and that patients could be treated accordingly with nephroureterectomy without the time, expense, and potential morbidity of a diagnostic ureteroscopy [45]. A urine sample for FISH requires placement in fixative prior to shipment to a laboratory setting. Urine sample acquired in the OR, therefore, would require coordination with pathology to ensure timely processing. FISH is used for diagnostic purposes but also has an important prognostic role in the management of bladder UC and potentially of UUC-UT [36, 46]. FISH tests may become positive up to 1 year prior to the identification of a resectable bladder tumor [32]. FISH may herald, therefore, a low-volume lesion in the upper tract far more amenable to nephron-sparing ureteroscopic techniques than ordinarily allowed when patients present with tumors >1 cm and within the threshold for positive imaging studies. BCG, which is commonly used in the treatment of high-grade nonmuscle-invasive disease and carcinoma in situ, has limited use in upper tract disease. However, a positive FISH test after the completion of BCG was associated in one study with recurrences in 12 of 12 patients [47]. A negative FISH after BCG revealed biopsy proven recurrence in half. Importantly, a positive FISH test after BCG implied a recurrence rate >3 times higher than for patients with a negative FISH test after BCG. FISH could then be similarly used in upper tract disease after the completion of endoscopic ablation of ureteral or renal pelvis tumors to predict for early recurrence and patient stratification for salvage therapies.

Microsatellite Mutation Analysis

Microsatellites are repeated sequences of DNA naturally found within the human genome that do not code for protein. Accordingly, as they acquire mutations, there appears to be no overt negative consequence for an individual and its progeny. Therefore, mutational analysis of DNA microsatellites is commonly used in the genetic evaluation of kinship and anthropological diversification. However, some microsatellite mutations occur near or within coding regions and these can lead to changes in protein expression or phenotype and disease. Microsatellite instability refers to condition in which there is hypermutability, often due to a defect in one of several DNA Mismatch Repair Enzymes. Microsatellite instability can be detected through PCR amplification and was first found in patients with the Lynch Syndrome or HNPCC [48]. MSI can be found in both normal and tumor tissues. Studies have shown microsatellite instability to be an independent molecular marker that has been shown to help identify those with hereditary susceptibility to UUT-UCC [12, 28].

Patients with known Lynch syndrome and three or more RBCs/high-power field on urinalysis should undergo further evaluation for UUT-UCC, since it is particularly associated with upper and less often lower tract urothelial malignancy. The Mismatch Repair gene MSH2 has been particularly associated with UUT-UCC. Therefore, high-risk features of Lynch Syndrome such as MSH2 mutations or family history of UUT-UCC may be candidates for surveillance of the upper urinary tract. Furthermore, patients presenting with upper tract urothelial cell carcinoma at a young age (anyone younger than age 60) should raise suspicion of Lynch Syndrome and a screening colonoscopy is often recommended if patients have not yet had one [49]. Additional factors that should warrant suspicion include any patient meeting the so-called 'Amsterdam criteria' (i.e., 3-2-1 rule) of three blood relatives affected with cancer spanning at least two generations with one of them being a first degree relative [50]. Finally any patient with bilateral UUT-UCC or a personal/family history of colorectal, endometrial, biliary, small bowel or ovarian carcinoma, as well as sebaceous adenoma of the skin should raise suspicion. Although PCR for the identification of molecular markers is the gold standard for Lynch Syndrome identification, patients with less tissue available (as is often the case with ureteroscopic biopsy) may undergo Immunohistochemistry testing first to check for protein markers that indicate a defective Mismatch Repair (e.g., MSH2, etc.). IHC testing, unlike PCR for MSI, has not been shown to be predictive of prognosis; therefore, IHC testing should be followed with eventual PCR once adequate tissue can be analyzed [28, 51, 52]. However, the value of MSI for UUT-UCCC goes beyond just detection of Lynch Syndrome patients. MSI can be detected in approximately 25% of patients with sporadic cancer. Since MSI has been shown to be a possible marker for better prognosis, some authors suggest checking for MSI in all intermediate risk patients in which treatment decisions may be altered based on outcome [28].

Other DNA-Based Mutation Assays

p53 family. Overexpression of Tumor Suppressor genes is one of the early common events in tumorigenesis for upper urinary tract-urothelial cell cancer. Overexpression of p53 was the first consistently recognized tumor oncogene mutated in urothelial carcinoma and its accumulation is a hallmark of an invasive phenotype [53]. P53 is a large gene, containing 11 exons and is located on the short or 'petite' arm of chromosome 17. Its genomic sequencing in pathologic samples in staging has little utility but has been evaluated with staining for its protein, TP53, in voided urine specimens. In an evaluation of upper tract urothelial carcinoma, however, staining revealed little benefit when broadly applied over a spectrum of stages and performed no better than cytology [54]. Another p53-related transcription factor, p63, and its protein TP63, have also been evaluated as a potential DNA- and protein-based biomarker. Expression of p63 may define a particularly aggressive tumor phenotype although in multivariable analysis may not prove to be an independent predictor of disease [19]. However, there does appear to be higher p63 expression in tumors derived from the upper urinary tract and TP63 mutation in voided cytology may therefore prove to be a useful method to distinguish between upper and lower urinary tract urothelial carcinomas [55].

Methylation. DNA methylation and silencing phenomenon are the hallmarks of epigenetic aberration that may underlie a large proportion of environmentally acquired DNA mutations [56]. Smoking may induce epigenetic changes in how DNA is transcribed allowing for more widespread genomic aberrations possible than with mutational events in specific driver genes. The use of known methylation 'hotspots' in cytology specimens could, therefore, provide a valuable method for diagnosis as well as predict which patients may have acquired an increased risk for the cancer phenotype. In fact, methylated biomarkers perform better in cytologic specimens than in whole tumor with receiver operating characteristics of 0.89 and 0.75, respectively [57].

FXYD3. Proteins derived from the FXYD3 gene are involved in transmembrane trafficking and is an important regulatory peptide that appears mutated in a variety of carcinomas including breast, upper urinary tract and bladder urothelial carcinomas. Its expression correlates with stage in bladder UC but not in UUT-UC and may be an important gene for analysis in differentiated upper from lower urinary tract disease [23].

Protein-Based Markers

There are hundreds of potential protein biomarkers of urothelial carcinoma that have been investigated as potential diagnostic or prognostic tools but few are clinically available. Clinical utility requires a test to be feasible, affordable, and reproducible in untrained hands and is largely limited to the use of ImmunoCyt, BTA, and NPM-22 (see Table 7.1).

Clinical

ImmunoCyt. ImmunoCyt uses 3 fluorescent monoclonal antibodies against two mucin-expressing peptides, M344, LDQ10 and a high molecular weight form of carcinoembryonic antigen (CEA) 19A211 to detect presence [58] of antigens in cells of voided urine samples. The assay requires cell fixation, filtration, staining, and then slide interpretation by an immune-histochemist. Its initial performance was encouraging and superior to cytology in that its sensitivity for grades 1, 2, and 3 disease was 67, 78, and 87%, respectively, compared to cytology (17.9, 46.3, and 63.8%,

Table 7.1 Performance comparison of common urinary biomarkers in the detection of upper urinary tract-urothelial carcinoma (UUT-UC)

	Cytology [36]	FISH [36]	Cytol + NPM22 [90]	BTA [69]	ImmunoCyt [61]
Sensitivity	80	85.7	83.3	65	86.1
Specificity	85.6	86.5	93.4	40	79.4
Pos Pred Val	10.7	23.1	84.7	83	54
Neg Pred Val	99.5	99.2	92.8	32	97

respectively) [59]. The enhanced sensitivity of ImmunoCyt came at the expense of specificity as urinary cytology of 94.5% was 10% higher than ImmunoCyt. Mowatt et al. reviewed several biomarker panels and found that the overall sensitivity (with 95% CI) of any one test was highest for ImmunoCyt [84% (77–91%)] and lowest for cytology [44% (38–51%)] and that the converse was true namely, that the specificity was highest for cytology [96% (94–98%)] and lowest for ImmunoCyt [75% (68–83%)] [60]. The utility of ImmunoCyt, however, was in its ability, as some writers describe, to avoid unnecessary cystoscopy and biopsy, which underlies the significant longitudinal cost of bladder cancer therapy. One of 23 patients with negative ImmunoCyt and cytology had a positive cystoscopy in one study leading the authors to suggest that in low-risk tumors, e.g., Ta or papillomas and no evidence of CIS, ImmunoCyt can be used to avoid cystoscopy [61, 62]. The experience with using ImmunoCyt for upper tract disease is limited. However, Lodde et al. found that the performance appeared similar to that of lower tract evaluation and included a sensitivity of 75% and a specificity of 95% [63]. The limitations of ImmunoCyt continue to be the reliance on outside trained reference laboratory processing and its consequent cost [64].

BTA (Bladder Tumor Antigen). BTA Stat and BTA TRAK are immunoassays that test for the Complement factor H and H-related peptide that can be found in the urine of patients with urothelial carcinoma. Unlike FISH and ImmunoCyt, BTA does not require a trained laboratory reader for result analysis. Instead, BTA assays are prepared in the ambulatory setting from a few drops of urine placed into the well of a supplied ELISA assay, similar to the technology and simplicity of most HCG Elisa assays used for pregnancy assessment. BTA assays are thus termed 'point of care' tests and their rapidity are a major positive attribute and with cystoscopy is the only FDA approved test in the management of urothelial carcinoma. BTA has significant sensitivity of >90% especially for low-grade Ta tumors and was better than UroVysion, dipstick, or telomerase testing [65]. However, of 80 negative cystoscopy patients, 21 had positive BTA results leading to a specificity of 74%. The BTA assay reacts against the complement antigens which would also be expected in samples with hematuria. Thus, a limitation of BTA would be in those patients who have significant enough hematuria from benign disease that a BTA test would be positive and unnecessarily lead to further investigation. In an analysis of 25 healthy volunteers, BTA was applied to urine with serial dilutions of 250, 1000, and 2500 red blood cells per high-powered field yielding false positive rates of 20, 44, and 76, respectively [66]. Guo et al. performed a pooled analysis of 13 studies of >3400 patients comparing BTA with cytology [67]. While cytology continued to have better specificity, BTA sensitivity of 67% (compared to cytology of 43%) suggests that clinicians' would be less likely to miss a patient with bladder cancer using BTA. For the detection of UUT-UC, BTA appears to be somewhat limited. Sensitivity and specificity of BTA alone, compared to cytology are quite poor with positive and negative predictive values of 83 and 32%, respectively, although its performance, as in bladder UC, appears to be tumor-grade dependent [68, 69]. The cost of each BTA unit is approximately $160 so despite its limitations as a qualitative assay, the speed of its result and feasibility contribute to its continued use in the clinic.

NMP-22. DNA transcription increases with the cancer phenotype and correlate with an increase in the nucleus:cytoplasm ratio. Thus, it is not surprising that the Nuclear Matrix Protein 22 (NMP22) is a useful biomarker in voided urines. As with other biomarkers with improved sensitivity over cytology, specificity continues to be an issue with NMP-22 testing. NPM-22 levels above 10.0 units per ml, for example, detected 18 of 18 patients with bladder cancer compared to only 6 with cytology [70]. The sensitivity of 100% (and specificity of 85%) is clearly better than cytology but, as with all biomarker studies, there is a trade-off for another performance attribute—low positive predictive values (PPV) of 30%. NMP-22 can be positive in conditions where there is high nuclear turnover including inflammatory conditions (e.g., cystitis, ureteral stents), urinary diversion, and pelvic radiation. Dong et al. found that healthy volunteer NMP22 levels averaged 0.01 ± 0 U/mL but averaged 16.61 ± 0.15 U/mL in patients with Bricker-type ileal conduits and 12.08 ± 0.10 U/mL in continent urinary diversions, all in patients with no known upper urinary tract recurrence of UC. Ishii et al. found that values of NMP-22 in 15 patients with ileal conduits were on average 335.6 ± 63.5 U/mL [71]. The use of NMP22 for the detection of upper urinary tract UC after urinary diversion, therefore, would be challenging unless a ureteral or renal pelvic wash, devoid of urinary diversion contaminants, or from a cutaneous ureterostomy was used [71].

Investigative Protein-Based Markers

A large number of proteins and biomarkers have been found that reliably detect the presence of malignant voided cells where cytology does not, none of which is available in a CLIA-approved capacity and have not been adequately assessed for their use in detecting upper urinary tract disease. Below is a concise summary of relevant biomarkers of interest to the clinician and known data regarding their use in upper urinary tract assessment.

Survivin. *Survivin* is an important inhibitor of proteins that induce cell death or apoptosis. *Survivin* stabilizes caspase, Bax, and Fas families of proteins all of which lead to decreased or regulated apoptosis. Mutations in *survivin* promote the anti-apoptosis phenotype and *survivin*-mutated cells thus escape programmed cell death, resist environmental stimuli to do so, and adopt chemoresistance. *Survivin* is detected in the voided urine of patients with superficial bladder cancer, performed better than NMP-22, and cytology, and is possibly a novel method to differentiate invasive from noninvasive bladder cancer phenotypes [72]. However, *survivin* is expressed at low levels in nearly half-sampled prostate tissues and urinary *survivin* levels decreased dramatically after radical prostatectomy [73]. In terms of upper tract disease, *survivin* may be useful in detecting recurrence because of the absence of the prostate in most men who undergo radical cystectomy and for low ambient levels of *survivin* expression in urine samples derived from urinary diversions [74]. The use of *survivin* in gauging the phenotype of UUT-UC appears to be somewhat limited. Nakanishi et al. found no *survivin* in normal renal pelvis urothelium and in 12.7% of samples with UUT-UC but could not correlate expression levels of *survivin* with tumor grade, stage, or patient survival [75]. *Survivin* is a nuclear protein and may thus be excluded from the urine after cytolysis. Indeed, *survivin* staining of UUT-UC specimens showed that only nuclear *survivin* levels predicted invasion and a poor patient prognosis (54% 5-year survival) where cytoplasm positive *survivin* and cytoplasm negative *survivin* level UUT-UC patients had no difference in survival [76].

Epithelial Cadherin (E-Cadherin). E-Cadherin is a protein involved with cellular attachment and interaction and its loss is thought to promote invasiveness and metastasis. Studies have shown an association of recurrent tumor and poor prognosis with E-cadherin loss [51]. This marker may therefore be useful as an adjunct test to identify patients who would benefit from more frequent follow-up or more aggressive treatment.

Hypoxia-inducible factor. Hypoxia-inducible factor is a protein involved in angiogenesis. It is not found in normal urothelium, but may be found in urothelial cancers of the upper and lower urinary tracts. Overexpression of HIF-1alpha in UUT-UCC has been shown to be associated with prognosis and poorer survival [77, 78]. Like E-cadherin, HIF levels can only be detected by immunohistochemistry and are thus subjected to user bias and processing error.

Telomerase. Telomerase is an enzyme that adds repeat sequences to ends of chromosomes and is important in chromosomal repair. Cancer, which is hallmarked by chromosomal breakage, has increased telomerase and levels of an important catalytic subunit, hTERT, have long been known to be activity in bladder cancer but not normal bladder [65]. Its use as a biomarker in voided urine is limited by the need for PCR-based DNA amplification and immediate refrigeration of samples but has been reliably predictable with quoted sensitivity of 46% and specificity of 91%. FISH can be used to determine Telomerase RNA activity in urothelial specimens after nephroureterectomy. Telomerase RNA is found to be generally active in most UUT-UCCC and increased expression was associated with poor prognosis. Wu et al. found increased telomerase in 97% of 31 tumors with UUT-UC and in 15 of 17 ureteral washings. Its sensitivity was far higher than voided cytology of 15% and ureteral washings for cytology of 53% in the same patients. Therefore, telomerase RNA activity may have prognostic and diagnostic capabilities where cytology has been equivocal for UUT-UC but suspicion remains high [79, 80].

L-Type amino acid transporter 1 (LAT 1). LAT 1 is a surface membrane protein that aids in amino acid transport. It is usually in its inactive form in normal urothelial tissue; however, it can be found in its active form in about half of UUT-UCCs and is prognostic for progression of UUT-UCC [81].

Other investigative biomarkers. The potential of additional biomarkers in the diagnosis of UUT-UC is potentially as long as a list of oncogenes, regulatory proteins, and mutations that could exist with the UUT-UC transcriptome. For any biomarker to be applicable, its detection must be reproducible and feasible regardless of its overall sensitivity and specificity. Numerous molecules have been assessed for their expression in UUT-UC and all have high sensitivity (and modest specificity) but almost all require whole tumor processing for staining, interpretation, and standardization against normal controls and include increased levels of Ki-67, BcL-2 oncoprotein, c-MET tyrosine kinase activity, deletions in 8q24 and 4p16.3, CEBPD, MIB1, and RON and low levels of the p27 [82–89].

Summary

Upper Urinary Tract-Urothelial Carcinoma (UUT-UC) can be survivable if tumors are recognized and treated early before the development of stage T3N0 or higher disease. Patients with UUT-UC often present with gross hematuria and may present with synchronous or metachronous tumors of the bladder in nearly a third of cases. Tests that can recognize UUT-UC early, and differentiate UUT-UC from bladder cancer, are not currently clinically available but lessons from biomarkers applied to bladder cancers are applicable to UUT-UC diagnosis and prognosis. Cytology continues to have high specificity but low sensitivity for low-stage, low-grade lesions of the upper tract but urinary FISH, especially from a ureterally catheterized sample, has high sensitivity, specificity, and predictive value, though not perfect. FISH may have value in the surveillance of patients with urinary diversions where the NMP-22 test has been shown to have little utility and where the BTA test may have difficulty in patients with >250 red blood cells per high-powered field. FGFR3 testing may help define a favorable subtype of UUT-UC and increased expression of TP53 or E-cadherin could suggest patients with disease that requires more intensive follow-up after nephrouretectomy. Some biomarkers appear to show higher expression in the upper urinary tract such as MSH2, MLH1, and FXYD3 and, where feasible, may have value in the interpretation of the positive cytology. The surveillance of UUT-UC after nephron-sparing approaches to low-volume or low-grade disease is challenging in that imaging studies may have low detectability and frequent ureteroscopy could be overly invasive. Detection of a suddenly positive BTA, NMP-22, or FISH test, MMR marker, or FGFR3 level in the voided urine could signal the need for ureteroscopic evaluation. Many hope that research into the genetics and molecular markers of each individual tumor will herald a new treatment paradigm in which tumors are treated less by the organ system in which they arise and more by the genetic and molecular fingerprint associated with the tumor. While no single tumor marker appears to be the perfect marker on its own with a high specificity and sensitivity, low cost and easy to obtain, perhaps further research will show that an individualized 'fingerprint approach' to the different markers will prove to be effective.

Summary Box

Upper Urinary Tract Urothelial Carcinoma (UUT-UC) may have genetic markers that are distinct from those of UC of the bladder and include mismatch repair genes like MSH2 and MLH1. Cytology continues to have high specificity but low sensitivity for low-stage, low-grade lesions of the Upper Urinary Tract. FISH has high sensitivity, specificity, and predictive value in the work up of UUT-UC with particular use in the surveillance of patients with urinary diversions. BTA testing is limited in UUT-UC samples with >250 red blood cells/hpf. FGFR3 testing may be help define a favorable subtype of UUT-UC Increased TP53 or E-cadherin expression may identify patients who require more intensive follow-up after nephroureterectomy.

References

1. Sidransky D, Frost P, Von Eschenbach A, et al. Clonal origin bladder cancer. N Engl J Med. 1992;326:737.
2. Burger M, Catto JW, Dalbagni G et al. Epidemiology and risk factors of urothelial bladder cancer. Eur Urol 2012.
3. Colli JL, Kolettis PN. Bladder cancer incidence and mortality rates compared to ecologic factors among states in America. Int Urol Nephrol. 2010;42:659.
4. Mitra AP, Alemozaffar M, Harris BN, et al. Outcomes after urothelial recurrence in bladder cancer patients undergoing radical cystectomy. Urology. 2014;84:1420.
5. Raman JD, Messer J, Sielatycki JA, et al. Incidence and survival of patients with carcinoma of the ureter and renal pelvis in the USA, 1973–2005. BJU Int. 2011;107:1059.
6. Kim M, Jeong CW, Kwak C, et al. Are urothelial carcinomas of the upper urinary tract a distinct entity from urothelial carcinomas of the urinary bladder? Behavior of urothelial carcinoma after radical surgery with respect to anatomical location: a case control study. BMC Cancer. 2015;15:149.
7. Patel N, Arya M, Muneer A, et al. Molecular aspects of upper tract urothelial carcinoma. Urol Oncol. 2014;32(28):e11.
8. Audenet F, Traxer O, Bensalah K, et al. Upper urinary tract instillations in the treatment of urothelial carcinomas: a review of technical constraints and outcomes. World J Urol. 2013;31:45.
9. Jebar AH, Hurst CD, Tomlinson DC, et al. FGFR3 and Ras gene mutations are mutually exclusive genetic events in urothelial cell carcinoma. Oncogene. 2005;24:5218.
10. Wang JK, Tollefson MK, Krambeck AE, et al. High rate of pathologic upgrading at nephroureterectomy for upper tract urothelial carcinoma. Urology. 2012;79:615.
11. Haddad M, Cloutier J, Cornu JN, et al. Immediate nephroureterectomy or after attempting conservative treatment, on elective indications, for upper urinary tract urothelial carcinoma: comparison of the pathology reports on a retrospective monocentric study. J Endourol. 2015;29:969.
12. Ho CL, Tzai TS, Chen JC, et al. The molecular signature for urothelial carcinoma of the upper urinary tract. J Urol. 2008;179:1155.
13. Hyams ES, Winer AG, Shah O. Retrograde ureteral and renal access in patients with urinary diversion. Urology. 2009;74:47.
14. Wang LJ, Lee SY, Teh BT, et al. Upper tract urothelial carcinomas in patients with chronic kidney disease: relationship with diagnostic challenge. Biomed Res Int. 2014;2014:989458.
15. Nison L, Roupret M, Bozzini G, et al. The oncologic impact of a delay between diagnosis and radical nephroureterectomy due to diagnostic ureteroscopy in upper urinary tract urothelial carcinomas: results from a large collaborative database. World J Urol. 2013;31:69.
16. Phillips JL, Hayward SW, Wang Y, et al. The consequences of chromosomal aneuploidy on gene expression profiles in a cell line model for prostate carcinogenesis. Cancer Res. 2001;61:8143.
17. van Rhijn BW, van der Kwast TH, Vis AN, et al. FGFR3 and P53 characterize alternative genetic pathways in the pathogenesis of urothelial cell carcinoma. Cancer Res. 2004;64:1911.

18. Lamy A, Gobet F, Laurent M, et al. Molecular profiling of bladder tumors based on the detection of FGFR3 and TP53 mutations. J Urol. 2006;176:2686.
19. Choi W, Shah JB, Tran M, et al. P63 expression defines a lethal subset of muscle-invasive bladder cancers. PLoS ONE. 2012;7:e30206.
20. Lyle SR, Hsieh CC, Fernandez CA, et al. Molecular grading of tumors of the upper urothelial tract using FGFR3 mutation status identifies patients with favorable prognosis. Res Rep Urol. 2012;4:65.
21. van Rhijn BW, van der Kwast TH, Liu L, et al. The FGFR3 mutation is related to favorable pT1 bladder cancer. J Urol. 2012;187:310.
22. Hanley KW, Viet SM, Hein MJ, et al. Exposure to o-toluidine, aniline, and nitrobenzene in a rubber chemical manufacturing plant: a retrospective exposure assessment update. J Occup Environ Hyg. 2012;9:478.
23. Zhang Z, Pang ST, Kasper KA, et al. FXYD3: a promising biomarker for urothelial carcinoma. Biomark Insights. 2011;6:17.
24. Zhang Z, Furge KA, Yang XJ, et al. Comparative gene expression profiling analysis of urothelial carcinoma of the renal pelvis and bladder. BMC Med Genomics. 2010;3:58.
25. Srinivasan R, Ricketts CJ, Sourbier C, et al. New strategies in renal cell carcinoma: targeting the genetic and metabolic basis of disease. Clin Cancer Res. 2015;21:10.
26. Stefanovic V, Polenakovic M, Toncheva D. Urothelial carcinoma associated with Balkan endemic nephropathy. A worldwide disease. Pathol Biol (Paris). 2011;59:286.
27. Audenet F, Colin P, Yates DR, et al. A proportion of hereditary upper urinary tract urothelial carcinomas are misclassified as sporadic according to a multi-institutional database analysis: proposal of patient-specific risk identification tool. BJU Int. 2012;110:E583.
28. Roupret M, Catto J, Coulet F, et al. Microsatellite instability as indicator of MSH2 gene mutation in patients with upper urinary tract transitional cell carcinoma. J Med Genet. 2004;41.e91.
29. Catto JW, Azzouzi AR, Amira N, et al. Distinct patterns of microsatellite instability are seen in tumours of the urinary tract. Oncogene. 2003;22:8699.
30. Sverrisson EF, Kim T, Espiritu PN, et al. The merits of cytology in the workup for upper tract urothelial carcinoma—a contemporary review of a perplexing issue. Int Braz J Urol. 2014;40:493.
31. Sakano S, Inamoto T, Inoue R et al. Positive voided urine cytology predicts worse pathological findings of nephroureterectomy specimens in patients with upper tract urothelial carcinoma: does selective ureteral cytology have an additional efficacy? Jpn J Clin Oncol 2015.
32. Sarosdy MF, Schellhammer P, Bokinsky G, et al. Clinical evaluation of a multi-target fluorescent in situ hybridization assay for detection of bladder cancer. J Urol. 2002;168:1950.
33. Wolinska WH, Melamed MR, Klein FA. Cytology of bladder papilloma. Acta Cytol. 1985;29:817.
34. Lodde M, Mayr R, Martini T, et al. Positive urine cytology and carcinoma in situ prior to second transurethral resection of the bladder correlate with positive second resection histology and the need for subsequent cystectomy. World J Urol. 2012;30:841.
35. Reynolds JP, Voss JS, Kipp BR, et al. Comparison of urine cytology and fluorescence in situ hybridization in upper urothelial tract samples. Cancer Cytopathol. 2014;122:459.
36. Fernandez MI, Parikh S, Grossman HB, et al. The role of FISH and cytology in upper urinary tract surveillance after radical cystectomy for bladder cancer. Urol Oncol. 2012;30:821.
37. Phillips JL, Richardson IC. Aneuploidy in bladder cancers: the utility of fluorescent in situ hybridization in clinical practice. BJU Int. 2006;98:33.
38. Sokolova IA, Halling KC, Jenkins RB, et al. The development of a multitarget, multicolor fluorescence in situ hybridization assay for the detection of urothelial carcinoma in urine. J Mol Diagn. 2000;2:116.
39. Knowles MA, Hurst CD. Molecular biology of bladder cancer: new insights into pathogenesis and clinical diversity. Nat Rev Cancer. 2015;15:25.
40. Halling KC, King W, Sokolova IA, et al. A comparison of cytology and fluorescence in situ hybridization for the detection of urothelial carcinoma. J Urol. 2000;164:1768.
41. Perlis N, Turker P, Bostrom PJ, et al. Upper urinary tract and urethral recurrences following radical cystectomy: review of risk factors and outcomes between centres with different follow-up protocols. World J Urol. 2013;31:161.
42. Picozzi S, Ricci C, Gaeta M, et al. Upper urinary tract recurrence following radical cystectomy for bladder cancer: a meta-analysis on 13,185 patients. J Urol. 2012;188:2046.
43. Sanderson KM, Cai J, Miranda G, et al. Upper tract urothelial recurrence following radical cystectomy for transitional cell carcinoma of the bladder: an analysis of 1,069 patients with 10-year followup. J Urol. 2007;177:2088.
44. Gruschwitz T, Gajda M, Enkelmann A, et al. FISH analysis of washing urine from the upper urinary tract for the detection of urothelial cancers. Int Urol Nephrol. 2014;46:1769.
45. Ho CC, Tan WP, Pathmanathan R, et al. Fluorescence-in-situ-hybridization in the surveillance of urothelial cancers: can use of cystoscopy or ureteroscopy be deferred? Asian Pac J Cancer Prev. 2013;14:4057.
46. Wang J, Wu J, Peng L, et al. Distinguishing urothelial carcinoma in the upper urinary tract from benign diseases with hematuria using FISH. Acta Cytol. 2012;56:533.

47. Kipp BR, Karnes RJ, Brankley SM, et al. Monitoring intravesical therapy for superficial bladder cancer using fluorescence in situ hybridization. J Urol. 2005;173:401.
48. Amira N, Rivet J, Soliman H, et al. Microsatellite instability in urothelial carcinoma of the upper urinary tract. J Urol. 2003;170:1151.
49. Mork M, Hubosky SG, Roupret M, et al. Lynch syndrome: a primer for urologists and panel recommendations. J Urol. 2015;194:21.
50. Umar A, Boland CR, Terdiman JP, et al. Revised Bethesda Guidelines for hereditary nonpolyposis colorectal cancer (Lynch syndrome) and microsatellite instability. J Natl Cancer Inst. 2004;96:261.
51. Fromont G, Roupret M, Amira N, et al. Tissue microarray analysis of the prognostic value of E-cadherin, Ki67, p53, p27, survivin and MSH2 expression in upper urinary tract transitional cell carcinoma. Eur Urol. 2005;48:764.
52. Roupret M, Coulet F, Azzouzi AR, et al. Accuracy of the routine detection of mutation in mismatch repair genes in patients with susceptibility to hereditary upper urinary tract transitional cell carcinoma. BJU Int. 2005;96:149.
53. Esrig D, Elmajian D, Groshen S, et al. Accumulation of nuclear p53 and tumor progression in bladder cancer. N Engl J Med. 1994;331:1259.
54. Mitchell S, Mayer E, Patel A. Expression of p53 in upper urinary tract urothelial carcinoma. Nat Rev Urol. 2011;8:516.
55. Langner C, Ratschek M, Tsybrovskyy O, et al. P63 immunoreactivity distinguishes upper urinary tract transitional-cell carcinoma and renal-cell carcinoma even in poorly differentiated tumors. J Histochem Cytochem. 2003;51:1097.
56. Miozzo M, Vaira V, Sirchia SM. Epigenetic alterations in cancer and personalized cancer treatment. Future Oncol. 2015;11:333.
57. Chen H, Yu Y, Rong S, et al. Evaluation of diagnostic accuracy of DNA methylation biomarkers for bladder cancer: a systematic review and meta-analysis. Biomarkers. 2014;19:189.
58. Eissa S, Swellam M, Sadek M, et al. Comparative evaluation of the nuclear matrix protein, fibronectin, urinary bladder cancer antigen and voided urine cytology in the detection of bladder tumors. J Urol. 2002;168:465.
59. Pfister C, Chautard D, Devonec M, et al. Immunocyt test improves the diagnostic accuracy of urinary cytology: results of a French multicenter study. J Urol. 2003;169:921.
60. Mowatt G, Zhu S, Kilonzo M, et al. Systematic review of the clinical effectiveness and cost-effectiveness of photodynamic diagnosis and urine biomarkers (FISH, ImmunoCyt, NMP22) and cytology for the detection and follow-up of bladder cancer. Health Technol Assess. 2010;14:1.
61. Mian C, Pycha A, Wiener H, et al. Immunocyt: a new tool for detecting transitional cell cancer of the urinary tract. J Urol. 1999;161:1486.
62. Mian C, Maier K, Comploj E, et al. uCyt+/ImmunoCyt in the detection of recurrent urothelial carcinoma: an update on 1991 analyses. Cancer. 2006;108:60.
63. Lodde M, Mian C, Wiener H, et al. Detection of upper urinary tract transitional cell carcinoma with ImmunoCyt: a preliminary report. Urology. 2001;58:362.
64. Mian C, Lodde M, Comploj E, et al. The value of the ImmunoCyt/uCyt+ test in the detection and follow-up of carcinoma in situ of the urinary bladder. Anticancer Res. 2005;25:3641.
65. Halling KC, King W, Sokolova IA, et al. A comparison of BTA stat, hemoglobin dipstick, telomerase and Vysis UroVysion assays for the detection of urothelial carcinoma in urine. J Urol. 2002;167:2001.
66. Oge O, Kozaci D, Gemalmaz H. The BTA stat test is nonspecific for hematuria: an experimental hematuria model. J Urol. 2002;167:1318.
67. Guo A, Wang X, Gao L, et al. Bladder tumour antigen (BTA stat) test compared to the urine cytology in the diagnosis of bladder cancer: a meta-analysis. Can Urol Assoc J. 2014;8:E347.
68. Jovanovic M, Hadzi-Djokic J, Dzamic Z, et al. Evaluation of the Bard BTA-test in the diagnosis of upper urinary tract tumours. Acta Chir Iugosl. 2007;54:19.
69. Zimmerman RL, Bagley D, Hawthorne C, et al. Utility of the Bard BTA test in detecting upper urinary tract transitional cell carcinoma. Urology. 1998;51:956.
70. Zippe C, Pandrangi L, Potts JM, et al. NMP22: a sensitive, cost-effective test in patients at risk for bladder cancer. Anticancer Res. 1999;19:2621.
71. Ishii T, Okadome A, Takeuchi F, et al. Urinary levels of nuclear matrix protein 22 in patients with urinary diversion. Urology. 2001;58:940.
72. Shariat SF, Casella R, Khoddami SM, et al. Urine detection of survivin is a sensitive marker for the noninvasive diagnosis of bladder cancer. J Urol. 2004;171:626.
73. Davies B, Chen J, Modugno F, et al. Contribution of the prostate limits the usefulness of survivin for the detection of bladder cancer. J Urol. 2005;174:1767.
74. Dong ZL, Lu ZP, Wang HZ, et al. Detection of nuclear matrix protein 22 and survivin baseline level in patients after radical cystectomy. Urol Int. 2011;87:445.
75. Nakanishi K, Tominaga S, Hiroi S, et al. Expression of survivin does not predict survival in patients with transitional cell carcinoma of the upper urinary tract. Virchows Arch. 2002;441:559.
76. Kitamura H, Torigoe T, Hirohashi Y, et al. Nuclear, but not cytoplasmic, localization of survivin as a negative prognostic factor for survival in upper urinary tract urothelial carcinoma. Virchows Arch. 2013;462:101.
77. Nakanishi K, Hiroi S, Tominaga S, et al. Expression of hypoxia-inducible factor-1alpha protein predicts survival in patients with transitional cell carcinoma of

the upper urinary tract. Clin Cancer Res. 2005;11:2583.

78. Ke HL, Wei YC, Yang SF, et al. Overexpression of hypoxia-inducible factor-1alpha predicts an unfavorable outcome in urothelial carcinoma of the upper urinary tract. Int J Urol. 2008;15:200.
79. Wu WJ, Liu LT, Huang CN, et al. The clinical implications of telomerase activity in upper tract urothelial cancer and washings. BJU Int. 2000;86:213.
80. Nakanishi K, Hiroi S, Kawai T, et al. Expression of telomerase catalytic subunit (hTERT) mRNA does not predict survival in patients with transitional cell carcinoma of the upper urinary tract. Mod Pathol. 2001;14:1073.
81. Nakanishi K, Ogata S, Matsuo H, et al. Expression of LAT1 predicts risk of progression of transitional cell carcinoma of the upper urinary tract. Virchows Arch. 2007;451:681.
82. Eltz S, Comperat E, Cussenot O, et al. Molecular and histological markers in urothelial carcinomas of the upper urinary tract. BJU Int. 2008;102:532.
83. Oku S, Higashi M, Imazono Y, et al. Overexpression of cyclooxygenase-2 in high-grade human transitional cell carcinoma of the upper urinary tract. BJU Int. 2003;91:109.
84. Kamai T, Takagi K, Asami H, et al. Prognostic significance of p27Kip1 and Ki-67 expression in carcinoma of the renal pelvis and ureter. BJU Int. 2000;86:14.
85. Comperat E, Roupret M, Chartier-Kastler E, et al. Prognostic value of MET, RON and histoprognostic factors for urothelial carcinoma in the upper urinary tract. J Urol. 2008;179:868.
86. Scarpini S, Roupret M, Renard-Penna R, et al. Impact of the expression of Aurora-A, p53, and MIB-1 on the prognosis of urothelial carcinomas of the upper urinary tract. Urol Oncol. 2012;30:182.
87. Roupret M, Drouin SJ, Cancel-Tassin G, et al. Genetic variability in 8q24 confers susceptibility to urothelial carcinoma of the upper urinary tract and is linked with patterns of disease aggressiveness at diagnosis. J Urol. 2012;187:424.
88. Yates DR, Roupret M, Drouin SJ et al. Genetic polymorphisms on 8q24.1 and 4p16.3 are not linked with urothelial carcinoma of the bladder in contrast to their association with aggressive upper urinary tract tumours. World J Urol 2013; **31**:53.
89. Wang YH, Wu WJ, Wang WJ et al. CEBPD amplification and overexpression in urothelial carcinoma: a driver of tumor metastasis indicating adverse prognosis. Oncotarget 2015.
90. Raina R, Pahlajani G, Ponsky LE, et al. The clinical utility of atypical cytology is significantly increased in both screening and monitoring for bladder cancer when indexed with nuclear matrix protein-22. BJU Int. 2008;102:297.

Upper Urinary Tract Carcinoma In Situ

8

Jay D. Raman, Joshua L. Warrick, Grant P. Redrow and Surena F. Matin

Introduction

Upper tract urothelial carcinoma (UTUC) is an uncommon genitourinary malignancy accounting for less than 5% of urothelial cancers and under 10% of renal tumors [1]. UTUC rates have continued to increase over the past thirty years with a recent population-based study from the United States highlighting an increase from 1.88 to 2.06 cases per 100,000 person/years [2]. Accompanying this increase in UTUC rates has been a corresponding rise in in situ disease (defined by the SEER summary staging system) from approximately 7 to 31% [2]. The focus of this chapter will focus on a subset of in situ disease namely upper tract CIS (UTCIS) with the goal of delving into diagnosis, pathologic interpretation, treatment algorithms, and survival outcomes. A notable caveat when interpreting data for UTCIS is that the uncommon presentation yields a paucity of level I data (i.e., randomized controlled trials), therefore necessitating review of an amalgam of smaller series to better understand disease outcomes particularly when related to therapeutic intervention.

Diagnosis of UTCIS

Definitions

A challenge in diagnosing UTCIS is the heterogeneous definition for this disease process as highlighted in the literature [3–12] (Table 8.1). The majority of published studies rely on the absence of a solid upper tract lesion accompanied by the presence of positive high-grade cytology from the ipsilateral upper tract (with or without a confirmatory biopsy) to define UTCIS. Additionally, some definitions also require negative bladder and prostatic urethral biopsies to conclusively exclude the potential for concurrent lower tract urothelial carcinoma. Finally, only one study used positive upper tract biopsy as inclusive diagnostic criteria highlighting the challenges in obtaining a tissue diagnosis for this

J. D. Raman (✉)
Division of Urology, Penn State Milton S. Hershey Medical Center, 500 University Drive, C4830F, Hershey 17033, PA, USA
e-mail: jraman@hmc.psu.edu

J. L. Warrick
Department of Pathology, Penn State Milton S. Hershey Medical Center, 500 University Drive, Hershey 17033, PA, USA
e-mail: jwarrick@hmc.psu.edu

G. P. Redrow
Department of Surgery (Urology), University of Texas Houston, 6410 Fannin Street, Houston 77030, TX, USA
e-mail: grant.p.redrow@uth.tmc.edu

S. F. Matin
Department of Urology, University of Texas MD Anderson Cancer Center, 1515 Holcomb Blvd, Houston 77030, TX, USA
e-mail: surmatin@mdanderson.org

M. Eshghi (ed.), *Urothelial Malignancies of the Upper Urinary Tract*,
https://doi.org/10.1007/978-3-319-51263-1_8

Table 8.1 Variable definitions of upper tract CIS (UTCIS) according to the published literature

Author (year)	Definition of UTCIS
Herr [3]	• Positive urine cytology • Positive excretory urogram • Positive retrograde pyelogram
Nishino et al. [4]	• Positive selective upper tract cytology and negative intravenous or retrograde pyelography
Nonomura et al. [5]	• Positive voided urine cytology with negative random biopsies of the bladder and prostatic urethra • No abnormality on excretory urogram • Two positive cytologies from samples collected by selective ipsilateral ureteral catheterization
Okubo et al. [6]	• Positive voided urine cytology with negative random biopsies of the bladder and prostatic urethra • No abnormality on excretory urogram • Two positive cytologies from samples collected by ureteral ipsilateral catheterization
Irie et al. [7]	• Two samples with positive cytology from lavage fluid during retrograde ureteral catheterization
Miyake et al. [8]	• Positive voided urine cytology with negative random biopsies of the bladder and prostatic urethra • No abnormality on excretory urogram • Two positive cytologies from samples collected by ureteral ipsilateral catheterization
Hayashida et al. [9]	• Positive urine cytology • Negative radiographic findings • Negative random biopsies of the bladder and prostate
Kojima et al. [10]	• Positive voided urine cytology with negative random biopsies of the bladder and prostatic urethra • No abnormality on excretory urogram • Three positive cytologies from samples collected by ureteral ipsilateral catheterization
Giannarini et al. [11]	• Positive cytology in selective upper tract washings • Negative bladder barbotage cytology • Negative multiple random biopsies of the bladder and prostatic urethra • No detectable lesions on upper tract imaging
Shapiro et al. [12]	• Confirmation on URS biopsy

entity. This lack of uniformity amongst studies regarding the definition of UTCIS clearly confounds the ability to determine treatment efficacy given the potential for inclusion of heterogeneous array of upper tract tumors under the UTCIS nomenclature.

We suggest that when possible histologic evidence of UTCIS either by brush or formal biopsy should be the referent standard for diagnosis. When brush or biopsy is not feasible or is non-diagnostic, selective ipsilateral ureteral and renal pelvis washings can serve as an adjunctive diagnostic procedure. Cytopathology confirmation of CIS in this setting coupled with visual confirmation of no other upper tract and lower tract cancers can be considered diagnostic for isolated UTCIS.

Diagnostic Modalities

Despite significant advances in endoscopic tools for evaluation of the upper urinary tract, limitations in biopsy tools and the flat nature of UTCIS render accurate diagnosis challenging. With respect to ureteroscopic visualization of the upper tract, some modifications to conventional white light examination have provided the opportunity for more refined diagnosis. In 2011, Traxer et al. [13] utilized narrow band imaging (NBI) for UTUC and noted an increased detection rate of almost 25% when compared to white light. In 2012, Aboumarzouk et al. [14] noted that the use of photodynamic diagnosis (PDD) with orally administered 5-aminolevulinic acid (5-ALA) yielded an incremented 5% gain in detection of UTUC compared to white light ureteroscopy. Although the sensitivity and specificity of PDD was not significantly greater than white light, the small sample size of 32 patients likely lacked statistical power to detect a true difference. In the future, more advanced real-time imaging techniques such as optical coherence tomography, endoluminal ultrasonography, and confocal laser microscopy all have the potential to emerge as options to improve detection and staging of upper tract tumors [13–20]. Nonetheless, at present, their role in diagnosis of UTCIS remains unexplored and largely speculative.

Tissue procurement is a key element for UTUC diagnosis particularly challenged by the flat nature of UTCIS. The optimal method for obtaining tissue from the upper tract remains incompletely defined although several groups have evaluated and compared techniques. In 2013, Kleinmann et al. [21] compared a flat wire basket and three French cup biopsy forceps for upper tract biopsies and noted that the basket yielded a significantly higher rate of specimens sufficient for diagnosis and grading. This tool, however, is most relevant for papillary tumors, whereas for sessile and flat lesions (i.e., UTCIS) basketing is not a viable option. Furthermore, biopsy of UTUC lesions is often valuable for assigning histologic grade but less so for histologic stage. Underscoring this point is data from Smith et al. who reviewed a series of upper tract biopsies noting upgrading or upstaging of tumor in 37% and 38%, respectively, on repeat biopsy or on definitive surgical management [22]. Clements et al. [23] further supported these observations by reporting that URS biopsy grade and not stage most predictive of adverse tumor pathology at RNU further supported these observations. Clearly, continued improvement of tissue procurement tools remains necessary for UTUC.

Imaging can also play a role in the diagnosis of UTUC with hydronephrosis accompanied by a soft tissue defect being a sensitive indicator for a locally advanced tumor [24]. However, axial cross-sectional imaging (CT or MRI) may not be effective at detecting small volume disease or recurrences. For example, a recent study by Sternberg et al. noted that CT urography detected only 29% of UT recurrences [25]. Therefore, we believe that given the nature of UTCIS, cross-sectional imaging serves mostly to evaluate for concurrent non-CIS papillary lesions while ruling out concurrent metastatic disease. The imaging is more limited in determination of urothelial thickening which may be more a hallmark of UTCIS.

Pathologic Characterization

UTCIS Primary Lesion

Grossly, areas of CIS are flat, may or may not be erythematous, and some will be imperceptible under white light endoscopic visualization. Microscopically these lesions usually do not grow beyond the urothelial basement membrane; however, they demonstrate high-grade nuclear atypia with loss of cellular polarity [26]. Five distinct subtypes have been identified; however, there is no difference in prognosis between groups [27, 28].

Flat urothelial carcinoma in situ (CIS) is characterized by cytological malignant cells involving the urothelial surface without formation of papillary structures (Fig. 8.1). These malignant cells uniformly have enlarged hyperchromatic nuclei with nucleoli that are often conspicuous. A subset of these cells has marked nuclear pleomorphism, though many cases are notable for nuclear monomorphism. In the prototypical UTCIS case, normal histologic maturation and cellularity polarity are lost, resulting in a jumbled, haphazard appearance of the surface urothelium. These changes are often recognizable at low-power magnification. Additionally, mitotic figures are usually easily identified, and atypical mitotic figures may be present.

Several named patterns of flat CIS are recognized, including large cell pleomorphic, large cell non-pleomorphic, small cell (which has not

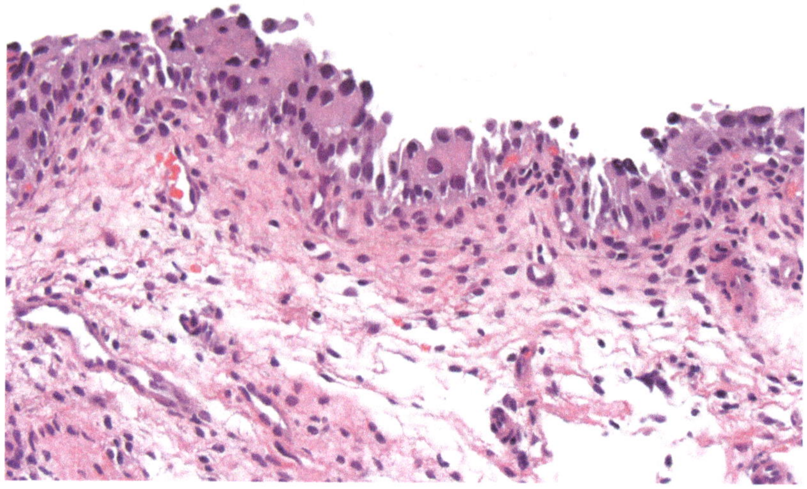

Fig. 8.1 Hematoxylin and eosin-stained sections (400× magnification). Sections of prototypical flat CIS show enlarge, hyperchromatic nuclei with a flat architecture. Nuclei are highly pleomorphic in this case

relationship to small cell neuroendocrine carcinoma), clinging, pagetoid, and undermining [29]. These subtypes are named to facilitate their recognition by pathologists, and at present have no direct bearing on clinical outcomes. The latter three patterns are often difficult to recognize histologically, particularly at frozen section or on small biopsies. This is of particular importance for the urologic surgeon whose management may be predicated on frozen section interpretation of margin status at time of extirpative upper tract surgery.

Flat CIS is frequently discohesive, with resulting denudation. Cases with prominent denudation define the clinging subtype (Fig. 8.2). Small biopsies in such cases may not sample cytological malignant cells, as these have been sloughed into the renal pelvis or ureteral lumen. A diagnosis of "denuded urothelium" in the setting of clinical suspicion for CIS should thus raise the concern for clinging CIS. Correlated with concurrent cytological sampling identifies the malignant cells in many such cases. Pagetoid CIS and undermining CIS are unusual in that they involve benign urothelium directly. Thus, while the majority of flat CIS have loss of maturation and polarity, these patterns have the appearance of benign urothelium on low power, and the diagnosis is based on the recognition of malignant cells involving otherwise benign urothelium. As mentioned early, identifying these malignant cells may be difficult, particularly on frozen sections.

The most important differential diagnosis in CIS is benign reactive urothelium, which may be seen in any insult to the urothelium, including stones, foreign bodies (i.e., ureteral stent), and infection. Communicating the presence of possible causes of reactive urothelial changes to the pathologist is thus of great importance.

Bladder Versus Upper Tract Cis

Clinical Course

Although histologically appearing similar, bladder CIS (BCIS) and UTCIS appear to be distinct entities with separate clinical courses. It is likely that these observed differences are not solely due to anatomical differences in the organ or origin, biases in detection, and differential follow-up algorithms, but potentially stem from distinct biologic differences as well [30].

Fig. 8.2 Hematoxylin and eosin-stained sections (400× magnification). Sections of clinging CIS show a predominantly denuded urothelium, with only scattered cytologically malignant cells remaining

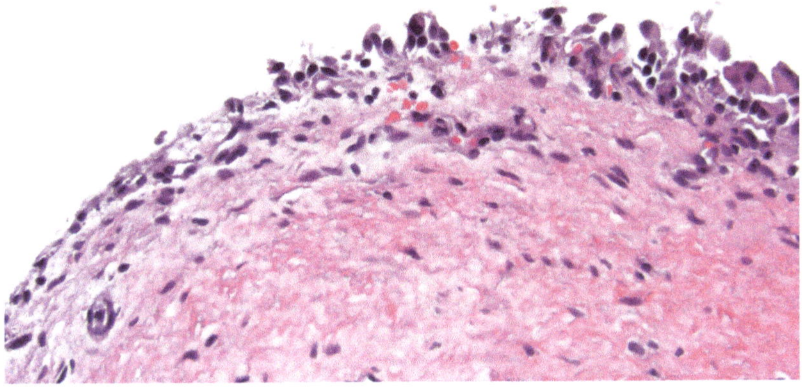

BCIS is known to progress to higher stage disease (muscle invasion or metastasis) in approximately 50% of untreated cases, and has a 10- and 15-year cancer-specific survival of 79 and 74%, respectively [31, 32]. BCIS also has the potential for progression to a higher stage disease despite intravesical therapy. For example, Chade and colleagues highlighted this fact in a series of 155 patients receiving Bacillus Calmette–Guerin (BCG) for BCIS while noting progression to cT1 or higher disease in 45% of patients, and cT2 or higher in 17% of patients. Furthermore, of those patients that initially responded to BCG, 88% developed a recurrence at 5 years [32].

Conversely, the progression rate of CIS of the upper tract managed by topical therapy appears to be significantly lower (~5%) and UTCIS has a 5-year cancer-specific survival rate of approximately 95% [2, 6, 7, 11, 33]. For example, one of the largest series of UTCIS treated with antegrade perfusion of BCG noted a progression rate of only 5% at a median follow-up of 42 months. Additionally, projected 5- and 10-year recurrence-free survival was 57 and 49%, respectively, although the cohort size of 42 renal units does render conclusions difficult to fully contextualize [11].

Despite these apparent differences, there does exist some degree of commonality between these disease processes. Indeed, the presence of multifocal UTCIS also increases the risk of developing high-risk bladder cancer [34]. Those with bladder cancer also present with an increased risk of UTUC [35]. Additionally, both BCIS and UTCIS are particularly sensitive to topical immunomodulators, with contemporary research showing long-term survival with these agents is equal to radical surgery [10]. However, due to the relative rarity of UTUC in general and the even more uncommon scenario of UTCIS, there is little guidance from the literature to definitively guide treatment strategies.

Molecular Alterations

Recent studies comparing gene expression profiles of bladder and upper tract urothelial carcinoma provide some insight on similar and distinct molecular signatures. Krabbe et al. [36] performed analysis by pathologic stage of bladder and upper tract urothelial cancers and found no difference in expression of cell cycle markers p21, p27, p53, cyclin E, and Ki-67. Other recent UTUC sequencing studies suggest that certain mutations may be absent or rare in these tumors when compared to bladder cancer UTUC [36–38]. For example, Safkianos et al. [38] used next-generation sequencing of high-grade urothelial tumors to identify FGFR3, HRAS, and CDKN2B that were more commonly mutated in UTUC while TP53 and ARID1A were less frequently altered when compared to high-grade bladder tumors. Of interest, RB1 mutations were not identified in their cohort of high-grade UTUC tumors compared to 21% of bladder cancer cases.

Despite these promising initial investigations, these studies focus on a homogenous array of papillary tumors. Therefore, at present, no molecular comparisons specifically focus on upper and lower tract CIS, and therefore such investigation remains a potential avenue of research.

Concomitant UTCIS and Papillary Tumors

While data regarding primary UTCIS is more limited, several studies have studied the impact of concomitant UTCIS occurring with primary UTUC tumors. In two contemporary studies, the coexisting presence of UTCIS with advanced primary UTUC tumors was significantly associated with inferior recurrence-free and cancer-specific survival [39, 40]. Furthermore, in a multi-institutional international retrospective analysis of 2681 patients who underwent radical nephroureterectomy (RNU) for UTUC, concomitant UTCIS was shown to be a significant risk factor for intravesical recurrence on multivariate analysis [34]. These observations were similarly noted in a cohort of 482 patients who underwent RNU for UTUC whereby the intravesical recurrence rate was 35% and concomitant CIS was associated with subsequent bladder recurrences. Of note, in this study, bladder tumor recurrence was not independently associated with higher cancer-specific mortality [41].

When considering the treatment of UTCIS in the subsequent section, we will focus exclusively on the presence of UTCIS as a single entity and not in the presence of concomitant solid tumors. This is an important consideration given the higher risk features and adverse disease outcomes observed when papillary tumors and UTCIS are present concomitantly.

Treatment of UTCIS

The gold standard management for UTUC including UTCIS is radical nephroureterectomy with an ipsilateral bladder cuff. Nonetheless, some patients have elective and imperative indications for kidney preservation and therefore endoscopic ablation (if possible) accompanied by topical intracavitary immunomodulating agents presents an option [42, 43]. Current evidence to date is somewhat limited as these studies are exclusively retrospective, single-center, and lack a comparative group. Nonetheless, despite these limitations, these studies represent the best available data in this setting. To illustrate this point, Kojima et al. retrospectively compared RNU to intracavitary BCG for UTCIS in 6 and 11 patients, respectively, and found no significant difference in 5-year recurrence-free or cancer-specific survival [10]. A much larger cohort can be evaluated through subgroup analysis of patients who underwent RNU for UTUC whereby those with pure UTCIS had a 3-year recurrence-free survival of 84.2% and 3-year disease-specific survival of 88.8% (similar to kidney preservation with topical therapy) [44, 45].

Intracavitary BCG is the most commonly utilized agent for UTCIS [3, 46]. Alternative medications such as mitomycin C, epirubicin, and thiotepa also have been evaluated in the adjuvant therapy setting although data is significantly more limited. Table 8.2 highlights the currently published studies that assess the success of topical therapy for pure UTCIS [3–12]. Delivery techniques varied with antegrade instillation via indwelling nephrostomy tube, retrograde instillation via a ureteral catheter, or

Table 8.2 Topical treatment regimens of UTCIS and reported outcomes

Author	Treatment algorithm	Outcome	Renal units treated	Median follow-up (months)
Herr [3]	Intravesical BCG × 6 weeks after surgical resection of primary tumor	Metastasis at 14 months Cytology and pyeloscopy negative for residual tumor	1	14
Nishino et al. [4]	BCG via ureteral stent or catheter × 4–8 weeks	Negative cytology—100%	8	22
		1 of 6 recurred in prostatic urethra		
Nonomura et al. [5]	Intravesical BCG with double pigtail stent × 6 weeks	Negative cytology—82%	11	NR
		recurrence—22%		
Okubo et al. [6]	BCG via retrograde ureteral catheter or nephrostomy tube × 6 weeks	Negative cytology—64%	14	20.5
		Recurrence—22%		
Irie et al. [7]	Intravesical BCG with double pigtail stent × 6 weeks	Negative cytology—100%	13	36
		UTUC recurrence—8%		
		Bladder recurrence—11%		
Miyake et al. [8]	BCG via retrograde ureteral catheter or nephrostomy tube × 6 weeks	Negative cytology—100%	17	30
		Recurrence—24%		
Hayashida et al. [9]	BCG via nephrostomy, indwelling ureteral stent, or ureteral catheter × 6 weeks	Negative cytology—100%	11	50.9
		Recurrence—50%		
Kojima et al. [10]	Intravesical BCG with double pigtail stent × 8 weeks	Negative cytology—77%	11	58.3
		Recurrence—23%		
Giannarini et al. [11]	BCG via nephrostomy × 8 weeks	Recurrence—40%	42	42
		Progression—5%		
		RNU—5%		
Shapiro et al. [12]	BCG/Interferon-a2B via open-ended ureteral catheter × 6 weeks Maintenance with 3 weekly instillations of BCG/Interferon-a2B at 3, 6, 12, 18 and 24 months	Complete response—82%	11	13.5
		No response—9%		
		Recurrence—9%		
		Overall survival 91%		
		Disease-specific survival—100%		

retrograde reflux via intravesical administration with indwelling ureteral stents. A recent porcine study has suggested that evaluation of the surface area of the upper tract collecting system as assessed by dye is superior using open-ended ureteral catheter with retrograde instillation versus nephrostomy tube and reflux with indwelling double pigtail stent [47]. A similarly designed human-based study has not been performed.

Response rates to treatment as assessed by ureteral or voided urine cytology vary between 64 and 100% (Table 8.2). Indeed, despite challenges in delivery of drug to the upper tract, this compares favorably to response rates for BCIS, which have been reported at 63–70% [3, 32]. BCG appears to be more effective for primary treatment of UTCIS than as an adjuvant following endoscopic treatment of Ta and/or T1 tumors. Highlighting this point is work from Giannarini et al. who found those treated for primary UTCIS had significantly lower rates of recurrence, progression, and RNU than those receiving adjuvant BCG after ablation of Ta/T1 tumors [11]. To date, one series of eleven patients utilized BCG in conjunction with interferon-a2B for six weekly instillations and five subsequent maintenance courses [12]. The initial complete response rate of 73% was comparable to other series, and there were no recurrences in patients who demonstrated initial response. As no other study to date has incorporated scheduled maintenance courses of intracavitary treatment, this is a highly relevant area requiring future exploration with precedent of success from the bladder cancer literature [48–50].

Clearly, the ability to predict a patient's response to BCG (or other immunomodulatory agents) would help in stratifying a patient to surgical or topical therapy management for UTCIS. In that regard, Nunez-Nateras and colleagues have evaluated the immunologic composition of bladder CIS prior to treatment [51]. Studies suggest that instillation of BCG creates an anti-neoplastic response by inciting a Th1 cytotoxic immune response [52]. In pathologic samples of BCIS prior to BCG treatment, those patients exhibiting predominantly a Th1 versus Th2 response were less likely to respond to BCG. Furthermore, work has highlighted that markers may be available to identify and segregate BCG non-responders with a sensitivity of 100% and specificity for BCG responders of 80% [51]. One postulates that a similar relationship would exist for UTCIS although such studies are clearly requisite.

BCG has notable risks and side effects that warrant considered when treating the bladder or upper tract. When considering the UTCIS treatment experience, notable reported side effects include the irritative voiding symptoms, hematuria, fever, as well as sepsis (which were fatal in one case) [3–12]. Low-grade temperatures may be managed conservatively, although temperatures over 39 °C may be a harbinger for systemic absorption and should be treated emergently [53]. Analogous to BCG instillation for bladder cancer, careful counseling on the potential side effects including the possibility of systemic disease should be undertaken.

Conclusions

The goal of the treatment of primary UTCIS should be, like in the treatment of BCIS, oncologic control along with organ preservation. The concern (albeit unlikely) exists that UTCIS could silently progress from a curable malignancy to a metastatic and incurable disease. With increasing awareness, standardization of definitions, and improved evidence-based treatment paradigms, the clinician's ability to identify and quantify primary and recurrent UTCIS will hopefully greatly improve subsequent patient care. At present, all current treatment and surveillance algorithms are extrapolated from bladder CIS experience. As a consequence, at this time UTCIS remains an orphan subtype of a rare malignancy, one that remains a clinical conundrum to the practicing urologist and due to low prevalence and technical constraints remains without dedicated research efforts. Indeed the next phases of UTCIS research must address current gaps such as improved diagnostic methods, effective delivery intracavitary agents, role of maintenance therapy, prediction of response to BCG, and refined genomics to better study the disease process. In this regard, future collaborative efforts between institutions will allow for larger, well-controlled, prospective trials.

Summary Box

- Upper tract carcinoma in situ (UTCIS) is a non-muscle invasive, high-grade cancer involving the epithelial lining of the renal pelvis, calyces, and ureter.
- UTCIS lesions may be erythematous and microscopically do not grow

beyond the urothelial basement membrane although they demonstrate high-grade nuclear atypia with loss of cellular polarity.
- Histologic evidence of UTCIS either by brush or formal biopsy should be the referent standard for diagnosis.
- Organ preservation remains a central goal in the management of UTCIS with topical intracavitary instillations (most well studied with BCG) playing a key role in achieving this goal.
- Despite challenges in delivery of drug to the upper tract, response rates assessed by ureteral or voided urine cytology are favorable ranging from 64 to 100%.
- Future UTCIS research should focus on improving diagnostic algorithms, better delivery systems of intracavitary agents to the upper tract, and refined genomics to better study the disease process.

References

1. Raman JD, Scherr DS. Management of patients with upper urinary tract transitional cell carcinoma. Nat Clin Pract Urol. 2007;4(8):432–43.
2. Raman JD, Messer J, Sielatycki JA, Hollenbeak CS. Incidence and survival of patients with carcinoma of the ureter and renal pelvis in the USA, 1973–2005. BJU Int. 2011;107(7):1059–64.
3. Herr HW. Durable response of a carcinoma in situ of the renal pelvis to topical bacillus Calmette-Guerin. J Urol. 1985;134(3):531–2.
4. Nishino Y, Yamamoto N, Komeda H, Takahashi Y, Deguchi T. Bacillus Calmette-Guerin instillation treatment for carcinoma in situ of the upper urinary tract. BJU Int. 2000;85(7):799–801.
5. Nonomura N, Ono Y, Nozawa M, Fukui T, Harada Y, Nishimura K, et al. Bacillus Calmette-Guerin perfusion therapy for the treatment of transitional cell carcinoma in situ of the upper urinary tract. Eur Urol. 2000;38(6):701–4; discussion 5.
6. Okubo K, Ichioka K, Terada N, Matsuta Y, Yoshimura K, Arai Y. Intrarenal bacillus Calmette-Guerin therapy for carcinoma in situ of the upper urinary tract: long-term follow-up and natural course in cases of failure. BJU Int. 2001;88 (4):343–7.
7. Irie A, Iwamura M, Kadowaki K, Ohkawa A, Uchida T, Baba S. Intravesical instillation of bacille Calmette-Guerin for carcinoma in situ of the urothelium involving the upper urinary tract using vesicoureteral reflux created by a double-pigtail catheter. Urology. 2002;59(1):53–7.
8. Miyake H, Eto H, Hara S, Okada H, Kamidono S, Hara I. Clinical outcome of bacillus Calmette-Guerin perfusion therapy for carcinoma in situ of the upper urinary tract. Int J Urol: Official Journal of the Japanese Urological Association. 2002;9(12):677–80.
9. Hayashida Y, Nomata K, Noguchi M, Eguchi J, Koga S, Yamashita S, et al. Long-term effects of bacille Calmette-Guerin perfusion therapy for treatment of transitional cell carcinoma in situ of upper urinary tract. Urology. 2004;63(6):1084–8.
10. Kojima Y, Tozawa K, Kawai N, Sasaki S, Hayashi Y, Kohri K. Long-term outcome of upper urinary tract carcinoma in situ: effectiveness of nephroureterectomy versus bacillus Calmette-Guerin therapy. Int J Urol: Official Journal of the Japanese Urological Association. 2006;13(4):340–4.
11. Giannarini G, Kessler TM, Birkhauser FD, Thalmann GN, Studer UE. Antegrade perfusion with bacillus Calmette-Guerin in patients with non-muscle-invasive urothelial carcinoma of the upper urinary tract: who may benefit? Eur Urol. 2011;60(5):955–60.
12. Shapiro EY, Lipsky MJ, Cha DY, McKiernan JM, Benson MC, Gupta M. Outcomes of intrarenal Bacillus Calmette-Guerin/interferon-α2B for biopsy-proven upper-tract carcinoma in situ. J Endourol/Endourol Soc. 2012;26(12):1645–50.
13. Traxer O, Geavlete B, de Medina SG, Sibony M, Al-Qahtani SM. Narrow-band imaging digital flexible ureteroscopy in detection of upper urinary tract transitional-cell carcinoma: initial experience. J Endourol/Endourol Soc. 2011;25(1):19–23.
14. Aboumarzouk OM, Ahmad S, Moseley H, Kata SG. Accuracy of photodynamic diagnosis in the detection and follow-up of patients with upper urinary tract lesions: initial 3-year experience. Arab J Urol. 2012;10(2):138–42.
15. Mueller-Lisse UL, Meissner OA, Babaryka G, Bauer M, Eibel R, Stief CG, et al. Catheter-based intraluminal optical coherence tomography (OCT) of the ureter: ex-vivo correlation with histology in porcine specimens. Eur Radiol. 2006;16(10):2259–64.
16. Matin SF, Kamat AM, Grossman HB. High-frequency endoluminal ultrasonography as an aid to the staging of upper tract urothelial carcinoma: imaging findings and pathologic correlation. J Ultrasound Med: Official Journal of the American Institute of Ultrasound in Medicine. 2010;29(9):1277–84.
17. Wu K, Liu JJ, Adams W, Sonn GA, Mach KE, Pan Y, et al. Dynamic real-time microscopy of the urinary tract using confocal laser endomicroscopy. Urology. 2011;78(1):225–31.
18. Ren H, Park KC, Pan R, Waltzer WC, Shroyer KR, Pan Y. Early detection of carcinoma in situ of the

bladder: a comparative study of white light cystoscopy, narrow band imaging, 5-ALA fluorescence cystoscopy and 3-dimensional optical coherence tomography. J Urol. 2012;187(3):1063–70.
19. Bus MT, Muller BG, de Bruin DM, Faber DJ, Kamphuis GM, van Leeuwen TG, et al. Volumetric in vivo visualization of upper urinary tract tumors using optical coherence tomography: a pilot study. J Urol. 2013;190(6):2236–42.
20. Chen SP, Liao JC. Confocal laser endomicroscopy of bladder and upper tract urothelial carcinoma: a new era of optical diagnosis? Curr Urol Rep. 2014;15 (9):437.
21. Kleinmann N, Healy KA, Hubosky SG, Margel D, Bibbo M, Bagley DH. Ureteroscopic biopsy of upper tract urothelial carcinoma: comparison of basket and forceps. J Endourol/Endourol Soc. 2013;27 (12):1450–4.
22. Smith AK, Stephenson AJ, Lane BR, Larson BT, Thomas AA, Gong MC, et al. Inadequacy of biopsy for diagnosis of upper tract urothelial carcinoma: implications for conservative management. Urology. 2011;78(1):82–6.
23. Clements T, Messer JC, Terrell JD, Herman MP, Ng CK, Scherr DS, et al. High-grade ureteroscopic biopsy is associated with advanced pathology of upper-tract urothelial carcinoma tumors at definitive surgical resection. J Endourol/Endourol Soc. 2012;26 (4):398–402.
24. Messer JC, Terrell JD, Herman MP, Ng CK, Scherr DS, Scoll B, et al. Multi-institutional validation of the ability of preoperative hydronephrosis to predict advanced pathologic tumor stage in upper-tract urothelial carcinoma. Urol Oncol. 2013;31(6):904–8.
25. Sternberg IA, Keren Paz GE, Chen LY, Herr HW, Donat SM, Bochner BH, et al. Upper tract imaging surveillance is not effective in diagnosing upper tract recurrence in patients followed for nonmuscle invasive bladder cancer. J Urol. 2013;190(4):1187–91.
26. Amin MB, Eble JN. Urological pathology. 1st ed., ix, 934 pp.
27. Epstein JI, Amin MB, Reuter VE, Epstein JI. Biopsy interpretation of the bladder. 2nd ed. Philadelphia: Wolters Kluwer/Lippincott Williams & Wilkins Health; 2010. vii, 355 pp.
28. Comperat E, Jacquet SF, Varinot J, Conort P, Roupret M, Chartier-Kastler E, et al. Different subtypes of carcinoma in situ of the bladder do not have a different prognosis. Virchows Arch: An International Journal of Pathology. 2013;462 (3):343–8.
29. McKenney JK, Gomez JA, Desai S, Lee MW, Amin MB. Morphologic expressions of urothelial carcinoma in situ: a detailed evaluation of its histologic patterns with emphasis on carcinoma in situ with microinvasion. Am J Surg Pathol. 2001;25(3):356–62.
30. Green DA, Rink M, Xylinas E, Matin SF, Stenzl A, Roupret M, et al. Urothelial carcinoma of the bladder and the upper tract: disparate twins. J Urol. 2013;189 (4):1214–21.
31. Cheng L, Cheville JC, Neumann RM, Leibovich BC, Egan KS, Spotts BE, et al. Survival of patients with carcinoma in situ of the urinary bladder. Cancer. 1999;85(11):2469–74.
32. Chade DC, Shariat SF, Godoy G, Savage CJ, Cronin AM, Bochner BH, et al. Clinical outcomes of primary bladder carcinoma in situ in a contemporary series. J Urol. 2010;184(1):74–80.
33. Munoz JJ, Ellison LM. Upper tract urothelial neoplasms: incidence and survival during the last 2 decades. J Urol. 2000;164(5):1523–5.
34. Xylinas E, Rink M, Margulis V, Karakiewicz P, Novara G, Shariat SF, et al. Multifocal carcinoma in situ of the upper tract is associated with high risk of bladder cancer recurrence. Eur Urol. 2012;61 (5):1069–70.
35. Wright JL, Hotaling J, Porter MP. Predictors of upper tract urothelial cell carcinoma after primary bladder cancer: a population based analysis. J Urol. 2009;181 (3):1035–9; discussion 9.
36. Krabbe LM, Lotan Y, Bagrodia A, Gayed BA, Darwish OM, Youssef RF, et al. Prospective comparison of molecular signatures in urothelial cancer of the bladder and the upper urinary tract—is there evidence for discordant biology? J Urol. 2014;191(4):926–31.
37. Zhang Z, Furge KA, Yang XJ, Teh BT, Hansel DE. Comparative gene expression profiling analysis of urothelial carcinoma of the renal pelvis and bladder. BMC Med Genomics. 2010;3:58.
38. Sfakianos JP, Cha EK, Iyer G, Scott SN, Zabor EC, Shah RH, et al. Genomic characterization of upper tract urothelial carcinoma. Eur Urol. 2015;68 (6):970–7.
39. Wheat JC, Weizer AZ, Wolf JS Jr, Lotan Y, Remzi M, Margulis V, et al. Concomitant carcinoma in situ is a feature of aggressive disease in patients with organ confined urothelial carcinoma following radical nephroureterectomy. Urol Oncol. 2012;30 (3):252–8.
40. Otto W, Shariat SF, Fritsche HM, Gupta A, Matsumoto K, Kassouf W, et al. Concomitant carcinoma in situ as an independent prognostic parameter for recurrence and survival in upper tract urothelial carcinoma: a multicenter analysis of 772 patients. World J Urol. 2011;29(4):487–94.
41. Xylinas E, Colin P, Audenet F, Phe V, Cormier L, Cussenot O, et al. Intravesical recurrence after radical nephroureterectomy for upper tract urothelial carcinomas: predictors and impact on subsequent oncological outcomes from a national multicenter study. World J Urol. 2013;31(1):61–8.
42. Roupret M, Babjuk M, Comperat E, Zigeuner R, Sylvester RJ, Burger M, et al. European association of urology guidelines on upper urinary tract urothelial cell carcinoma: 2015 update. Eur Urol. 2015;68 (5):868–79.
43. Raman JD. Kidney sparing surgery for upper-tract urothelial carcinoma. Minerva urologica e

nefrologica (The Italian Journal of Urology and Nephrology). 2016.
44. Margulis V, Shariat SF, Matin SF, Kamat AM, Zigeuner R, Kikuchi E, et al. Outcomes of radical nephroureterectomy: a series from the upper tract urothelial carcinoma collaboration. Cancer. 2009;115 (6):1224–33.
45. Karam JA, Margulis V, Montorsi F, Karakiewicz PI, Lotan Y, Kikuchi E, et al. Carcinoma in situ of the upper urinary tract treated with radical nephroureterectomy—results from a multicenter study. Eur Urol. 2008;54(4):961–3.
46. Morales A, Eidinger D, Bruce AW. Intracavitary bacillus Calmette-Guerin in the treatment of superficial bladder tumors. J Urol. 1976;116(2):180–3.
47. Pollard ME, Levinson AW, Shapiro EY, Cha DY, Small AC, Mohamed NE, et al. Comparison of 3 upper tract anticarcinogenic agent delivery techniques in an ex vivo porcine model. Urology. 2013;82(6):1451 e1–6.
48. Lamm DL. Preventing progression and improving survival with BCG maintenance. Eur Urol. 2000;37 (Suppl 1):9–15.
49. Lamm DL, Blumenstein BA, Crissman JD, Montie JE, Gottesman JE, Lowe BA, et al. Maintenance bacillus Calmette-Guerin immunotherapy for recurrent TA, T1 and carcinoma in situ transitional cell carcinoma of the bladder: a randomized Southwest Oncology Group Study. J Urol. 2000;163(4):1124–9.
50. Sylvester RJ, van der MA, Lamm DL. Intravesical bacillus Calmette-Guerin reduces the risk of progression in patients with superficial bladder cancer: a meta-analysis of the published results of randomized clinical trials. J Urol. 2002;168(5):1964–70.
51. Nunez-Nateras R, Castle EP, Protheroe CA, Stanton ML, Ocal TI, Ferrigni EN, et al. Predicting response to bacillus Calmette-Guerin (BCG) in patients with carcinoma in situ of the bladder. Urol Oncol. 2014;32(1):45 e23–30.
52. Ponticiello A, Perna F, Maione S, Stradolini M, Testa G, Terrazzano G, et al. Analysis of local T lymphocyte subsets upon stimulation with intravesical BCG: a model to study tuberculosis immunity. Respir Med. 2004;98(6):509–14.
53. Schnapp DS, Weiss GH, Smith AD. Fever following intracavitary bacillus Calmette-Guerin therapy for upper tract transitional cell carcinoma. J Urol. 1996;156(2 Pt 1):386–8.

From Bedside to Endoscopy to Microscopy to Diagnosis: Samples Collection and Processing

9

Esther Chaewon Yoon and Minghao Zhong

Urine Cytology

Urine cytology is a non-invasive method for detecting urothelial carcinoma by identifying abnormal urothelial cells in the voided urine or bladder washes. This technique was initiated by George Papanicolaou in the 1940s as a way to detect and follow patients with bladder cancer [1]. It took approximately 20 years of practice and adjustments to establish a technique that is highly accurate and have good correlation among the cytology, histologic, and clinical features and diagnosis of high-grade urothelial carcinoma (UC) [2–5]. Even in present days, cytology remains an inexpensive, quick, and reliable method to diagnose high-grade UC [4, 6–8]. The most common indication for urine cytology is hematuria [7]. Another indication is surveillance for recurrent UC [7] since patients with a prior diagnosed and treated urothelial cancer are at risk for recurrence or a de novo primary elsewhere in the urinary tract. Urine cytology is not used for screening asymptomatic individuals, because the benefits outweigh the considerable cost [2, 5]. It is used, however, for high-risk patients, such with those who have occupational exposure to aniline dye, the aromatic amines, or receiving cyclophosphamide treatment for diseases like multiple sclerosis.

E. C. Yoon · M. Zhong (✉)
Department of Pathology, Westchester Medical Health Network/New York Medical College, 100 Woods Road, Valhalla 10595, NY, USA
e-mail: Minghao.Zhong@wmchealth.org

E. C. Yoon
e-mail: EstherChaewon.Yoon@wmchealth.org

Specimen Collection

There are three types of urinary specimens for work up upper urinary malignancy, and each method has its own advantages and disadvantages [9, 10].

Voided Urine

Voided urine should be obtained 3–4 h after the patient's last urine. First morning voided urine specimens should be avoided, because cells are in a stagnant, low pH, and hypertonic environment which causes degenerative changes, making cytological assessment difficult. The minimum volume of urine required for adequate cellularity is variable, but it may be as high as 25–100 ml. In women, voided urine can be contaminated by vaginal epithelial cells, but in most instances this does not compromise a diagnosis. Still, to help ensure the adequacy of the sample, a midstream clean-catch specimen is recommended. Additional consideration of voided urine for upper urinary malignancy is false

M. Eshghi (ed.), *Urothelial Malignancies of the Upper Urinary Tract*,
https://doi.org/10.1007/978-3-319-51263-1_9

negative due to hydronephroureterosis, which further dilutes the sample from bladder urine. However, voided urine is still an initial work up for upper urinary malignancy, because of its simplicity [11, 12].

Catheterized Urine

Specimens obtained by catheterization have disadvantages for both the patient and the cytopathologist. First, for the patient, catheterization carries a risk of urinary tract infection. Second, urine collected from an indwelling catheter is often a pooled specimen that has been in room temperature for many hours, and cellular degeneration can be more pronounced. Third, the tip of the catheter often scrapes off benign urothelial cell clusters, which mimic a low-grade papillary neoplasm in cyto-morphology (Fig. 9.1). Therefore, greater diagnostic caution is advised: the diagnosis of carcinoma should not be made unless the cytological evidence is unequivocal. Retrograde catheterization, a selective catheterization procedure, could be used for purpose of localization of high-grade UC of either the left or right ureter or renal pelvis [13–16].

Upper Tract Washings and Brushings

When an upper urinary tract malignancy is suspected, directed washings, brushings, and/or biopsies of a ureter or renal pelvis lesion should be performed. Although brushings obtained by direct visualization using an endoscope were introduced in 1973, they are rarely obtained. The sensitivity and specificity of brushings compare favorably with those of other cytological methods (voided, catheterized, irrigation). The most common upper tract specimen is the directed washing with or without an upper tract biopsy. Directed washing specimens are particularly challenging for both urologists and cytologists. Urologists often cannot visualize the lesions in the upper tract as compared to those in the bladder; hence, they often rely on cyto-morphology of the cells from the washing specimen more than actual biopsy of lesions in the bladder. Furthermore, when they try to obtain a biopsy; often these specimens are small and crushed. The stakes are higher, because the operation of choice for a tumor in the upper tract is removal of the kidney and/or ureter. In most cases, the significant imaging finding is only a lifting defect, and the differential diagnosis is a tumor or a stone. Unfortunately, some stones can produce benign cytologic atypia which can mimic urothelial neoplasms. Finally, because of mechanical manipulation of the environment, even some normal specimens from the upper tract often show diffuse nuclear enlargement, an increased nuclear-to-cytoplasmic ratio, and very high cellularity. These entirely benign changes can suggest a tumor in an already suspicious setting and can lead to a false–positive diagnosis. For these reasons, it is impossible to accurately diagnose low-grade lesions in upper tract specimens. For high-grade tumors, the sensitivity rate of ureteral washing and ureteral

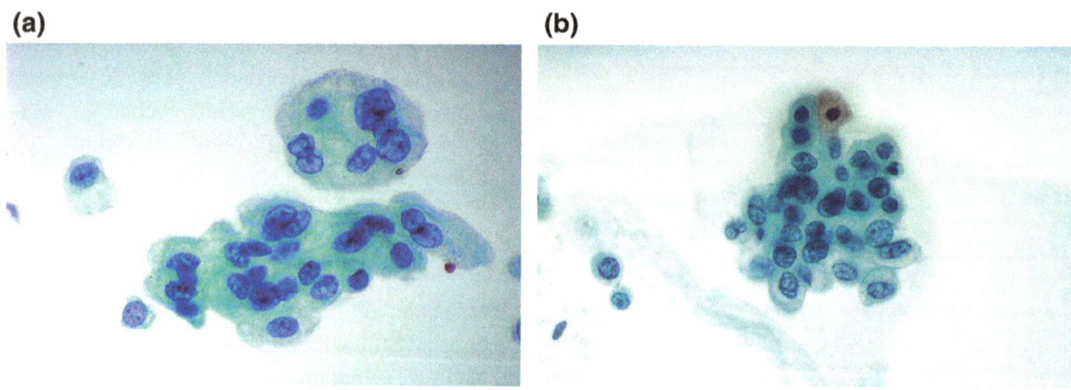

Fig. 9.1 Urine cytology of reactive urothelium and low-grade urothelial carcinoma has many overlapping characteristics. **a** Large clusters of reactive urothelial cells from retrograde urine brushing, can easily be mistaken for low-grade urothelial carcinoma. **b** Loosely structured cluster of low-grade urothelial carcinoma cells with minimal nuclear enlargement and hyperchromasia

biopsy for the detection of malignancy are similar and approach ~70%. With bilateral specimens, one can compare subtle changes between a lesion (on one side) and a presumably normal specimen (on the other side). The preparation of a "cell block" (a formalin-fixed, paraffin-embedded sediment of the urine sample) can be particularly useful because small pieces of tumor are often easier to evaluate with this preparation method [17, 18].

Sample Processing

Fresh specimens, less than 12 hours old, do not need fixation. If it takes a specimen 12–24 h to reach the laboratory, refrigeration is recommended. If the specimen processing time is delayed for more than 24 h, preservation with equal volume of 50–70% ethanol +2% carbowax is required to avoid degeneration. To achieve best results, the patient should be provided with a 250–300ml-wide mouth glass or plastic container which is one-third filled with fixative. This makes the collection more convenient and reliable. The urinary sediment can be processed in a variety of ways. The specimen can be centrifuged for 10 min at moderate speed and then a direct smear of sediment can be made on adhesive-coated slides. The urine can be filtered using one of the commercially available filtering devices, either for direct viewing of cells on the surface of the filter, or after transferring the filtered cells to a glass slide by imprinting them (reverse filtration). Alternatively, the cellular sediment can be placed on an adhesive-coated slide by use of a cytocentrifuge. Several commercially available method of preparation of the urinary sediment in liquid base have been developed within recent year. Both ThinPrep and SurePath have received FDA approval and are widely used in clinical laboratories [19–22].

Ancillary Tests

Great efforts have been made to develop a test that will either improve cytology in detecting UC or better predict carcinoma progression. The hope is that a more accurate test will eliminate the need for costly and uncomfortable cystoscopy in the follow-up of patients with superficial cancers who were treated conservatively [2, 7]. Because upper urinary tract UC is not as easily accessible as bladder UC, these ancillary tests may play more important role. Many of these tests have greater sensitivity than cytology alone, but their less-than-ideal specificity remains a problem. Like cytologic examination, these tests have difficulties distinguishing reactive conditions, such as stone-induced urothelial atypia, from low-grade UC.

FISH/UroVysion

Deletion of the p16 gene at chromosome 9p21 is one of the most common early alterations in low-grade carcinomas. High-grade carcinomas are associated with aberrations of chromosomes 1, 3, 7, 9, 11, and 17. FISH technology can be applied to cytologic preparations to detect such cytogenetic abnormalities. Because no single abnormality is present in all cancers, the success of the technique depends on using several probes. UroVysion (Abbott Molecular, Des Plaines, IL), a multi-target FISH assay, combines centromeric probes to chromosomes 3, 7, and 17 with a locus-specific probe to band 9p21 (Fig. 9.2). UroVysion has been approved for the surveillance of patients treated for bladder cancer and as a screening tool in patients with hematuria [23, 24]. In preclinical trials, for Food and Drug Administration (FDA) approval, the sensitivity of the test for low-grade lesions ranged from 48 to 61% (specificity 88–95%) and for high-grade UC from 88 to 93% (specificity 80–95%) [24]. This method is reportedly more accurate than concurrent cytology, although the performance of cytology in these trials was significantly worse than has been reported in almost all previous large series. Recent studies suggest that the benefit of UroVysion is greatest for superficial tumors [25, 26].

UroVysion has its limitations. First, its performance (like that of cytology) varies considerably among laboratories. Sensitivity and

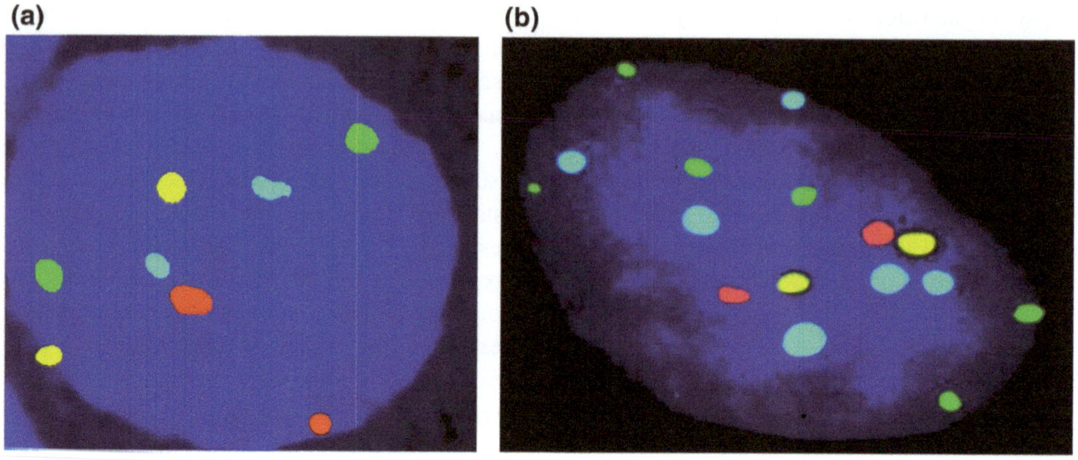

Fig. 9.2 Detection of urothelial carcinoma by the UroVysion FISH analysis. **a** Normal urothelial cells showing two signals from each probe for CEP3 (*red*), CEP7 (*green*), CEP17 (*aqua*), and 9p21 (*gold*); **b** Urothelial carcinoma cells showing aneuploid cell image with >2 signals CEP3 (*red*), CEP7 (*green*), CEP17 (*aqua*), and 9p21 (*gold*). Four or more such cells out of 25 analyzed cells would be a positive FISH result

specificity range from 50 to 89%, and from 29 to 89%, resepectively. Although this performance has improved over 10 years, recent studies continue to show significant variation. More importantly, the proportion of patients with truly false–positive results (i.e., no tumor on follow-up) versus those with "anticipatory positives" (i.e., tumor eventually found on extended follow-up) is still debated. Second, there is disagreement on the criteria for a positive result. Studies have shown that revised criteria, especially for tetraploid cells, can result in greater specificity than the original criteria used in the FDA trial. Third, many laboratories now use computer-assisted screening (e.g., BioView and Ikonisys) to interpret test results, a technology that was not available during the initial FDA trials. The degree to which this method has altered the performance of this test is not well defined. Fourth, the performance of the test for upper tract lesions, where help is perhaps most needed, has been poor. Finally, the value of UroVysion in clinical practice depends not only on the characteristics of the test itself and the patient population studied, but also the performance characteristics of the urine cytology to which it is compared. In other words, it might be most useful where cytological evaluation is least reliable. Taken together, the data suggest that where the quality of urine cytology is high, ancillary tests in general (and UroVysion particular) provide little added benefit except in highly selected groups like high-risk patients [27–29].

Cytology Combined with Immunostain

In order to improve diagnostic sensitivity of urine cytology, immunostaining of urothelial cells was developed and was applied to urine specimens [30]. ImmunoCyt (DiagnoCure, Inc., Quebec, Canada) is a multiplex immunocytofluorescence bladder cancer detection assay that combines fluorescently labeled monoclonal antibodies for M344, LDQ10, 19A211, and a glycosylated form of the carcinoembryonic antigen (CEA). A minimum evaluation of 500 epithelial cells is required, and the presence of one fluorescent cell is considered positive. However, microhematuria, cystitis and benign prostatic hyperplasia can lead to false–positive results [31–33].

Urine Protein Markers

Many soluble protein markers in voided urine have been explored for bladder cancer diagnosis and screening. These markers include blood group antigens, tumor-associated antigens, proliferating antigens, oncogenes, peptide growth factors and their receptors, cell adhesion molecules, tumor angiogenesis and angiogenesis inhibitors, and cell cycle regulator proteins. Several of these markers, including bladder tumor antigen (BTA-stat, BTA-TRAK), nuclear matrix protein-22 (Bladder Check and Bladder Cancer Test), and fibrinogen degradation products (ACCU-DX), have been approved by the FDA for clinical use. NMP22 is a structural component of the nucleus that determines nuclear morphology, organizes DNA 3-dimensionally, and is implicated in replication and gene expression. Fibronectin is an extracellular matrix component widely distributed on cells and is involved in the mechanism of human bladder cancer cell invasion. The bladder tumor antigen (BTA) stat test (Polymedco Inc., NY, USA) is a qualitative, point-of-care test capable of detecting human complement factor H-related protein, known to be produced by several human bladder cell lines but not by other epithelial cell lines [34, 35]. Cytokeratins 8 and 18 are frequently overexpressed in tumor cells and excreted as fragmented urinary proteins. Such proteins can be readily detected in urine by immunoassay and can be used as an aid to the diagnosis and monitoring of bladder cancer patients in conjunction with cystoscopy. The combined use of all three markers increase the sensitivity of cytology from 44.0 to 95.3%. NMP22 may also be useful in improving detection of low-grade and non-muscle-invasive tumors as the sensitivity for low-grade tumors was higher (83.9%) than for high-grade tumors (62.5%). Sensitivity of NMP22 for non-muscle-invasive versus muscle-invasive disease was also higher (81.8% vs. 57.1%, respectively). However, these tests have high false positivity rates due to the presence of inflammatory cells and other contaminated cells. The ultimate goals of biomarkers for bladder cancer diagnosis and surveillance would be to provide sufficient negative predictive value to allow patients to forgo more invasive tests such as cystoscopy or to risk stratify patients with indolent versus aggressive disease [36–38]. Currently, clinically available tests such as described above have their limitations including complexity, cost, sensitivity, and specificity. Therefore, identification of better biomarkers to improve the diagnostic sensitivity and specificity is of a top priority.

Somatic Mutations

Prior research has shown that different genetic defects generally underlie the two pathways of urothelial tumorigenesis [39, 40]. Low-grade papillary non-muscle-invasive tumors are generally characterized by constitutive activation of the receptor tyrosine kinase-Ras pathway, such as activating mutations in the HRAS and fibroblast growth factor receptor 3 (FGFR3) genes. In contrast, high-grade muscle-invasive tumors are characterized by alterations in the tumor suppressor protein p53 (TP53) and retinoblastoma 1 (RB1) pathways. While these initial studies served as a critical foundation for understanding the mechanisms underpinning the different clinical phenotypes of urothelial cancer, the era of high throughput genomics platforms have revealed that urothelial cancer is much more complex and heterogeneous than the prior somewhat "simplistic" genomic subsets. Two recent studies reported genome-wide analysis of bladder cancer by both whole-genome and whole-exome sequencing. One consisted of 99 urothelial tumors from an Asian population. The other consisted of 131 chemotherapy-naive, muscle-invasive, high-grade urothelial tumors as part of The Cancer Genome Atlas (TCGA) bladder cancer project. The two studies identified 37 and 32 significantly mutated genes, respectively. Despite obvious differences between the two studies (e.g., the former contains the low-grade non-muscle-invasive tumors while the latter does not), the two biomarkers for bladder cancer reported gene lists share a lot in common. For example, among the 19 significantly mutated genes with mutation frequency >5% in the TCGA dataset, 12 are also identified as significantly mutated by the Asian study. Many of them have not previously been reported as statistically significantly mutated in bladder cancer. Pathway analysis showed that somatic mutations are enriched in p53/Rb pathway, RTK/RAS/PI(3)K pathway, and histone modification genes. Several of these alterations, particularly those involving the PI(3)K/AKT/mTOR, CDKN2A/CDK4/CCND1 and RTK/RAS pathways, are amenable in principle to therapeutic targeting. The frequent mutations of chromatin remodeling genes, such as ARID1A and EP300, were confirmed by both studies, and were also reported by another independent study of smaller scale from one of the above two groups. The nature of the mutations in these chromatin modification genes indicates that many of them are tumor suppressors. The observation that 76% of the tumors analyzed by TCGA had an inactivating mutation in one or more of the chromatin regulatory genes suggests new possibilities for bladder cancer treatment. Besides these well-known cancer-relevant pathways, new genes and pathways were also identified. For example, the study also revealed frequent genomic alterations in genes involved in the process of sister chromatid cohesion and segregation (SCCS), including STAG2, ESPL1, and NIPBL [41].

More recently, *TERT* promoter mutations have been discovered to associate with UC [42, 43]. The *TERT* gene, located on chromosome 5, consists of 16 exons and 15 introns. The core promoter of *TERT* including 330 base pairs upstream of the translation start site (ATG) is GC-rich and contains many sites for transcription factors including oncoproteins such as c-Myc, HIF-1, AP2, estrogen receptor, and tumor suppressors such as p53, WT1, and Menin. Two highly recurrent and mutually exclusive somatic mutations were found in melanoma and bladder cancer at two residues at −124 (1295228) and −146 (1295250) bp from the ATG start site in the *TERT* promoter. The C > T (G > A) transition at both sites also resulted in creation of the Ets/TCF binding motifs [44, 45]. In recent reports, patients with urothelial cell carcinoma of the bladder found that these somatic mutations occurred in ~70% of the bladder cancer. The high frequency of these mutations in UC and simple point mutations in relative conservative region (~100 bp) make *TERT* promoter mutations to be a better biomarker for UC.

With the increasing understanding of genomic alterations in bladder cancer, we anticipate that new genetic and epigenetic biomarkers will be discovered and validated. Furthermore, rapid progress in proteomics and metabolomics would add additional markers to improve the usefulness and accuracy of diagnostic, prognostic, and predictive markers. To validate these potential biomarkers, it requires large cohorts of patients with high-quality biologic samples and complete clinical annotation. Therefore, the formation of multicenter consortia is necessary to accumulate enough patients with multiple clinical samples and longitudinal follow-up. The areas of further development include urine sample collection and preservation, simple low-volume and low cost assay format, and sensitivity and specificity improvement for individual markers. Finally, it will be necessary to combine different types of urine biomarkers including exfoliated cells, DNAs, RNAs, proteins, metabolites using bioinformatic tools into integrated biomarker signatures of risk, prognosis, and prediction. This will achieve better sensitivity and specificity compared to separate individual markers. Such signatures will eventually lead to the development of panel of highly predictive markers which can be applied in clinical practice through multiplex approaches.

Large Specimen Processing

Large sample processing of endoscopically resected ureteral or collecting system tumors are similar to processing TURBT specimen. In case of ureteral resection due to the small size of ureter resectoscope, the specimen size is usually small and may have artifacts due to electrocautery. Therefore, it is ideal to obtain some undisturbed tissues initially before definitive resection. Renal pelvis biopsies obtained with cold cup by large resectoscopes are almost always adequate. Non-endoscopic specimen from upper tract such as a segment of ureter or a nephroureterectomy is processed like all other large specimens and may require special stainings. It is very critical to assess if the ureteral tumor has penetrated into the periureteral tissue. In the collecting system the depth of invasion and margins should be assessed by sending separate tissue samples marked specifically such as base of tumor after resection, medial margin of resection, or resection at the UPJ area. Such additional sampling and markings help the pathologist to provide a more accurate report and true representation of staging which plays an important role in decision making about adjuvant treatment.

Summary Box

- The value of urine cytology for detecting high-grade urothelial carcinoma is high, but the quality of urine cytology varies among laboratories.
- The cytological criteria for low-grade urothelial carcinoma lack specificity and should not be used.
- Upper urinary tract specimens should be diagnosed conservatively.
- Urologists should be aware that different methods of sample collection and processing could cause different cytological appearances.
- In defined clinical settings, UroVysion is a useful adjunct to cytology for detection of urothelial carcinoma.
- Cold Cup Biopsy is essential in the renal pelvic calyceal area for accurate staging.

References

1. Papanicolaou GN, Marshall VF. Urine sediment smears as a diagnostic procedure in cancers of the urinary tract. Science. 1945;101(2629):519–20. Epub 1945/05/18. doi:10.1126/science.101.2629.519. PubMed PMID: 17775845.
2. Sullivan PS, Chan JB, Levin MR, Rao J. Urine cytology and adjunct markers for detection and surveillance of bladder cancer. Am J Transl Res. 2010;2(4):412–40. Epub 2010/08/25. PubMed PMID: 20733951; PubMed Central PMCID: PMC2923865.
3. Mowatt G, Zhu S, Kilonzo M, Boachie C, Fraser C, Griffiths TR, et al. Systematic review of the clinical effectiveness and cost-effectiveness of photodynamic diagnosis and urine biomarkers (FISH, ImmunoCyt, NMP22) and cytology for the detection and follow-up of bladder cancer. Health Technol Assess. 2010;14(4):1–331, iii–iv. Epub 2010/01/20. doi:10.3310/hta14040. PubMed PMID: 20082749.
4. Halachmi S, Linn JF, Amiel GE, Moskovitz B, Nativ O. Urine cytology, tumour markers and bladder cancer. Br J Urol. 1998;82(5):647–54. Epub 1998/12/05. PubMed PMID: 9839578.
5. Xie Q, Huang Z, Zhu Z, Zheng X, Liu J, Zhang M, et al. Diagnostic value of urine cytology in bladder cancer. A meta-analysis. Anal Quant Cytopathol Histopathol. 2016;38(1):38–44. Epub 2016/07/02. PubMed PMID: 27363065.
6. Tahoun NS, Abdel Maksoud AM, Mohamed DB. Evaluation of the value of combined urine cytology and cystoscopy for follow-up of superficial transitional cell carcinoma of the urinary bladder. J Egypt Natl Cancer Ins. 2010;22(2):105–11. Epub 2010/06/01. PubMed PMID: 21860467.
7. Alameddine M, Nassir A. The influence of urine cytology on our practice. Urol Ann. 2012;4(2):80–3. Epub 2012/05/26. doi:10.4103/0974-7796.95550. PubMed PMID: 22629001; PubMed Central PMCID: PMC3355705.
8. Falebita OA, Lee G, Sweeney P. Urine cytology in the evaluation of urological malignancy revisited: is it still necessary? Urol Int. 2010;84(1):45–9. Epub 2010/02/23. doi:10.1159/000273465. PubMed PMID: 20173368.
9. Vap LM, Shropshire SB. Urine cytology: collection, film preparation, and evaluation. Vet Clin North Am Small Anim Pract. 2016. Epub 2016/08/27. doi:10.1016/j.cvsm.2016.07.009. PubMed PMID: 27562934.
10. Hundley AF, Maygarden S, Wu JM, Visco AG, Connolly A. Adequacy of urine cytology specimens: an assessment of collection techniques. Int Urogynecol J Pelvic Floor Dysfunct. 2007;18(9):997–1001. Epub 2007/01/06. doi:10.1007/s00192-006-0277-5. PubMed PMID: 17205220.
11. Konety BR, Metro MJ, Melham MF, Salup RR. Diagnostic value of voided urine and bladder barbotage cytology in detecting transitional cell carcinoma of the urinary tract. Urol Int. 1999;62(1):26–30. Epub 1999/08/07. doi:30350. PubMed PMID: 10436427.
12. Raab SS, Grzybicki DM, Vrbin CM, Geisinger KR. Urine cytology discrepancies: frequency, causes, and outcomes. Am J Clin Pathol. 2007;127(6):946–53. Epub 2007/05/19. doi:10.1309/XUVXFXMFPL7TELCE. PubMed PMID: 17509992.
13. Gogus C, Baltaci S, Sahinli S, Turkolmez K, Beduk Y, Gogus O. Value of selective upper tract cytology for recognition of upper tract tumors after treatment of superficial bladder cancer. Int J Urol: Official Journal of the Japanese Urological

Association. 2003;10(5):243–6. Epub 2003/04/16. PubMed PMID: 12694462.
14. Sadek S, Soloway MS, Hook S, Civantos F. The value of upper tract cytology after transurethral resection of bladder tumor in patients with bladder transitional cell cancer. J Urol. 1999;161(1):77–9; discussion 9–80. Epub 1999/02/26. PubMed PMID: 10037373.
15. Zincke H, Aguilo JJ, Farrow GM, Utz DC, Khan AU. Significance of urinary cytology in the early detection of transitional cell cancer of the upper urinary tract. J Urol. 1976;116(6):781–3. Epub 1976/12/01. PubMed PMID: 1003651.
16. Barry JM, Pitre TM, Hodges CV. Ureteroileourethrostomy: 16-year followup. J Urol. 1976;115(1):29–31. Epub 1976/01/01. PubMed PMID: 1246108.
17. Yonekawa M, Hoshida Y, Hanai J, Tuboniwa N, Katayama K, Kishimoto T, et al. Catheterized urine cytology of mucinous carcinoma arising in the renal pelvis. A case report. Acta Cytol. 2000;44(3):442–4. Epub 2000/06/02. PubMed PMID: 10834008.
18. Layfield LJ, Jones C, Rowe L, Gopez EV. Institutional review of outside cytology materials: a retrospective analysis of two institutions' experiences. Diagn Cytopathol. 2002;26(1):45–8. Epub 2002/01/10. PubMed PMID: 11782087.
19. Straccia P, Bizzarro T, Fadda G, Pierconti F. Comparison between cytospin and liquid-based cytology in urine specimens classified according to the Paris system for reporting urinary cytology. Cancer Cytopathol. 2016;124(7):519–23. Epub 2016/03/19. doi:10.1002/cncy.21709. PubMed PMID: 26989867.
20. Zardawi IM, Duncan J. Evaluation of a centrifuge method and thin-layer preparation in urine cytology. Acta Cytol. 2003;47(6):1038–42. Epub 2003/12/17. PubMed PMID: 14674075.
21. Wright RG, Halford JA. Evaluation of thin-layer methods in urine cytology. Cytopathology: Official Journal of the British Society for Clinical Cytology. 2001;12(5):306–13. Epub 2001/11/28. PubMed PMID: 11722510.
22. Nicol TL, Kelly D, Reynolds L, Rosenthal DL. Comparison of TriPath thin-layer technology with conventional methods on nongynecologic specimens. Acta Cytol. 2000;44(4):567–75. Epub 2000/08/10. PubMed PMID: 10934950.
23. Halling KC. Vysis UroVysion for the detection of urothelial carcinoma. Expert Rev Mol Diagn. 2003;3 (4):507–19. Epub 2003/07/25. doi:10.1586/14737159.3.4.507. PubMed PMID: 12877389.
24. New clinical data further supports accuracy of the Vysis UroVysion test. Expert Rev Mol Diagn. 2002;2(2):93–4. Epub 2002/04/19. PubMed PMID: 11962341.
25. Gudjonsson S, Isfoss BL, Hansson K, Domanski AM, Warenholt J, Soller W, et al. The value of the UroVysion assay for surveillance of non-muscle-invasive bladder cancer. Eur Urol. 2008;54(2):402–8. Epub 2007/12/18. doi:10.1016/j.eururo.2007.11.051. PubMed PMID: 18082934.
26. Bubendorf L, Piaton E. UroVysion(R) multiprobe FISH in the triage of equivocal urinary cytology cases. Ann Pathol. 2012;32(6):e52–6, 438–43. Epub 2012/12/19. doi:10.1016/j.annpat.2012.09.207. PubMed PMID: 23244486.
27. Denice Smith G, Sangle NA, Wilson A, Chadwick BE, Bentz JS, Gopez EV, et al. A retrospective review of UroVysion fish interpretations over 8.6 years: a major shift in the patient test population. Diagn Cytopathol. 2013;41(5):437–47. Epub 2012/08/07. doi:10.1002/dc.22881. PubMed PMID: 22865746.
28. Nguyen CT, Litt DB, Dolar SE, Ulchaker JC, Jones JS, Brainard JA. Prognostic significance of nondiagnostic molecular changes in urine detected by UroVysion fluorescence in situ hybridization during surveillance for bladder cancer. Urology. 2009;73 (2):347–50. Epub 2008/11/22. doi:10.1016/j.urology.2008.09.042. PubMed PMID: 19022486.
29. Halling KC, Kipp BR. Bladder cancer detection using FISH (UroVysion assay). Adv Anat Pathol. 2008;15 (5):279–86. Epub 2008/08/30. doi:10.1097/PAP.0b013e3181832320. PubMed PMID: 18724101.
30. Mian C, Pycha A, Wiener H, Haitel A, Lodde M, Marberger M. Immunocyt: a new tool for detecting transitional cell cancer of the urinary tract. J Urol. 1999;161(5):1486–9. Epub 1999/04/21. PubMed PMID: 10210378.
31. He H, Han C, Hao L, Zang G. ImmunoCyt test compared to cytology in the diagnosis of bladder cancer: a meta-analysis. Oncol Lett. 2016;12(1):83–8. Epub 2016/06/28. doi:10.3892/ol.2016.4556. PubMed PMID: 27347104; PubMed Central PMCID: PMC4906922.
32. Yang M, Zheng Z, Zhuang Z, Zhao X, Xu Z, Lin H. ImmunoCyt and cytology for diagnosis of bladder carcinoma: a meta analysis. Chin Med J. 2014;127 (4):758–64. Epub 2014/02/19. PubMed PMID: 24534237.
33. Li HX, Li M, Li CL, Ma JH, Wang MR, Rao J, et al. ImmunoCyt and cytokeratin 20 immunocytochemistry as adjunct markers for urine cytologic detection of bladder cancer: a prospective study. Anal Quant Cytol Histol/Int Acad Cytol Am Soc Cytol. 2010;32 (1):45–52. Epub 2010/08/13. PubMed PMID: 20701087.
34. Sarosdy MF, deVere White RW, Soloway MS, Sheinfeld J, Hudson MA, Schellhammer PF, et al. Results of a multicenter trial using the BTA test to monitor for and diagnose recurrent bladder cancer. J Urol. 1995;154(2 Pt 1):379–83; discussion 83–4. Epub 1995/08/01. PubMed PMID: 7609102.
35. Guo A, Wang X, Gao L, Shi J, Sun C, Wan Z. Bladder tumour antigen (BTA stat) test compared to the urine cytology in the diagnosis of bladder cancer: a meta-analysis. Can Urol Assoc J (Journal de l'Association des urologues du Canada). 2014;8(5–6):E347–52. Epub 2014/06/19. doi:10.5489/cuaj.1668. PubMed PMID: 24940462; PubMed Central PMCID: PMC4039599.

36. Soloway MS, Briggman V, Carpinito GA, Chodak GW, Church PA, Lamm DL, et al. Use of a new tumor marker, urinary NMP22, in the detection of occult or rapidly recurring transitional cell carcinoma of the urinary tract following surgical treatment. J Urol. 1996;156(2 Pt 1):363–7. Epub 1996/08/01. PubMed PMID: 8683680.
37. Giannopoulos A, Manousakas T, Mitropoulos D, Botsoli-Stergiou E, Constantinides C, Giannopoulou M, et al. Comparative evaluation of the BTAstat test, NMP22, and voided urine cytology in the detection of primary and recurrent bladder tumors. Urology. 2000;55(6):871–5. Epub 2000/06/07. PubMed PMID: 10840098.
38. Onal B, Han U, Yilmaz S, Koybasioglu F, Altug U. The use of urinary nuclear matrix protein 22 (NMP22) as a diagnostic adjunct to urine cytology for monitoring of recurrent bladder cancer—institutional experience and review. Diagn Cytopathol. 2015;43(4):307–14. Epub 2014/12/10. doi:10.1002/dc.23239. PubMed PMID: 25488052.
39. Al Hussain TO, Akhtar M. Molecular basis of urinary bladder cancer. Adv Anat Pathol. 2013;20(1):53–60. Epub 2012/12/13. doi:10.1097/PAP.0b013e31827bd0ec. PubMed PMID: 23232572.
40. Mhawech-Fauceglia P, Cheney RT, Schwaller J. Genetic alterations in urothelial bladder carcinoma: an updated review. Cancer. 2006;106(6):1205–16. Epub 2006/02/14. doi:10.1002/cncr.21743. PubMed PMID: 16470587.
41. Solomon DA, Kim JS, Waldman T. Cohesin gene mutations in tumorigenesis: from discovery to clinical significance. BMB Rep. 2014;47(6):299–310. Epub 2014/05/27. PubMed PMID: 24856830; PubMed Central PMCID: PMC4163871.
42. Vinagre J, Almeida A, Populo H, Batista R, Lyra J, Pinto V, et al. Frequency of TERT promoter mutations in human cancers. Nat Commun. 2013;4:2185. Epub 2013/07/28. doi:10.1038/ncomms3185. PubMed PMID: 23887589.
43. Kurtis B, Zhuge J, Ojaimi C, Ye F, Cai D, Zhang D, et al. Recurrent TERT promoter mutations in urothelial carcinoma and potential clinical applications. Ann Diagn Pathol. 2016;21:7–11. Epub 2016/04/05. doi:10.1016/j.anndiagpath.2015.12.002. PubMed PMID: 27040924.
44. Huang FW, Hodis E, Xu MJ, Kryukov GV, Chin L, Garraway LA. Highly recurrent TERT promoter mutations in human melanoma. Science. 2013;339(6122):957–9. Epub 2013/01/26. doi:10.1126/science.1229259. PubMed PMID: 23348506; PubMed Central PMCID: PMC4423787.
45. Horn S, Figl A, Rachakonda PS, Fischer C, Sucker A, Gast A, et al. TERT promoter mutations in familial and sporadic melanoma. Science. 2013;339(6122):959–61. Epub 2013/01/26. doi:10.1126/science.1230062. PubMed PMID: 23348503.

10 Pathology of Urothelial Malignancies of the Upper Urinary Tract

Sabina Hajiyeva and Minghao Zhong

Overview of Normal Structure and Urothelial Malignancy from Upper Urinary Tract

The kidneys are the functional unit of the urinary system. Within the kidneys, millions of nephrons maintain body water, salt, and pH balance and eliminate solutes from the blood. The kidneys accomplish these functions by filtering blood plasma into urine, which is eliminated from the body via the upper and lower urinary tract. The upper urinary tract includes calyces, renal pelvis, and ureter; the lower urinary tract includes urinary bladder and urethra. The whole urinary tract is lined by urothelium (previously called transitional epithelium), which rests on a basement membrane. Compared to the lower urinary tract, the upper urinary tract demonstrates significant histoanatomy variation. The ureter (Fig. 10.1a) presents with similar histoanatomy structures: urothelium, laminar propria, muscularis propria, and serosa/adventitia. On the other hand, in the renal sinus and the calyces (Fig. 10.1b), the muscularis is absent to sometimes indiscernible. Urothelium directly contacts with renal parenchyma at renal sinus and minor calyces without subepithelial connective tissue. This distinction determines the different treatment and staging system for urothelial malignancies between upper and lower urinary tract.

Upper urinary tract (UUT) urothelial carcinomas (UC) are defined as malignant urothelial neoplasms involving the urinary tract from the renal calyces to the distal ureter. UC of the renal pelvis and the ureter are relatively uncommon and account for approximately 7–8% of all renal malignancies and only 5% of all urothelial tumors of the urinary tract [1–4]. Tumors affect 0.7 to 1.1/100,000 individuals with a male-to-female incidence of 1.7:1 [1, 2]. The tumors are more common in older individuals with the mean age of incidence of 70 years [1–3]. Ureteral tumors occur about one half as often as tumors located in the renal pelvis. Urothelial carcinoma accounts for more than 95% of urothelial tumors of the upper urinary tract [2, 3]. Upper urinary tract (UUT) urothelial tumors are more common in men, with a male-to-female ratio of 3:1. UUT urothelial tumors are twice as common in white people as in people of African descent. Unlike in bladder cancer in which 80% of tumors are noninvasive, only 40% of upper tract tumors are noninvasive.

Grade and stage are the most important prognostic factors in urothelial carcinoma of the upper tract [5, 6]. The grading system is identical to that applied in the bladder. In 2004, a current

S. Hajiyeva · M. Zhong (✉)
Department of Pathology, Westchester Medical Health Network/New York Medical College, 100 Woods Road, Valhalla, NY 10530, USA
e-mail: Minghao.Zhong@wmchealth.org

S. Hajiyeva
e-mail: sabinanb@gmail.com

M. Eshghi (ed.), *Urothelial Malignancies of the Upper Urinary Tract*,
https://doi.org/10.1007/978-3-319-51263-1_10

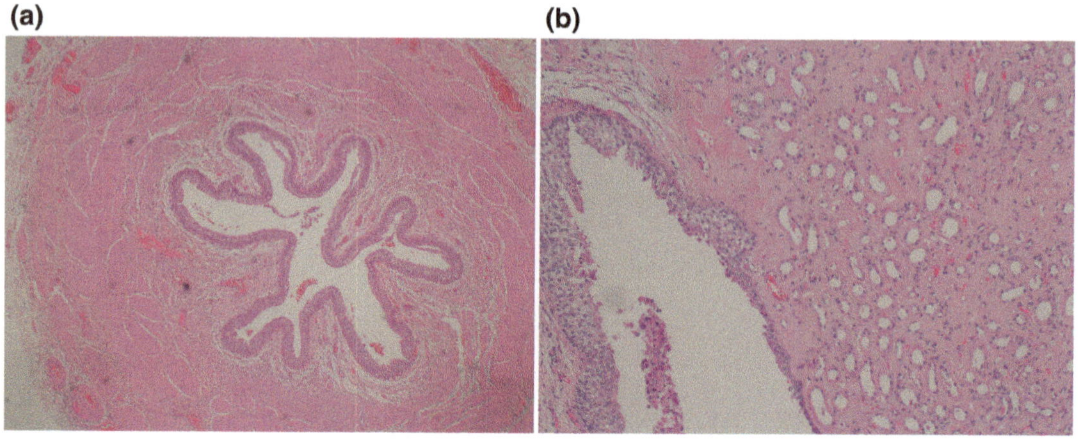

Fig. 10.1 Normal microscopic structure of *upper* urinary tract. **a**, cross section of ureter shows urothelium, lamina propria, muscularis propria, and adventia. **b**. renal pelvis demonstrates the direct contact of urothelium and renal parenchyma without lamina propria or muscularis propria

classification system for noninvasive papillary urothelial neoplasms, identical to the 1998 WHO/ISUP classification system, was adopted in Pathology and Genetics of Tumours of the Urinary System and Male Genital Organs, one of a series of WHO "Blue Books" for the classification of tumors. This new system separates noninvasive papillary urothelial neoplasms into four categories, designated papilloma, papillary urothelial neoplasm of low malignant potential (PUNLMP), low-grade carcinoma, and high-grade carcinoma. The incoming (2016) WHO "Blue Books" will lump PUNLMP and low-grade carcinoma together as low-grade carcinoma. The American Joint Committee on Cancer tumor, node, and metastasis (TNM) staging system has been used extensively and is shown in Table 10.1.

Noninvasive Urothelial Carcinoma

Noninvasive malignancies include (low and high grade) papillary urothelial carcinoma(UC) and urothelial carcinoma in situ (CIS). Low-grade papillary urothelial carcinoma (Fig. 10.2a) features with some degree of cytoarchitectural disorder and distinct but low-grade cytological abnormality. HG-UC (Fig. 10.2b) is characterized by an overall disordered appearance, with both architectural and cytological abnormalities that are recognizable at low-power magnification. Papillae are frequently fused, and neoplastic cells are irregularly clustered and disorganized, with moderate to marked pleomorphism, clumped chromatin, and occasional prominent nucleoli. Mitotic figures, frequently atypical, are seen at all levels of the urothelium [7, 8]. The biopsy specimen of UUT-UC is usually small and superficial which is insufficient for evaluation of invasion [9].

Urothelial carcinoma in situ (CIS) (Fig. 10.2c) is a preinvasive flat lesion comprising malignant cells with nucleomegaly, irregular chromatin distribution/hyperchromatism, pleomorphism, and frequent mitoses [7]. It has the biologic potential for aggressive behavior with a high risk of recurrence and progression to muscle-invasive urothelial carcinoma [10–12]. It is very rare to see isolated CIS in upper urinary tract. CIS of upper urinary tract generally does not induce symptom and get medical attention early. Urothelial carcinoma in situ (CIS) is usually seen to be associated with multifocal UC in bladder or high-grade UC with lateral extension. Additionally, noninvasive urothelial carcinoma with glandular differentiation (previously called adenocarcinoma—in situ) (Fig. 10.2d) has also been described in kidney.

Table 10.1 The American Joint Committee on Cancer tumor, node, and metastasis (TNM) staging system

Primary tumor (T)	
TX	Primary tumor cannot be assessed
T0	No evidence of primary tumor
Ta	Papillary noninvasive carcinoma
Tis	Carcinoma in situ
T1	Tumor invades the subepithelial connective tissue
T2	Tumor invades the muscularis
T3	(For renal pelvis only) tumor invades beyond muscularis into peripelvic fat or the renal parenchyma T3
	(For ureter only) tumor invades beyond muscularis into periureteric fat
T4	Tumor invades adjacent organs or through the kidney into the perirenal fat
Regional lymph nodes (N)*	
NX	Regional lymph nodes cannot be assessed
N0	No regional lymph node metastasis
N1	Metastasis in a single lymph node ≤2 cm in greatest dimension
N2	Metastasis in a single lymph node >2 cm but not >5 cm in greatest dimension; or in multiple lymph nodes, none >5 cm in greatest dimension
N3	Metastasis in a lymph node, >5 cm in greatest dimension
Distant metastasis (M)	
M0	No distant metastasis
M1	Distant metastasis

Upper Urinary Tract Urothelial Carcinoma with Intratubular Spread

Urothelial carcinoma with intratubular spread (retrograde spread within renal tubules) is well-known and peculiar histopathological finding in UUT-UC. It is fairly common phenomenon in UUT-UC and is associated with a variety of clinical-pathological features. High-grade UUT-UC tends to have more extensive intratubular spread and secondary invasion into renal parenchyma. Based on histopathological patterns, intratubular spread has been classified into four different types (Table 10.2): pagetoid, typical, florid, and secondary invasion from intratubular spread [13]. The example of four different types of intratubular spread with the cocktail stain of p63, PAX8, and PAS is shown in (Fig. 10.3).

Invasive Urothelial Carcinoma

By definition, invasion is that carcinoma has penetrated the basement membrane and invaded into the lamina propria or deeper tissue. It can arise anywhere in upper urinary tract. Due to the significant histoanatomy variation which was discussed earlier, different staging systems (Table 10.1) are used for upper and lower urinary tract. Please note that there is no T1 or T2 in some invasive UC at renal pelvis, due to the absence of lamina propria and muscularis propria in this area. Poor fixation of large and friable tumors and processing artifacts may cause the difficulties in accurate staging. Another important staging issue is that UC invading to peripelvic or periureteric fat is considered as T3 disease; UC invading to perirenal fat is considered as T4 disease. Therefore, carefully dissecting and sampling are crucial for this matter [6, 10, 14–16].

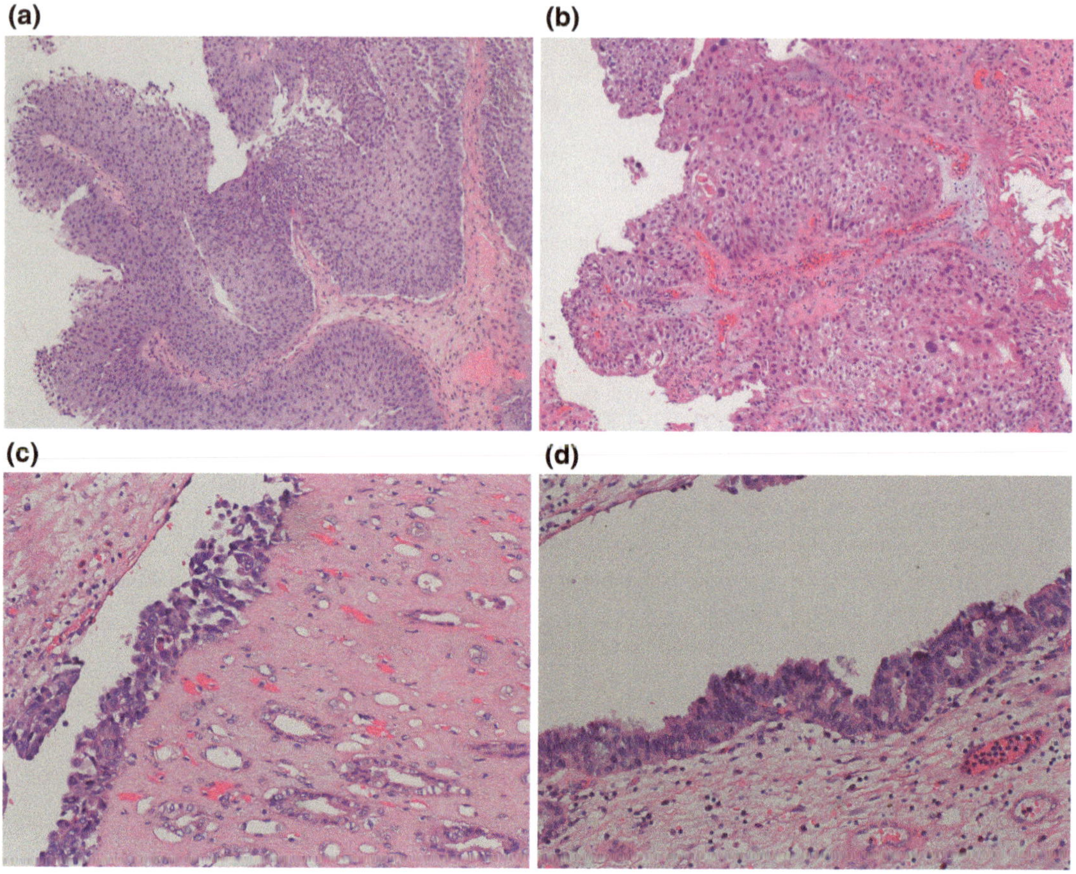

Fig. 10.2 Noninvasive urothelial carcinoma. **a** Low-grade papillary urothelial carcinoma **b** High-grade papillary urothelial carcinoma **c** Urothelial carcinoma in situ **d** Noninvasive urothelial carcinoma with glandular differentiation

Table 10.2 Pathological features of different types of intratubular spread of UUT-UC

Type	Location	# of tubules involvement	Recognizable on H&E	Architecture	Association of grade	Association of invasion
Typical	Close to calyx	Few	Yes	Tubular, pseudoglandular	High/low	Invasion and noninvasion
Pagetoid	Close to calyx	Few	Maybe	Pagetoid, few cells	High/low	Invasion and noninvasion
Florid	Extended to medulla/cortex junction	More than 10	Yes	Pseudoglandular, solid nest with smooth contour	High	Invasion
Invasion from tubular spread	May reach cortex	Multi-foci, more than 10 on each focus	Yes	Solid nest with irregular contour	High	Invasion

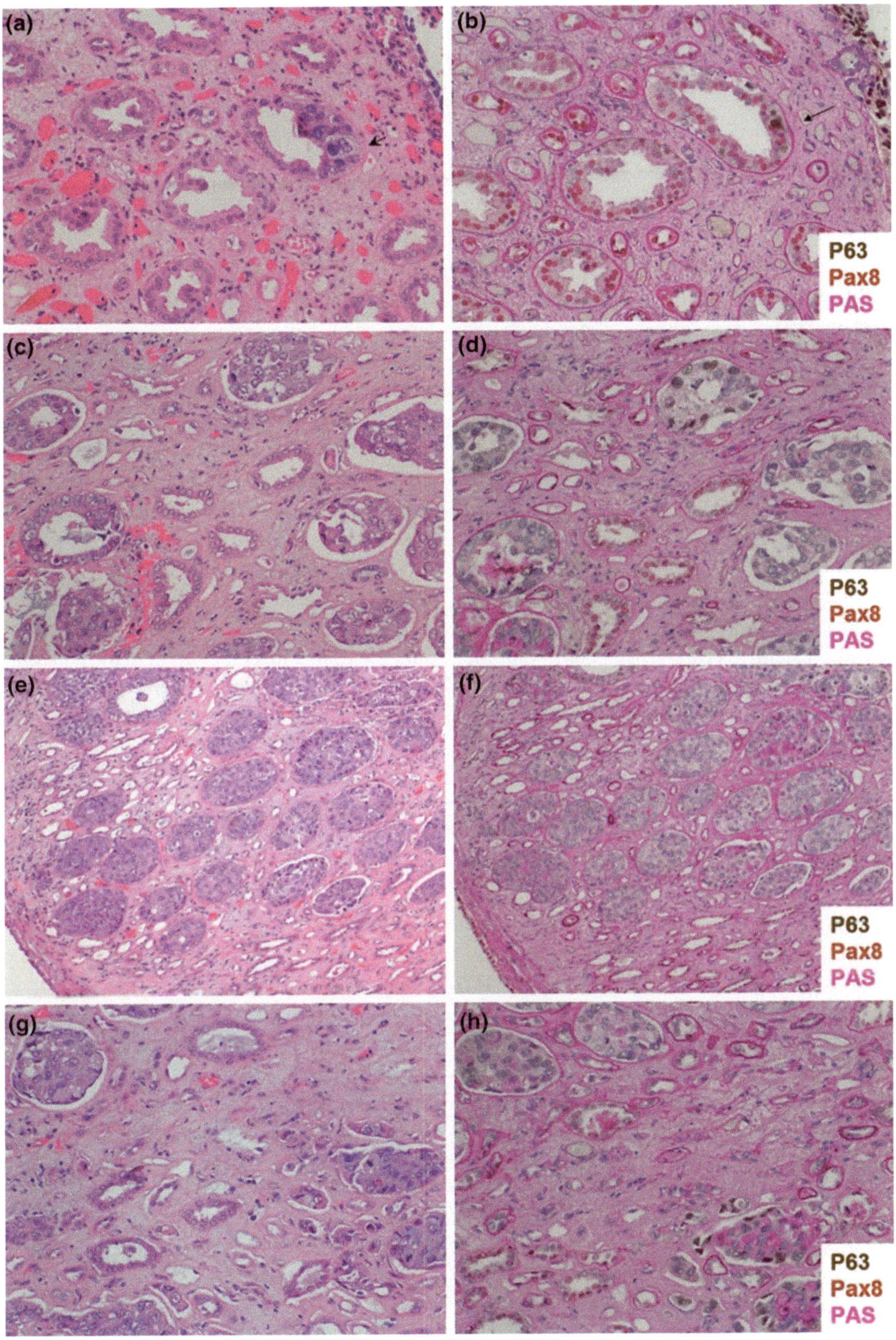
(a)
(b)
P63
Pax8
PAS
(c)
(d)
P63
Pax8
PAS
(e)
(f)
P63
Pax8
PAS
(g)
(h)
P63
Pax8
PAS

◀ **Fig. 10.3** Histopathological features and cocktail stains of 4 different types intratubular spreading (IS). **a,b** Pagetoid IS. The involved tubules contain predominantly renal tubule cells with only a few urothelial carcinoma cells. The renal tubules maintain the usual morphology without dramatic distortion or expansion. **c,d** Classical IS. The involved tubules are extended and contain predominantly urothelial carcinoma cells with the architecture ranging from tubular, pseudoglandular to solid nest and some showing contraction effect around the smooth renal tubular space. **e,f**: Florid IS. The involved tubules are significantly enlarged and exclusively occupied by urothelial carcinoma with solid nest pattern and smooth contour. **g,h**: Secondary invasion from IS compose of both noninvasive IS and invasive component. The invasive component is usually single cell or small cluster cells with irregular contour and desmoplastic reaction. **b, d, f** and **h**: Are cocktail stain (*brown*: P63; *Red*: Pax8 and PAS stain) of corresponding IS

Histologically, majority of invasive UC is classical urothelial morphology. Owning to the morphologic plasticity of UC, different differentiation components are quit common in high-grade UC. Distinguishing differentiation components may have clinical significance [17–19]. Additionally, those differentiations can be very extensive and need to be distinguished from pure carcinoma (such as, squamous, adenocarcinoma), which are rare.

UC with squamous differentiation (Fig. 10.4a) is the most common variant and usually associated with calculi, urinary catheter, chronic infection, and congenital defect (horseshoe kidney, et al.). The histopathology of this tumor is similar to that of UC with squamous differentiation in the bladder [20, 21]. Generous sampling and ruling out classical urothelial morphology are necessary for diagnosis of pure squamous cell carcinoma (SCC). SCC also should be distinguished from metastatic squamous cell carcinoma, which usually is straightforward when clinical and pathologic features are considered.

UC with glandular differentiation (Fig. 10.4b) is the second most common form of divergent differentiation. The diagnosis of primary adenocarcinoma should only be made when a tumor exhibits pure (100%) glandular differentiation. Urothelial carcinoma with glandular differentiation is the preferred term for a lesion that exhibits a mixture of typical urothelial carcinoma and adenocarcinoma. In addition to metastatic adenocarcinoma, renal cell carcinoma, particularly, collecting duct carcinoma should be distinguished from UC with glandular differentiation at kidney [19, 21].

High-grade UC is well known for sarcomatoid differentiation (Fig. 10.4d), which is the third most common differentiation variant. On the other hand, renal cell carcinoma also has been associated with sarcomatoid differentiation [22]. In this situation, identification of relative low-grade carcinoma component and IHC stains is essential for the accurate diagnosis. The spindle cell sarcoma is the most common form of sarcomatoid differentiation; osteosarcoma, chondrosarcoma, and leiomyosarcoma are also reported.

UC with small cell differentiation (Fig. 10.4c) is the least common differentiation variant. In fact, small cell carcinoma component is frequently found in conjunction with conventional urothelial carcinoma and/or other histologic variants: squamous and glandular differentiation [23, 24].

In addition to UC with different differentiation components, histologic variants of UC are also reported [25–27]. These include: nested, invasive micropapillary (Fig. 10.4e), plasmacytoid (Fig. 10.4f), lymphoepithelima-like, microcystic variants.

Renal cell carcinoma, much more common in kidney than urothelial carcinoma, is not in the scope of discussion in this book and should be always in the differential diagnosis. Furthermore, malignant involvement of upper GU tract may occur by direct local extension or metastasis, such as cervix, prostate, or bladder, breast, and colon.

Other Non-Urothelial Malignancy

Several other rare malignant entities [28–31] in UUT may mimic urothelial carcinoma. Urologist and pathologist should be aware of the existence of these entities.

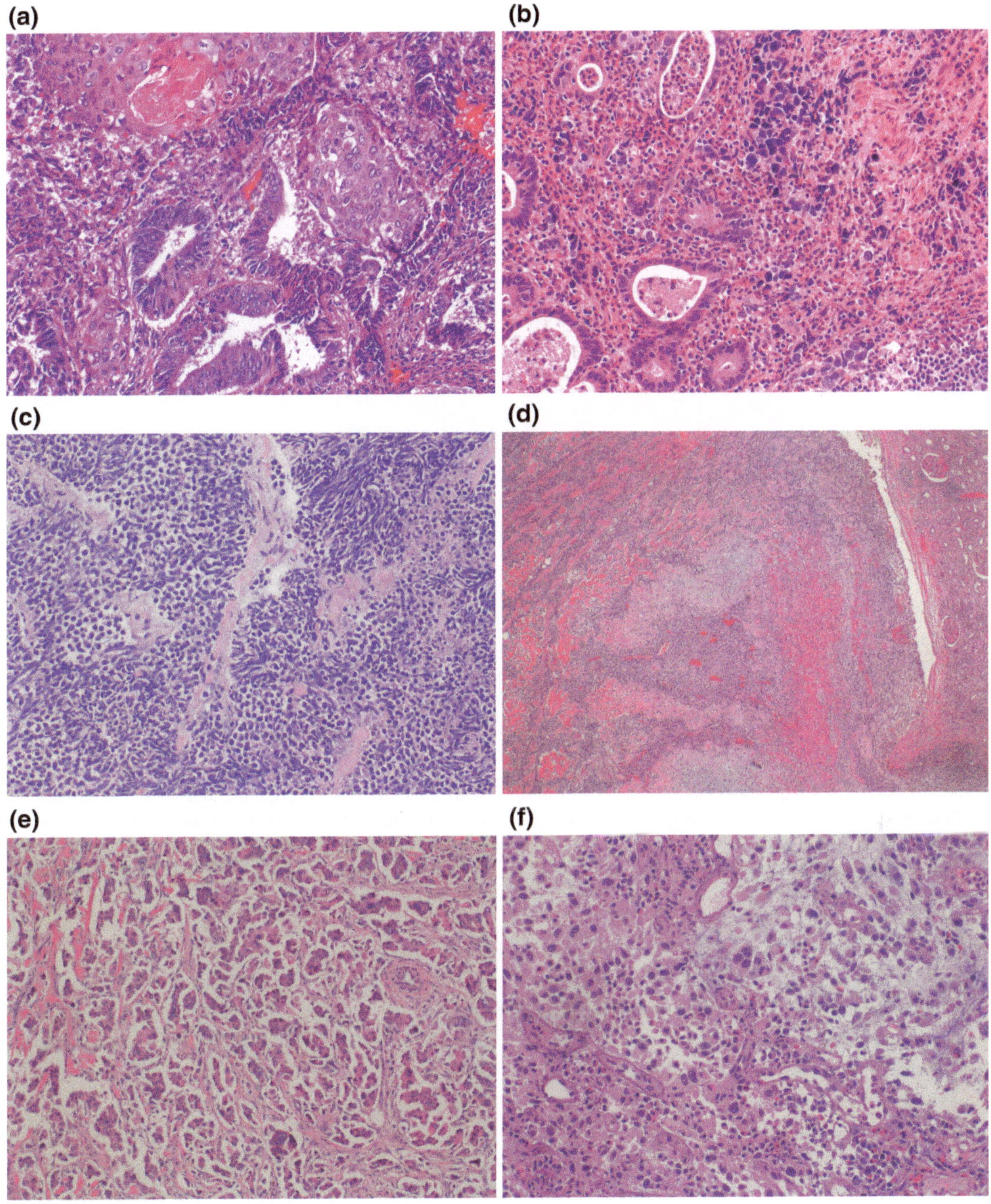

Fig. 10.4 Invasive urothelial carcinoma with different differentiation components and histological variants. **a** UC with both squamous and glandular differentiation; **b** UC with glandular differentiation; **c** UC with small cell differentiation; **d** UC with sarcomatoid differentiation (both osteosarcoma and chondrosarcoma components) **e** invasive micropapillary UC **f** plasmacytoid UC

Inflammatory myofibroblastic tumor (IMT) (Fig. 10.5a) of the UUT is extremely rare and only a few case reports are available in the literature. IMT of the kidney and the renal mass, in many patients, was discovered incidentally. Clinical examination and radiological

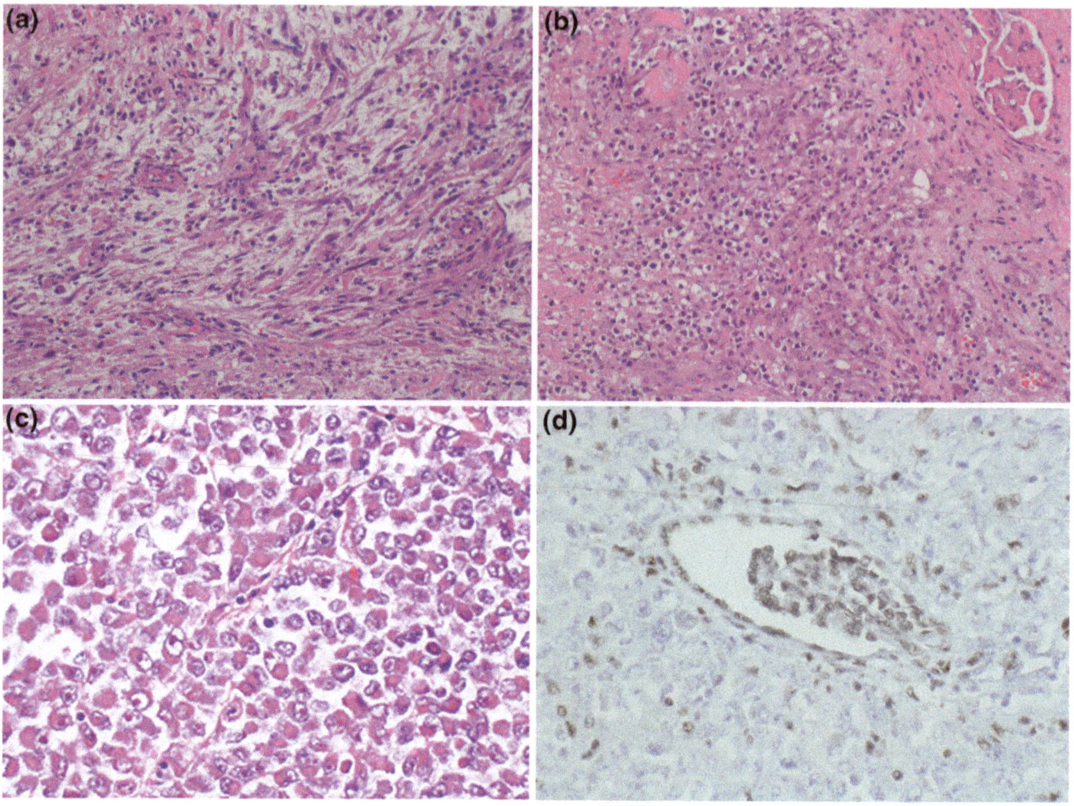

Fig. 10.5 Other non-urothelial malignancy in upper urinary tract. **a** Inflammatory myofibroblastic tumor (IMT) shows plump spindle cells with lymphoplasmacytic infiltration; **b** Diffuse large B-cell lymphoma of kidney shows renal parenchyma with large atypical lymphocytes which may mimic high-grade urothelial carcinoma; **c** Rhabdoid tumor (RT) of the kidney is characterized with *pink* cytoplasm, eccentric nuclei and intracytoplasmic inclusions of eosinophilic hyaline globules. This may mimic sarcomatoid or plasmacytoid urothelial carcinoma. **d** loss of INI1 expression is one of diagnosis criteria for RT

investigations are often inconclusive. Histologically, a proliferation of spindle cells with elongated eosinophilic cytoplasmic processes in a loose edematous or myxoid background is seen. The nuclei may be large with occasional atypia. Occasional mitotic figures are seen, none of which is atypical. The inflammatory background is prominent and usually is lymphoplasmacytic infiltrate. Some lesions have infiltrates of eosinophils or neutrophils. Pancytokeratin reactivity, which may be patchy, is seen in many cases of inflammatory myofibroblastic tumor. Recognizing this spindle cell lesion and differentiating them from sarcomatoid carcinoma is important because these two diagnostic categories have differing therapeutic and prognostic implications.

Lymphoma (Fig. 10.5b) may occur in the UUT as a primary lesion or as part of a systemic disease. Diffuse large B-cell lymphoma (DLBCL) is the single most frequent histologic subtype. It can mimic poorly differentiated carcinoma at histological level. Additionally, portion of DLBCL cells can be positive for P63 which can lead the misdiagnosis of UC. However, DLBCL are always negative for CK stain. Therefore, careful morphology evaluation and IHC panel examination (not single IHC) are essential for an accurate diagnosis.

Rhabdoid tumor of the kidney (Fig. 10.5c) is a rare, highly aggressive malignancy of early childhood, closely related to atypical teratoid/rhabdoid tumor (AT/RT) of the brain.

Local symptoms and signs include haematuria and loin/flank mass. Additionally, patients may develop hypercalcemia secondary to elevated parathormone levels. The term "rhabdoid" stems from the histologic appearance, pink cytoplasm with eccentric nuclei due to intracytoplasmic inclusions of eosinophilic hyaline globules, which resembles that of a tumor of skeletal muscle origin. All rhabdoid tumors share deletions in the long arm of chromosome 22, mapped to the INI1 gene. Loss of INI1 IHC stain (Fig. 10.5d) has been used to confirm the diagnosis of rhabdoid tumor.

Non-Neoplastic, Tumor-like Conditions

Ureteropelvic junction (UPJ) obstruction (Fig. 10.6a) is defined as an obstruction of the flow of urine from the renal pelvis to the proximal ureter. The condition is frequently encountered by both adult and pediatric population [31, 32], is the most common cause of neonatal and antenatal hydronephrosis. Most patients with UPJ obstruction presented with pain, hematuria, urosepsis, failure to thrive, or a palpable mass, which may mimic UC, clinically. The UPJ obstruction area is usually inflamed and markedly thickened due to varying degrees of perifascicular fibrosis and/or muscular hypertrophy.

Immunoglobulin G4-related kidney disease (Fig. 10.6b) usually affects middle-aged or elderly patients and shows a definite male predominance (73–90%), which is similar in patients with IgG4-SD involving other organs [33–35]. The disease in kidney manifests most commonly as tubulointerstitial nephritis, followed by glomerular disease such as membranous glomerulonephritis. Other less frequent conditions, including IgG4-related chronic sclerosing pyelitis, IgG4-related plasma-cell arteritis, and IgG4-related inflammatory pseudotumors of the ureter, have also been reported. The key histologic findings of IgG4-KD are dense lymphoplasmacytic infiltration with increased IgG4-positive plasma cells, and storiform fibrosis, both of which are identical to the findings of IgG4-SD involving other organs. In addition, the characteristic microscopic features of IgG4-related tubulointerstitial nephritis are nests of inflammatory cells with irregular fibers surrounding them, and immune complex deposition in the tubular basement membrane. Fibro epithelial tumor is a perdunculated benign lesion seen mostly in the ureter.

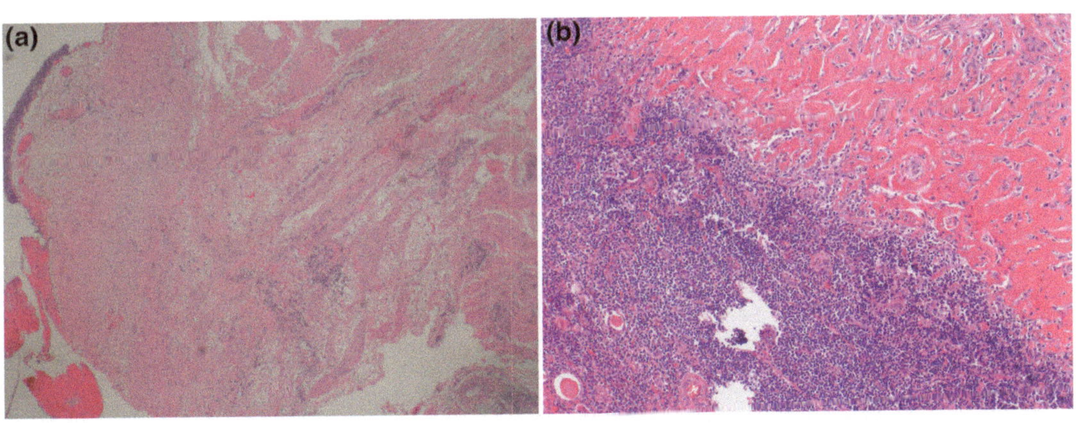

Fig. 10.6 Non-neoplastic, tumor-like conditions. **a** Ureteropelvic junction (UPJ) obstruction shows submucosal fibrosis and muscularis propria hypertyophy: **b** Immunoglobulin G4-related kidney disease shows dense lymphoplasmacytic infiltration and extensive fibrosis and sclerosis, IgG4 positive plasma cells were increase. Both condition are benign and may cause mass formation mimicking urothelial carcinoma

Summary Box

- Compare to the lower urinary tract, the upper urinary tract demonstrates significant histoanatomy variation.
- The upper urinary tract may be involved by distinct entities which have different prognosis and diverse treatment options.
- Urothelial carcinoma with intratubular spread (retrograde spread within renal tubules) is well-known and peculiar histopathological finding in UUT-UC.
- Several other rare malignant entities in UUT may mimic urothelial carcinoma.
- Non-neoplastic, tumor-like conditions may mimic urothelial carcinoma both clinically and pathologically

References

1. Melzer M, Braf Z, Beyar H, Rakowszczyk M. Primary tumors of the renal pelvis and ureter. Int Surg. 1972;57(9):699–702 Epub 1972/09/01.
2. Patel N, Arya M, Muneer A, Powles T, Sullivan M, Hines J, et al. Molecular aspects of upper tract urothelial carcinoma. Urologic oncology. 2014;32 (1):28 e11-20 Epub 2013/02/23. doi:10.1016/j.urolonc.2012.10.002. PubMed PMID: 23428541.
3. Green DA, Rink M, Xylinas E, Matin SF, Stenzl A, Roupret M, et al. Urothelial carcinoma of the bladder and the upper tract: disparate twins. J Urology. 2013;189(4):1214–21. Epub 2012/10/02. doi:10.1016/j.juro.2012.05.079. PubMed PMID: 23023150.
4. Azemar MD, Comperat E, Richard F, Cussenot O, Roupret M. Bladder recurrence after surgery for upper urinary tract urothelial cell carcinoma: frequency, risk factors, and surveillance. Urologic Oncology. 2011;29(2):130–6. Epub 2009/09/19. doi:10.1016/j.urolonc.2009.06.003. PubMed PMID: 19762256.
5. Leow JJ, Orsola A, Chang SL, Bellmunt J. A contemporary review of management and prognostic factors of upper tract urothelial carcinoma. Cancer Treatment Rev. 2015;41(4):310–9. Epub 2015/03/05. doi:10.1016/j.ctrv.2015.02.006. PubMed PMID: 25736461.
6. Cosentino M, Palou J, Gaya JM, Breda A, Rodriguez-Faba O, Villavicencio-Mavrich H. Upper urinary tract urothelial cell carcinoma: location as a predictive factor for concomitant bladder carcinoma. World J Urology. 2013;31(1):141–5. Epub 2012/05/04. doi:10.1007/s00345-012-0877-2. PubMed PMID: 22552732.
7. Hofstadter F, Delgado R, Jakse G, Judmaier W. Urothelial dysplasia and carcinoma in situ of the bladder. Cancer. 1986;57(2):356–61 Epub 1986/01/15.
8. Humphrey PA. Urothelial carcinoma in situ of the bladder. J Urology. 2012;187(3):1057–8. Epub 2012/01/24. doi:10.1016/j.juro.2011.12.020. PubMed PMID: 22265997.
9. Rojas CP, Castle SM, Llanos CA, Santos Cortes JA, Bird V, Rodriguez S, et al. Low biopsy volume in ureteroscopy does not affect tumor biopsy grading in upper tract urothelial carcinoma. Urologic Oncology. 2013;31(8):1696–700. Epub 2012/07/24. doi:10.1016/j.urolonc.2012.05.010. PubMed PMID: 22819696.
10. Mazzucchelli R, Scarpelli M, Galosi AB, Di Primio R, Lopez-Beltran A, Cheng L, et al. Pathology of upper tract urothelial carcinoma with emphasis on staging. Int J Immunopath Pharmacol. 2014;27 (4):509–16 Epub 2015/01/13.
11. Gillan A, El-Mokadem I, Rai B, Lang S, Alcorn J, Shams Ud Din A, et al. Carcinoma in situ is significantly underdetected by prenephroureterectomy ureteroscopy in the management of upper tract urothelial cancers. BioMed Res Int. 2015;2015:547586. Epub 2015/02/06. doi:10.1155/2015/547586. PubMed PMID: 25654112; PubMed Central PMCID: PMC4310489.
12. Otto W, Shariat SF, Fritsche HM, Gupta A, Matsumoto K, Kassouf W, et al. Concomitant carcinoma in situ as an independent prognostic parameter for recurrence and survival in upper tract urothelial carcinoma: a multicenter analysis of 772 patients. World J Urology. 2011;29(4):487–94. Epub 2011/01/21. doi:10.1007/s00345-011-0645-8. PubMed PMID: 21249372.
13. Sarungbam J, Kurtis B, Phillips J, Cai D, Zhang D, Humayun I, et al. Upper urinary tract urothelial carcinoma with intratubular spread. Am J Clini Experimental urology. 2014;2(2):102–10. Epub 2014/11/07. PubMed PMID: 25374911; PubMed Central PMCID: PMC4219305.
14. Gupta R, Paner GP, Amin MB. Neoplasms of the upper urinary tract: a review with focus on urothelial carcinoma of the pelvicalyceal system and aspects related to its diagnosis and reporting. Advances in Anatomic Pathology. 2008;15(3):127–39. Epub 2008/04/25. doi:10.1097/PAP.0b013e31817145a9. PubMed PMID: 18434765.
15. Raman JD, Ng CK, Scherr DS, Margulis V, Lotan Y, Bensalah K, et al. Impact of tumor location on prognosis for patients with upper tract urothelial carcinoma managed by radical nephroureterectomy. European Urology. 2010;57(6):1072–9. Epub 2009/07/22. doi:10.1016/j.eururo.2009.07.002. PubMed PMID: 19619934.
16. Yates DR, Catto JW. Distinct patterns and behaviour of urothelial carcinoma with respect to anatomical location: how molecular biomarkers can augment clinico-pathological predictors in upper urinary tract tumours. W J Urology. 2013;31(1):21–9. Epub 2012/09/19. doi:10.1007/s00345-012-0946-6. PubMed PMID: 22986906.

17. Sakano S, Matsuyama H, Kamiryo Y, Hayashida S, Yamamoto N, Kaneda Y, et al. Impact of variant histology on disease aggressiveness and outcome after nephroureterectomy in Japanese patients with upper tract urothelial carcinoma. Int J Clini Oncology. 2015;20(2):362–8. Epub 2014/06/27. doi:10.1007/s10147-014-0721-3. PubMed PMID: 24964974.
18. Hsieh MC, Sung MT, Chiang PH, Huang CH, Tang Y, Su YL. The Prognostic Impact of Histopathological Variants in Patients with Advanced Urothelial Carcinoma. PloS one. 2015;10(6):e0129268. Epub 2015/06/27. doi:10.1371/journal.pone.0129268. PubMed PMID: 26114748; PubMed Central PMCID: PMC4482548.
19. Rink M, Robinson BD, Green DA, Cha EK, Hansen J, Comploj E, et al. Impact of histological variants on clinical outcomes of patients with upper urinary tract urothelial carcinoma. J urology. 2012;188(2):398–404. Epub 2012/06/16. doi:10.1016/j.juro.2012.04.009. PubMed PMID: 22698626.
20. Makise N, Morikawa T, Kawai T, Nakagawa T, Kume H, Homma Y, et al. Squamous differentiation and prognosis in upper urinary tract urothelial carcinoma. International journal of clinical and experimental pathology. 2015;8(6):7203–9. Epub 2015/08/12. PubMed PMID: 26261615; PubMed Central PMCID: PMC4525949.
21. Lee YJ, Moon KC, Jeong CW, Kwak C, Kim HH, Ku JH. Impact of squamous and glandular differentiation on oncologic outcomes in upper and lower tract urothelial carcinoma. PloS one. 2014;9(9):e107027. Epub 2014/09/06. doi:10.1371/journal.pone.0107027. PubMed PMID: 25191845; PubMed Central PMCID: PMC4156382.
22. Shanks JH, Iczkowski KA. Divergent differentiation in urothelial carcinoma and other bladder cancer subtypes with selected mimics. Histopathology. 2009;54(7):885–900. Epub 2009/01/31. doi:10.1111/j.1365-2559.2008.03167.x. PubMed PMID: 19178589.
23. Ouzzane A, Ghoneim TP, Udo K, Verhasselt-Crinquette M, Puech P, Betrouni N, et al. Small cell carcinoma of the upper urinary tract (UUT-SCC): report of a rare entity and systematic review of the literature. Cancer Treatment Rev. 2011;37(5):366–72. Epub 2011/01/25. doi:10.1016/j.ctrv.2010.12.005. PubMed PMID: 21257269.
24. Koga F, Yokoyama M, Fukushima H. Small cell carcinoma of the urinary bladder: a contemporary review with a special focus on bladder-sparing treatments. Expert Rev anticancer therapy. 2013;13(11):1269–79. Epub 2013/10/31. doi:10.1586/14737140.2013.851605. PubMed PMID: 24168010.
25. Loghin A, Chibelean C, Orsolya M, Nechifor-Boila A, Borda A. Micropapillary urothelial carcinoma: an aggressive variant of urothelial carcinoma. Romanian journal of morphology and embryology =. Revue roumaine de morphologie et embryologie. 2014;55(3):939–45 Epub 2014/10/21.
26. Porten SP, Willis D, Kamat AM. Variant histology: role in management and prognosis of nonmuscle invasive bladder cancer. Current Opinion Urology. 2014;24(5):517–23. Epub 2014/06/13. doi:10.1097/MOU.0000000000000089. PubMed PMID: 24921905.
27. Venyo AK. Nested variant of urothelial carcinoma. Advances in urology. 2014;2014:192720. Epub 2014/03/04. doi:10.1155/2014/192720. PubMed PMID: 24587796; PubMed Central PMCID: PMC3920611.
28. Montgomery EA, Shuster DD, Burkart AL, Esteban JM, Sgrignoli A, Elwood L, et al. Inflammatory myofibroblastic tumors of the urinary tract: a clinicopathologic study of 46 cases, including a malignant example inflammatory fibrosarcoma and a subset associated with high-grade urothelial carcinoma. Am J Sur Pathology. 2006;30(12):1502–12. Epub 2006/11/24. doi:10.1097/01.pas.0000213280.35413.1b. PubMed PMID: 17122505.
29. Bozas G, Tassidou A, Moulopoulos LA, Constandinidis C, Bamias A, Dimopoulos MA. Non-Hodgkin's lymphoma of the renal pelvis. Clini Lymphoma Myeloma. 2006;6(5):404–6. Epub 2006/04/28. doi:10.3816/CLM.2006.n.018. PubMed PMID: 16640818.
30. Vujanic GM, Sandstedt B, Harms D, Boccon-Gibod L, Delemarre JF. Rhabdoid tumour of the kidney: a clinicopathological study of 22 patients from the International Society of Paediatric Oncology (SIOP) nephroblastoma file. Histopathology. 1996;28(4):333–40 Epub 1996/04/01.
31. Hu G, Luo M, Xu Y. Giant hydronephrosis secondary to ureteropelvic junction obstruction in adults: report of a case and review of literatures. Int J clini Experimental Med. 2015;8(3):4715–7. Epub 2015/06/13. PubMed PMID: 26064410; PubMed Central PMCID: PMC4443244.
32. Khan F, Ahmed K, Lee N, Challacombe B, Khan MS, Dasgupta P. Management of ureteropelvic junction obstruction in adults. Nature Rev Urology. 2014;11(11):629–38. Epub 2014/10/08. doi:10.1038/nrurol.2014.240. PubMed PMID: 25287785.
33. Lei WH, Xin J, Shao CX, Mao MF, Zhu CY, Wu CF, et al. IgG4-related kidney disease mimicking malignant ureter tumor: case report and literature review. Medicine. 2016;95(3):e2550. Epub 2016/01/29. doi:10.1097/MD.0000000000002550. PubMed PMID: 26817905; PubMed Central PMCID: PMC4998279.
34. Divatia M, Kim SA, Ro JY. IgG4-related sclerosing disease, an emerging entity: a review of a multi-system disease. Yonsei medical journal. 2012;53(1):15–34. Epub 2011/12/22. doi:10.3349/ymj.2012.53.1.15. PubMed PMID: 22187229; PubMed Central PMCID: PMC3250325.
35. Nishi S, Imai N, Yoshida K, Ito Y, Saeki T. Clinicopathological findings of immunoglobulin G4-related kidney disease. Clini Experimental nephrology. 2011;15(6):810–9. Epub 2011/08/27. doi:10.1007/s10157-011-0526-x. PubMed PMID: 21870078.

Part III

Operative Techniques and Outcomes

Characteristics of Semirigid and Flexible Ureteroscopes for Upper Tract Tumors

11

Arash Akhavein and Manoj Monga

Introduction

At the dawn of nineteenth century, Bozzini invented the first endoscope for the examinations of the canals and cavities of the human body [1]. Endoscopic visualization of the upper urinary tract was described in early twentieth century by Hugh Hampton Young, who passed a pediatric cystoscope into the ureter of a child with posterior urethral valves. By late 1950s fiberoptics were incorporated in endoscopy. This allowed replacement of the optical rod lens systems in "rigid" ureteroscopes with more flexible optical fibers leading to development of "semirigid" scopes which can be gently bent for navigation through the urethra and the ureter. Marshall reported the first use of optical fibers in ureteroscopy in 1964 [2]. The ureteroscopic approach to tumors was first described by Goodman in 1984 [3]. Today both non-flexible (semirigid) and flexible (optical or digital) ureteroscopes are commonly utilized in diagnosis, management, and surveillance of upper urinary tract tumors.

A. Akhavein (✉) · M. Monga
Glickman Urological and Kidney Institute,
Cleveland Clinic, Cleveland, OH, USA
e-mail: akhavea@ccf.org

A. Akhavein
Cedar Sinai Medical Center, Los Angeles, CA, USA

Semirigid Ureteroscopes

The basic elements of a semirigid ureteroscope (SRU) include the containing metallic tube, the relay lens system, the light delivery system (typically optical fiber), the irrigation and working channels, and the eyepiece which can be attached to a video camera. The application of the SRU in management of upper tract urothelial carcinomas (UTUCs) involves mainly the distal and some lower mid ureteral tumors.

Commonly Utilized SRUS

Most commonly available SRUs are 33–43 cm in length. The outer diameter of most scopes is tapered and is narrowest at the tip, usually around 6.9–7.5 French (Fr) depending on the manufacturer and the model. The shape of the tip also varies to some degree between these models and usually is beveled in a way to protect the ureteral orifice from trauma upon entry. They most commonly incorporate two channels: one with smaller caliber usually used to run the irrigation fluid (approximately 2.5 Fr) and the other one used as a dedicated working channel for instruments and laser fibers (~3.5 Fr). Richard Wolf offers an ultrathin SRU (4.5 Fr) with narrower caliber (e.g., "Needle" ureteroscope). The manufacturer-reported physical characteristics of some commonly available SRUs are summarized in Table 11.1.

M. Eshghi (ed.), *Urothelial Malignancies of the Upper Urinary Tract*,
https://doi.org/10.1007/978-3-319-51263-1_11

Table 11.1 Commonly used semirigid ureteroscopes

Brand	Model	Lens angle (°)	Working length (cm)	Diameter (tip/base) (Fr)	Working channels	Working channel diameter (Fr)
Gyrus ACMI	MR-6A/MR-6LA	5	33/41	6.9/10.2	2	3.4 + 2.3
Olympus	OES Pro	7	33/43	6.4/7.8	1	4.2
	OES 4000 Double	7	33/43	7.5	2	3.4 + 2.4
	WA29042	7	43	8.6/9.8	1	6.4
Richard Wolf	8702	5	33/43	6/7.5	1	4
	8708 "DOC"	5	33/43	6.5/8.5	2	4 + 2.4
	8701 ("Needle")	5	31.5/43	4.5/6.5	1	3
Karl Storz	27000 L/K	6	43/34	6.5/9.9	1	4.8 (Max 4 Fr instrument)
	27001 L/K	6	43/34	7/12	1	5 (Max 4 Fr instrument)
	27002 L/K	6	43/34	8/12	1	6 (Max 4 Fr instrument)
	27003 L	6	43	9.5/12	2	(Simultaneous 2 and 3 Fr instruments)
Stryker	SRU-6X	6	33/43	6.9/10	2	3.4 + 2.5

Flexible Ureteroscopes (Ureterorenoscopes)

Flexible ureteroscope applications transitioned from diagnostic to therapeutic in the mid-1990s. The flexible endoscope is more versatile at maneuvering the angulated and curved course of the ureters proximal to the iliac vessels and pelvic inlet. As mentioned earlier, tumors that are located above the distal ureter may not be routinely accessed via a semirigid ureteroscope in a safe and reliable manner, in particular in male patients.

Deflection of the Scope Tip

Flexible ureteroscopes can passively follow the curved course of the ureter and also have a thumb-controlled active deflection mechanism that allows directing of the tip of the scope toward the desired direction in a single plane. Most flexible ureteroscopes provide a single active deflection mechanism with about 180–275° of turning of the tip. All scopes are available with active deflection in an "intuitive" (American) orientation, meaning the tip of the scope turns to the same direction the lever is pushed, or in a reverse deflection mechanism (European), with the tip of the scope turning up when the lever is pushed down and vice versa.

In addition to active tip deflection, some flexible scopes have a "softer" passive deflection area at a short distance from the tip, allowing secondary turning and navigation of multiple angles using both active and passive deflection. Gyrus ACMI (now a subsidiary of Olympus, Center Valley, PA) and Stryker (Stryker, San Jose, CA) have provided flexible ureteroscope models with a secondary active (dual-lever) deflection mechanism.

Flexible Ureteroscope Tip Design

The shape and configuration of the tip of the flexible ureteroscopes vary. Some flexible scopes feature a beveled tip design which facilitates self-dilation of the ureteral orifice and ureter when the scope is advanced (e.g., Richard Wolf Viper and Karl Storz Flex-X^2 among others). The configuration of tips is different among respective makes and models as well. It is important for the operator to be aware of the relationship of the location of working channel(s) with respect to the position of the image-acquiring unit (optic bundle/video chip) and thus the center of the image, to know where the instruments or laser fiber would exit when passed out of the scope tip. Flexible ureteroscopes that feature a rotating shaft (e.g., Olympus URF-P5 and URF-P6) allow for relative ease in adjusting the location of the instrument or laser fiber around the target for better and safer access, alleviating the need for actual manual rotation of the entire scope handle by the operator. Lastly, the field of view of the lens is critical as this will impact the perceived size of a stone or lesion on the video monitor; when switching from one scope to another it is important to be cognizant of this change.

Optical Fiber and Distal Sensor Digital Ureteroscope

Both optical fiber "conventional" flexible ureteroscopes and newer "digital" flexible scopes are commercially available. The digital ureteroscopes utilize a CCD (charge-coupled device) or CMOS (complementary metal-oxide semiconductor) "camera" chip at the tip of the scope which generates the image, thus obviating the need for a bulky camera head while providing higher resolution as will be discussed below. Digital ureterorenoscopes routinely utilize illuminating LEDs (light emitting diodes) at the tip of the scope next to the CMOS/CCD as well, which allows elimination of bulky illumination fibers and therefore leading to a narrower diameter of the scope. Table 11.2 summarizes the physical properties of commonly available flexible ureteroscopes, both conventional fiberoptic and digital. The latest addition is Lithovue, a disposable ureteroscope from Boston Scientific.

Table 11.2 Commonly used flexible ureterorenoscopes

Brand	Model	Type (OF/DS)[a]	Working length (cm)	Diameter (tip/shaft) (Fr)	Field of view (°)	Active deflection up/down (°)	Working channels	Working channel diameter (Fr)
Gyrus ACMI	DUR-8	OF	65	6.75/8.6	80	175/185	1	3.6
	DUR-D	DS	65	8.7/9.3	80	250/250	1	3.6
Olympus	URF-P6	OF	67	4.9/7.95	90	275/275	1	3.6
	URF-V	DS	67	8.5/9.9	80	180/275	1	3.6
	URF V2	DS	67	8.5/8.4	80	275/275	1	3.6
Richard Wolf	Viper	OF	68	6/8.8	85	270/270	1	3.6
	Cobra	OF	68	6/9.9	85	270/270	2	3.3/3.3
	Boa vision	DS	68	6.6/8.7	90	270/270	1	3.6
	Cobra Vision	DS	68	5.2/9.9	90	270/270	2	3.6/2.4
Karl Storz	Flex-X^2	OF	67	7.5/8.5	88	270/270	1	3.6
	Flex-X^c	DS	70	8.5/8.4	90	270/270	1	3.6
Stryker	URT-7000S/Si	DS	65	9.6	90	240/240	1	3.6

[a] *OF* Optical Fiber, *DS* Digital Sensor

Image Quality: Digital Flexible (DFU) Versus Fiberoptic Ureteroscopes (FFU)

The DFUs offer higher image resolution (ability to distinguish between two points) compared to FFUs by virtue of having many more pixels compared to number of optical optic bundles in FFUs that form the image. Optical quality as defined by parameters such as low optical distortion, higher resolution, and larger field of view was tested among 4 FFUs (ACMI Dur-8 Elite®, Storz Flex-X2®, Olympus XURF-P5®, and Wolf 7325.076®) in an in vitro comparative study and found to be best in the Olympus and Wolf scopes tested [4]. The image size is also 1.5–3x larger in the digital scopes [5]. In a mainly in vitro study comparing the Storz Flex-X^2 and Flex-X^c (FFU and DFU respectively, Karl Storz, Tuttlingen, Germany), Lusch and colleagues demonstrated better resolution, color representation, and visualization in the upper urinary with the digital Flex-X^c [6]. The superior visual characteristics of the DFU will result in better detection of lesions, including small upper tract urothelial tumors which could be missed with a FFU.

Other technological developments may facilitate detection of subtle lesions. Narrow band imaging (NBI) is currently offered by Olympus as an integrated feature of their DFUs (Olympus, Center Valley, PA). In bladder cancer NBI improves the visualization of urothelial surface detail especially tumoral microvasculature and increased angiogenesis compared to surrounding normal urothelium and has been shown to increase tumor detection rate [7]. Traxer and colleagues also report a 22.7% increase in upper tract urothelial tumor detection by using NBI compared to white light ureteroscopy. They objectively showed that NBI can help detect additional tumors that would be missed by white light imaging in 14.2% of cases, and true extent of the lesions not visualized by white light in 8.5% of the cases [8].

Ease of Navigation in Pyelocalyceal System

All modern flexible ureterorenoscopes incorporate an active deflection mechanism of the tip to allow better navigation and access to different calyces, especially the lower pole ones with infundibuli at acute angles from the ureteropelvic junction. As mentioned in Table 11.2, different flexible scopes are capable of different degrees of upward/downward flexion. This is an important factor that can affect the ease of navigating the collecting system. An in vitro study in a model of a moderately hydronephrotic kidney with long infundibuli and relatively limited room for passive deflection, scopes with exaggerated active deflection showed better access to lower pole [9]. Historically, with older generation instrumentation, it was shown that about half the time (51%) some degree of passive deflection of the scope inside the kidney was needed in addition to the active mechanism to gain access to some inferior pole calyces [10]. A factor that influences the ease of passage of the ureteroscope over a guidewire into the ureteral orifice and subsequently through the ureter is the shaft stiffness. This has been studied previously and found to vary between different flexible ureteroscopes and found to be different among different models [11]. Although it may be easier to pass stiffer scopes into a tight ureter due to less likelihood of buckling, they may be harder to maneuver into lower pole calyces by use of secondary passive deflection. Therefore manufacturers of flexible scopes have tried to maintain shaft stiffness while a softer deflectable segment close to the tip of the scope.

The strength of the active deflection mechanism to maintain the angle of scope deflection with passage of laser fibers or other instruments can play a major role in successful access to the tumors located in lower pole calyces, where maximum deflection often is required to encounter the lesion. It has been shown that passage of various instruments can decrease the deflection to about half (53%) [12]. It should be also emphasized that the operator can maximize the scope deflection by simple maneuvers to minimize bending the shaft such as holding the ureteroscope in a straight line and as taut as possible, passage of a super-stiff guidewire in the working channel, or just by utilizing a ureteral access sheath which will externally support the shaft [13].

When comparing 2 DFUs (Gyrus ACMI DUR-D and Olympus URF-V) to the Olympus URF-P5 fiberoptic scope for maneuverability, the DFUs were unable to reach the target in 3 of 45 (6.6%) and in 6 of 56 (10.7%) cases, respectively; however, the smaller URF-P5 fiberoptic scope could reach the target (stone) in all cases [14].

Channel Size and Irrigation Adequacy of Ureteroscopes

The size of the working channel for most SRUs is roughly in the 3–6 Fr range (see Table 11.1), most commonly a 3.4 Fr channel for instruments and a dedicated, smaller (~2.5 Fr) channel for running the irrigation fluid. Flexible ureteroscopes very commonly have a single 3.6 Fr working channel (for both the instrument and irrigation fluid). Therefore insertion of a larger instrument or laser fiber in single channel scopes (i.e., almost all flexible and few SRUs) will reduce the available space for passage of irrigation fluid and in effect makes it harder to maintain a good flow rate to clear the blood and the debris.

The development of a dual channel flexible ureteroscope (Richard Wolf Cobra) has allowed for a dedicated irrigation port. In vitro comparison of irrigate flow rate in this ureteroscope with the single channel model from the same manufacturer (Richard Wolf Viper) showed up to 37 times increase in overall flow speed (ranging from 1.5 to 37x) depending on various instrument inserted in the working channel of both scopes [15]. This corroborates with a recently published in vivo study comparing the evacuation of a standard bloody filed in a middle calyx of a porcine kidney which reports a significantly shorter evacuation time (about half) for the dual channel Cobra scope compared to various single channel scopes [16].

Generally speaking, the larger the diameter of a SRU the more space it occupies in the ureteral lumen, leaving less room for back flow of the irrigate (despite having a larger channel for inflow). This in turn may result in more pressure build up in upper urinary tract. With flexible scopes, utilization of a ureteral access sheath will provide a space around the shaft allowing return of fluid with ease and better flow of irrigation. Without the use of an access sheath during flexible ureteroscopy, one has to be mindful that the irrigation pressure required to clear the field of view from blood, tumor, and associated calcification debris may easily exceed not only the normal renal pyelocalyceal pressure (approximately 10 mmHg), but also significantly the threshold of pyelovenous backflow (about 30–45 mmHg) [17].

Durability of Flexible Ureteroscopes

Compared to SRUs, flexible scopes are more fragile and have shorter life span. The life span of a scope can be influenced by its design and build, frequency of use, surgeon's experience, difficulty, and types of procedures, utilization of laser energy or stiff-end wires, and potentially the cleaning/sterilization techniques.

Different studies have reported a reduction in the active deflection mechanism of the scope with continued use, anywhere from 28% in older series [18] to about 10% with modern scopes [19] while citing it a major source of failure. Multiple series over time have reported on longevity of flexible ureteroscopes and the time period or number of cases before a major repair was required. As one would imagine, these numbers in fact have improved in recent series [20]. In 2010, Knudsen and colleagues assessed the durability of four contemporary FFUs from four major manufacturers in a prospective, randomized, and multicenter trial. This study showed a difference (albeit not statistically significant) in number of cases before a major repair was required for each scope, which ranged from 5.3 to 18. The most frequent cause for repair in this study was to poor visibility followed by

Table 11.3 Fiberoptic and digital ureteroscope durability [21]

	Average cases before repair
Fiberoptic ureteroscopes:	
Richard wolf viper	17.3
Olypmus URF-P5	18
Stryker flex vision	17.6
Gyrus ACMI DUR-8E	5.3
Digital ureteroscopes:	
Gyrus ACMI DUR-D	11.25
Olympus URF-V	14

lowered maneuverability [21]. The average number of cases before repair was required for the FFus and DFUs in this study are shown in Table 11.3.

DFUs seem to have the advantage of consistent image quality with multiple use by eliminating the issue of fiber optic bundle losses that frequently happen in FFUs. A recent study by Multescu of the digital Storz Flex-X^{c} scope (Karl Storz Endoscopy, El Segundo, CA) reported increased durability as measured by number of procedures before repairs, attributed to both improvement of the build quality and cautious handling of the scope by operator and involved personnel [22]. Larger, multicenter studies with different DFUs are needed to further elucidate their durability, variability between each manufacturer's model, as well as common patterns of failure.

Cost of Flexible Ureteroscopes

Majority of upper tract urothelial tumors will require diagnostic and therapeutic interventions which require flexible ureterorensoscopes. Cost of obtaining and maintenance of flexible ureteroscopes and accessories clearly will have a major impact on institutions that perform ureteroscopy. When taking into account the initial price of smaller than 9 Fr flexible ureteroscopes from major manufacturers (Storz 11274AA, Olympus URF-P3, Wolf 7325.172, Gyrus ACMI AUR-7, and Gyrus ACMI DUR-8), repair costs, warranty coverage, and also the published durability outcomes of these scopes at that time, one meta-analysis showed significant variability of 95% (~31,000–60,000 US Dollars in 2003) in cost for first year of ownership and performing 100 ureteroscopic cases [23].

Repair costs can be significant with flexible ureteroscopes, estimated to be about 600 U.S. dollars per case by Tosoian and colleagues at their institution in 2013. They calculated a net loss of $455 (−4%) for each inpatient ureteroscopy case, while OP cases generated a net profit of $659 (13%) per case. Overall the ureteroscopy cases were associated with a net profit of close to $600 in their study [24]. Ureteroscopy appears to be sustainable financially, and emphasis should be placed on minimizing scope damage and safe handling of the equipment by surgeon and other personnel. It should also be noted that the stress placed on flexible ureteroscopes is likely greater for urinary lithiasis procedures compared to urothelial tumor cases. In a recent study, Carey et al. [25] showed that refurbished flexible ureteroscopes that had undergone major repair were much more fragile compared to identical brand new scopes in a tertiary care center with multiple surgeons. Refurbished ureteroscope by an outsourced vendor showed a very high frequency of damage and repair requirement, which should be considered when obtaining flexible ureteroscopes for a high-volume hospital.

Summary Box

- Semirigid ureteroscopes are valuable tools for assessment of distal/mid ureter for tumors. Due to their tapered shaft, passing the scope into the ureter will also gently dilate the ureteral orifice and distal ureter and allowing easier advancement for access sheaths or flexible scopes.

- Fexible ureteroscopes provide active deflection mechanism of the tip for 180–275°. Most flexible ureteroscopes also have a soft passive deflection area close to the tip, allowing better access to lower-most calyces. Optimal scope configuration would include a stiffer shaft (easier threading over a guidewire with less buckling in the ureter) and a soft passive deflection zone (ease of access for difficult angles).
- The digital flexible ureteroscopes offer higher image resolution compared to fiberoptic scopes. The image size is also 1.5–3x larger in digital scopes. At least one study has shown better visualization of upper urinary tract with a digital compared to a fiberoptic scope by same manufacturer.
- Narrow band imaging is becoming popular and is proving to be a valuable tool for accurate visualization and increased detection rate of upper tract urothelial tumors.
- Use of ureteral access sheaths allows for better flow of irrigate and clearing of the visualized field, lesser risk of pyelocalyceal over-pressurization, and easier in-and-out movement of flexible ureteroscope for multiple biopsies. Ureter must be cleared of lesions and determined to be of appropriate caliber prior to access sheath placement.
- Refurbished flexible ureteroscopes have been shown to have a higher frequency of damage requiring repairs, which should be considered when obtaining scopes for a high-volume hospital.

References

1. Bozzini P. Lichtleiter, eine Erfindung zur Anschauung innerer Teile und Krankheiten, nebst der Abbildung (Light conductor, an invention for examining internal parts and diseases, together with illustrations). J der practischen Arzneykunde und Wundarzneykunst (J Practical Med Surgery). 1806;24:107–24.
2. Marshall VF. Fiber Optics in Urology. J Urol. 1964;91:110–4.
3. Goodman TM. Ureteroscopy with rigid instruments in the management of distal ureteral disease. J Urol. 1984;132:250–3.
4. Paffen ML, Keizer JG, de Winter GV, Arends AJ, Hendrikx AJ. A comparison of the physical properties of four new generation flexible ureteroscopes: (de)flection, flow properties, torsion stiffness, and optical characteristics. J Endourol. 2008;22 (10):2227–34.
5. Razvan M, Geavlete B, Georgescu D, Geavlete P. Conventional fiberoptic flexible ureteroscope versus fourth generation digital flexible ureteroscope: a critical comparison. J Endourol. 2010;24(1):17–21.
6. Lusch A, Abdelshehid C, Hidas G, Osann KE, Okhunov Z, McDougall E, Landman J. In vitro and in vivo comparison of optics and performance of a distal sensor Ureteroscope versus a standard fiberoptic Ureteroscope. J Endourol. 2013;27(7):896–902.
7. Li K, Lin T, Fan X, Duan Y, Huang J. Diagnosis of narrow-band imaging in non-muscle-invasive bladder cancer: a systematic review and meta-analysis. Int J Urol. 2013;20(6):602–9.
8. Traxer O, Geavlete B, de Medina SG, Sibony M, Al-Qahtani S. Narrow-band imaging digital flexible ureteroscopy in detection of upper urinary tract transitional-cell carcinoma: initial experience. J Endourol. 2011;25(1):19–23.
9. Monga M, Weiland D, Pedro RN, Lynch AC, Anderson K. Intrarenal manipulation of flexible ureteroscopes: a comparative study. BJU Int. 2007; 100(1):157–9.
10. Bagley DH. Intrarenal access with the flexible ureteropyeloscope: effects of active and passive tip deflection. J Endourol. 1993;7(3):221–4.
11. Monga M, Anderson K, Durfee W. Physical properties of flexible Ureteroscopes: implications for clinical practice. J Endourol. 2004;18(5):462–5.
12. Poon M, Beaghler M, Baldwin D. Flexible endoscope deflectability: changes using a variety of working instruments and laser fibers. J Endourol. 1997;11:247–9.
13. Monga M, Dretler SP, Landman J, Slaton JW, Conradie MC, Clayman RV. Maximizing ureteroscope deflection: play it straight. Urology. 2002;60 (5):902–5.

14. Shah K, Monga M, Knudsen B. Prospective randomized trial comparing 2 flexible digital ureteroscopes: ACMI/Olympus invisio DUR-D and Olympus URF-V. Urology. 2015;85(6):1267–71.
15. Haberman K, Ortiz-Alvarado O, Chotikawanich E, Monga M. A dual-channel flexible ureteroscope: evaluation of deflection, flow, illumination, and optics. J Endourol. 2011;25(9):1411–4.
16. Lusch A, Okhunov Z, del Junco M, Yoon R, Khanipour R, Menhadji A, Landman J. Comparison of optics and performance of single channel and a novel dual-channel fiberoptic ureteroscope. Urology. 2015;85(1):268–72.
17. Jung H, Osther P. Intraluminal pressure profiles during flexible ureterorenoscopy. SpringerPlus. 2015;4:373.
18. Afane JS, Olweny EO, Bercowsky E, Sundaram CP, Dunn MD, Shalhav AL, McDougall EM, Clayman RV. Flexible ureteroscopes: a single center evaluation of the durability and function of the new endoscopes smaller than 9Fr. J Urol. 2000;164(4):1164–8.
19. Multescu R, Geavlete B, Geavlete P. A new era: performance and limitations of the latest models of flexible ureteroscopes. Urology. 2013;82(6):1236–9.
20. Payne DA, Keeley Jr FX. Rigid and Flexible Ureteroscopes: Technical Features. Smith's Textbook of Endourology. 3rd ed. West Sussex, United Kingdom: Wiley-Blackwell; 2012.
21. Knudsen B, Miyaoka R, Shah K, Holden T, Turk TM, Pedro RN, Kriedberg C, Hinck B, Ortiz-Alvarado O, Monga M. Durability of the next-generation flexible fiberoptic Ureteroscopes: a randomized prospective multi-institutional clinical trial. Urology. 2010;75(3):534–8.
22. Multescu R, Geavlete B, Georgescu D, Geavlete P. Improved durability of flex-Xc digital flexible ureteroscope: how long can you expect it to last? Urology. 2014;84(1):32–5.
23. Landman J, Lee DI, Lee C, Monga M. Evaluation of overall costs of currently available small flexible ureteroscopes. Urology. 2003;62(2):218–22.
24. Tosoian JJ, Ludwig W, Sopko N, Mullins JK, Matlaga BR. The effect of repair costs on the profitability of a ureteroscopy program. J Endourol. 2015;29(4):406–9.
25. Carey RI, Martin CJ, Knego JR. Prospective evaluation of refurbished flexible ureteroscope durability seen in a large public tertiary care center with multiple surgeons. Urology. 2014;84(1):42–5.

12 Narrow Band Imaging in the Evaluation of Upper Tract Urothelial Cancer

Barak Rosenzweig, Harry Herr and Jonathan A. Coleman

Introduction

Urothelial carcinomas (UC) represent a field disease of the urothelium and can involve multiple sites throughout the lower (bladder and urethra) or upper (renal pelvis and ureters) urinary tract. The vast majority of UCs are located in the bladder (90–95%) which is disproportionate relative to the total surface area of the entire urinary tract. Upper urinary tract urothelial carcinomas (UTUC) are relatively rare constituting 5–10% of UCs only [1–4]. Patients with upper tract cancer are generally older than patients with bladder tumors. Upper tract tumors are rarely present before the age of 40 years, and the mean age at presentation is 65 years [5, 6]. Based on the SEER database, the incidence of ureteral and renal pelvis tumors in the United States increased from 0.73 to 1.0 per 100,000 person-years in between 1985 and 1994, respectively [1]. This increase may also be associated with a slight stage migration in renal pelvis and ureteral carcinomas as shown by David et al. [7], with the proportion of stage 0a tumors increasing and stage I tumors decreasing. Despite these observed trends, there has been no change in survival outcomes yet reported suggesting that the increasing incidence of upper tract tumors may be related to aging in the general population and the growing prevalence of incidentally detected cancers. Additional explanation may be linked to the survival improvement of bladder UC patients, length time bias associated with slower growing tumors and increasing at-risk time for development of upper tract involvement.

Clinical Characteristics and the Role of Conservative Management

The biologic behavior of UTUC appears to differ from that of bladder cancer based on clinical features. Tumors in the upper tract are more often high grade and over 60% of UTUCs are found to be invasive at diagnosis compared with only 15–25% for bladder cancer [4, 8]. UTUCs that invade the muscle wall usually have a very poor prognosis. The 5-year cancer specific survival is <50% for pT2/pT3 and <10% for pT4 [4, 9]. Radical nephroureterectomy (RNU) is considered the gold standard treatment for UTUC although may be overly aggressive as treatment for selected cancers [4]. The most recent guidelines by the European Association of Urology (EAU) support

B. Rosenzweig · H. Herr · J. A. Coleman (✉)
Department of Surgery, Urology, Memorial Sloan Kettering Cancer Center, 1275 York Avenue, New York, NY 10065, USA
e-mail: colemanj@mskcc.org

B. Rosenzweig
e-mail: rosenzwb@mskcc.org

H. Herr
e-mail: herrh@mskcc.org

M. Eshghi (ed.), *Urothelial Malignancies of the Upper Urinary Tract*,
https://doi.org/10.1007/978-3-319-51263-1_12

the indication for conservative management of UTUC in low-risk cases when the contralateral kidney is functional, it can also be considered in all imperative cases (i.e., renal insufficiency or solitary kidney) [10]. Kidney-sparing surgery for low-risk UTUC prevents the morbidity associated with open radical surgery without compromising oncologic outcome and kidney function [11].

Concurrent bladder cancer is found in 17% of UTUCs [12]. Bladder recurrence is found in 22–47% of UTUC patients whereas contralateral UTUC in 2–6% only [13–16]. Based on SEER data, Rabbani et al. [17] identified stable incidence for UTUC in primary bladder cancer patients on long-term surveillance indicating the need for continuing follow-up and surveillance in this site. More recent analysis has suggested that routine imaging alone may not be effective and use of urine cytology, careful history, and physical examination may be equally important [18]. Indeed, imaging alone may not be adequate for the following patients with UTUC as reflected in current follow-up guidelines by the EAU that recommends cystoscopy, ureteroscopy, and cytology at 3 and 6 months, and then every 6 months over 2 years and then yearly [4].

Considering the natural history of UTUC, its potentially aggressive clinical course, and accordingly, the rigorous recommendations for follow-up, serious effort has been made in the clinical and technological arena in order to optimize diagnostic approaches with endoscopic evaluation. Ureteroscopy can improve diagnostic accuracy from 75 to 85–90% comparing to excretory or retrograde urography [19, 20]. Additional advantages of ureteroscopy include the ability to visually inspect the tumor for invasive characteristics and to perform simultaneous biopsy and selective cytology allowing for histologic correlation [21, 22]. In spite of these multiple methodological approaches, there are limitations to the accuracy of identifying and accurately characterizing tumors in the upper tract with endoscopy. Due to anatomic orientation of tubular structures like the ureter and calyces, imaging with ureteroscope is often oblique to the urothelial surface and not as close to perpendicular as in bladder endoscopy. Flat appearing lesions, such as carcinoma in situ (CIS), are hard to identify, can be easily mistaken for inflammation or missed due to other challenges in visualization. The ability to obtain adequate tissue from single or multiple/random sampling is another factor affecting the reliability of histologic tissue evaluation [23]. Consistent with these findings, a high rate of upgrading and upstaging in nephroureterectomy specimens has been reported by Wang et al. [24], attributed largely to the limitations in adequate visual inspection and sampling.

Novel diagnostic tools have the potential to improve UTUC visualization and diagnosis. Optical properties based on the interaction between light and tissue includes scattering, absorption, and fluorescence which can be used to characterize certain tissue types. Narrow band imaging (NBI), photodynamic diagnosis (PDD), and Storz professional imaging enhancement system (SPIES) are aimed at improving visualization of UTUC while optical coherence tomography (OCT), and confocal laser endomicroscopy (CLE) aim to provide real-time prediction of histopathology [25]. This chapter will focus on the NBI technology and its use in evaluating tumors in the upper urinary tract.

Technology and Technique of Narrow Band Imaging (NBI)

Most video endoscopes use white light from a xenon source for illumination. The reflected light is captured by a charge-coupled device (CCD) chip on the tip of the instrument in order to reconstruct the images [26]. The reflectance spectrum differs from the emission spectrum of the light source; during live observation, the spectral composition of the reflected light is influenced by the structure of the tissue and the blood flow [27–29]. The visualized image can be further altered by filtering and processing software to match surgeon preference, yet may remove information contained within the raw signal. The depth of penetration into the illuminated mucosa depends on the wave length applied—deep for the red, superficial for blue, and green for intermediate. Hemoglobin is the major agent responsible for the absorption of visible light, with a principle peak in the blue part of the spectrum (415 nm) which explains the red color of vessels [26].

Narrow band imaging is an optical image enhancement technology introduced in the early 2000s [27]. The NBI technology uses optical filters for RGB (Red, Green, and Blue) sequential illumination and narrows its bandwidth of the spectral transmittance [27, 28]. Gaps exist between the three narrow bands so they do not fully cover the range of visible light, which causes different depths of penetration (Fig. 12.1). The reconstructed images are therefore slightly different from each of the three channels (R, G, and B) and correspond to different layers of the mucosa. The displayed image combines the morphology of the three narrowed bands.

Preliminary testing of this three-band NBI was conducted on the vessels of human tongue mucosa [28]. Soon thereafter it was clinically applied to the inspection of gastrointestinal (GI) tissues for disease processes, such as identification of Barrett's esophagus and colonic polyps [26] and then late to applications in ear, nose, and throat (ENT) with some promising results [30, 31]. Application of NBI imaging for genitourinary applications is slightly different and based on only two narrow band wavelengths (blue at 415 nm and green at 540 nm, Fig. 12.2), as opposed to the three previously described wavelengths applied to the GI pathologies [32].

The shorter wavelength (415 nm) penetrates only the superficial layers of the mucosa. This light is absorbed by superficial capillary vessels and shows a brownish-black on the video image. The longer wavelength (540 nm) penetrates deeper and absorbed by vessels located in the deep mucosa and submucosa layers, it appears green on imaging. NBI improves visualization of tumors by enhancing the contrast between well-vascularized lesions and normal pink-white mucosa. The exclusion of red wavelengths has been chosen by the development team as representing the most effective imaging in urologic applications.

Use of NBI imaging during upper tract endoscopy is similar to the approach utilized with flexible cystoscopy and requires the use of appropriate video processor hardware and equipped ureteroscopic instruments. Most typically, this is done with flexible ureteroscope units

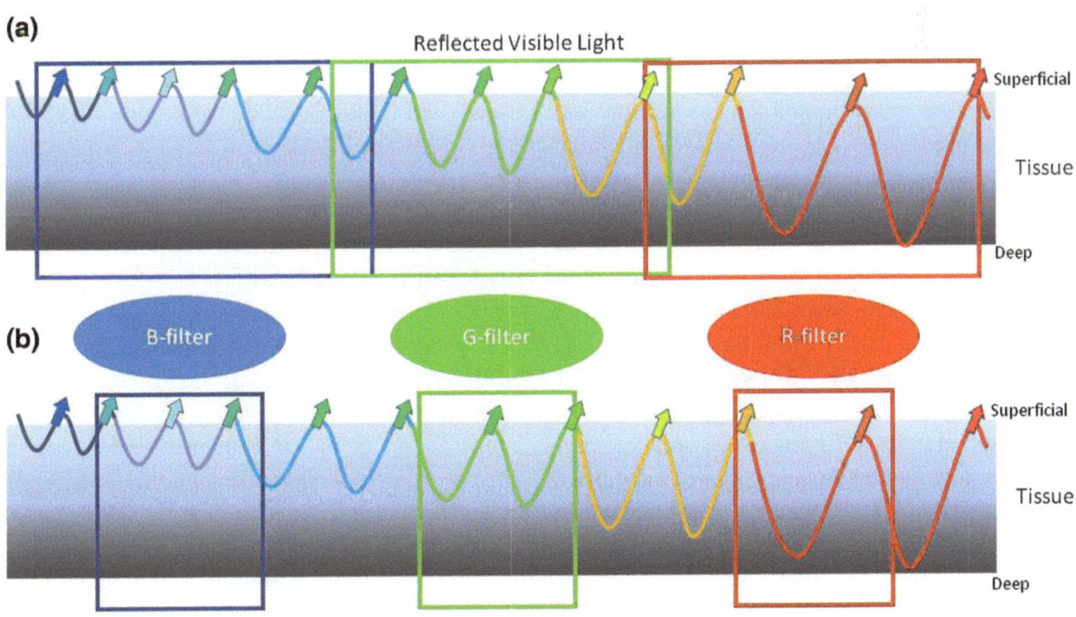

Fig. 12.1 Schematic representation of the interactions between tissue and light with the broadband (**a**) or narrow band (**b**) R/G/B interference filter

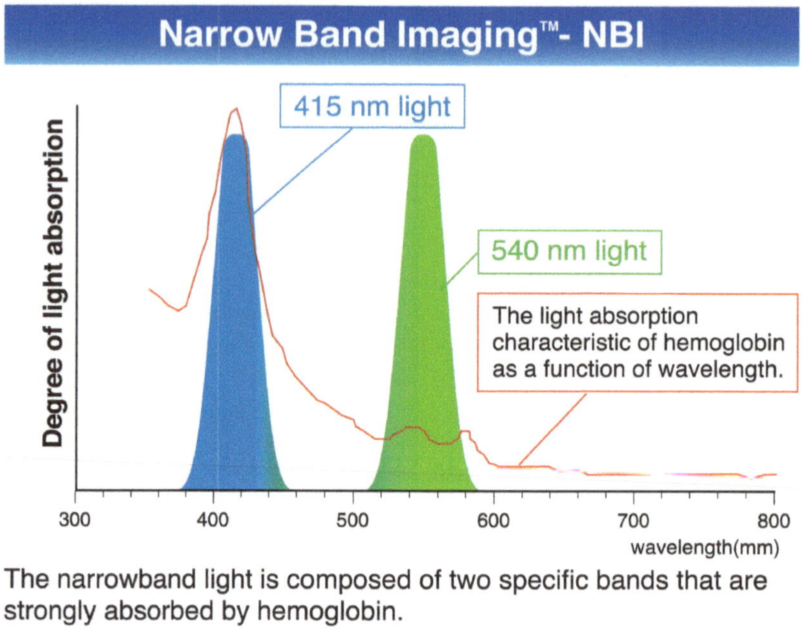

Fig. 12.2 Narrow band imaging for urothelial applications including transitional cell carcinoma. Two narrow band wavelengths (*blue* at 415 nm and *green* at 540 nm) are used. Hemoglobin is the major agent responsible for the absorption of visible light, with a principle peak in the blue part of the spectrum (415 nm). (Courtesy of Olympus Corporation, Japan.)

that have a tip diameter of 9.9 or 8.4 French, depending on the generation of equipment being used. Camera heads equipped with NBI technology are also available that permit this form of imaging with traditional rigid cystoscopy and semirigid ureteroscopy although imaging resolution may be more limited in this setting and less often used.

In flexible endoscopic equipment, the technical component utilizes a CCD mounted on the distal end of the flexible scope that is used for both narrow band and "normal" white light imaging (WLI). The instrument is calibrated at the beginning of use to white balance the scope for both WLI and NBI just as performed for standard, camera-based endoscopic procedures. Toggling between WLI and NBI can be performed at any time by having the surgeon press a button assigned on the camera head or by an assistant activating a toggle button on the bedside video processor unit. This simple process is considered equivalent to standard endoscopic imaging technique and does not require specialized instruction.

Experience with NBI for upper tract endoscopy is highly selective with few objective measures available for comparing results to standard WLI. The NBI technique is considered simple and easy to use, with no different tumor detection rate or learning curve comparing new users' to experienced urologists [32–34] (Figs. 12.3 and 12.4).

Narrow Band Imaging Application and Bladder Cancer

NBI enhancement of vascularization aids in discriminating several types of bladder tumors from normal surrounding tissue; papillary tumors appear dark green or brownish green due to fibrovascular stalk enhancement, they are usually quite distinct and contrast sharply. Flat lesions, such as carcinoma in situ (CIS) which are "easy to miss" lesions, constitute dense capillaries hence better identified by NBI.

The role of NBI in cystoscopy and bladder cancer was subject to several publications in the

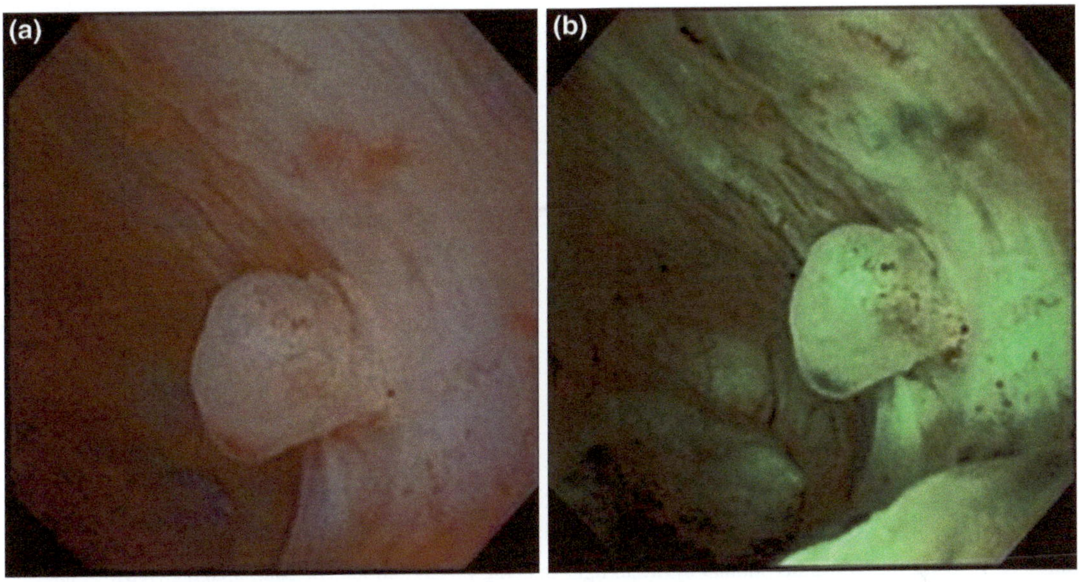

Fig. 12.3 Renal pelvis urothelium and nodule as shown by white light ureteroscopic endoscopy (**a**) and Narrow Band Imaging (**b**) in a patient with history of kidney stones and recent laser lithotripsy with stent placement. Note the lack of vascularity and bland interface between the nodule and normal urothelium characteristic of benign tissue

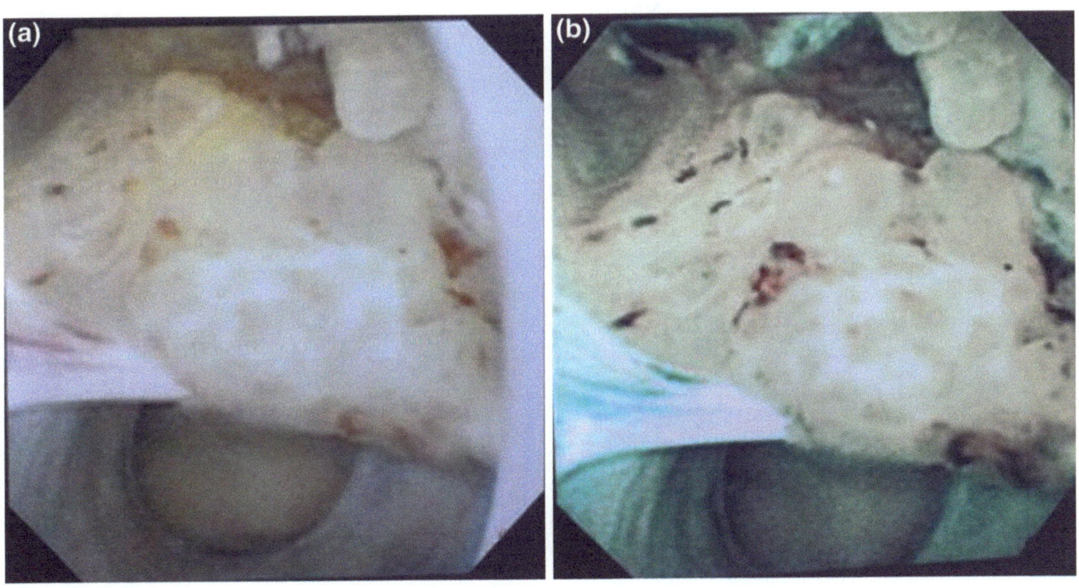

Fig. 12.4 Renal pelvis urothelium and low-grade urothelial tumor as shown by white light ureteroscopic endoscopy (**a**) and narrow band imaging (**b**) in a patient with history of Lynch Syndrome (Hereditary Non-Polyposis Colorectal Cancer syndrome or HNPCC) and recurrent low-grade urothelial tumors. NBI is useful in demonstrating low level vascular changes within the tumor; sharp interface between neoplastic and normal urothelium; and absence of neovascularity in the normal urothelium surrounding the tumor

past decade. Questions such as detection rate of tumors and CIS, BCG response evaluation, therapeutic impact, surgeon's ease of use, and even combining NBI with other therapeutic procedures were addressed. Dr. Herr's recent excellent review wonderfully organized the current literature's answers to these clinical questions.

Detection rate was shown to be higher with superior sensitivity and negative predicting value (>90%) for NBI over white light cystoscopy (Table 12.1). Lower specificity, leading to higher rate of negative biopsies, was accordingly reported with NBI, believed not to be significant or detrimental with no increased toxicity. The use of NBI also improved detection rate for CIS (Table 12.2) and was proved efficient confirming negative (complete) resection margins as well.

Evaluating response to Bacille Calmette-Guérin (BCG) therapy using white light cystoscopy can be challenging. Intense inflammatory reaction can be induced by this treatment with diffuse red and friable mucosal appearance mimicking CIS. NBI was used in order to cope with that challenge. Dr. Herr used NBI to evaluate 61 patients 3 months after BCG, reporting better identification of residual tumors [35].

The therapeutic impact of NBI still needs to be proven. Better cystoscopic visualization seems to be a key component of achieving complete resection, lower recurrence rates, and

Table 12.1 Detection of bladder tumors by white light imaging (WLI) and narrow band imaging (NBI) cystoscopy

Series [Au] + Refs.	No. of cases	Cystoscopy (WLI/NBI)	Sensitivity (%)	Specificity (%)	PPV	NPV
Bryan et al. [55]	29	WLI	82	79	70	81
		NBI	96	85	61	92
Herr and Donat [52]	427	WLI	87	85	66	96
		NBI	100	82	63	100
Cauberg et al. [56]	95	WLI	79	75	NA	NA
		NBI	95	69	NA	NA
Tatsugami et al. [57]	104	WLI	57	86	69	79
		NBI	93	71	63	95
Shen et al. [58]	78	WLI	78	83	NA	79
		NBI	93	73	NA	87
Xiaodong and Zhangqun [59]	64	WLI	79	76	NA	NA
		NBI	97	86	NA	NA
Geavlete et al. [60]	95	WLI	84	NA	NA	NA
		NBI	95	NA	NA	NA
Zhu et al. [61]	12	WLI	50	91	NA	NA
		NBI	78	80	NA	NA
Chen et al. [62]	179	WLI	97	81	NA	NA
		NBI	79	79	NA	NA
Jecu et al. [63]	23	WLI	86	NA	NA	NA
		NBI	94	NA	NA	NA
Song et al. [64]	47	WLI	90	62	53	93
		NBI	100	16	36	100
Ye et al. [65]	384	WLI	75	59	76	98
		NBI	99	61	70	66

PPV Positive predictive value, *NPV* Negative predictive value

Table 12.2 Detection of carcinoma in situ (CIS) by white light imaging (WLI) and narrow band imaging (NBI) cystoscopy

Series [Au] + Ref	No. of cases	Cystoscopy (WLI/NBI)	Sensitivity (%)	Specificity (%)	PPV	NPV
Herr and Donat [52]	67	WLI	83	76	36	97
		NBI	100	72	36	100
Tatsugami et al. [57]	30	WLI	50	83	76	61
		NBI	90	75	79	87
Cauberg et al. [56]	11	WLI	55	NA	NA	NA
		NBI	69	NA	NA	NA
Shen et al. [58]	11	WLI	68	83	NA	75
		NBI	88	77	NA	83
Naya et al. [66]	10	WLI	NA	NA	NA	NA
		NBI	75	81	NA	NA
Jecu et al. [63]	23	WLI	60	NA	NA	NA
		NBI	95	NA	NA	NA

PPV Positive predictive value, *NPV* Negative predictive value

better outcomes. Indeed lower recurrence rates were reported after NBI-assisted transurethral resection of bladder tumors (TURBT), transurethral outpatient fulguration of tumors as well as after Re-TURBT's [36–38]. Alongside TURBT, NBI was suggested to enhance other transurethral interventions. Geavlete et al. and Stănescu et al. used NBI cystoscopy in association with bipolar plasma vaporization (BPV). They both showed significant improvement in diagnostic accuracy of large non-muscle invasive bladder tumors as well as superior efficacy and safety compared with TURBT. The combined approach provided a lower residual tumor rate at repeat TUR and a reduced recurrence rate [39, 40]. Multicenter, randomized, international trial has been set to clarify the role of NBI in lowering bladder cancer recurrence rate [41].

Narrow Band Imaging Application and Upper Urinary Tract Urothelial Carcinoma (UTUC)

Computed tomography (CT) urography has the highest diagnostic accuracy in high-risk patients [4, 42]. Invasive diagnostic procedures such as flexible ureteroscopy were suggested by the most recent EAU guidelines for diagnostic uncertainty, when conservative treatment is considered, or in patients with a solitary kidney [10]. Flexible ureteroscopy is used to visualize and biopsy the ureter, renal pelvis, and collecting system. The grade of UTUC on ureteroscopic biopsy was shown to closely associate with the pathological stage, and provide accurate diagnostic information [43, 44]. Ureteroscopic biopsies can determine tumor grade in 90% of cases with a low false-negative rate, regardless of sample size [45]. Higher detection rate exemplified in bladder cancer using NBI raise the potential of applying this technique in hope for similar outcomes in UTUC detection and follow-up.

Unfortunately, the available evidence in order to determine NBI advantage in this setting is extremely scarce. Updated literature review for NBI in UTUC revealed six papers [25, 46–50] with only one English written original paper describing detection rates [49]. This paper describes 27 cases, out of which 14 were previously diagnosed with UTUC, going through NBI as part of their follow-up, and 13 newly diagnosed patients. The NBI followed a preliminary performed white light ureteroscopy. In the previously diagnosed group, NBI additionally diagnosed two tumors out of seven tumors in total, and extended tumor limits in one patient.

In the newly diagnosed group, NBI detected three additional tumors sometimes in the same patient, e.g., out of three tumors in the same patient, two only were detected by white light ureteroscopy. It also showed extended margins detection. In total, out of 35 diagnosed tumors, five (14.2%) were solely diagnosed by NBI, and in additional three (8.5%) tumors NBI identified extended limits compared with white light ureteroscopy. The authors summarized their findings to show 22.7% improvement in detection rate using NBI. They concluded NBI to be a valuable diagnostic technology for UTUC showing considerable improvement of tumor visual accuracy as well as tumor detection rate. This paper furthermore described NBI advantages as enabling the urologist to determine the exact limits of tumors, thereby facilitating complete surgical treatment [49]. In spite of these encouraging results two critical points come in mind regarding the described manuscript. The lack of pathological analysis for the "extended margins of tumors" which were visible only by NBI, miss the definitive diagnosis for the presumed increased visualization. Another criticism concerns NBI performed immediately after white light ureteroscopy. Performing NBI immediately after white light ureteroscopy raises the concern of higher detection rate due to "second look" and not as a result of better diagnostic tool usage (observer bias). Similar concerns were raised regarding NBI bladder cancer detection rate [51]. This dilemma was previously negotiated and nicely settled in Dr. Herr's paper stating one should look at the combination of modalities and not whether one is better than the other [52]. Other papers supported the possible role of NBI improving ureteroscopic visualization of UTUC [25, 48], even further defined by some as the most promising technique serving this purpose [4, 50].

Despite performing no control trials regarding NBI imaging of UTUC, the authors of this chapter share the impression of NBI handing the urologist with better detection and tumor extension diagnosis. Sharing that impression with the readers, we can look at the tumor visibility on NBI as shown in Figs. 12.5, 12.6 and 12.7.

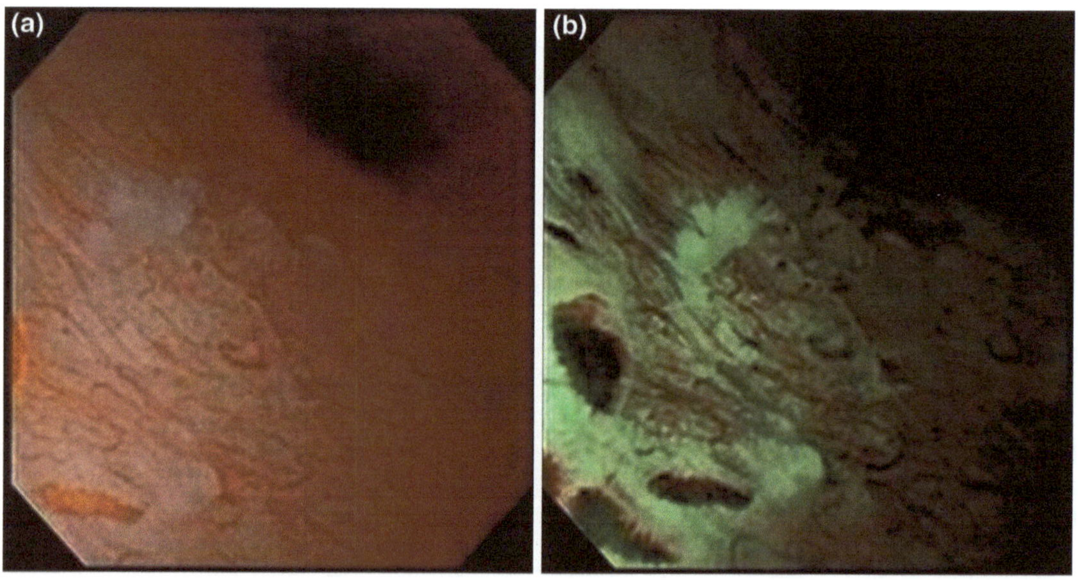

Fig. 12.5 Renal pelvis urothelium and high-grade urothelial tumor as shown by white light ureteroscopic endoscopy (**a**) and narrow band imaging (**b**) in a patient with history of bladder carcinoma in situ. Renal pelvis aspiration cytologies in this case were positive and biopsies of nearby tumor revealed high-grade tumor. NBI is useful in demonstrating subtle papillary architecture with associated vascularity in neoplastic tissue (*arrow*) as well as accentuating aberrant neovascular changes in the underlying urothelial layers

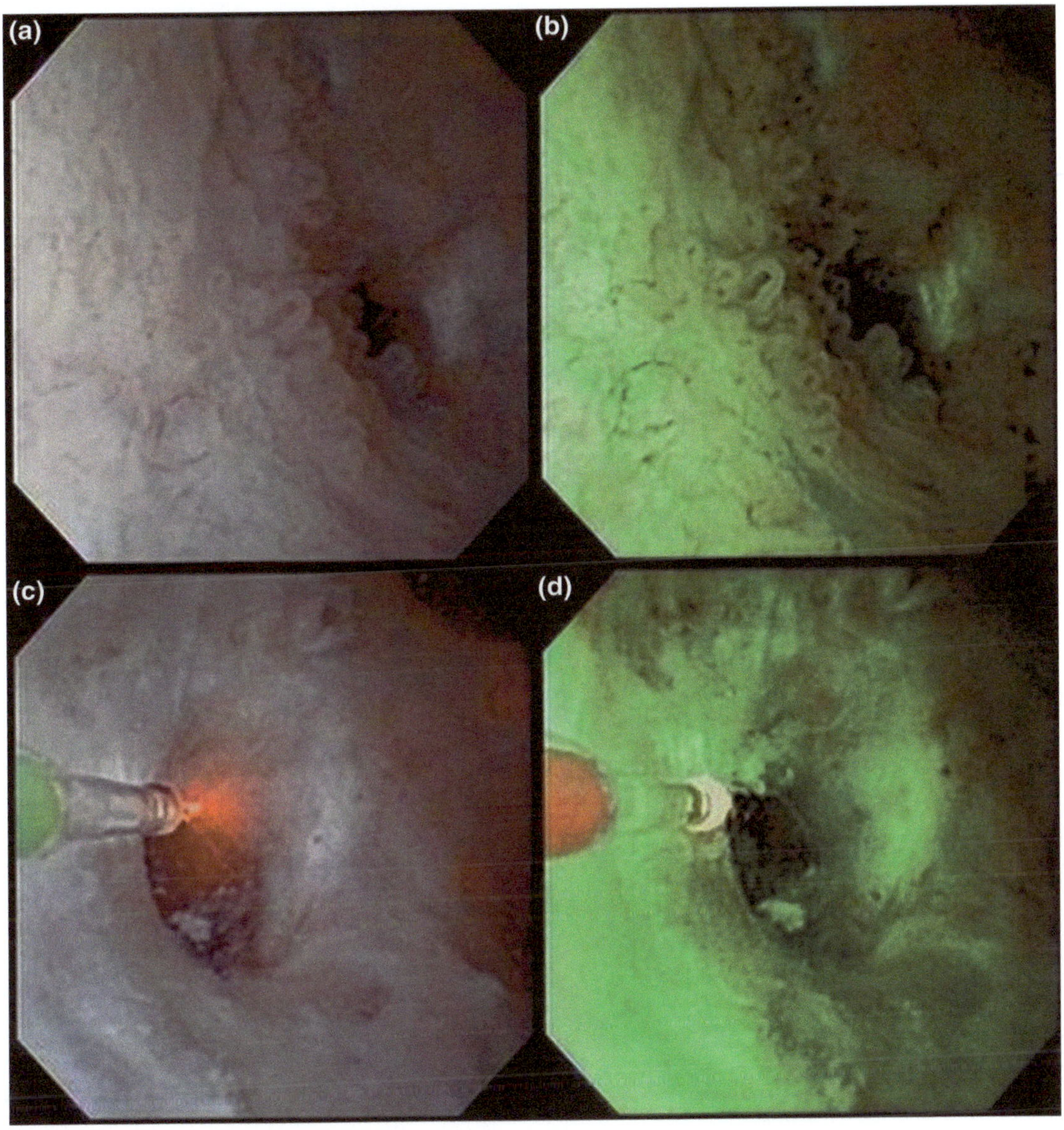

Fig. 12.6 Renal pelvis urothelium and high-grade urothelial tumor as shown by white light ureteroscopic endoscopy (**a**) and narrow band imaging (**b**) in a patient with solitary kidney and recurrent high-grade bladder cancer. Treatment with laser ablation is performed under alternating white light and NBI to evaluate for treatment effect. NBI may be useful for the following denuding effects to the surface urothelium and identifying areas of thinning muscularis (*arrow*). Care should be taken to avoid overtreatment to discolored areas seen on NBI where blood may be trapped in previously ablated tissue

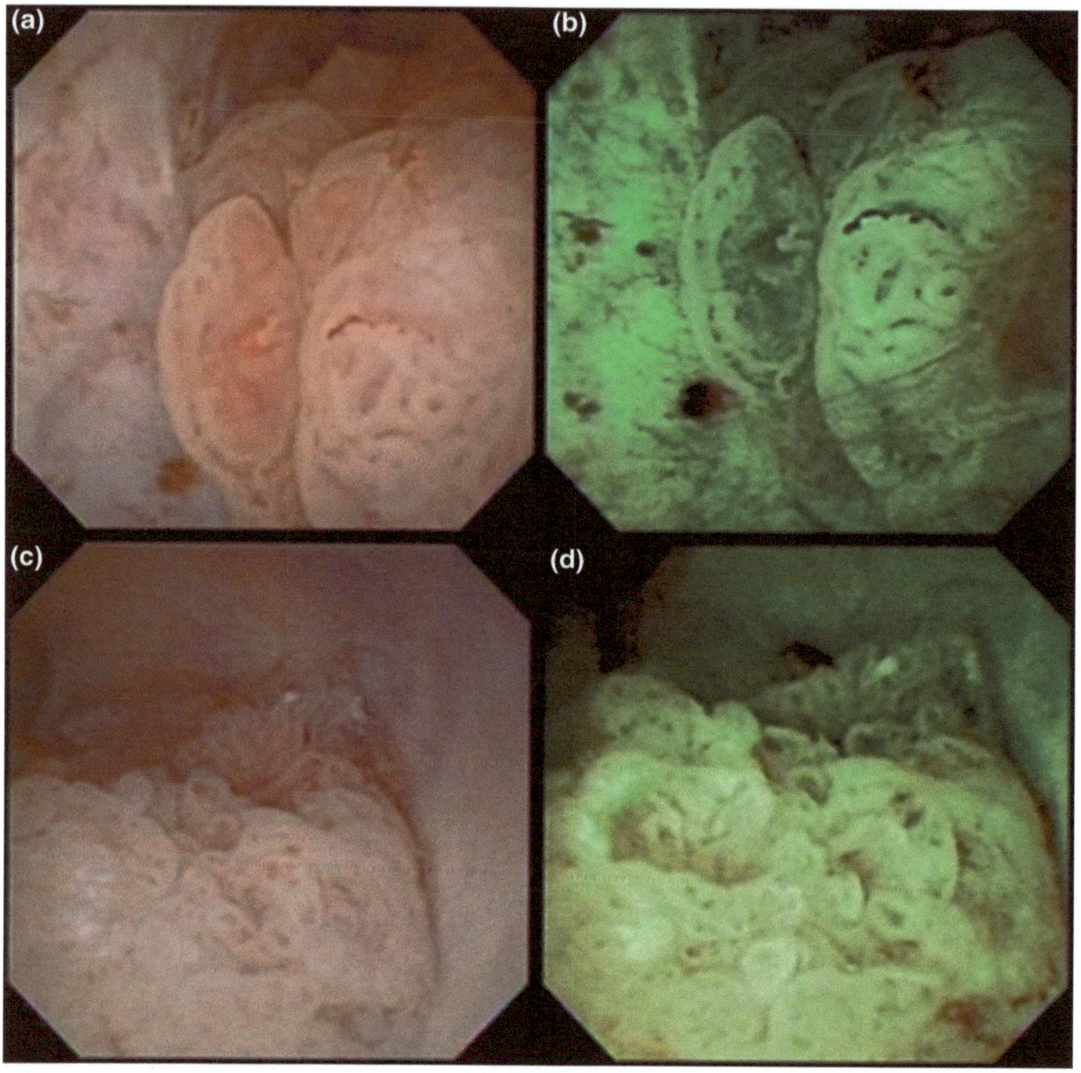

Fig. 12.7 UTUC mucosa and tumor as shown by white light ureteroscopy (*left panel*) and narrow band imaging (*right panel*)

Conclusions

Conservative endoscopic management for UTUC is becoming a more standard and viable option for patients. The incorporation of new, advanced technologies into the field is enhancing the capabilities of these approaches in areas of diagnosis, tumor characterization, and treatment. An important key component is the opportunity for incremental improvement in visualization of tumors, such as manifested by digital imaging and NBI, that may provide the surgeon with the potential for better detection, treatment, follow-up, and oncologic outcomes. Great challenges lie in developing prospective studies to determine the clinical benefits that may be associated with these technologies. Yet, just as a viewer may feel a strong preference for high-definition LCD television image over standard definition when watching the same program, a surgeon may just as easily understand that anything that enhances visualization of tissue anatomy can be considered advantageous.

UTUC are rare tumors, a fact illustrated by lack of robust evidence-based medicine even in the most updated clinical recommendations [1, 2, 4]. Acquisition of evidence-based data and gold standard trials can be challenging while treating rare diseases [53]. Indeed current literature supporting NBI superiority for detecting UTUC is sparse. Drifting away from the secure land of evidence-based medicine, we need to put in mind the potential for foreign influences of therapeutic decisions, especially when technology is involved [54].

Standing where we are now we believe the best practical approach will be to cautiously use urothelial bladder cancer NBI data, assuming similar biologic tumor behavior, alongside our best clinical judgment. We must consult our patients accordingly and make sure we all fully understand the limitations we confront adopting this technology. As clinical researchers we are obligated to make an effort and find the evidence needed for taking well-based decisions in the future.

Summary Box

- Tumors in the upper tract are more often high grade with over 60% of upper urinary tract urothelial carcinomas found to be invasive at diagnosis. Rigorous follow-up is therefore recommended.
- Narrow band imaging (NBI) is an optical image enhancement technology which uses optical filters for RGB (Red, Green, and Blue) sequential illumination and narrows its bandwidth of the spectral transmittance. The reconstructed images are slightly different from each of the three channels (R, G, and B) and correspond to different layers of the mucosa.
- Cystoscopy using NBI exemplified higher detection rate of bladder cancer in several clinical scenarios.
- NBI ureteroscopy was suggested to improve detection rate of upper urinary tract urothelial carcinomas, although confined by scarce evidence.
- Further research is needed to establish the role for NBI in detection of upper urinary tract urothelial carcinomas.

References

1. Munoz JJ, Ellison LM. Upper tract urothelial neoplasms: incidence and survival during the last 2 decades. J Urol [Internet]. 2000 Nov [cited 2015 Jul 20];164(5):1523–5. Available from: http://www.ncbi.nlm.nih.gov/pubmed/11025695.
2. Siegel R, Naishadham D, Jemal A. Cancer statistics, 2012. CA Cancer J Clin [Internet]. Jan [cited 2014 Jul 9];62(1):10–29. Available from: http://www.ncbi.nlm.nih.gov/pubmed/22237781.
3. Ploeg M, Aben KKH, Kiemeney LA. The present and future burden of urinary bladder cancer in the world. World J Urol [Internet]. 2009 Jun [cited 2015 Jul 2];27(3):289–93. Available from: http://www.pubmedcentral.nih.gov/articlerender.fcgi?artid=2694323&tool=pmcentrez&rendertype=abstract.
4. Rouprêt M, Babjuk M, Compérat E, Zigeuner R, Sylvester R, Burger M, et al. European guidelines on upper tract urothelial carcinomas: 2013 update. Eur Urol [Internet]. 2013 Jun [cited 2015 Jul 2];63(6):1059–71. Available from: http://www.ncbi.nlm.nih.gov/pubmed/23540953.
5. Melamed MR, Reuter VE. Pathology and staging of urothelial tumors of the kidney and ureter. Urol Clin North Am [Internet]. 1993 May [cited 2015 Jul 20];20(2):333–47. Available from: http://www.ncbi.nlm.nih.gov/pubmed/8388136.
6. Anderström C, Johansson SL, Pettersson S, Wahlqvist L. Carcinoma of the ureter: a clinicopathologic study of 49 cases. J Urol [Internet]. 1989 Aug [cited 2015 Jul 20];142(2 Pt 1):280 3. Available from: http://www.ncbi.nlm.nih.gov/pubmed/2486233.
7. David KA, Mallin K, Milowsky MI, Ritchey J, Carroll PR, Nanus DM. Surveillance of urothelial carcinoma: stage and grade migration, 1993–2005 and survival trends, 1993-2000. Cancer [Internet]. 2009 Apr 1 [cited 2015 Jul 20];115(7):1435–47. Available from: http://www.ncbi.nlm.nih.gov/pubmed/19215030.
8. Margulis V, Shariat SF, Matin SF, Kamat AM, Zigeuner R, Kikuchi E, et al. Outcomes of radical nephroureterectomy: a series from the Upper Tract Urothelial Carcinoma Collaboration. Cancer [Internet]. 2009 Mar 15 [cited 2015 Jul 2];115(6):1224–33. Available from: http://www.ncbi.nlm.nih.gov/pubmed/19156917.
9. Lughezzani G, Burger M, Margulis V, Matin SF, Novara G, Roupret M, et al. Prognostic factors in upper urinary tract urothelial carcinomas: a

comprehensive review of the current literature. Eur Urol [Internet]. 2012 Jul [cited 2015 Jul 27];62 (1):100–14. Available from: http://www.ncbi.nlm.nih.gov/pubmed/22381168.

10. Rouprêt M, Babjuk M, Compérat E, Zigeuner R, Sylvester RJ, Burger M, et al. European Association of Urology Guidelines on Upper Urinary Tract Urothelial Cell Carcinoma: 2015 Update. Eur Urol [Internet]. 2015 Jul 15 [cited 2015 Jul 27]; Available from: http://www.ncbi.nlm.nih.gov/pubmed/26188393.
11. Yakoubi R, Colin P, Seisen T, Léon P, Nison L, Bozzini G, et al. Radical nephroureterectomy versus endoscopic procedures for the treatment of localised upper tract urothelial carcinoma: a meta-analysis and a systematic review of current evidence from comparative studies. Eur J Surg Oncol [Internet]. 2014 Dec [cited 2015 Jul 6];40(12):1629–34. Available from: http://www.ncbi.nlm.nih.gov/pubmed/25108813.
12. Cosentino M, Palou J, Gaya JM, Breda A, Rodriguez-Faba O, Villavicencio-Mavrich H. Upper urinary tract urothelial cell carcinoma: location as a predictive factor for concomitant bladder carcinoma. World J Urol [Internet]. 2013 Feb [cited 2015 Jul 2];31(1):141–5. Available from: http://www.ncbi.nlm.nih.gov/pubmed/22552732.
13. Zigeuner RE, Hutterer G, Chromecki T, Rehak P, Langner C. Bladder tumour development after urothelial carcinoma of the upper urinary tract is related to primary tumour location. BJU Int [Internet]. 2006 Dec [cited 2015 Jul 2];98(6):1181–6. Available from: http://www.ncbi.nlm.nih.gov/pubmed/17125475.
14. Novara G, De Marco V, Dalpiaz O, Gottardo F, Bouygues V, Galfano A, et al. Independent predictors of metachronous bladder transitional cell carcinoma (TCC) after nephroureterectomy for TCC of the upper urinary tract. BJU Int [Internet]. 2008 Jun [cited 2015 Jul 21];101(11):1368–74. Available from: http://www.ncbi.nlm.nih.gov/pubmed/18241252.
15. Li W-M, Shen J-T, Li C-C, Ke H-L, Wei Y-C, Wu W-J, et al. Oncologic outcomes following three different approaches to the distal ureter and bladder cuff in nephroureterectomy for primary upper urinary tract urothelial carcinoma. Eur Urol [Internet]. 2010 Jun [cited 2015 Jul 2];57(6):963–9. Available from: http://www.ncbi.nlm.nih.gov/pubmed/20079965.
16. Novara G, De Marco V, Dalpiaz O, Galfano A, Bouygues V, Gardiman M, et al. Independent predictors of contralateral metachronous upper urinary tract transitional cell carcinoma after nephroureterectomy: Multi-institutional dataset from three European centers. Int J Urol [Internet]. 2009 Feb 27 [cited 2015 Jul 2];16(2):187–91. Available from: http://www.ncbi.nlm.nih.gov/pubmed/19054165.
17. Rabbani F, Perrotti M, Russo P, Herr HW. Upper-tract tumors after an initial diagnosis of bladder cancer: argument for long-term surveillance. J Clin Oncol [Internet]. 2001 Jan 1 [cited 2015 Jul 21];19(1):94–100. Available from: http://www.ncbi.nlm.nih.gov/pubmed/11134200.
18. Sternberg IA, Keren Paz GE, Chen LY, Herr HW, Donat SM, Bochner BH, et al. Upper tract imaging surveillance is not effective in diagnosing upper tract recurrence in patients followed for nonmuscle invasive bladder cancer. J Urol [Internet]. 2013 Oct [cited 2016 Mar 24];190(4):1187–91. Available from: http://www.ncbi.nlm.nih.gov/pubmed/23680310.
19. Streem SB, Pontes JE, Novick AC, Montie JE. Ureteropyeloscopy in the evaluation of upper tract filling defects. J Urol [Internet]. 1986 Aug [cited 2015 Jul 22];136(2):383–5. Available from: http://www.ncbi.nlm.nih.gov/pubmed/3735500.
20. Blute ML, Segura JW, Patterson DE, Benson RC, Zincke H. Impact of endourology on diagnosis and management of upper urinary tract urothelial cancer. J Urol [Internet]. 1989 Jun [cited 2015 Jul 22];141 (6):1298–301. Available from: http://www.ncbi.nlm.nih.gov/pubmed/2724425.
21. Keeley FX, Kulp DA, Bibbo M, McCue PA, Bagley DH. Diagnostic accuracy of ureteroscopic biopsy in upper tract transitional cell carcinoma. J Urol [Internet]. 1997 Jan [cited 2015 Jul 22];157 (1):33–7. Available from: http://www.ncbi.nlm.nih.gov/pubmed/8976209.
22. Guarnizo E, Pavlovich CP, Seiba M, Carlson DL, Vaughan ED, Sosa RE. Ureteroscopic biopsy of upper tract urothelial carcinoma: improved diagnostic accuracy and histopathological considerations using a multi-biopsy approach. J Urol [Internet]. 2000 Jan [cited 2015 Jul 22];163(1):52–5. Available from: http://www.ncbi.nlm.nih.gov/pubmed/10604312.
23. Tavora F, Fajardo DA, Lee TK, Lotan T, Miller JS, Miyamoto H, et al. Small endoscopic biopsies of the ureter and renal pelvis: pathologic pitfalls. Am J Surg Pathol [Internet]. 2009 Oct [cited 2015 Jul 22];33 (10):1540–6. Available from: http://www.ncbi.nlm.nih.gov/pubmed/19654502.
24. Wang JK, Tollefson MK, Krambeck AE, Trost LW, Thompson RH. High rate of pathologic upgrading at nephroureterectomy for upper tract urothelial carcinoma. Urology [Internet]. 2012 Mar [cited 2015 Jul 22];79(3):615–9. Available from: http://www.ncbi.nlm.nih.gov/pubmed/22386411.
25. Bus MTJ, de Bruin DM, Faber DJ, Kamphuis GM, Zondervan PJ, Laguna Pes MP, et al. Optical diagnostics for upper urinary tract urothelial cancer: technology, thresholds, and clinical applications. J Endourol [Internet]. 2015 Feb [cited 2015 Jul 22];29(2):113–23. Available from: http://www.ncbi.nlm.nih.gov/pubmed/25178057.
26. Kuznetsov K, Lambert R, Rey J-F. Narrow-band imaging: potential and limitations. Endoscopy [Internet]. 2006 Jan [cited 2015 Jul 22];38(1):76–81. Available from: http://www.ncbi.nlm.nih.gov/pubmed/16429359.
27. Gono K, Yamaguchi MON. Improvement of image quality of the electroendoscopy by narrowing

spectral shapes of observation light. Proc Int Congr Imaging Sci. 2002;5:399–400.
28. Gono K, Yamazaki K, Doguchi N, Nonami T, Obi T, Yamaguchi M, Ohyama N, Machida H, Sano Y, Yoshida S, Hamamoto Y. Endoscopic Observation of Tissue by Narrowband Illumination. Opt Rev. 2003;10(4):211–5.
29. Gono K, Obi T, Yamaguchi M, Ohyama N, Machida H, Sano Y, et al. Appearance of enhanced tissue features in narrow-band endoscopic imaging. J Biomed Opt [Internet]. Jan [cited 2015 Jul 22];9(3):568–77. Available from: http://www.ncbi.nlm.nih.gov/pubmed/15189095.
30. Takenaka R, Kawahara Y, Okada H, Hori K, Inoue M, Kawano S, et al. Narrow-band imaging provides reliable screening for esophageal malignancy in patients with head and neck cancers. Am J Gastroenterol [Internet]. 2009 Dec [cited 2015 Jul 22];104(12):2942–8. Available from: http://www.ncbi.nlm.nih.gov/pubmed/19623169.
31. Wang W-H, Lin Y-C, Lee K-F, Weng H-H. Nasopharyngeal carcinoma detected by narrow-band imaging endoscopy. Oral Oncol [Internet]. 2011 Aug [cited 2015 Jul 22];47(8):736–41. Available from: http://www.ncbi.nlm.nih.gov/pubmed/21393053.
32. Herr HW. Narrow-band imaging evaluation of bladder tumors. Curr Urol Rep [Internet]. 2014 Apr [cited 2015 Jul 22];15(4):395. Available from: http://www.ncbi.nlm.nih.gov/pubmed/24652533.
33. Herr H, Donat M, Dalbagni G, Taylor J. Narrow-band imaging cystoscopy to evaluate bladder tumours–individual surgeon variability. BJU Int [Internet]. 2010 Jul [cited 2015 Jul 23];106(1):53–5. Available from: http://www.pubmedcentral.nih.gov/articlerender.fcgi?artid=3137239&tool=pmcentrez&rendertype=abstract.
34. Bryan RT, Shah ZH, Collins SI, Wallace DMA. Narrow-band imaging flexible cystoscopy: a new user's experience. J Endourol [Internet]. 2010 Aug [cited 2015 Jul 23];24(8):1339–43. Available from: http://www.ncbi.nlm.nih.gov/pubmed/20629569.
35. Herr HW. Narrow-band imaging cystoscopy to evaluate the response to bacille Calmette-Guérin therapy: preliminary results. BJU Int [Internet]. 2010 Feb [cited 2015 Jul 24];105(3):314–6. Available from: http://www.ncbi.nlm.nih.gov/pubmed/19793381.
36. Cauberg ECC, Mamoulakis C, de la Rosette JJMCH, de Reijke TM. Narrow band imaging-assisted transurethral resection for non-muscle invasive bladder cancer significantly reduces residual tumour rate. World J Urol [Internet]. 2011 Aug [cited 2015 Jul 24];29(4):503–9. Available from: http://www.pubmedcentral.nih.gov/articlerender.fcgi?artid=3143329&tool=pmcentrez&rendertype=abstract.
37. Herr HW, Donat SM. Reduced bladder tumour recurrence rate associated with narrow-band imaging surveillance cystoscopy. BJU Int [Internet]. 2011 Feb [cited 2015 Jul 24];107(3):396–8. Available from: http://www.ncbi.nlm.nih.gov/pubmed/20707789.
38. Herr HW. Randomized trial of narrow-band versus white-light cystoscopy for restaging (second-look) transurethral resection of bladder tumors. Eur Urol [Internet]. 2015 Apr [cited 2015 Jul 30];67(4):605–8. Available from: http://www.ncbi.nlm.nih.gov/pubmed/25041849.
39. Geavlete B, Multescu R, Georgescu D, Stanescu F, Jecu M, Geavlete P. Narrow band imaging cystoscopy and bipolar plasma vaporization for large nonmuscle-invasive bladder tumors–results of a prospective, randomized comparison to the standard approach. Urology [Internet]. 2012 Apr [cited 2015 Jul 24];79(4):846–51. Available from: http://www.ncbi.nlm.nih.gov/pubmed/22342408.
40. Stănescu F, Geavlete B, Georgescu D, Jecu M, Moldoveanu C, Adou L, et al. NBI—plasma vaporization hybrid approach in bladder cancer endoscopic management. J Med Life [Internet]. 2014 Jun 15 [cited 2015 Jul 24];7(2):155–9. Available from: http://www.pubmedcentral.nih.gov/articlerender.fcgi?artid=4197500&tool=pmcentrez&rendertype=abstract.
41. De la Rosette J, Gravas S. A multi-center, randomized international study to compare the impact of narrow band imaging versus white light cystoscopy in the recurrence of bladder cancer. J Endourol [Internet]. 2010 May [cited 2015 Jul 24];24(5):660–1. Available from: http://www.ncbi.nlm.nih.gov/pubmed/20443701.
42. Cowan NC, Turney BW, Taylor NJ, McCarthy CL, Crew JP. Multidetector computed tomography urography for diagnosing upper urinary tract urothelial tumour. BJU Int [Internet]. 2007 Jun [cited 2015 Jun 28];99(6):1363–70. Available from: http://www.ncbi.nlm.nih.gov/pubmed/17428251.
43. Furukawa J, Miyake H, Sakai I, Fujisawa M. Significance of ureteroscopic biopsy grade in patients with upper tract urothelial carcinoma. Curr Urol [Internet]. 2013 Jan [cited 2015 Aug 3];6(3):156–9. Available from: http://www.pubmedcentral.nih.gov/articlerender.fcgi?artid=3783279&tool=pmcentrez&rendertype=abstract.
44. Skolarikos A, Griffiths TRL, Powell PH, Thomas DJ, Neal DE, Kelly JD. Cytologic analysis of ureteral washings is informative in patients with grade 2 upper tract TCC considering endoscopic treatment. Urology [Internet]. 2003 Jun [cited 2015 Aug 3];61(6):1146–50. Available from: http://www.ncbi.nlm.nih.gov/pubmed/12809884.
45. Clements T, Messer JC, Terrell JD, Herman MP, Ng CK, Scherr DS, et al. High-grade ureteroscopic biopsy is associated with advanced pathology of upper-tract urothelial carcinoma tumors at definitive surgical resection. J Endourol [Internet]. 2012 Apr [cited 2015 Jul 27];26(4):398–402. Available from: http://www.ncbi.nlm.nih.gov/pubmed/22192113.
46. Ishioka J, Kihara K, Higuchi S, Nakayama T, Takeshita H, Yoshida S, et al. New head-mounted

display system applied to endoscopic management of upper urinary tract carcinomas. Int Braz J Urol [Internet]. Jan [cited 2015 Jul 27];40(6):842–5. Available from: http://www.ncbi.nlm.nih.gov/pubmed/25615254.
47. Nison L, Bozzini G, Rouprêt M, Traxer O, Colin P. [Clinical, ureteroscopic and photodynamic diagnosis of urothelial carcinomas of the upper tract: state-of-the art for the yearly scientific report of the French National Association of Urology]. Prog Urol [Internet]. 2014 Nov [cited 2015 Jul 27];24(15):977–86. Available from: http://www.ncbi.nlm.nih.gov/pubmed/25199724.
48. Meyer F, Al Qahtani S, Gil-Diez de Medina S, Geavlete B, Thomas A, Traxer O. [Narrow band imaging: description of the technique and initial experience with upper urinary tract carcinomas]. Prog Urol [Internet]. 2011 Sep [cited 2015 Jul 27];21(8):527–33. Available from: http://www.ncbi.nlm.nih.gov/pubmed/21872155.
49. Traxer O, Geavlete B, de Medina SGD, Sibony M, Al-Qahtani SM. Narrow-band imaging digital flexible ureteroscopy in detection of upper urinary tract transitional-cell carcinoma: initial experience. J Endourol [Internet]. 2011 Jan [cited 2015 Jul 27];25(1):19–23. Available from: http://www.ncbi.nlm.nih.gov/pubmed/21247287.
50. Audenet F, Traxer O, Yates DR, Cussenot O, Rouprêt M. Potential role of photodynamic techniques combined with new generation flexible ureterorenoscopes and molecular markers for the management of urothelial carcinoma of the upper urinary tract. BJU Int [Internet]. 2012 Feb [cited 2015 Jun 18];109(4):608–13; discussion 613–4. Available from: http://www.ncbi.nlm.nih.gov/pubmed/21985291.
51. Cauberg ECC, de la Rosette JJMCH, de Reijke TM. How to improve the effectiveness of transurethral resection in nonmuscle invasive bladder cancer? Curr Opin Urol [Internet]. 2009 Sep [cited 2015 Jul 29];19(5):504–10. Available from: http://www.ncbi.nlm.nih.gov/pubmed/19571756.
52. Herr HW, Donat SM. A comparison of white-light cystoscopy and narrow-band imaging cystoscopy to detect bladder tumour recurrences. BJU Int [Internet]. 2008 Nov [cited 2015 Jul 23];102(9):1111–4. Available from: http://www.ncbi.nlm.nih.gov/pubmed/18778359.
53. Behera M, Kumar A, Soares HP, Sokol L, Djulbegovic B. Evidence-based medicine for rare diseases: implications for data interpretation and clinical trial design. Cancer Control [Internet]. 2007 Apr [cited 2015 Jul 30];14(2):160–6. Available from: http://www.ncbi.nlm.nih.gov/pubmed/17387301.
54. Lepor H. Does the medical evidence justify robotic assisted laparoscopic radical prostatectomy as the new gold standard for radical prostatectomy? Urol Oncol [Internet]. 2013 Mar [cited 2015 Jul 30];31(2):137–9. Available from: http://www.ncbi.nlm.nih.gov/pubmed/23586101.
55. Bryan RT, Billingham LJ, Wallace DMA. Narrow-band imaging flexible cystoscopy in the detection of recurrent urothelial cancer of the bladder. BJU Int [Internet]. 2008 Mar [cited 2015 Jul 23];101(6):702–5; discussion 705–6. Available from: http://www.ncbi.nlm.nih.gov/pubmed/18005206.
56. Cauberg ECC, Kloen S, Visser M, de la Rosette JJMCH, Babjuk M, Soukup V, et al. Narrow band imaging cystoscopy improves the detection of non-muscle-invasive bladder cancer. Urology [Internet]. 2010 Sep [cited 2015 Jul 23];76(3):658–63. Available from: http://www.ncbi.nlm.nih.gov/pubmed/20223505.
57. Tatsugami K, Kuroiwa K, Kamoto T, Nishiyama H, Watanabe J, Ishikawa S, et al. Evaluation of narrow-band imaging as a complementary method for the detection of bladder cancer. J Endourol [Internet]. 2010 Nov [cited 2015 Jul 23];24(11):1807–11. Available from: http://www.ncbi.nlm.nih.gov/pubmed/20707727.
58. Shen Y-J, Zhu Y-P, Ye D-W, Yao X-D, Zhang S-L, Dai B, et al. Narrow-band imaging flexible cystoscopy in the detection of primary non-muscle invasive bladder cancer: a "second look" matters? Int Urol Nephrol [Internet]. 2012 Apr [cited 2015 Jul 23];44(2):451–7. Available from: http://www.ncbi.nlm.nih.gov/pubmed/21792663.
59. Xiaodong S, Zhangqun YSB. Application of narrow band imaging in the early diagnosis and recurrent monitoring of bladder cancer. J Contemp Urol Reprod Oncol. 2009;6:325–7.
60. Geavlete B, Jecu M, Multescu R, Geavlete P. Narrow-band imaging cystoscopy in non-muscle-invasive bladder cancer: a prospective comparison to the standard approach. Ther Adv Urol [Internet]. 2012 Oct [cited 2015 Jul 23];4(5):211–7. Available from: http://www.pubmedcentral.nih.gov/articlerender.fcgi?artid=3441134&tool=pmcentrez&rendertype=abstract.
61. Zhu Y-P, Shen Y-J, Ye D-W, Wang C-F, Yao X-D, Zhang S-L, et al. Narrow-band imaging flexible cystoscopy in the detection of clinically unconfirmed positive urine cytology. Urol Int [Internet]. 2012 Jan [cited 2015 Jul 23];88(1):84–7. Available from: http://www.ncbi.nlm.nih.gov/pubmed/22104957.
62. Chen G, Wang B, Li H, Ma X, Shi T, Zhang X. Applying narrow-band imaging in complement with white-light imaging cystoscopy in the detection of urothelial carcinoma of the bladder. Urol Oncol [Internet]. 2013 May [cited 2015 Jul 23];31(4):475–9. Available from: http://www.ncbi.nlm.nih.gov/pubmed/22079940.
63. Jecu M, Geavlete B, Mulţescu R, Stănescu F, Moldoveanu C, Adou L, et al. NBI cystoscopy in routine urological practice - from better vision to improve therapeutic management. J Med Life [Internet]. 2014 Jul 15 [cited 2015 Jul 31];7(2):282–6. Available from: http://www.pubmedcentral.nih.gov/articlerender.fcgi?artid=4197490&tool=pmcentrez&rendertype=abstract.

64. Song PH, Cho S, Ko YH. Decision Based on Narrow Band Imaging Cystoscopy without a Referential Normal Standard Rather Increases Unnecessary Biopsy in Detection of recurrent Bladder Urothelial Carcinoma Early after Intravesical Instillation. Cancer Res Treat [Internet]. 2015 Mar 2 [cited 2015 Jul 31]; Available from: http://www.ncbi.nlm.nih.gov/pubmed/25761489.
65. Ye Z, Hu J, Song X, Li F, Zhao X, Chen S, et al. A comparison of NBI and WLI cystoscopy in detecting non-muscle-invasive bladder cancer: A prospective, randomized and multi-center study. Sci Rep [Internet]. 2015 Jan [cited 2015 Jul 31];5:10905. Available from: http://www.pubmedcentral.nih.gov/articlerender.fcgi?artid=4456941&tool=pmcentrez&rendertype=abstract.
66. Naya Y, Oishi M, Yamada Y, Ueda T, Fujihara A, Nakanishi H, et al. Initial experience of combined use of photodynamic diagnosis and narrow band imaging for detection of flat urothelial lesion. Int J Clin Oncol [Internet]. 2015 Jul [cited 2015 Jul 31];20(3):593–7. Available from: http://www.ncbi.nlm.nih.gov/pubmed/25228479.

13 Blue Light Endoscopy

Saman Moazami, Mark P. Schoenberg and Joshua M. Stern

Introduction

Upper tract urothelial cell carcinoma (UTUC) comprises 5% of all urothelial malignancies [1]. The ability to accurately predict pathologic stage and grade of UTUC is crucial for prognostication and selection of appropriate therapeutic intervention. The advent of high definition flexible ureteroscopy has increased the use of minimally invasive endoscopic evaluation and treatment of UTUC [2]. Nonetheless, accurate endoscopic staging of upper tract tumors remains challenged by difficult visualization and the limited size of the pathologic specimen obtained. Specifically, 45% of papillary tumors are upstaged at final definitive resection [3]. Consequently, definitive counseling of patients after endoscopic biopsy remains difficult. Using the latest endoscopic equipment in a high volume center, Gupta et al. evaluated pathology reports of 76 patients collected after radical nephroureterectomy (NU) to determine the accuracy of upper tract ureteroscopic (URS) biopsy. Ureteroscopic mapping was accurate in 75% of patients, failing to identify 25% of the lesions seen on final resection. 36% of low-grade tumors on endoscopic biopsy were upgraded to high grade, while there was 65% upstaging of ureteroscopic biopsies [1]. Several other authors have found similar discordance between NU pathology and URS biopsy. In a cohort of 56 patients who underwent multiple ureteroscopic biopsies followed by nephroureterectomy, Smith et al. found 18/65 (28%) specimens underwent grade reclassification, while 32% were upstaged from noninvasive to invasive disease [4]. Selective cytology, advanced imaging, and endoluminal ultrasound are useful adjuncts to endoscopic staging, yet there continues to be high rates of upgrading and upstaging of ureteroscopic biopsies following nephroureterectomy [5]. Given the limitations of traditional histology after endoscopic biopsy, and in an effort to more accurately phenotype UTUC tumors, Margulis et al. recently demonstrated the concordance of a biomarker panel obtained after endoscopic biopsy to that obtained after NU [6]. Molecular markers in UTUC may be a beneficial adjunct to individualizing treatment regimens and may augment the current predictive capability of endoscopic biopsy. The identification and biopsy of the tumor remains the first step in the diagnosis of an upper tract lesion. As such, continued evolution of the endoscopic evaluation is warranted for patients with UTUC.

S. Moazami · M. P. Schoenberg · J. M. Stern (✉)
Department of Urology, Montefiore Medical Center/Albert Einstein College of Medicine, 1250 Waters Place, Tower 1, Suite 706, Bronx, NY, USA
e-mail: jstern@montefiore.org

S. Moazami
e-mail: smoazami@montefiore.org

M. P. Schoenberg
e-mail: mschoenb@montefiore.org

M. Eshghi (ed.), *Urothelial Malignancies of the Upper Urinary Tract*,
https://doi.org/10.1007/978-3-319-51263-1_13

Blue light endoscopy (HAL-BLC) is a recently adopted adjunct to standard white light endoscopy in bladder cancer management. Data on HAL-BLC collected from bladder cancer patients show increasing rates of tumor detection, with subsequent decrease in residual tumor at follow-up. Blue light endoscopy for UTUC may have similar benefit in the diagnosis and treatment of patients with upper tract disease.

Mechanism of Photodynamic Therapy

Photodynamic therapy is a process that involves the administration of a photosensitizing agent and its activation via a specific wavelength of light. This interaction leads to a transfer of energy resulting in a triplet-electron state. The energy from this electron is then transferred to oxygen, producing a photodynamic reaction, and the production of reactive oxygen species [7]. The most common photosensitizers (PS) used in urologic surgery are Aminolevulinic acid (5-ALA) and Hexaminolevulinate (HAL). HAL is currently the only sensitizer approved for use in the United States [8]. Photosensitizers can be administered intravenously, orally, topically or intraluminally. Intravesical instillation for blue light cystoscopy and oral administration with subsequent ureteroscopy are the standards in urology. Instillation of Intravesical HAL is done 1 h prior to blue light cystoscopy, while oral administration of 5-ALA requires administration approximately 3–4 h prior to ureteroscopy [9]. The PS enters the cell via a variety of proposed mechanisms. Increased tumor vasculature permeability to macromolecules is thought to be an important step in the accumulation of PS within the targeted tissue. Administering 5-ALA through an alkyl ester such as HAL makes the PS more lipophilic which will increase cellular uptake [10]. Once photosensitizer extravasation into the tumor interstitium occurs, cellular uptake is thought to be via binding to low-density lipoproteins (LDL), which have been shown to be upregulated in many malignancies. When using PS for therapeutic purposes, activation of a porphyrin derivative via light energy triggers the release of reactive oxygen species that leads to a cascade of events, resulting in Bcl-2 mediated apoptosis. The effects of PDT are not strictly limited to the induction of apoptosis, but are also thought to involve necrosis, autophagy, and cytotoxic T cell activation [11].

PDT can also be an adjunct to tumor detection. While tissue destruction through reactive oxygen species can be achieved with laser irradiation of a PS, fluorescent detection is a diagnostic use of a PS. This occurs through an alternate pathway resulting in energy loss from the activated PS when exposed to blue light (360–450 nm), leading to fluorescent emission [7]. The use of PDT in urology currently employs this mechanism. HAL produces 2.5 times the amount of fluorescence as 5-ALA at 45 times lower concentration [12].

History of Modern Photodynamic Therapy

The use of "concentrated light beams" ("koncentrerade ljusstrålar") for the treatment of human disease began in 1903 when Niels Finsen was awarded the Nobel Prize for his discovery of red light in the treatment of smallpox and ultraviolet light as a therapeutic option for cutaneous tuberculosis [13]. The combination of light therapy with chemical agents occurred in the same year when Herman Von Tappeiner and A. Jesionek used topical eosin and white light to treat skin lesions [13]. Lipson et al. [14] first described the use of hematoporphyrin derivatives at the Mayo Clinic in the 1960s. They demonstrated that localization and accumulation of these derivatives in tumors with high vascularity resulted in fluorescent emission [14]. The first clinical trials involving hematoporphyrin derivatives began in 1976 when Kelly and Snell described the use of hematoporphyrin derivatives to assist in the identification and treatment of bladder cancer [15]. From these trials stemmed the utilization of hematoporphyrins for the diagnosis and treatment of lesions of the skin, brain, tracheobronchial tree, and gastrointestinal tract [16].

Photodynamic Therapy in the Urinary Tract

The majority of evidence surrounding the use of photosensitizers in diagnosing urothelial cell carcinoma comes from studies of bladder tumors. Zaak et al. reported a large study of 1,012 fluorescent endoscopies after intravesical administration of 5-ALA. 34.2% of tumors seen with PDT were missed by standard white light. Of these lesions, 38.7% were high grade. Additionally, 88 cases of CIS were identified and standard cystoscopy missed nearly ½ of those lesions. [17]. Recent advances in porphyrin development have led to the use of a more lipophilic ester of 5-ALA known as Hexaminolevulinate (HAL) [18]. The main advantage of HAL over 5-ALA is its ability to produce an increased amount of photoactive substance in less time and at lower doses. HAL is currently the only photoactive compound approved by the Food and Drug Administration for use in the United States [19].

The rational for the adoption of blue light endoscopy to UTUC comes from evidence collected in bladder cancer over the past decade. A large international randomized control trial of 814 patients with non-muscle invasive bladder cancer compared HAL-BLC to white light cystoscopy (WLC) at the time of transurethral resection. 16% of tumors seen with fluorescent cystoscopy were not detected by standard WLC ($p = 0.001$). 41 patients were diagnosed with carcinoma in situ (CIS) and 32% of those CIS lesions were completely missed by WLC ($p < 0.0001$). At 9 months follow-up there were fewer recurrences in the BLC group as compared to the WLC group (47% vs. 56%, $p = 0.026$), and a follow-up study at 55 months showed that patients resected with HAL-BLC had a delay in the median time to recurrence (16.4 months vs. 9.4 months, $p = 0.04$) [20]. A meta-analysis of five prospective studies including 1,345 patients with non-muscle invasive disease compared HAL-BLC to WLC. HAL-BLC found significantly more Ta tumors (14.7%; $p < 0.001$; [OR]: 4.898; 95% CI, 1.937–12.390) and CIS lesions (40.8%; $p < 0.001$; OR: 12.372; 95% CI, 6.343–24.133) compared to WLC. Recurrence rates were significantly lower with blue light (34.5% vs. 45.4% ($p = 0.006$)) at 12 months [21]. Regarding the safety of intravesical porphyrin use, an analysis of six studies suggest its use posed little additional risk other than that expected during standard white light endoscopy. Adverse events based on laboratory findings, vital signs, and physical examinations were rare [22]. While the role of HAL-BLC in bladder cancer is more established, its use in upper tract disease remains in its infancy (Fig. 13.1).

Endoscopic Management of Upper Tract Tumors

While advances in endoscopic technology have enabled urologists to perform simultaneous diagnostics and treatment of UTUC, accurate endoscopic staging of upper tract tumors remains challenging in light of difficult visualization, and

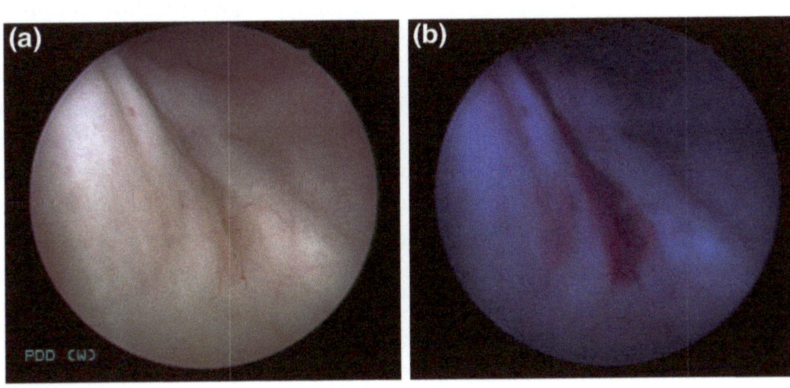

Fig. 13.1 **a** Surveillance cystoscopy with *white* light. **b** *Blue* light cystoscopy demonstrating a lesion consistent with high-grade papillary urothelial cell carcinoma

the limited size of the pathologic specimen obtained [23]. Numerous studies have established tumor stage as the most important prognostic factor in UTUC [24–26]. In a series of 252 patients with median follow-up of 64 months, Hall et al. reported 5-year disease-specific survival rates as 100% for Ta, 91.7% for T1, 72.6% for T2, and 40.5% for T3. On multivariate analysis, patient age ($p = 0.042$) and tumor stage ($P < 0.0001$) were the only significant predictors of disease-specific survival [27]. Tumor upstaging after endoscopic biopsy is highly prevalent and as such represents one of the deficiencies of contemporary endoscopic management of UTUC. Guarnizo et al. [3] observed that approximately 45% of tumors in their series were upstaged from Ta to T1–T3 at the time of definitive resection. The explanation for such upstaging includes tumors that were originally missed endoscopically, and the difficulty in obtaining deep biopsies ureteroscopically.

Given such limitations, endoscopic management often relies on tumor grade to guide management decisions. While there are reports suggesting biopsy grade may correlate well with final grade and in select cases with final stage, the sum of the data is equivocal and improved accuracy is still needed. Keeley et al. compared tumor grade on ureteroscopic biopsy to final pathology in 42 specimens. 27/30 (90%) low or moderate grade and 11/12 (91.6%) high-grade biopsy specimens correlated with final pathologic grade ($p < 0.0001$). None of the 10 patients with low-grade biopsies had invasive disease on final pathology. 8/12 (66.7%) patients with high-grade disease on biopsy had pT2 or pT3, while 34% of patients, final stage correlated poorly with biopsy grade ($p = 0.0006$) [28]. Skolarikos et al. reported on 51 cases of ureteroscopic biopsy to determine how well they compared to final pathology. Ureteroscopic biopsy G3 tumors ($n = 13$) correlated with final pathologic grade in 92% of cases. Similarly, the six patients with ureteroscopic biopsy grade 1 correlated well with final pathologic grade. However, there was poor grade correlation among the 32 G2 tumors on final pathology with 28% upgraded to G3. In those biopsies that were clearly low or high grade, tumor grade correlated well with stage, such that none of the G1 tumors were found to have muscle invasion while 11/13 G3 tumors had tumor invasion into muscle or parenchyma (pT2 or greater; $P < 0.0001$). The G2 tumor biopsies did not correlate well with final stage [29]. Furukawa et al. also evaluated biopsy and NU specimen in 40 patients. In 88%, biopsy grade correlated well with final pathologic grade. This series showed good correlation between tumor biopsy grade and final pathologic stage with 18/19 patients with low-grade tumor biopsies having no invasion on final pathology [30]. Nonetheless, other series mentioned earlier, suggest there is high-grade upstaging, and up to 25% missed tumors with endoscopic management [1, 4].

In addition to endoscopic diagnosis, many centers routinely use endoscopic management of low-grade UTUC as a good option for select patients. Lucas et al. looked at 48 low-grade tumors, 27 treated conservatively, and 21 managed with immediate nephroureterectomy. The 5-year disease-specific survival for low-grade disease was 86.2% versus 87.4% in the endoscopic versus NU group ($p = 0.909$) [31]. Roupret et al. also compared NU to endoscopic treatment in 97 patients. The 5-year disease-specific survival rate was 84 and 80.7%, for low-grade tumors receiving NU or endoscopic management ($p = 0.89$). The 5-year recurrence free survival rates for low-grade disease was 75.3 and 72% respectively ($p = 0.78$) [32].

Long-term follow-up of patients undergoing endoscopic management relies on accurate identification of tumors. In a cohort of 73 patients with UTUC followed for a median period of 54 months upper tract recurrence occurred in 68% of cases, with 19% progressing to nephroureterectomy. Overall and disease-specific survival at 5 years were 69.7 and 88.9%, with mean disease-specific survival of 190 months [33]. While oncologic outcomes demonstrated the feasibility of endoscopic management for a select group of patients, it is not known what percent of "recurrences" were actually missed tumors. Given the heterogeneity of the data on endoscopic evaluation and tumor staging of UTUC, an adjunct that could increase accurate detection of tumors would be of great importance.

Photodynamic Diagnosis of Upper Urinary Tract Lesions

The use of photodynamic therapy for endoscopic management of UTUC dates back to the late 1990s when Waidelich et al. reported on the use of oral 5-aminolevulinic acid (5-ALA) in a series of four patients with widespread superficial papillary in both renal units or a solitary kidney. They administered 40 mg/kg oral 5-ALA dissolved in 200 mL of water, 3–6 h prior to irradiation, followed by endoscopic irradiation of these tumors. All four patients had tumors confirmed to be pTaG1–2 on ureteroscopic biopsy completed 1-week prior to photodynamic therapy. Irradiation was carried out with 514 nm (green) or 645 nm (red) wavelength laser. Complete response was shown in two patients, with partial response in two subjects [34]. Since this early report, the data on photodynamic therapy in urology has focused on diagnosis rather then ablation. Aboumarzouk et al. compared the detection rate of blue light endoscopy using oral 5-ALA to CT urogram and white light ureteroscopy in 30 patients. Patients received 20 mg/kg of oral 5-ALA, 3–4 h prior to their procedure, based on the pharmacokinetics of protoporphyrin IX induced by 5 ALA. Of the 17 lesions identified, blue light ureteroscopy detected 16/17 (94%) tumors compared to 14/17 (82%) and 13/17 (76.5%) in white light ureteroscopy and CT urogram respectively. Importantly, only blue light endoscopy identified the three patients with CIS [35]. Ahmad et al. reported on results from 26 biopsies of UTUC. 11/26 tumors were detected by both white and blue light, with all biopsies being positive for malignancy. 10/26 biopsies (38.5%) were identified just with blue light, and consisted of 7 Ta lesions, 2 dysplastic lesions, and 1 benign lesion. Five random biopsies were taken from mucosa with normal appearance, listed as suspicious regions on CT urogram. All of these biopsies returned negative for malignancy. One of the dysplastic lesions was subsequently biopsied again and confirmed to be pTaG2 [9]. Similar to its efficacy in detecting small or flat lesions of the bladder mucosa that are undetected by white light cystoscopy, this small series demonstrates that blue light photodynamic endoscopy in the upper urinary tract has the potential to improve the detection of UTUC [9, 16]. This same group recently published their cohort of 106 upper tract units. 48/106 units were found to have lesions on ureteroscopy. 32/48 had confirmed UTUC, with 11 patients having CIS, and five patients having a predominance of CIS mixed with other pathology. The detection rate for malignant lesions was 47.9% for white light, and 95.8% for blue light ($p < 0.0001$). The results showed a sensitivity for detecting upper tract lesions of [95.8% (CI: 85.7–99.5)] with blue light, compared to [53.3% (CI: 37.7–68.8)] with white light ureteroscopy ($p < 0.0001$). Detection of CIS was similarly more significant with blue light (93.75% vs. 18.75%, $p = 0.0006$) [36]. While these results are promising, larger series are needed to clarify its oncologic outcomes with regards to recurrence and progression free survival.

While the current protocol for HAL-BLC requires intravesical instillation an hour prior to cystoscopy, there is currently no standard procedure for the administration of photoactive substances prior to upper tract endoscopy. Although instillation via percutaneous nephrostomy tube and or ureteral catheter is feasible, the duration of exposure to the agent remains unknown and the required dwell time to maximize cellular uptake has not been established [2]. Administration of chemotherapy and immunotherapy to the upper tract suffers from similar lack of standardization and as such does not provide a benchmark from which blue light endoscopy can build upon. Studies examining adjuvant administration of BCG or Mitomycin to the upper tract have varying results. Studies have shown high rates of recurrence and progression, and partial/complete response in only a limited number of patients [37–39]. Nonetheless, small series have demonstrated success with BCG

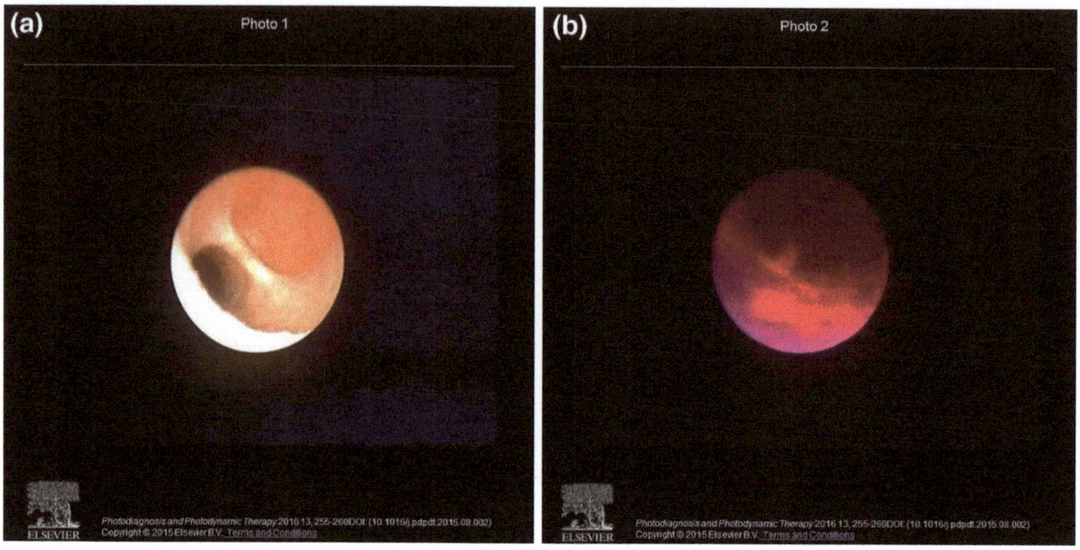

Fig. 13.2 **a** Standard *white* light ureteroscopy of the collecting system and **b** Fluorescent tumor in the collecting system, with biopsy revealing carcinoma in situ. From Kata et al. [36]

instillation to the upper tract for patients with known CIS [40–42].

Efforts to increase the efficacy of agent delivery to the upper tract are ongoing in an attempt to improve endoscopic management of this disease. Wang et al. investigated the use of a reverse thermosensitive polymer (RTP) injected in the distal ureter through a 3F retrograde catheter. A 6F open-ended ureteral catheter was introduced into the renal pelvis prior to injection of the RTP, and used to administer mitomycin after occlusion of the distal ureter. At body temperature the polymer remains viscous, and allows for injection of chemotherapeutic agents into the upper tract. The polymer acts as an occlusion device to increase dwell time, and remains viscous at body temperature. The gel is subsequently liquefied through injection of room temperature saline through the ureteral catheter. The mitomycin used in this porcine model was combined with 50% contrast in order to visualize its presence in the upper tract over time. Drainage of contrast in the control groups occurred at a mean of 5 min, while the experimental group had no contrast drainage after 60 min [43]. Mean renal pressures were maintained at safe levels, between 60 and 75 cm H20, which is lower in comparison to average pressures of 110–136 cm H_2O during flexible ureteroscopy without the use of an access sheath [43–45]. The use of reverse thermosensitive polymers has potential to provide a novel adjunct to increase dwell time of topical porphyrin derivatives prior to blue light ureteroscopy (Fig. 13.2).

Future Directions

The future of PDT involves a better understanding of the basic science and underlying mechanisms at the cellular level, with improvements in the current delivery systems to target tissue [7]. The field of nanotechnology is one that may enhance PDT, by increasing delivery of PS to target tissue. Many agents that are delivered intravenously are bound to plasma proteins thus limited drug deposition to the target tissue [46]. Poly (D,Llactide-co-glycolide) (PLGA) is a Food and Drug Administration approved nanoparticle that is biodegradable, biocompatible, and non-immunogenic. In a recent study, the efficacy of PLGA as a delivery agent was analyzed. Results showed that PLGA nanoparticles coated with polyethylene glycol (PEG) and delivered with a PS, produced faster and more efficient apoptosis when exposed to a specified wavelength. The presence of both PLGA and PEG increased stability of the agent, and prevented clearance by macrophages. Endocytosis of these particles enables delivery of the PS to lysosomes, which are then activated on exposure to light, with subsequent induction of apoptosis. [47].

Photochemical internalization is another future application of PDT, and involves combining photosensitizers with a chemotherapeutic agent. This technique attempts to minimize the morbidity of chemotherapy by delivery of low dose chemotherapeutic/PDT combination agent into target tissue. Site specific illumination of the PS releases the chemotherapeutic at the target site, thereby offering a focal delivery option [7]. PDT has also been studied in combination with oncolytic viral therapy. Khaled et al. recently examined the effect of reovirus in combination with 5-ALA on pancreatic cancer cell lines in -vitro. They found that combination therapy resulted in a significantly increased cytotoxic effect compared to monotherapy ($p = 0{\cdot}042$) with 100% cell death [48]. Liposomes have also been studied in vitro as a means of delivery PDT. Choi et al. looked at liposomes containing 5-ALA as a target against human cholangiocarcinoma cells. Compared to 5-ALA itself, liposome carriers increased both the uptake efficiency and phototoxic effect within these cell lines [49]. Further development of these technologies may enable urologist to not only use this modality as a means of improved tumor detection, but as a potential therapeutic intervention with increasing tissue sparing techniques.

Summary Box

- The ability to accurately predict pathologic stage and grade of upper tract urothelial cell carcinoma (UTUC) is crucial for prognostication and selection of appropriate therapeutic intervention.
- Accurate endoscopic staging of upper tract tumors remains challenged by difficult visualization and the limited size of the pathologic specimen obtained, with tumor upstaging being highly prevalent.
- While there are reports suggesting biopsy grade may correlate well with final grade and in select cases with final stage, the sum of the data is equivocal and improved accuracy is still needed.
- The use of blue light cystoscopy for detection in bladder cancer has resulted in higher tumor detection and lower rates of recurrence.
- While data is limited, blue light ureteroscopy demonstrates significantly higher rates of tumor detection in the upper urinary tract, when compared to both white light ureteroscopy and CT urogram.

References

1. Yamany T, van Batavia J, Ahn J, Shapiro E, Gupta M. Ureterorenoscopy for upper tract urothelial carcinoma: how often are we missing lesions? Urology. 2015;85(2):311–5.
2. Audenet F, Traxer O, Yates DR, Cussenot O, Roupret M. Potential role of photodynamic techniques combined with new generation flexible ureterorenoscopes and molecular markers for the management of urothelial carcinoma of the upper urinary tract. BJU Int. 2012;109(4):608–13; discussion 13–4.
3. Guarnizo E, Pavlovich CP, Seiba M, Carlson DL, Vaughan ED Jr, Sosa RE. Ureteroscopic biopsy of upper tract urothelial carcinoma: improved diagnostic accuracy and histopathological considerations using a multi-biopsy approach. J Urol. 2000;163(1):52–5.
4. Smith AK, Stephenson AJ, Lane BR, Larson BT, Thomas AA, Gong MC, et al. Inadequacy of biopsy for diagnosis of upper tract urothelial carcinoma: implications for conservative management. Urology. 2011;78(1):82–6.
5. Bus MT, de Bruin DM, Faber DJ, Kamphuis GM, Zondervan PJ, Laguna Pes MP, et al. Optical diagnostics for upper urinary tract urothelial cancer: technology, thresholds, and clinical applications. J Endourol Endourol Soc. 2015;29(2):113–23.
6. Gayed BA, Bagrodia A, Gaitonde M, Krabbe LM, Meissner M, Kapur P, et al. Feasibility of obtaining biomarker profiles from endoscopic biopsy specimens in upper tract urothelial carcinoma: preliminary results. Urol Oncol. 2015;33(1):18 e21–6.

7. Allison RR. Photodynamic therapy: oncologic horizons. Future Oncol. 2014;10(1):123–4.
8. Allison RR, Moghissi K. Photodynamic therapy (PDT): PDT mechanisms. Clin Endosc. 2013;46(1):24–9.
9. Ahmad S, Aboumarzouk O, Somani B, Nabi G, Kata SG. Oral 5-aminolevulinic acid in simultaneous photodynamic diagnosis of upper and lower urinary tract transitional cell carcinoma—a prospective audit. BJU Int. 2012;110(11 Pt B):E596–600.
10. Kloek J, Akkermans W. Beijersbergen van Henegouwen GM. Derivatives of 5-aminolevulinic acid for photodynamic therapy: enzymatic conversion into protoporphyrin. Photochem Photobiol. 1998;67(1):150–4.
11. Mroz P, Yaroslavsky A, Kharkwal GB, Hamblin MR. Cell death pathways in photodynamic therapy of cancer. Cancers. 2011;3(2):2516–39.
12. Marti A, Lange N, van den Bergh H, Sedmera D, Jichlinski P, Kucera P. Optimisation of the formation and distribution of protoporphyrin IX in the urothelium: an in vitro approach. J Urol. 1999;162(2):546–52.
13. Dolmans DE, Fukumura D, Jain RK. Photodynamic therapy for cancer. Nat Rev Cancer. 2003;3(5):380–7.
14. Lipson RL, Baldes EJ, Olsen AM. Hematoporphyrin derivative: a new aid for endoscopic detection of malignant disease. J Thorac Cardiovasc Surg. 1961;42:623–9.
15. Kelly JF, Snell ME. Hematoporphyrin derivative: a possible aid in the diagnosis and therapy of carcinoma of the bladder. J Urol. 1976;115(2):150–1.
16. Somani BK, Moseley H, Eljamel MS, Nabi G, Kata SG. Photodynamic diagnosis (PDD) for upper urinary tract transitional cell carcinoma (UT-TCC): evolution of a new technique. Photodiagn Photodyn Ther. 2010;7(1):39–43.
17. Zaak D, Kriegmair M, Stepp H, Stepp H, Baumgartner R, Oberneder R, et al. Endoscopic detection of transitional cell carcinoma with 5-aminolevulinic acid: results of 1012 fluorescence endoscopies. Urology. 2001;57(4):690–4.
18. Jocham D, Witjes F, Wagner S, Zeylemaker B, van Moorselaar J, Grimm MO, et al. Improved detection and treatment of bladder cancer using hexaminolevulinate imaging: a prospective, phase III multicenter study. J Urol. 2005;174(3):862–6; discussion 6.
19. Lotan Y. Promises and challenges of fluorescence cystoscopy. Urologic Oncol. 2015.
20. Grossman HB, Stenzl A, Fradet Y, Mynderse LA, Kriegmair M, Witjes JA, et al. Long-term decrease in bladder cancer recurrence with hexaminolevulinate enabled fluorescence cystoscopy. J Urol. 2012;188(1):58–62.
21. Burger M, Grossman HB, Droller M, Schmidbauer J, Hermann G, Dragoescu O, et al. Photodynamic diagnosis of non-muscle-invasive bladder cancer with hexaminolevulinate cystoscopy: a meta-analysis of detection and recurrence based on raw data. Eur Urol. 2013;64(5):846–54.
22. Daneshmand S, Schuckman AK, Bochner BH, Cookson MS, Downs TM, Gomella LG, et al. Hexaminolevulinate blue-light cystoscopy in non-muscle-invasive bladder cancer: review of the clinical evidence and consensus statement on appropriate use in the USA. Nat Rev Urol. 2014;11(10):589–96.
23. Smith P, Mandel J, Raman JD. Conservative nephron-sparing treatment of upper-tract tumors. Curr Urol Rep. 2013;14(2):102–8.
24. Margulis V, Shariat SF, Matin SF, Kamat AM, Zigeuner R, Kikuchi E, et al. Outcomes of radical nephroureterectomy: a series from the Upper Tract Urothelial Carcinoma Collaboration. Cancer. 2009;115(6):1224–33.
25. Langner C, Hutterer G, Chromecki T, Winkelmayer I, Rehak P, Zigeuner R. pT classification, grade, and vascular invasion as prognostic indicators in urothelial carcinoma of the upper urinary tract. Mod Pathol. 2006;19(2):272–9.
26. Li CC, Chang TH, Wu WJ, Ke HL, Huang SP, Tsai PC, et al. Significant predictive factors for prognosis of primary upper urinary tract cancer after radical nephroureterectomy in Taiwanese patients. Eur Urol. 2008;54(5):1127–34.
27. Hall MC, Womack S, Sagalowsky AI, Carmody T, Erickstad MD, Roehrborn CG. Prognostic factors, recurrence, and survival in transitional cell carcinoma of the upper urinary tract: a 30-year experience in 252 patients. Urology. 1998;52(4):594–601.
28. Keeley FX, Kulp DA, Bibbo M, McCue PA, Bagley DH. Diagnostic accuracy of ureteroscopic biopsy in upper tract transitional cell carcinoma. J Urol. 1997;157(1):33–7.
29. Skolarikos A, Griffiths TR, Powell PH, Thomas DJ, Neal DE, Kelly JD. Cytologic analysis of ureteral washings is informative in patients with grade 2 upper tract TCC considering endoscopic treatment. Urology. 2003;61(6):1146–50.
30. Furukawa J, Miyake H, Sakai I, Fujisawa M. Significance of ureteroscopic biopsy grade in patients with upper tract urothelial carcinoma. Curr Urol. 2013;6(3):156–9.
31. Lucas SM, Svatek RS, Olgin G, Arriaga Y, Kabbani W, Sagalowsky AI, et al. Conservative management in selected patients with upper tract urothelial carcinoma compares favourably with early radical surgery. BJU Int. 2008;102(2):172–6.
32. Roupret M, Hupertan V, Traxer O, Loison G, Chartier-Kastler E, Conort P, et al. Comparison of open nephroureterectomy and ureteroscopic and percutaneous management of upper urinary tract transitional cell carcinoma. Urology. 2006;67(6):1181–7.
33. Cutress ML, Stewart GD, Wells-Cole S, Phipps S, Thomas BG, Tolley DA. Long-term endoscopic management of upper tract urothelial carcinoma:

20-year single-centre experience. BJU Int. 2012;110(11):1608–17.
34. Waidelich R, Hofstetter A, Stepp H, Baumgartner R, Weninger E, Kriegmair M. Early clinical experience with 5-aminolevulinic acid for the photodynamic therapy of upper tract urothelial tumors. J Urol. 1998;159(2):401–4.
35. Aboumarzouk OM, Mains E, Moseley H, Kata SG. Diagnosis of upper urinary tract tumours: is photodynamic diagnosis assisted ureterorenoscopy required as an addition to modern imaging and ureterorenoscopy? Photodiagn Photodyn Ther. 2013;10(2):127–33.
36. Kata SG, Aboumarzouk OM, Zreik A, Somani B, Ahmad S, Nabi G, et al. Photodynamic diagnostic ureterorenoscopy: a valuable tool in the detection of upper urinary tract tumour. Photodiagnosis and photodynamic therapy. Photodiagn Photodyn Ther. 2016;13:255–60. doi:10.1016/j.pdpdt.2015.08.002 Epub 2015 Aug 6.
37. Jarrett TW, Sweetser PM, Weiss GH, Smith AD. Percutaneous management of transitional cell carcinoma of the renal collecting system: 9-year experience. J Urol. 1995;154(5):1629–35.
38. Keeley FX Jr, Bagley DH. Adjuvant mitomycin C following endoscopic treatment of upper tract transitional cell carcinoma. J Urol. 1997;158(6):2074–7.
39. Thalmann GN, Markwalder R, Walter B, Studer UE. Long-term experience with bacillus Calmette-Guerin therapy of upper urinary tract transitional cell carcinoma in patients not eligible for surgery. J Urol. 2002;168(4 Pt 1):1381–5.
40. Patel A, Fuchs GJ. New techniques for the administration of topical adjuvant therapy after endoscopic ablation of upper urinary tract transitional cell carcinoma. J Urol. 1998;159(1):71–5.
41. Nonomura N, Ono Y, Nozawa M, Fukui T, Harada Y, Nishimura K, et al. Bacillus Calmette-Guerin perfusion therapy for the treatment of transitional cell carcinoma in situ of the upper urinary tract. Eur Urol. 2000;38(6):701–4;discussion 5.
42. Nishino Y, Yamamoto N, Komeda H, Takahashi Y, Deguchi T. Bacillus Calmette-Guerin instillation treatment for carcinoma in situ of the upper urinary tract. BJU Int. 2000;85(7):799–801.
43. Wang AJ, Goldsmith ZG, Neisius A, Astroza GM, Oredein-McCoy O, Iqbal MW, et al. Increasing dwell time of mitomycin C in the upper tract with a reverse thermosensitive polymer. J Endourol Endourol Soc. 2013;27(3):288–93.
44. Kohler R. Investigations on backflow in retrograde pyelography; a roentgenological and clinical study. Acta Radiol. 1953;39(99):1–92.
45. Auge BK, Pietrow PK, Lallas CD, Raj GV, Santa-Cruz RW, Preminger GM. Ureteral access sheath provides protection against elevated renal pressures during routine flexible ureteroscopic stone manipulation. J Endourol Endourol Soc. 2004;18(1):33–6.
46. Chatterjee DK, Fong LS, Zhang Y. Nanoparticles in photodynamic therapy: an emerging paradigm. Adv Drug Deliv Rev. 2008;60(15):1627–37.
47. Boix-Garriga E, Acedo P, Casado A, Villanueva A, Stockert JC, Canete M, et al. Poly(D, L-lactide-co-glycolide) nanoparticles as delivery agents for photodynamic therapy: enhancing singlet oxygen release and phototoxicity by surface PEG coating. Nanotechnology. 2015;26(36):365104.
48. Khaled YS, Wright K, Melcher A, Jayne D. Anti-cancer effects of oncolytic viral therapy combined with photodynamic therapy in human pancreatic cancer cell lines. Lancet. 2015;385(Suppl 1):S56.
49. Choi KH, Chung CW, Kim CH, Kim do H, Jeong YI, Kang DH. Effect of 5-aminolevulinic acid-encapsulate liposomes on photodynamic therapy in human cholangiocarcinoma cells. J Nanosci Nanotechnol. 2014;14(8):5628–32.

Instruments for Upper Tract Biopsy and Treatment

14

Ariel Schulman and Majid Eshghi

Clinical Evaluation

Upper tract urothelial carcinoma (UTUC) accounts for 4% of urothelial malignancies and 7% of tumors found in the kidney [1]. It occurs most commonly in males in the sixth and seventh decades and most often presents with hematuria [2, 3]. Tumors are also detected during the evaluation of flank pain or abnormal imaging findings. Since the 1970s, the incidence of UTUC has risen with the increased use of abdominal imaging and more rigorous bladder cancer follow-up [4].

Standard clinical evaluation of the upper urinary tract includes cross-sectional imaging of the abdomen and pelvis with urographic follow-through, selective urine tumor markers and endoscopic inspection and biopsy of abnormal lesions [5]. Most important is a complete visual examination of all lesions and procurement of sufficient tissue for pathologic diagnosis, grading, and staging. The identification of one lesion should not preclude complete inspection of the entire urothelium as multifocal disease is common [6].

Despite advances in endoscopic techniques, undergrading and understaging of upper tract tumors remains a significant concern [7]. Small volume tissue samples and the technical difficulty of obtaining adequate specimen from beyond the mucosal surface limit the accuracy of upper tract biopsy. It is prudent to submit multiple specimens with more than one type of instrument to improve the diagnostic yield [8]. One may consider intraoperative pathology examination at the time of ureteroscopy to confirm adequate tissue collection. A nondiagnostic biopsy should prompt further investigation, particularly in the presence of positive cytology or visualized mucosal abnormality.

Electronic supplementary material The online version of this chapter (doi:10.1007/978-3-319-51263-1_14) contains supplementary material, which is available to authorized users.

A. Schulman (✉)
Division of Urology, Duke University School of Medicine, Durham, NC, USA
e-mail: schulmana@wcmc.com

A. Schulman
Department of Urology, New York Medical College, Valhalla, NY, USA

M. Eshghi
Department of Urology, Westchester Medical Health Network/New York Medical College, Valhalla, NY 10595, USA
e-mail: majid_eshghi@nymc.edu

M. Eshghi (ed.), *Urothelial Malignancies of the Upper Urinary Tract*,
https://doi.org/10.1007/978-3-319-51263-1_14

The Retrograde Approach

Examination of the Lower Urinary Tract

The retrograde approach is preferred for the initial endoscopic inspection of the upper urinary tract [9]. It is familiar to Urologists well tolerated and provides access to all areas of the collecting system. Evaluation begins with a bimanual examination under anesthesia to identify any palpable abnormalities of the urethra or bladder. A 30° rigid cystoscope is then used for visualization of the urethra and systematic circumferential inspection of the bladder. Dedicated bladder washings for cytology are submitted. For complete visualization, a 70° lens and flexible cystoscope can be used adjunctively for inspection of the anterior wall and bladder neck [10]. Abnormal lesions of the bladder and urethra are completely resected and sent for pathologic analysis. We typically use a 26 French bipolar resectoscope with saline irrigation for bladder tumors. Dedicated samples are sent from the base of the tumor to define depth of invasion.

Ureteral Access

Following examination and treatment of lesions of the bladder, the ureters are approached. A six-French open-ended or cone-tipped catheter is placed at the ureteral orifice and contrast is injected to opacify the ureter to identify filling defects (Fig. 14.1). Abnormal regions are correlated to bony landmarks for anatomic localization. We consider ureteral lesions above the iliac crest as proximal, below the pelvic brim as distal, and those in between as mid ureter. If there is pre-operative suspicion of tumor in the intramural ureter, a small diameter, semi-rigid ureteroscope can be used for direct inspection and pyelography before the passage of wires or catheters (Fig. 14.2).

In the absence of disease in the distal ureter, the ureteral orifice is cannulated with a guide wire that is advanced several centimeters proximally to allow for atraumatic delivery of an open-ended catheter into the distal ureter. We typically use a Sensor™ wire (Boston Scientific, Natick, MA) for initial entry. The proximal floppy tip is ideal for initial access to gently navigate the ureteral lumen while the nitinol shaft provides rigidity for advancement [11]. Selective cytology is obtained and submitted for dedicated examination and additional contrast is injected with continuous, gentle pressure to opacify the length of the ureter (Fig. 14.3).

Following pyelography, the ureter is accessed with an ureteroscope. We prefer to visually inspect the upper tract mucosa before the passage of instruments for undisturbed native inspection and to avoid specimen dislodgement. This

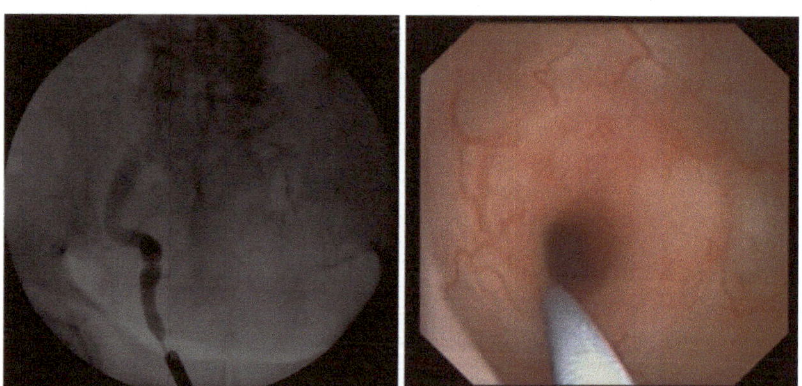

Fig. 14.1 Right retrograde pyelography with an annular, constrictive defect of the distal ureter. Inspection revealed a sessile, hyperemic structured region, and biopsy was consistent with high-grade urothelial carcinoma

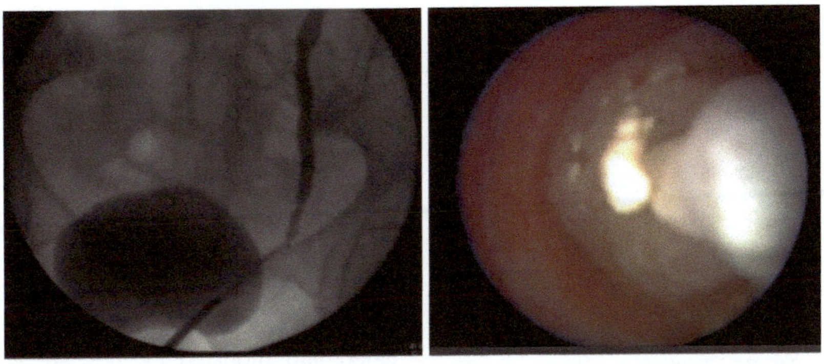

Fig. 14.2 Direct inspection of the left distal ureter with a semi-rigid ureteroscope of an obstructive, papillary tumor of the intramural and distal ureter. Pyelography through the scope noted a long filling defect with proximal hydronephrosis

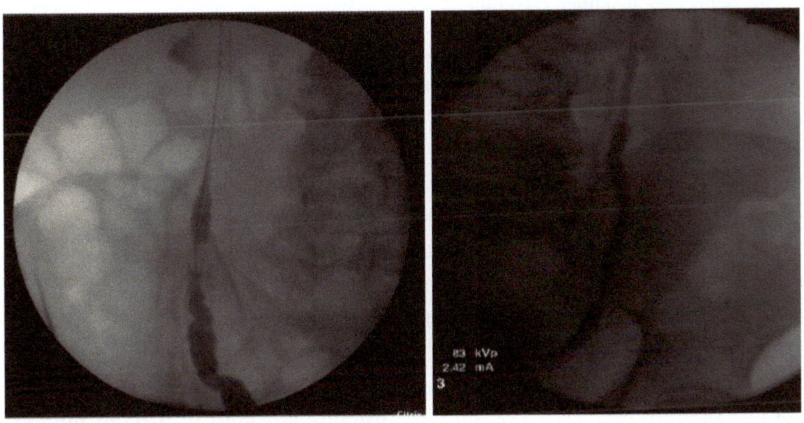

Fig. 14.3 Pyelography of the proximal and mid ureter. *Left* An obstructive 3 cm defect is noted in the mid ureter. *Right* A long region of multifocal, irregular is noted in the proximal ureter

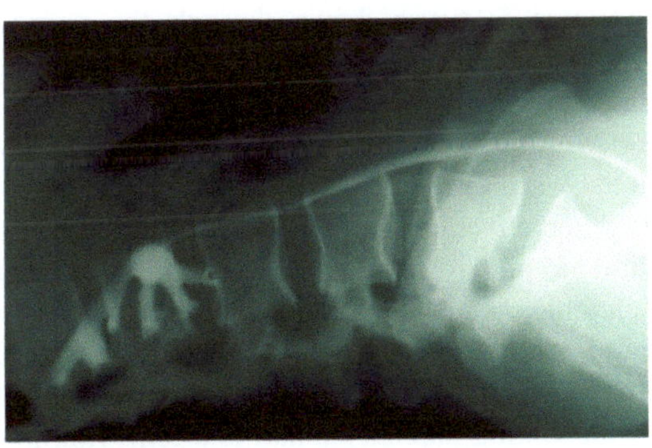

Fig. 14.4 Cross-table fluoroscopy accentuates the normal arc taken by the native ureter across the bony pelvis

“no-touch” technique is particularly important to identify carcinoma-in situ or sessile lesions and has proven safe in large series [12]. Current generation flexible scopes offer improved flexible tip control to accommodate the natural curvature of the ureter with the requisite stiffness to advance without a traveling wire (Figs. 14.4 and 14.5) [13]. Lesions of the distal and mid ureter may initially be inspected with a semi-rigid ureteroscope while lesions of the proximal ureter and renal pelvis typically require flexible ureteroscopy.

The most significant update to ureteroscope technology has been the transition from fiberoptic image transmission to digital, “chip on the tip” technology with improved quality, magnification, and self-focus [14]. While digital scopes weigh less and do not require an external light source, they have a larger shaft diameter that may limit scope passage in some cases [15].

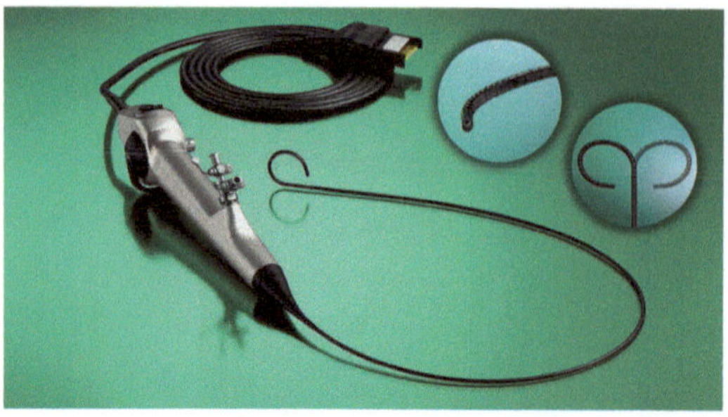

Fig. 14.5 The flexible Video-Uretero-Renoscope Flex-Xc (KARL STORZ, Tuttlingen, Germany) utilizes a digital CMOS chip for excellent image quality with built in LED illumination which ensures homogenous illumination. The distal tip circumference is 8.4 Fr and the scope has a 270° distal tip deflection in either direction. The handle is lightweight and ergonomically designed with no camera head or external light source required. ©KARL STORZ GmbH & Co. KG Germany; used with permission

Difficult Ureteral Access

Primary entry into the ureteral orifice with an ureteroscope is usually well tolerated but up to 10% of patients do not accommodate initial scope passage [16]. Complicating patient factors to consider include a history of pelvic radiation or previous ureteral reimplantation. Patients with an indwelling stent, previous ipsilateral manipulation, and older age seem to better tolerate initial entry [17]. If the scope cannot enter the ureter, adjunctive techniques to gain entry include the use of angled or glide wires, titration of bladder volume, and digital manipulation of the trigone from the rectum.

If a wire can be passed into the ureter but the scope cannot be advanced across the orifice, balloon dilation, or sequential dilators can be used under fluoroscopic guidance to gain ease entry. Additionally, a small diameter semi-rigid scope can be advanced dorsal to the guide wire while circumferentially rotating to move the beak of the spoke beyond the ventral lip of the orifice (Fig. 14.6). In the absence of disease in the distal ureter, a ureteral access sheath may be used in select cases [18].

In rare instances where the ureter cannot be accessed despite adjunctive techniques, a small-bore (4.8–5.0 Fr) stent is placed to allow for passive ureteral dilation and a second attempt at ureteroscopy is performed several weeks later [19]. Stent placement can impact endoscopic findings and this can be tempered with pre-operative removal of the stent several days prior to the second attempt at ureteroscopy.

Ureteroscopic Biopsy

Once access to the ureter is obtained, the scope is advanced proximally. Mucosal lesions are evaluated and biopsied as they are encountered to prevent dislodgement and traumatic bleeding from the advancing scope. The lesion is visually inspected and correlated with filling defects seen on imaging. For obstructive lesions, gentle proximal pyelography can help to define the length and intraluminal volume of the tumor.

Following visual inspection, specimen collection is initiated. Initial biopsies are performed with a flexible, cold-cup ureteral biopsy forceps. The forceps are opened, advanced into the tumor, and the tissue is grasped (Fig. 14.7). The forceps are withdrawn with a brisk snapping motion to sharply avulse specimen from the surrounding tissue.

For complete specimen retrieval, the biopsy forceps are held in a fixed position at the tip of the scope and forceps are removed in tandem from the patient. The specimen is then submitted for pathologic analysis. In this manner, the specimen is never drawn through the narrow working channel of the scope. Directed biopsies from the base of the tumor should be performed for identification of mucosal invasion and additional washings are sent for cytologic analysis.

Alternative commercial forceps include the Piranha ureteroscopic biopsy forceps (Boston Scientific, Natick, MA) and 2.4 French BIGopsy biopsy forceps (Cook Medical, Bloomington, IN). Ureteroscopic baskets are particularly useful for debulking papillary tumor and removing larger volumes of tissue. We commonly use the ZeroTip™ and Segura™ stone retrieval baskets (Boston Scientific, Natick, MA) for larger tumors (Fig. 14.8). In some cases, a semi-rigid ureteral resectoscopes can be advanced to an upper tract tumor for complete removal with deep intramural resection (Fig. 14.9).

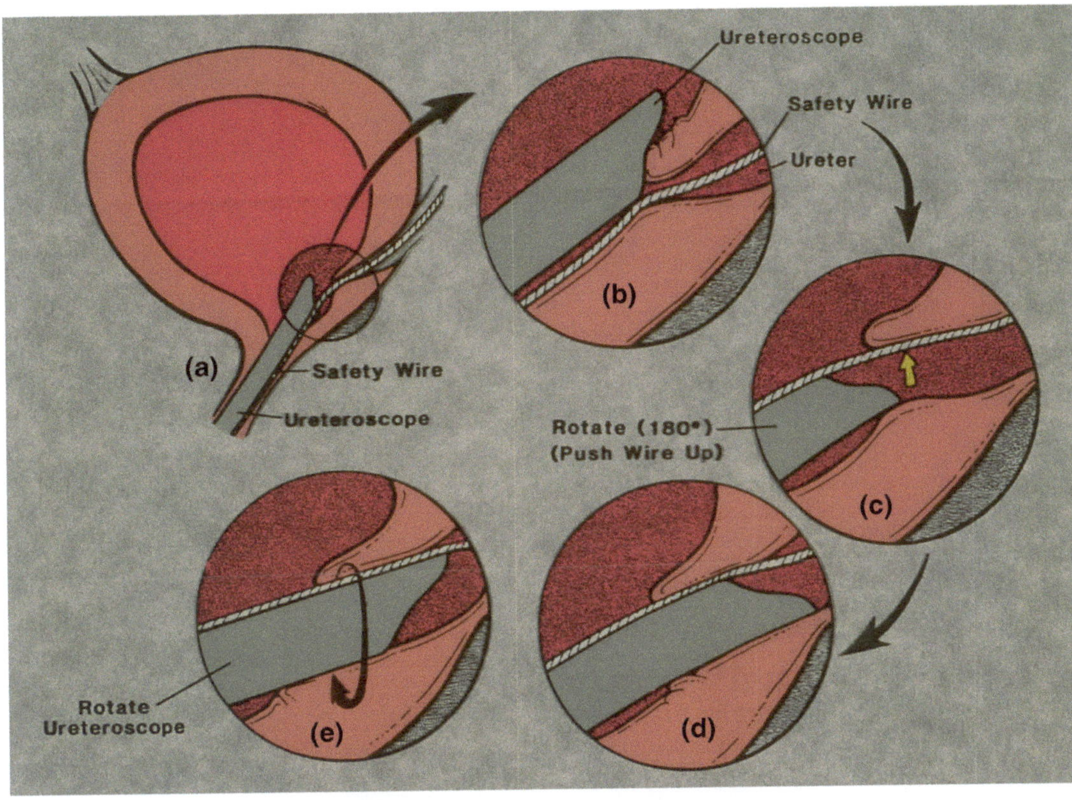

Fig. 14.6 When advancing anterior to the wire, the superior beak of a semi-rigid scope is limited by the ventral lip of the orifice (**a+b**). To enter the ureter, the scope is positioned "under the wire" and circumferentially rotated (**c**) while advancing proximally to allow the beak to bypass the orifice (**d+e**)

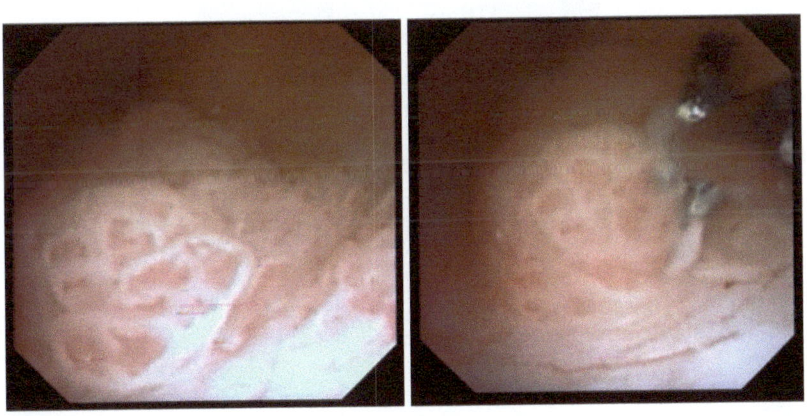

Fig. 14.7 A flexible, ureteroscopic cold-cup forceps is directed at the base of a papillary lesion for biopsy

Comparative performance features of biopsy instruments include the size and depth of specimen collected, tissue fragmentation, and most importantly feasibility of pathologic grading and staging [20, 21]. We advocate submitting multiple samples with several instruments to optimize diagnostic yield.

After biopsy and debulking, the base of the tumor is fulgurated with a ureteral cautery electrode or laser fiber. The holmium (Ho:YAG)

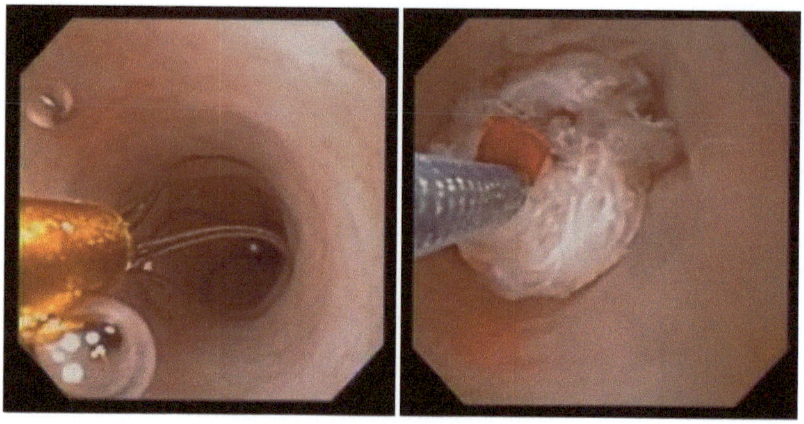

Fig. 14.8 A Segura™ flatwire basket (Boston Scientific) can collect large volumes of intraluminal tissue for pathologic review and debulking

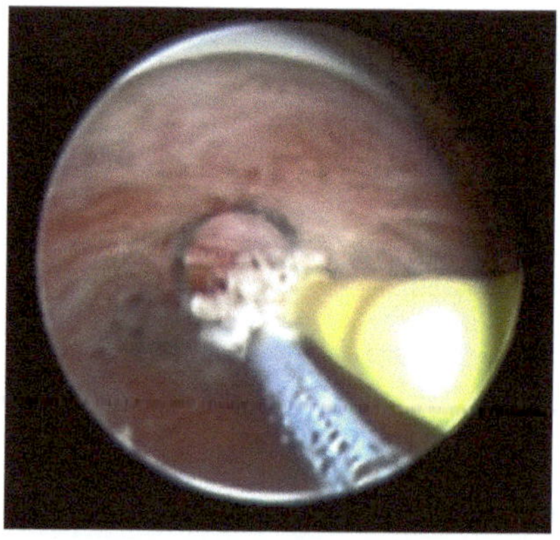

Fig. 14.9 A monopolar ureteral resectoscope resects deeply into the wall of the distal ureter for complete tumor removal and accurate staging

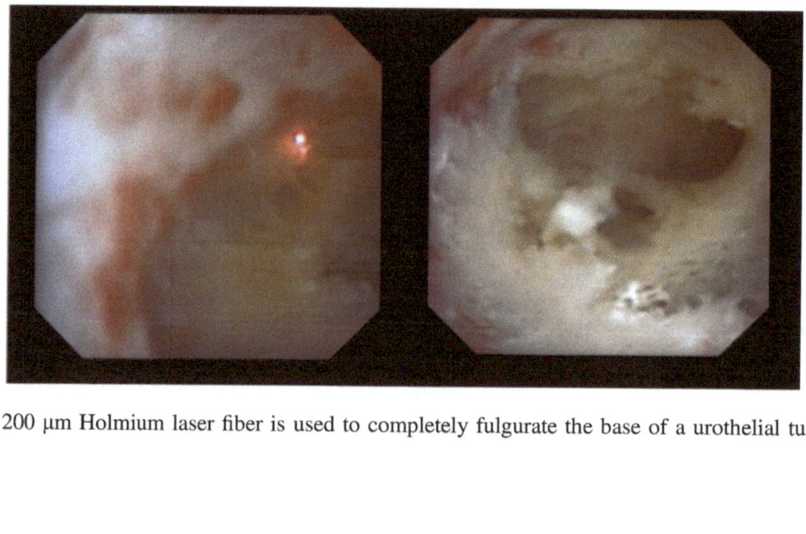

Fig. 14.10 A 200 μm Holmium laser fiber is used to completely fulgurate the base of a urothelial tumor

laser is used with direct tissue contact and creates ablation up to 0.5 mm of tissue depth. The shallow penetration makes it the preferred laser energy source to minimize ureteral stricture and nearby organ injury. Typical settings are 0.5 kJ of energy with a rate of 10–15 Hz (Fig. 14.10).

Assessment of the Pelvicalyceal System

After examination and treatment of ureteral lesions, the scope is advanced to the renal pelvis. Cytology washings are submitted for examination and a pyelogram is performed to outline a roadmap for inspection and to identify filling defects (Figs. 14.11 and 14.12). Complete pyeloscopy is performed in systematic fashion with inspection of both anterior and posteriorly directed calyces. Lower pole lesions pose the greatest challenge for inspection and biopsy due to the required scope angulation. The placement of instruments through the working channel can further limit maximal deflection. If complete visualization and treatment of a lower pole lesion is not feasible ureteroscopically, an antegrade approach should be considered.

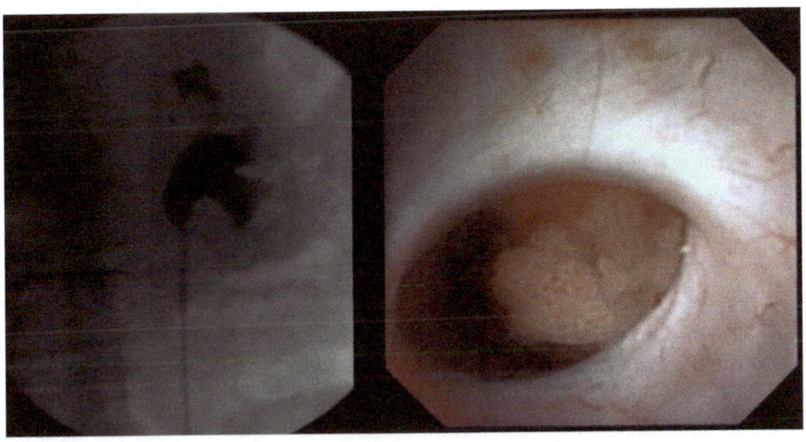

Fig. 14.11 Retrograde pyelography shows irregular narrowing of the upper pole infundibulum. Inspection revealed a stenotic infundibulum and multiple papillary tumors located circumferentially around the entry to the calyx

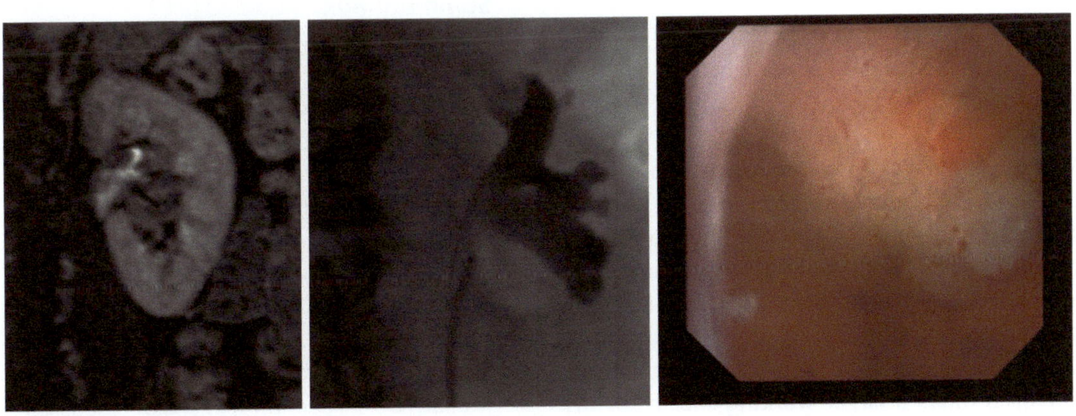

Fig. 14.12 A broad-based sessile lesion is noted in the upper pole papilla on MRI and pyelogram. Inspection revealed a bulky, papillary tumor

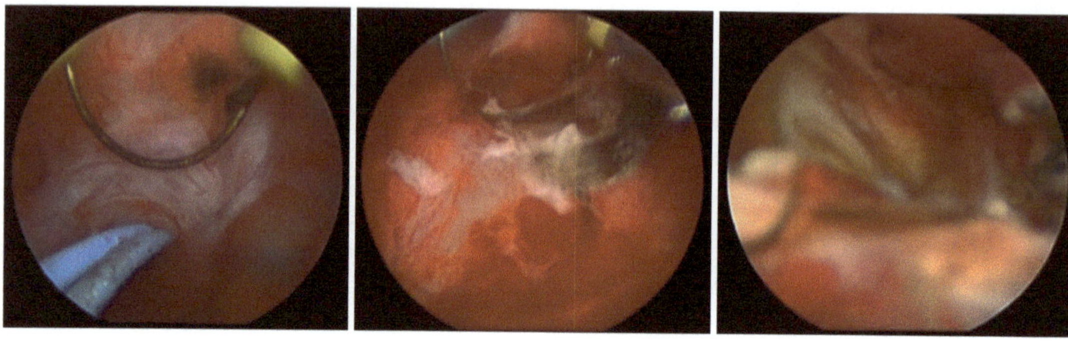

Fig. 14.13 Percutaneous access for re-resection of multiple papillary tumors of the upper pole. A 24 Fr transurethral resectoscope is used through a 30 Fr clear access sheath to obtain deep specimens. *Yellow* sinus fat is visible at the base of the resection. The tumor was upgraded and upstaged following pathologic examination of percutaneous specimens

Biopsy and fulguration of pelvicalyceal tumors is approached in similar fashion to ureteral tumors with the use of forceps and baskets for biopsy. The capacious nature of the renal collecting system may produce larger volume tumors compared to the ureter and more debulking is sometimes required. Within the renal pelvis and calyces, the Neodymium (Nd: YAG) laser is used to safely ablate intraluminal tumor efficiently [22]. The laser is positioned 2–3 mm away from the tumor and delivers energy to 5–10 mm of tissue depth. Efficacy is visually monitored by progressive white blanching of the tumor. We typically use a 30 W continuous power setting. Following debulking, additional biopsies are taken from the base of the tumor and the holmium laser is used for fulguration and hemostasis. Videos 14.1 and 14.2.

The Antegrade, Percutaneous Approach

While retrograde ureteroscopy is the initial approach, some patients benefit from an antegrade, percutaneous approach for biopsy and treatment. Indications include lesions not amenable to a retrograde treatment and anatomic variation such as a urinary diversion that prevents retrograde access. The percutaneous approach offers a larger working sheath for irrigation of clots and removal of a larger volume of disease. A 26 Fr transurethral resectoscope is used for deep specimen collection (Fig. 14.13). One disadvantage of percutaneous access is the risk of retroperitoneal and tract seeding, although this is limited to select case reports [23].

Percutaneous renal access is obtained in standard fashion, with preferred entry through the papilla of a posterior calyx. The selection of polar entry into the kidney is dependent on the location of the lesion, with an upper pole puncture providing the best access to the ureteropelvic junction and lower pole. In addition to the standard 30 Fr percutaneous access sheath (Boston Scientific, Natick, MA), a "mini-perc" technique (Mini-PERC) can be used for insertion of a 13 Fr sheath into the collecting system for passage of a flexible cystoscope for inspection and biopsy.

Summary Box

- The clinical evaluation of suspected urothelial carcinoma of the upper urinary tract includes cross-sectional imaging of the abdomen and pelvis with urographic follow-through, urine tumor markers and endoscopic inspection, and biopsy of suspicious lesions.
- Ideally, the upper tract urothelium is inspected before the passage of guidewires or instruments to obtain a true native inspection of the mucosal surface.

- Clinical history may suggest a ureteral orifice that is difficult to identify or cannulate and adjunctive endoscopic techniques are sometimes required for ureteral access.
- Despite technical improvements, undergrading and understaging remains a significant concern. Multiple samples with forceps and baskets should be obtained to improve the diagnostic yield and selective cytology at various stages of examination and biopsy should be submitted.
- While retrograde access is the preferred first line approach, percutaneous antegrade access may be required in some cases.

Acknowledgements Author acknowledges the contribution of Denton Allman, MD, and Jonathan Wagmaister, MD, Westchester Medical Health Network, New York Medical College, Valhalla, NY and thanks him for his helpful comments and feedback.

References

1. Transitional cell cancer of the renal pelvis and ureter treatment—for health professionals (PDQ) Bethesda (MD): National Cancer Institute; 2015. Available at: http://www.cancer.gov/types/kidney/hp/transitional-cell-treatment-pdq. Accessed 12 Oct 2015.
2. Kates M, Badalato GM, Gupta M, McKiernan JM. Secondary bladder cancer after upper tract urothelial carcinoma in the US population. BJU Int. 2012;110(9):1325–9.
3. Lucca I, Leow JJ, Shariat SF, Chang SL. Diagnosis and management of upper tract urothelial carcinoma. Hematol Oncol Clin North Am. 2015;29(2):271–88.
4. Raman JD, Messer J, Sielatycki JA, Hollenbeak CS. Incidence and survival of patients with carcinoma of the ureter and renal pelvis in the USA, 1973–2005. BJU Int. 2011;107(7):1059–64.
5. Davis R, Jones JS, Barocas DA, Castle EP, Lang EK, Leveillee RJ, Messing EM, Miller SD, Peterson AC, Turk TMT, Weitzel W. Diagnosis, evaluation and follow-up of asymptomatic microhematuria (AMH) in adults: AUA guideline. Linthicum (MD): American Urological Association; 2012. Available at: https://www.auanet.org/education/guidelines/asymptomatic-microhematuria.cfm. Accessed 15 Oct 2015.
6. Yafi FA, Novara G, Shariat SF, Gupta A, Matsumoto K, Walton TJ, et al. Impact of tumour location versus multifocality in patients with upper tract urothelial carcinoma treated with nephroureterectomy and bladder cuff excision: a homogeneous series without perioperative chemotherapy. BJU Int. 2012;110(2 Pt 2):E7–13.
7. Wang JK, Tollefson MK, Krambeck AE, Trost LW, Thompson RH. High rate of pathologic upgrading at nephroureterectomy for upper tract urothelial carcinoma. Urology. 2012;79(3):615–9.
8. Guarnizo E, Pavlovich CP, Seiba M, Carlson DL, Vaughan ED Jr, Sosa RE. Ureteroscopic biopsy of upper tract urothelial carcinoma: improved diagnostic accuracy and histopathological considerations using a multi-biopsy approach. J Urol. 2000;163(1):52–5.
9. Roupret M, Babjuk M, Comperat E, Zigeuner R, Sylvester RJ, Burger M, et al. European association of urology guidelines on upper urinary tract urothelial cell carcinoma: 2015 update. Eur Urol. 2015;68:868–79.
10. Nieder AM, Manoharan M. The role of the surgeon and transurethral resection in the treatment of superficial bladder cancer. SciWorld J. 2006;7(6):2626–31.
11. Clayman M, Uribe CA, Eichel L, Gordon Z, McDougall EM, Clayman RV. Comparison of guide wires in urology. Which, when and why? J Urol. 2004;171(6 Pt 1):2146–50.
12. Patel SR, McLaren ID, Nakada SY. The ureteroscope as a safety wire for ureteronephroscopy. J Endourol. 2012;26(4):351–4.
13. Johnson GB, Portela D, Grasso M. Advanced ureteroscopy: wireless and sheathless. J Endourol. 2006;20(8):552–5.
14. Bird V. Flexible ureteroscopes: fiberoptic and digital. In: Monga M, editor. Ureteroscopy. Indications, instrumentation and technique. New York: Humana Press; 2013. p. 111.
15. Hudson RG, Conlin MJ, Bagley DH. Ureteric access with flexible ureteroscopes: effect of the size of the ureteroscope. BJU Int. 2005;95(7):1043–4.
16. Ji C, Gan W, Guo H, Lian H, Zhang S, Yang R, Zhao X. A prospective trial on ureteral stenting combined with secondary ureteroscopy after an initial failed procedure. Urol Res. 2012;40(5):593–8.
17. Mogilevkin Y, Sofer M, Margel D, Greenstein A, Lifshitz D. Predicting an effective ureteral access sheath insertion: a bicenter prospective study. J Endourol. 2014;28(12):1414–7.
18. Gorin MA, Santos Cortes JA, Kyle CC, Carey RI, Bird VG. Initial clinical experience with use of ureteral access sheaths in the diagnosis and treatment of upper tract urothelial carcinoma. Urology. 2011;78(3):523–7.
19. Ambani SN, Faerber GJ, Roberts WW, Hollingsworth JM, Wolf JS Jr. Ureteral stents for impassable ureteroscopy. J Endourol. 2013;27(5):549–53.
20. Wason SE, Seigne JD, Schned AR, Pais VM Jr. Ureteroscopic biopsy of upper tract urothelial

carcinoma using a novel ureteroscopic biopsy forceps. Can J Urol. 2012;19(6):6560–5.
21. Kleinmann N, Healy KA, Hubosky SG, Margel D, Bibbo M, Bagley DH. Ureteroscopic biopsy of upper tract urothelial carcinoma: comparison of basket and forceps. J Endourol. 2013;27(12):1450–4.
22. Cohen JH, Cohen SD, Grasso M. Flexible ureteroscopy: wireless and sheathless. In: Monga M, editor. Ureteroscopy. Indications, instrumentation and technique. New York: Humana Press; 2013. p. 297.
23. Goel MC, Mahendra V, Roberts JG. Percutaneous management of renal pelvic urothelial tumors: long-term followup. J Urol. 2003;169(3):925–9 discussion 929–30.

15 Semirigid and Flexible Ureteroscopy

Arash Akhavein and Manoj Monga

Introduction/Indications

As briefly mentioned in previous chapter, the least invasive method for direct visualization of any upper urinary tract urothelial tumor is ureteroscopy (URS). URS allows for diagnostic, therapeutic, as well as surveillance measures for these lesions. Semirigid URS is indicated mainly for distal and some mid-ureteral masses, while flexible ureterorenoscopy should be utilized for proximal ureter, renal pelvis, and calyces [1, 2].

Semirigid Ureteroscopy

After identification of the patient and transfer to the operating room, a brief pause is taken to verify the correct patient, procedure, laterality, and peri-operative quality indicators such as proper antibiosis, normothermia, and deep venous thrombosis prophylaxis. For ureteroscopic procedures, we usually utilize general anesthesia with full neuromuscular blockade (zero "twitches" on the monitor). Patient is then placed in dorsal lithotomy position and pressure points are carefully padded. Standard aseptic preparation and draping then follows. Table 15.1 lists the commonly utilized items for semirigid ureteroscopy for upper tract tumors as we describe.

We begin the procedure by rigid cystoscopy to completely visualize the entire urothelial surface of the bladder. Any suspicious lesions that are found are biopsied (a cold cup biopsy forceps for smaller lesions followed by monopolar fulguration, or possibly formal transurethral resection by a bipolar loop for larger lesions).

At this point if a retrograde ureteropyelogram (RPG) is desired to better delineate the upper tract and identify the filling defects, it will be performed. This is done mainly if we lack sufficient visualization on prior radiographic studies, seldom performed if computerized tomography (CT) ureterogram has provided the necessary information with regard to the urinary tract anatomy and location of the lesions. A cone-tip ureteral catheter provides sufficient occlusion of the ureteral orifice, and we utilize 1:2 diluted contrast medium injections by a 10 ml syringe and low pressure. Care must be taken not to over-pressurize the upper tract and renal pelvis.

We routinely utilize the "no-touch technique" and avoid placing a safety guidewire initially, prior to performing URS. This prevents any traumatization of the urothelium and tumor(s) by the wire, thus avoiding bleeding and poor visualization during the procedure. This is in contrast to urinary lithiasis cases where safety wires are routinely placed.

A. Akhavein (✉) · M. Monga
Glickman Urological and Kidney Institute, Cleveland Clinic, Cleveland, OH 44195, USA
e-mail: akhavea@ccf.org

A. Akhavein
Cedar Sinai Medical Center, Los Angeles, CA, USA

M. Eshghi (ed.), *Urothelial Malignancies of the Upper Urinary Tract*,
https://doi.org/10.1007/978-3-319-51263-1_15

Table 15.1 List of utilized instruments for semirigid ureteroscopy

In addition to a regular cystoscopy setup which includes the following:
Rigid cystoscope with 30° lens (70° available)
Camera and light cord
Irrigation tubing and metal stopcock
Drapes, C-arm cover, sterile towels
Hemostats, pan set, lubrication, Saline solution
10 mL syringe ×2
Sterile cup for specimens
Light source, video equipment, monitors
Fluoroscopy equipment (C-arm)
Items to be opened on the field:
Initial safety guidewire (e.g., a 0.038″ Sensor wire, Boston Scientific)
Semirigid ureteroscope
Single action pumping system (SAPS®, Boston Scientific)
Working port seals (e.g., rubber nipples, Adjustable Biopsy Port Seal by various manufacturers)
Nonadherent dressing pads for biopsy specimen collection (e.g., Covidien Telfa)
Items to have readily available to be opened:
Contrast medium (dilute to ~30–50% strength with Saline on the field)
5 Fr open-ended ureteral catheter
Stiff guidewire (e.g., Amplatz Super Stiff®, Boston Scientific)
Cone-tip ureteral catheter
Biopsy forceps (e.g., Piranha®, Boston Scientific)
BIGopsy biopsy forceps (Cook Medical, Bloomington, IN)
Ureteroscopic brush
A nitinol tipless basket for biopsy (e.g., Halo® 1.5 Fr, Sacred Heart)
Ureteroscopic monopolar electrode for fulguration
200–365 μm laser fibers, Ho:YAG laser machine
Double-J ureteral stents of different sizes
10 Fr dual lumen ureteral catheter

Semirigid ureteroscopy is then performed to examine the distal ureter. We use the Wolf Dual Channel "D.O.C" scope or the Wolf "needle scope" in case of small caliber ureteral orifice (Richard Wolf, Vernon Hills, IL). The technical specifications of these scopes as well as other manufacturer models are presented in detail in Chap. 11. For the irrigation system, we use the single action pumping system (SAPS, Boston Scientific, Marlborough, Massachusetts) which allows for good control over irrigation pressure, with possibility of rapid response to changes in the environment.

Depending on the patient's anatomy the distal ureter, or sometimes the entire length to the level of the ureteropelvic junction can be inspected with this method. If any lesions are encountered, biopsy can be done via a biopsy forceps or a tipless basket, among other instruments. A 200–350 μm laser fiber with Ho:YAG (holmium-doped yttrium aluminum garnet) laser is commonly used to ablate the tumor if needed. A thorough discussion of available instruments will be provided in a separate chapter. We try to utilize low irrigation pressures only to keep the visualized field clear. Gentle RPG may be performed by injecting the diluted contrast through the ureteroscope. Since the ureter is often not pre-stented and may be difficult to navigate due to anatomic reasons, careful utilization of a wire inserted through the scope to guide the tip may help with its passage. Again this depends also on proximity to the lesions and caution should be exercised not to pass the wire too far inside or injure the tumor with the tip.

If the ureter appears too tight and we cannot pass a ureteroscope safely, we do not dilate the ureter (balloon, etc.) but rather will place a ureteral stent and allow the ureter to dilate for 1–2 weeks before revisiting.

Flexible Ureterorenoscopy

The semirigid ureteroscope can safely access variable lengths in the ureter, from the distal ureter only to the entire length. Passage of the semirigid scope not only "clears" the visualized parts, but also helps with gentle and gradual dilation of the ureteral orifice and ureter proximally. After the limit has been reached with this scope, we gently place a wire, usually a 0.038 inch hydrophilic tip Sensor wire® (Boston Scientific, Marlborough, Massachusetts) or a double floppy tip super-stiff wire, just to the visualized level of the ureter and not beyond that. The semirigid scope is then withdrawn with wire in place. Please refer to Table 15.2 for the list of commonly utilized items in flexible ureteroscopy for upper tract tumors.

A narrow caliber flexible ureteroscope such as Olympus P6 (Olympus, Center Valley, PA) is then back-loaded over the wire and gently advanced into the ureter. Also, ureteroscopes that offer Narrow Band Imaging (NBI) such as the Olympus digital ureteroscope can be utilized for improved visualization of tumors and increased diagnostic accuracy [3]. In pre-stented cases or when the ureter appears to be of good caliber with no significant lesions, we utilize a Wolf Viper (Richard Wolf, Vernon Hills, IL) ureteroscope, which is slightly larger in caliber compared to the narrowest flexible scopes but does offer better ergonomics and better image quality [4]. Examination of the ureter proximal to the inspected parts is done after the wire is removed, and the flexible scope is then advanced into the renal pelvis. If a renal pelvis barbotage is needed for cytoanalysis, we collect it through the scope by injection of 5–10 ml of normal saline solution and withdrawing the barbotage fluid. This is done prior to potential use of any contrast medium, to avoid potential effects of the contrast over urothelial cells and interference with the cytology results due to contrast effect on cells [5].

Known lesions or areas of concern are located and inspected first, and fluoroscopy can be used to help guide our navigation if necessary. If no lesions are identified at those locations or once the desired intervention (e.g., biopsy, fulguration, etc.) is performed for, all calyces are then systematically inspected and all encountered tumors/lesions are addressed. Irrigation and maneuvering of the scope are done gently to avoid bleeding and also over distention of the collecting system.

After this step, the Sensor wire is replaced through the ureteroscope and gently coiled inside the renal pelvis or desired location for stent placement. The scope is then withdrawn. We routinely place a double-J stent for approximately 1 week following this procedure. This will be removed at the time of follow up in urology clinic, or deferred to later depending on future surgical treatment.

Summary Box

- Ureteroscopy (URS) is the least invasive method of directly visualizing upper tract tumors. Semirigid URS is indicated mainly for distal and mid-ureteral masses, while flexible URS is utilized for lesions in the proximal ureter, renal pelvis, and calyces.
- The "no-touch technique" (avoidance of initial guidewire placement prior to performing URS) should be utilized for upper tract tumor evaluation. This prevents any traumatization of the urothelium and the lesion(s) by the wire, thus avoiding artifacts, bleeding, and poor visualization.

Table 15.2 List of utilized instruments for flexible ureteroscopy

Items to be opened on the field:
Initial safety guidewire (e.g., a 0.038″ Sensor wire, Boston Scientific)
Stiff guidewire (e.g., Amplatz Super Stiff®, Boston Scientific)
Single action pumping system (SAPS®, Boston Scientific)
Working port seals (e.g., rubber nipples, adjustable biopsy port seal by various manufacturers)
Nonadherent dressing pads for biopsy specimen collection (e.g., Covidien Telfa)
10 Fr dual lumen ureteral catheter
Flexible ureteroscope (e.g., Olympus P6, Wolf Viper, etc.)
Items to have readily available to be opened:
Contrast medium (dilute to ~30–50% strength with Saline on the field)
Semirigid ureteroscope
5 Fr open-ended ureteral catheter
Cone-tip ureteral catheter
Ureteral access sheaths (e.g., Flexor®, Cook)
Biopsy forceps (e.g., Piranha®, Boston Scientific)
A nitinol tipless basket for biopsy (e.g., Halo® 1.5 Fr, Sacred Heart)
Ureteroscopic monopolar electrode for fulguration
200–365 μm laser fibers, Ho:YAG laser machine
Double-J ureteral stents of different sizes
Ureteral access sheath (e.g., Cook Flexor® or Boston Scientific Navigator®)[a]

[a]12–14 Fr or smaller ×35 cm for females or ×45 cm for males

- Generally, the ureter is cleared initially with semirigid URS and any suspicious lesions are addressed. Low pressure irrigation and "no-touch technique" should be used as much as possible. If a guidewire is needed to navigate tighter areas of the ureter, caution should be exercised not to pass the wire too far or injure the tumor with it.
- For tight ureters that cannot be navigated easily, we recommend placing a ureteral stent and revisiting in 1–2 weeks, as opposed to immediate dilation (balloon, etc.), to minimize risk of injury/perforation.
- Once the limit of semirigid URS is reached, a guidewire is gently placed and kept only at the previously visualized level while the scope is removed. A narrow flexible ureteroscope is then back-loaded over this wire and advanced gently only to the level which has already been visualized. The wire is then removed and the rest of the upper tract is evaluated with flexible URS. Known lesions or areas of concern are inspected first. Fluoroscopy can help to guide the navigation if necessary.
- After URS is done and all lesions are addressed, we recommend placing a JJ stent for 1 week following the procedure. This can be removed at follow-up appointment or kept for potential repeat URS or other interventions, if needed.

References

1. Huffman JL, Bagley DH, Lyon ES, Morse MJ, Herr HW, Whitmore WF Jr. Endoscopic diagnosis and treatment of upper-tract urothelial tumors. A preliminary report. Cancer. 1985;55(6):1422–8.

2. Bagley DH. Ureteroscopic diagnosis and treatment of upper urinary tract neoplasms. Smith's textbook of endourology. 3rd ed. West Sussex, United Kingdom: Wiley-Blackwell; 2012.
3. Traxer O, Geavlete B, de Medina SG, Sibony M, Al-Qahtani SM. Narrow-band imaging digital flexible ureteroscopy in detection of upper urinary tract transitional-cell carcinoma: initial experience. J Endourol. 2011;25(1):19–23.
4. Abdelshehid C, Ahlering MT, Chou D, Park HK, Basillote J, Protsenko D, et al. Comparison of flexible ureteroscopes: deflection, irrigant flow and optical characteristics. J Urol. 2005;173(6):2017–21.
5. McClennan BL, Oertel YC, Malmgren RA, Mendoza M. The effect of water soluble contrast material on urine cytology. Acta Cytol. 1978 Jul–Aug;22(4):230–3.

Distal and Segmental Ureterectomy

16

Ahmed A. Aboumohamed and Reza Ghavamian

Indications and Contraindications

The decision of Distal Ureterectomy (DU) versus Segmental Ureterectomy (SU) is a complex process that requires very detailed pre-operative work-up, informed discussion with the patient regarding individual patient and tumor-related factors, current status of evidence in the literature for its utilization, and the need for more stringent follow-up regimens.

- Indications
  - Patient related
    Solitary kidney
    Renal function impairment
    Need for post-operative platinum-based chemotherapy
  - Tumor related
    Low grade tumors
    Ureteral-only disease
    No evidence of invasive disease on CTU
    Single small tumor or locally confined tumors
    Synchronous bilateral disease
- Contraindications
  - Multiple or high grade unilateral tumors
  - Synchronous ureteral and pelvicalyceal tumors
  - Large lesions (>1 cm)
  - Evidence of infiltrative lesion on CTU

Patient Pre-operative Evaluation and Preparation

Extensive pre-operative evaluation is needed before making a final decision to proceed with DU/SU. The patient should also be counseled regarding the need for more stringent follow-up regimen.

Lab Work-Up

Full laboratory work-up is needed before surgery which include complete metabolic panel, complete blood count, and urine cytology.

Radiologic Evaluation

Complete radiologic evaluation of the entire urinary tract is needed. Preferably CT abdomen and pelvis without and with IV contrast is

A. A. Aboumohamed
Urology Department, Montefiore Medical Center, 3400 Bainbridge Avenue, 5th Floor, Bronx, NY 10467, USA
e-mail: a_elreheem@hotmail.com

R. Ghavamian (✉)
Department of Urology, Northwell Health, Northwell Hofstra School of Medicine, Hempsted, NY, USA
e-mail: reza.ghavamian@gmail.com

M. Eshghi (ed.), *Urothelial Malignancies of the Upper Urinary Tract*,
https://doi.org/10.1007/978-3-319-51263-1_16

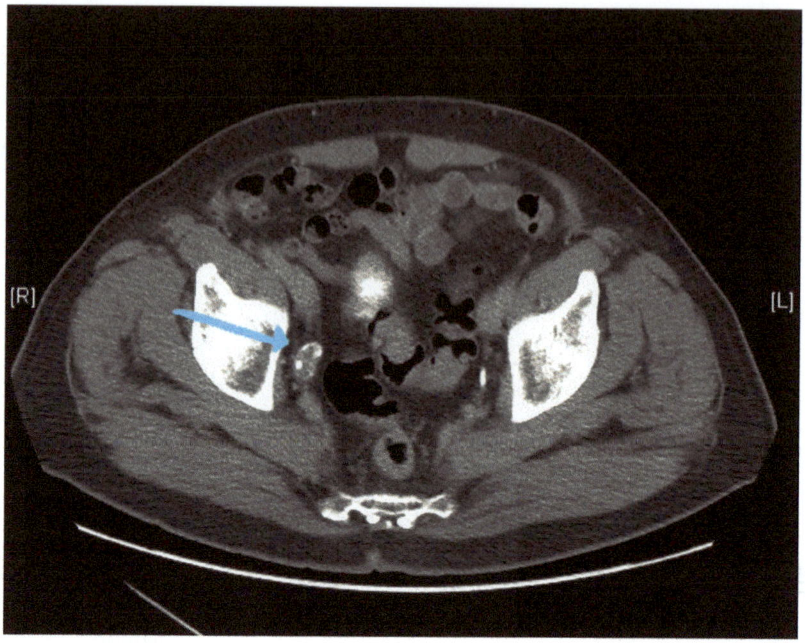

Fig. 16.1 Pre-operative Cat Scan, arrow showing a mass filling defect in the right distal ureter on delayed images

performed (Fig. 16.1). In patients who are unable to get IV contrast, a noncontrast CT, or MRU is performed.

The presence of hydronephrosis is highly suggestive of locally advanced disease.

Endoscopic Evaluation and Biopsy

Cystoscpic evaluation of the bladder must be performed in all cases to exclude synchronous bladder urothelial lesions.

Ureteroscopic evaluation of the ureter, renal pelvis and collecting system should be performed, and extent of the disease should be assessed, along with ureteroscopic biopsy of the tumor.

Retrograde ureteropyelogram is an option for upper tract evaluation.

Operative Technical Details

DU/SU can be done through a standard open approach or through a minimally invasive laparoscopic/robotic approach.

Patient positioning and subtle surgical steps differ according to the surgical approach and tumor location/intended surgery (DU vs. SU).

Different kidney-sparing extirpative surgery can be offered to those patients depending on various factors as tumor location, extent of ureteral involvement, and the length of defect in the urinary system after ureterectomy.

Accordingly, various options exist for urinary reconstruction:

- Distal ureterectomy with ureteral reimplantation.
- Distal ureterctomy with ureteral reimplanation with utilization of psoas hitch with or without bladder flap.
- Segmental ureterectomy with ureteroureterostomy.
- Segmental ureterectomy with trans-ureteroureterostomy.
- Segmental/total ureterectomy with ileal ureter replacement.
- Segmental/total ureterectomy with renal auto-transplantation.

Patient Positioning

For tumors in the distal ureter where DU is planned, the patient is usually placed dorsally in supine position (for open approach) or dorsal lithotomoy position in laparoscopic/robotic surgery.

For tumors more proximally located in the ureter where SU is planned, the patient is usually placed in lateral position with diseased side up.

Procedure Details

Distal Ureterectomy

Lesions in the distal ureter can be accessed through an extraperitoneal approach through a Gibson incision, if utilizing an open technique, or a transperitoneal laparoscopic or robotic approach.

The proximal and distal extents of the lesion within the ureter need to be accurately identified through pre-operative work-up (imaging and diagnostic ureteroscopy). Intraoperative flexible ureteroscopy may be needed for more accurate excision of the entire lesion. Intraoperative ultrasound helps in accurate identification of the mass inside the ureter (Figs. 16.2 and 16.3).

Intraoperative frozen section biopsies are helpful for more certain negative margins.

Lesions in the distal ureter can be managed by excision of the distal part of the ureter with the mass inside making sure to maintain at least 1 cm grossly negative safety margin on the proximal side of the lesion. Removal of a bladder cuff en-bloc with the ureteral segment is done for distal disease control (Fig. 16.4).

Ureter is usually re-implanted in the dome of the bladder (Fig. 16.5). Large defects in the urinary system after ureterectomy that would interfere with tension free anastomosis during closure of the urinary system can be managed by bladder psoas hitch with or without bladder flap.

Double Pigtail Ureteral stent is usually left in for 4–6 weeks. Foley catheter is left in for 1–2 weeks depending on extent of work done on bladder during reconstruction. Drain is usually left for a few days and removed when output is minimal.

Segmental Ureterectomy

Segmental ureterectomy follows the same oncologic principles as distal ureterectomy that

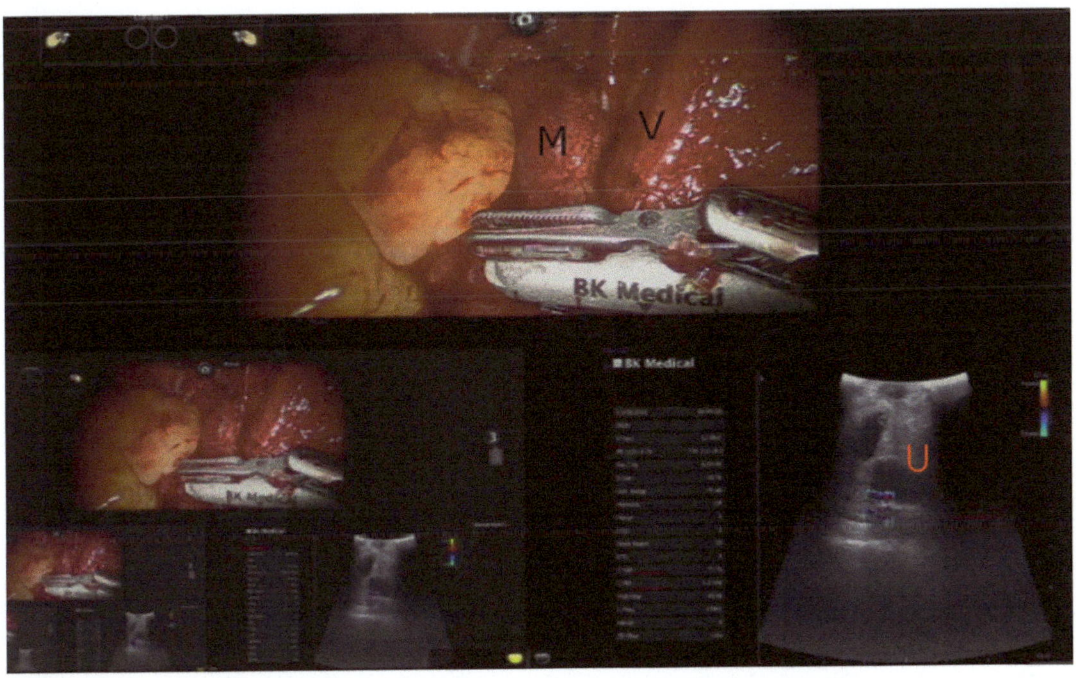

Fig. 16.2 Cross-sectional intraoperative ultrasound view during a robotic distal ureterectomy clearly identifies the tumor extent (*M* mass filled ureter; *V* iliac vessels; *U* urine filled ureter)

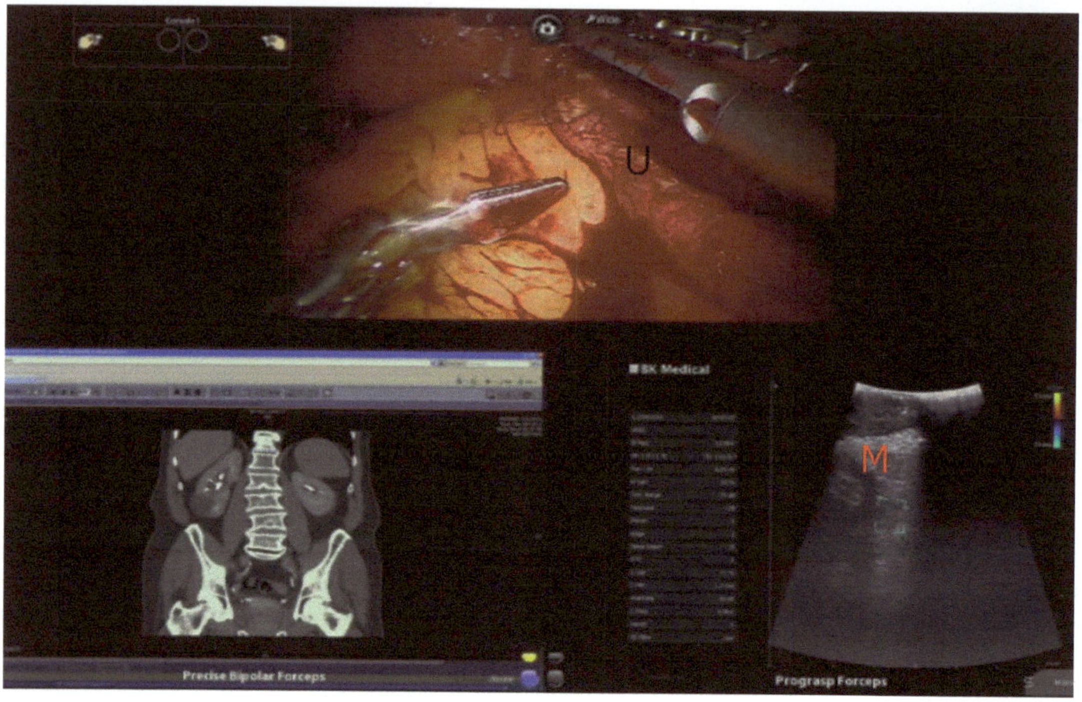

Fig. 16.3 Longitudinal intraoperative ultrasound view during a robotic distal ureterectomy clearly identifies the tumor inside the ureter (*U* ureter; *M* mass inside the ureter)

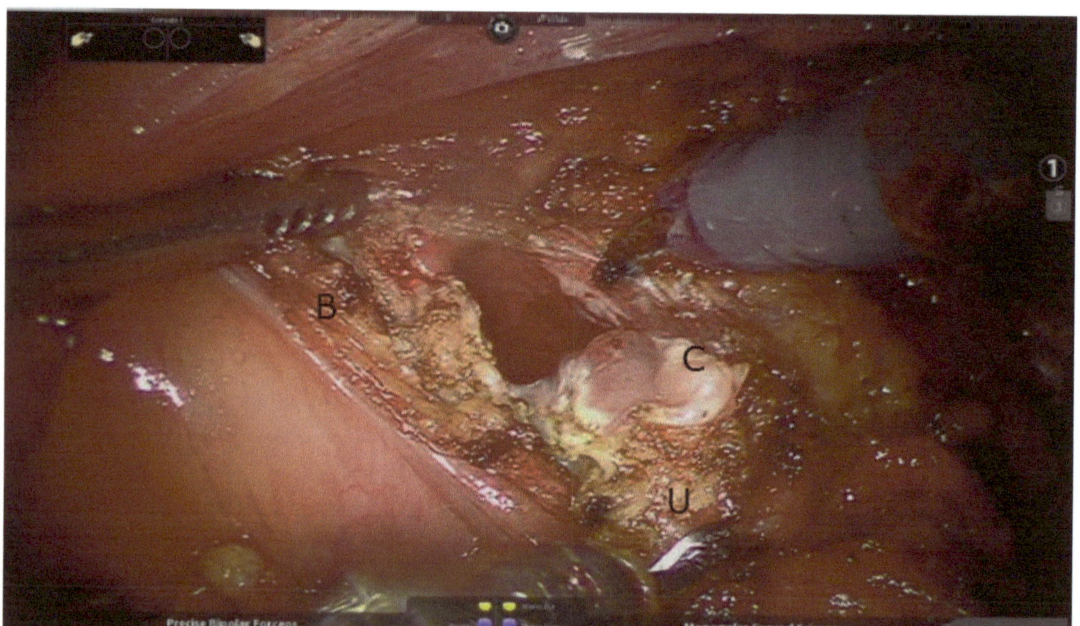

Fig. 16.4 A bladder cuff is excised during robotic distal ureterectomy (*B* urinary bladder; *U* ureter; *C* bladder cuff)

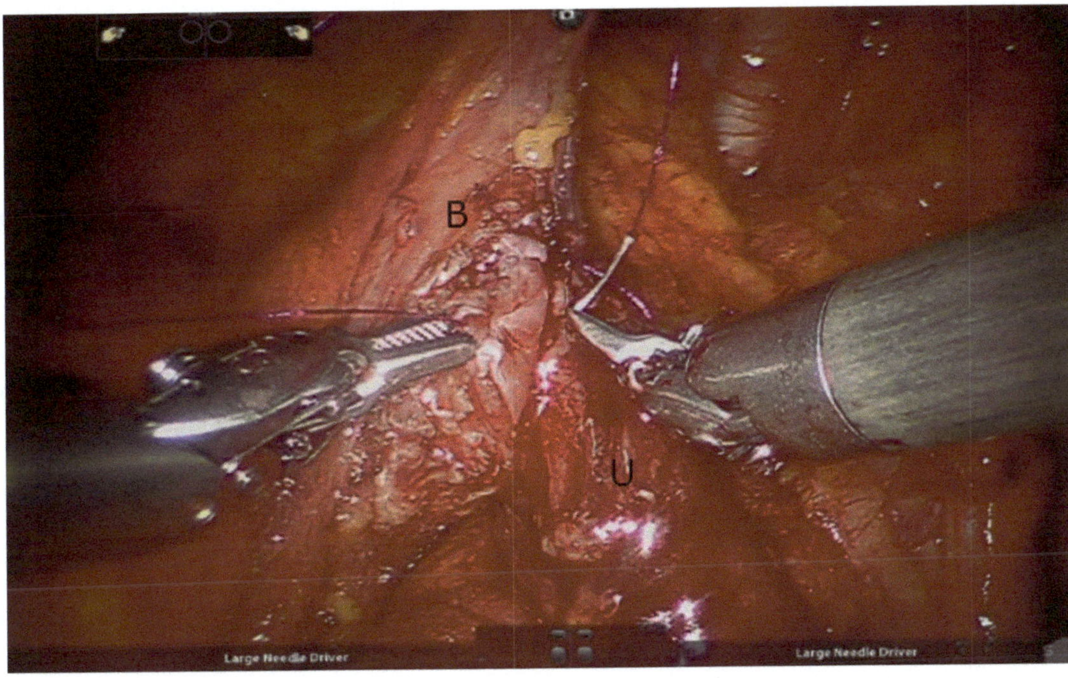

Fig. 16.5 Ureter is re-implanted in the dome of the bladder (*B* urinary bladder; *U* ureter)

includes removal of the part of the ureter containing the mass while maintaining negative margins through pre-operative identification of extent of the lesion, maintaining at least 1 cm safety margin, use of intraoperative flexible ureteroscopy, intraoperative ultrasound, and intraoperative frozen section biopsies.

Urinary reconstruction following segmental ureterectomy can be more challenging. Resection of more than 4 cm of the ureter may interfere with tension free ureteroureterostomy, and more complicated reconstructive technique may need to be utilized. Alternative reconstructive techniques include trans-ureteroureterostomy or ileal segment replacement of the ureter. Rarely, when a long segment of the ureter is to be excised or total ureterectomy is planned, an alternative to ileal ureter can be renal autotransplantation into the pelvis along with pyelovesicostomy [1].

Double Pigtail ureteral stent is similarly placed for 4–6 weeks post-operatively. JP drain is left for a few days and a Foley catheter is left for approximately a week to ensure adequate drainage.

Lymph Node Dissection

There is no high level evidence for the value of lymph node dissection for these cases; however, most reports would advocate regional lymphadenectomy of lymph nodes in the draining area of the part of the ureter harboring the mass.

Lesions in the distal ureter would advocate ipsilateral pelvic lymphadenectomy.

Lesions in the middle ureter would advocate ipsilateral common iliac lymphadenectomy.

Lesions in the proximal ureter would advocate ipsilateral retroperitoneal lymphadenectomy.

Ureterectomy of more than one segment of the ureter may advocate more extensive lymphadenectomy.

Complications and Management Recommendations

General nonspecific operative and peri-operative complications that may happen include intraoperative bleeding, surgical site infection, cardiovascular/pulmonary complications, and injury to adjacent organs such as, bowel, vascular injuries.

Early Post-operative Complications

Urinary Leakage

- Ensure maximal urine drainage through adequate caliber Foley catheter.
- Vital checks to exclude infected urinoma.
- Fluid restriction.
- Frequent imaging to exclude urinoma collection (CT scan is usually preferred in this setting).
- Percutaneous nephrostomy in cases that fail conservative management.

Urinary Tract Infection

- Ensure adequate hydration and urine output.
- Urine culture.
- Culture specific antibiotics.

Delayed Post-operative Complications

The main possible long-term complication is stricture formation either at site of uretero ureterostomy or ureteroneocystotomy with subsequent hydronephrosis. This may require frequent interventions, and possible impact on ipsilateral renal unit.

Basic Management Strategy

- Early endoscopic dilation and stenting.
- Surgical repair in refractory cases.
- Nephroureterectomy in refractory cases with poorly functional renal unit.

Urothelial Carcinoma Recurrence

Urothelial carcinoma recurrence post DU/SU is a challenging scenario. Small low grade lesions can be managed by endoscopic laser ablation. Large, multiple or high grade lesions would mostly need completion nephroureterectomy.

Post-operative Management and Follow-up

Standard Post-operative Management

Standard post-operative management includes serial vital signs checks, peri-operative IV hydration, monitoring of urine and drain outputs, pain control, and early ambulation.

Foley catheter is usually needed for 3–5 days to ensure maximal urine drainage, unless more complex urinary reconstruction was done which necessitates longer Foley catheter drainage.

Drain may be left for 2–3 days, particularly for extraperitoneal approach. Ureteral stent may be removed in 4–6 weeks.

Oncologic Follow-up

The oncologic surveillance protocol is usually more frequent and intense than after nephroureterectomy.

Most follow-up regimens would advocate:

- CT Urogram and urine cytology every 3–6 months for the first year, every 6 months for the subsequent 2 years, and yearly afterward.
- Cystoscopy, ureteroscopy, and selective cytology follow a similar protocol.

Brief Literature Review/Oncologic Efficacy

Upper tract urothelial carcinoma is a rare tumor. To date, level 1 evidence of the oncologic efficacy of radical nephroureterectomy versus DU/SU does not exist. However, multiple comparative retrospective studies have been published and reported comparable oncologic control for DU/SU as compared to the gold standard radical nephroureterectomy, when used selectively (Table 16.1) [2–7].

Table 16.1 Selected series reporting on oncologic outcomes after SU, TU, and NU

Study	Year	Study design	No of patients	Follow-up "months"	Survivals
Jeldres et al. [2] "*multicenter*"	2010	Retrospective SEER data, comparative	(2044) * 569 SU * 1475 NU "1222 had NUC"	30	No significant difference in 2- and 5-year CSS
Colin et al. [3] "*multicenter*"	2012	Retrospective, comparative	(468) * 52 SU * 416 RNU	26 (10–48)	No significant difference in 5-year RFS, CSS, or MFS
Bagrodia et al. [4] "*multicenter*"	2013	Retrospective UTUC collaboration, comparative	(835) * 81 PU * 754 RNU	34 (1–246)	No significant difference in 5-year RFS or CSS
Dalpiaz et al. [5] "*single center*"	2014	Retrospective, comparative	(91) * 49 DU * 42 RNU	51.5 (4–290)	No significant difference in 5-year RFS or CSS
Pedrosa et al. [6] "*single center*"	2015	Retrospective, comparative	(141) * 35 SU * 10 TU * 96 NU	56.9 (0.2–181.1)	No significant difference in 3-year RFS, CSS, or OS

SU segmental ureterectomy; *TU* total ureterectomy; *NU* nephroureterectomy; *RFS* recurrence free survival; *CSS* cancer specific survival; *OS* overall survival; *NUC* nephroureterectomy with bladder cuff excision; *PU* partial ureterectomy; *RNU* radical nephroureterectomy; *MFS* metastasis free survival; *UTUC* upper tract urothelial carcinoma

Summary Box

- DU/SU can be a valid management option for select cases of ureteral urothelial cancer.
- Strict patient and tumor characteristics are needed to ensure adequate oncologic outcomes.
- When appropriately selected, oncologic outcomes of DU/SU are comparable to the gold standard nephroureterectomy.
- More stringent surveillance regimens are needed after DU/SU.

References

1. Cheng YT, Flechner SM, Chiang PH. The role of laparoscopy-assisted renal autotransplantation in the treatment of primary ureteral tumor. Ann Surg Oncol. 2014;21:3691.
2. Jeldres C, Lughezzani G, Sun M, et al. Segmental ureterectomy can safely be performed in patients with transitional cell carcinoma of the ureter. J Urol. 2010;183:1324.
3. Colin P, Ouzzane A, Pignot G, et al. Comparison of oncological outcomes after segmental ureterectomy or radical nephroureterectomy in urothelial carcinomas of the upper urinary tract: results from a large French multicentre study. BJU Int. 2012;110:1134.
4. Bagrodia A, Kuehhas FE, Gayed BA, et al. Comparative analysis of oncologic outcomes of partial ureterectomy vs radical nephroureterectomy in upper tract urothelial carcinoma. Urology. 2013;81:972.
5. Dalpiaz O, Ehrlich G, Quehenberger F et al. Distal ureterectomy is a safe surgical option in patients with urothelial carcinoma of the distal ureter. Urol Oncol. 2014;32:34 e1.
6. Pedrosa JA, Masterson TA, Rice KR, et al. Oncologic outcomes and prognostic impact of urothelial recurrences in patients undergoing segmental and total ureterectomy for upper tract urothelial carcinoma. Can Urol Assoc J. 2015;9.E187.
7. Abouassaly R, Alibhai SM, Shah N, et al. Troubling outcomes from population-level analysis of surgery for upper tract urothelial carcinoma. Urology. 2010;76:895.

Open Nephroureterectomy

17

Reza Mehrazin and Carl A. Olsson

Upper tract urothelial carcinoma (UTUC) represents 5% of all urothelial tumors and around 5–7% of all renal tumors, with a peak incidence occurring in the eighth decade of life. UTUC is a rare disease and is associated with high rate of recurrence and progression. Tumor stage and grade tend to be parallel with one another, with low grade UTUC mostly Ta or T1, while high grade UTUC is more commonly T2 or higher. The 5-year overall disease-specific survival is 75%, ranging from 95–100% for stage Ta or Tis to 40% for T3 tumors [1]. UTUC occurs more frequently in the lower ureter than in the upper ureter (70% distal, 25% mid, and 5% ureteropelvic junction) [1]. Moreover, patients with UTUC are at high risk (30–50%) of developing intravesical concurrence and/or recurrence [2]. This downstream phenomenon of tumor seeding is the reason why the entire length of the ureter from the level of the lesion and extending to include a bladder cuff surrounding the ureteral orifice is removed at the time of radical nephroureterectomy (RNU). Open radical nephroureterectomy (ONU) with resection of the ipsilateral bladder cuff has been the standard treatment for several decades. Since the introduction of minimally invasive surgery (MIS), laparoscopic and robotic assisted nephroureterectomy have been increasingly utilized for management of UTUC. Given the low incidence of UTUC, oncologic efficacy of MIS is still a standing concern, with institutional and population studies suggesting that perhaps laparoscopic nephroureterectomy should be performed only in patients with favorable tumor characteristics. In this chapter, we review the specific indications and techniques for ONU in management of patients with UTUC.

ONU can be performed through a variation of approaches and the type of incision depends on surgeon's experience, size of the specimen, extent of the disease, and patient's body habitus. During ONU for renal UTUC, the ureter and ureteral orifice are removed en bloc with the kidney and perinephric fat. The surgery can be performed through either a long midline transabdominal incision or, preferably, through a subcostal or flank incision along with a lower midline, Gibson, or Pfannenstiel incision, for excision of the bladder cuff. A third option is combining the upper flank approach with a Gibson-like lower extension in a continuous, single retroperitoneal incision (Fig. 17.1).

R. Mehrazin · C. A. Olsson (✉)
Department of Urology and Oncological Science, Icahn School of Medicine at Mount Sinai, New York, NY 10029, USA
e-mail: carl.olsson@mountsinai.org; colsson@imppllc.com

R. Mehrazin
e-mail: reza.mehrazin@mountsinai.org; reza.mehrazin@gmail.com

C. A. Olsson
John K Lattimer, Emeritus, Professor, Columbia University Medical Center, New York, NY, USA

M. Eshghi (ed.), *Urothelial Malignancies of the Upper Urinary Tract*,
https://doi.org/10.1007/978-3-319-51263-1_17

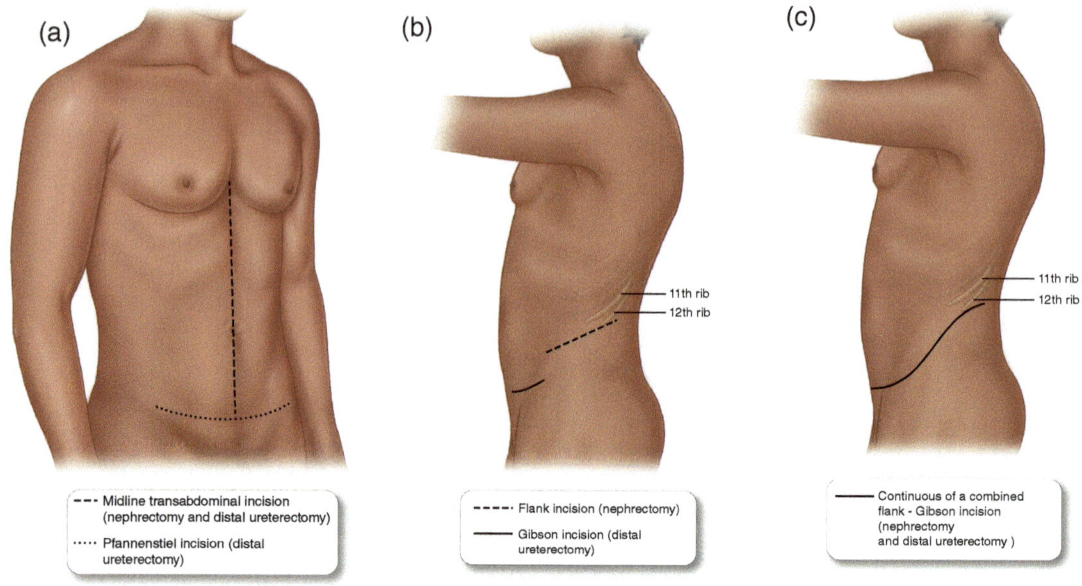

Fig. 17.1 **a** Midline transabdominal incision (nephrectomy and distal ureterectomy) and pfannenstiel incision (distal ureterectomy). **b** Flank incision (nephrectomy) and gibson incision (distal ureterectomy). **c** Continuous or combined flank-gibson incision (nephrectomy and distal ureterectomy)

Some mention must be made of the use of neo-adjuvant chemotherapy using platinum-based regimens. The National Comprehensive Cancer Network (NCCN) guidelines suggest considering this in high grade or stage patients facing ONU as their post-operative creatinine levels may interdict against adjuvant treatment. The appropriate use of peri-operative antimicrobial and deep venous thrombosis prophylaxis is paramount. First or second-generation cephalosporin, fluoroquinolone, or ampicillin/sulbactam are the recommended pre-operative antibiotics and should be continued for 24 h. For thromboprophylaxis, use of intermittent pneumatic compression devices and pharmacological venous thromboembolism prophylaxis (e.g., subcutaneous heparin) prior to the incision and throughout the length of hospital stay is important.

Access to the renal hilum and upper pole of the kidney are usually limited through a midline incision and more easily approached from the flank. The thoracoabdominal approach provides great exposure to the kidney for tumors that are very large but renal UTUCs (unlike renal parenchymal tumors) rarely progress to sizes requiring a thoracoabdominal approach. Further, thoracoabdominal surgery adds chest tube management to post-operative care. If nephrectomy is performed through a flank incision, then it may be necessary to reposition the patient for lower midline or Pfannenstiel incision. In contrast, the patient approached with an upper flank approach with Gibson-like lower extension can be placed into a simple oblique, extended position. Regardless of the approach, it is critical that the ureter must be removed in its entirety; failure to do so puts the patient at-risk of distal recurrence.

Managing the Nephrectomy

If the adrenal gland appears normal on pre-operative imaging, adrenal sparing is preferred. It is always useful to know the status of the adrenal glands when retroperitoneal surgery is planned. During an ONU, the kidney should be removed with its surrounding perinephric fat and Gerota's fascia. The hilar vessels are individually dissected, controlled, and transected in the standard open nephrectomy fashion. Preferably, two

O-silk ties are placed proximally and one distally for individual arteries and veins. The outermost silk on the patient's side is best a suture ligature. If lymphatic vessels are encountered at the time of dissection, they should meticulously be cauterized, clipped, or tied.

Abnormalities of the renal vein are not uncommon, particularly on the left side. The surgeon should be aware of the circumaortic venous plexus surrounding the aorta in many patients with (often sizable) left renal vein branching posteriorly, as lumbar veins drain directed to the azygos system [3].

Open Nephron-Sparing Surgery for UTUC

Nephron-sparing surgery (NSS) for management of UTUC might be considered in highly select patients. Since cancer staging for UTUC is mostly established by endoscopic biopsy, inaccuracy of grading and, more particularly staging of the lesion is always a concern. However, in individuals with low grade and low stage disease who have synchronous bilateral tumors, solitary kidney, or have increased predisposition to recurrence of disease, NSS is an option. Open pyelotomy, segmental ureterectomy, and partial nephrectomy are commonly utilized renal preserving approaches. For pyelotomy or partial nephrectomy, the renal hilum and pelvis are exposed and the field is packed with laparotomy pads to isolate the kidney before making an intrarenal incision. All measures to minimize the risk of tumor spillage should be considered. For renal pelvic tumor, a curvilinear incision is made in the renal pelvis, the tumor is excised along with its base to allow proper pathologic determination of tumor stage; if this is rendered impossible by the position of the lesion, the base is vigorously cauterized, employing laser, or electrocautery fulguration. After tumor excision, the pelvis should be closed using a 4–0 monofilament suture or other absorbable material, following which the potentially contaminated laparotomy pads are removed and the entire wound site copiously irrigated with sterile water (not saline). Placement of ureteral stent after open pyelotomy is optional; however, placement of a suction drain is recommended. If a formal partial nephrectomy is elected, after the tumor bearing part of the kidney is removed, the collecting system is closed using absorbable suture material and edges of the renal capsule are re-approximated when possible to complete the renorrhaphy [4].

The reported incidence of isolated tumors of the ureter represents about 30% of all UTUC [5]. Segmental ureterectomy has been reported in cases of isolated low grade tumors in the proximal-to-mid ureter, in patients wherein NSS is considered beneficial. It is generally better accepted than endoscopic management, as it has the advantage of providing a definitive pathological stage and grade. Prior to open segmental ureterectomy, the approximate location of the tumor should be known from the pre-operative endoscopic and imaging evaluations. Similar to an open renal surgery, the ureter is best accessed through a retroperitoneal incision, with the resection site operative field packed with laparotomy pads (and handled as with renal UTUC cases). The tumor is palpated and ureter is then transected, proximal, and distal to the tumor, with a 1–2 cm margin. The excised segment should be sent for frozen section to confirm negative margins on each side of the ureteral lesion. The edges of the ureter are then spatulated, stented, and anastomosed in a tension-free manner. It should be emphasized that proximal-to-mid-ureteral resection and reanastomosis may be hazardous in that distal ureteral recurrence remains a future issue, often demanding serial ureteroscopy in follow-up.

The classic situation in which NSS is performed for ureteral UTUC is when the lesion is confined to the distal ureter. In cases where the UTUC is isolated to the distal ureter, distal ureterectomy (with a bladder cuff surrounding the ureteral orifice) can be performed, insuring against distal ureteral recurrence, and avoiding the need for serial ureteroscopy for follow-up. Further, this procedure is considered appropriate for lesions regardless of grade of the tumor; when resecting distal ureteral high grade UTUC, ipsilateral pelvic lymphadenectomy should be strongly considered.

Depending on the proximal extent of the ureterectomy, if direct ureteroneocystostomy is not possible, either psoas hitch, Boari flap or combined psoas-Boari reconstruction can be performed. The latter can bridge gaps up to the lower pole of the kidney (and sometimes to the renal pelvis), but in cases of total ureterectomy, construction of an ileal neo-ureter should be considered.

Management of Distal Ureter and Bladder Cuff

Resection of the intramural segment of the ureter with the bladder cuff is the standard of care during nephroureterectomy. The distal ureter and the bladder cuff can be managed by several different techniques; if not managed appropriately, cancer recurrence rate can be as high as 33–64% [6]. Historically, compared to endoscopic distal ureteral UTUC management, open intravesical approaches are associated with improved recurrence free survival and less risk of intravesical recurrence [6].

During an ONU, depending on the type of incision (1 incision vs. 2 incisions), to eliminate the risk of tumor spillage, the ureter should be kept in continuity with the kidney specimen. However, if the kidney specimen has to be removed for any reason before completing the distal ureterectomy, the ureter may be divided by cautery in a nontumor bearing area, carefully applying surgical clips or suture ties above and below the transection point and cauterizing both free ends.

Open distal ureterectomy may be performed extravesically, by dissecting the distal ureter precisely to (and beyond) the orifice level in the bladder, tenting the ureter on traction, and securing the cuff of the bladder with a right-angle clamp. However, this technique is often fraught with failure to remove the entire ureter with bladder cuff when the distal ureteral traction results in tearing of tissues. The preferred approach to distal ureterectomy is transvesical through an anterior cystotomy.

In a two-incision ONU, after the nephrectomy and dissection of proximal-to-mid ureter are performed, the proximal subcostal incision is closed and covered with dressing. The specimen is left inside the abdomen unless the surgeon decides in favor of ureteral transection despite the risk of tumor spread (qv above).

To access the distal ureter, bladder, and the ureteral orifice, a lower midline, Gibson or Pfannenstiel is recommended as the second incision (or else the flank incision extended in a Gibson-like manner may suffice). If the ureter is being approached transperitoneally through a midline incision, the sigmoid or cecum colon is mobilized medially, and the posterior peritoneum is opened. With a Gibson or combined Gibson-flank approach, the entire length of ureter down to and including the bladder are exposed retroperitoneally. The distal ureter is best accessed and identified at or above the bifurcation of the common iliac artery. A vessel loop or Penrose drain is placed around the ureter, which is then dissected toward the bladder. In the course of this dissection, the proximal and distal vesical artery branches of the hypogastric artery are encountered, doubly ligated and divided. When the actual vesical muscularis is reached, attention is re-directed to the anterior bladder wall, where an oblique anterior cystotomy is made.

The ureteral orifices are both identified (to insure protection of the contralateral orifice) and the ipsilateral orifice is intubated with a 5 Fr or 8 Fr feeding tube, taking care not to spill tumor cell-bearing urine. This latter is simple in the case of ONU wherein the kidney has already been totally devascularized, but more difficult when an isolated distal ureterectomy is planned. For distal ureterectomy where the kidney is still functional, a clamp is advised on a portion of the ureter above the lesion but below the planned transection point before intubation. The orifice is then circumcised with electrocautery and a tagging suture is placed across the orifice, inclusive of the feeding tube which is used as a tractor aiding the proximal intramural dissection. The circumcised peri-orificeal incision is carried down to the ureteral wall, unless the location of the tumor is at the intramural tunnel, wherein a wide dissection amply surrounding the cancer is carried out. With more proximal lesions, the dissection may be safely confined to entire diameter of the ureter alone. Typically, following the ureteral wall circumferentially from anterior to posterior allows the surgeon to free all attachments to detrusor muscle so the specimen can be removed intact. The hiatus is closed in two layers, using 2–0 interrupted absorbable sutures to close the posterior muscularis, following which a 3–0 running absorbable suture is used to close the bladder mucosa, taking care to avoid damage to the contralateral orifice. The anterior cystotomy is closed using a running 3–0 absorbable suture to re-approximate the cystotomy mucosal edges, and 2–0 absorbable interrupted sutures to close the muscle and adventitia. The bladder is filled with 180–240 ml of sterile water to test the closure.

Lymphadenectomy

Although lymphadenectomy improves cancer staging, its therapeutic role in management of UTUC remains controversial. Some retrospective studies report a correlation between improved survival and lymphadenectomy performed at the time of nephroureterctomy [7], others found no difference in cancer-specific mortality among pathologic NO and Nx patients. Much of the controversy regarding lymphadenectomy for UTUC has revolved around the extent and the template of lymphadenectomy. However, if one decides to perform lymphadenectomy, generally, the recommended template for renal or proximal tumors is hilar and para-aortic or para-caval lymph nodes. On the other hand, for distal ureteral tumors, pelvic node dissection is the suggested template for dissection. This varies with the level of the lesion, so that the distal para-aortic or para-caval nodes may be the upper extent; in contrast, a totally pelvic ureteral cancer location suggests the need for an extended dissection extending from the ipsilateral common iliac vessels to the node of Cloquet and laterally to the genitofemoral nerve to below the obturator nerve medially.

Wound Closure and Drainage

Even though bladder is closed in a water-tight manner, placement of a pelvic suction drain is recommended. If NSS is performed, a suction drain should also be placed in the renal fossa near the closure of urothelium. Regardless of the type of incision, tight closure of the musculofacial wall, without compromising tissue perfusion is important. If fascia is closed with great tension, the tissue will become ischemic and result in dehiscence or hernia formation. Flank incision can be closed in three layers: transversus abdominis, internal oblique fascia, and external oblique fascia or more quickly with a running heavy nylon single stitch taken to all layers at once. If a midline abdominal incision is made, the closure can again be accomplished with a single running heavy suture closing the fascial layers without necrosing the rectus abdominis muscle. On average, a Foley catheter is left in for 5–7 days and a 3-view cystogram can be obtained prior to removing the catheter. A single dose of intravesical instillation of Mitomycin-C should be considered prior to removing the foley, as it has shown to reduce the risk of bladder tumor recurrence within the first year following nephroureterectomy.

Follow-up of the patient is not well defined. Clearly, regardless of final tumor pathology, the patient will have to tolerate 3-month cystoscopy for at least a year, with increasing intervals thereafter presumably determined by the first year findings. No adjunctive chemotherapy or radiation is required by any low grade T0 or T1 patient. In contrast, the NCCN suggests that, in patients with high grade T2–4 cancers, adjuvant chemotherapy should be considered. The authors feel strongly that adjunctive chemotherapy should be initiated in men with lymph node involvement and in those whose tumors show lymphovascular involvement. Imaging consisting of CT or MRI of the abdomen and chest X-ray should be done at intervals of 6–12 months, for an undefined duration that will depend on findings that usually present in the first 2–3 years.

Summary Box

- ONU with resection of the ipsilateral bladder cuff is the gold-standard treatment for UTUC.
- All measures to minimize the risk of tumor cell spillage should be considered at all times.
- The distal ureter and the bladder cuff can be managed by several different techniques; however, if not managed appropriately, cancer cell spillage and recurrence rate can spoil a good cancer operation.

References

1. Hall MC, Womack S, Sagalowsky AI, et al. Prognostic factors, recurrence, and survival in transitional cell carcinoma of the upper urinary tract: a 30-year experience in 252 patients. Urology. 1998;52:594.
2. Zigeuner RE, Hutterer G, Chromecki T, et al. Bladder tumour development after urothelial carcinoma of the upper urinary tract is related to primary tumour location. BJU Int. 2006;98:1181.
3. Mitty HA. Circumaortic renal collar. A potentially hazardous anomaly of the left renal vein. Am J Roentgenol Radium Ther Nucl Med. 1975;125:307.
4. Uzzo RG, Novick AC. Nephron sparing surgery for renal tumors: indications, techniques and outcomes. J Urol. 2001;166:6.
5. Jeldres C, Sun M, Isbarn H, et al. A population-based assessment of perioperative mortality after nephroureterectomy for upper-tract urothelial carcinoma. Urology. 2010;75:315.
6. Xylinas E, Rink M, Cha EK, et al. Impact of distal ureter management on oncologic outcomes following radical nephroureterectomy for upper tract urothelial carcinoma. Eur Urol. 2014;65:210.
7. Roscigno M, Shariat SF, Margulis V, et al. The extent of lymphadenectomy seems to be associated with better survival in patients with nonmetastatic upper-tract urothelial carcinoma: how many lymph nodes should be removed? Eur Urol. 2009;56:512.

Surgical Advances in Nephroureterectomy: Laparoscopic and Robotic Approaches

18

Jonathan Bloom and John L. Phillips

Introduction

Radical nephroureterectomy represents the gold standard in the surgical management of upper urinary tract urothelial carcinoma (UUT-UC). The premise of the surgery has remained the same since the concept was first introduced by Howard Kelly (1858–1943) with the aim of removing all potential sites of urothelial disease and ipsilateral sites of recurrence. Upper tract urothelial carcinoma is an aggressive disease that despite surgery has a significant mortality and recurrence rate, especially for invasive (i.e., $\geq$T2) disease [1, 2]. New advances in endoscopic, laparoscopic, and robot-assisted technologies have reduced the morbidity of this procedure as well as given urologists new tools to improve upon the traditional results of surgery. Laparoscopic nephrectomy has emerged to become the gold standard for appropriate cases related to renal cell carcinoma [3]. The resection of the distal ureter, the bladder cuff, and its repair, however, are more challenging and have been surgically addressed in multiple publications [4]. Regional ureteral resection and primary repair have been applied to isolated ureteral UC, facilitated by robotic technology, and the results of these cases have demonstrated that there are nephron-sparing approaches that can be applied to UUT-UC [5]. Derived from the experience with UC of the bladder, neoadjuvant chemotherapy prior to nephroureterectomy (or in lieu of it) has shown promise but is limited by the paucity of clinical trial outcome data [6, 7]. This chapter will focus on the technique of nephroureterectomy and nephron-sparing approaches and review the current data of neoadjuvant therapies prior to nephroureterectomy.

History of Nephroureterectomy

Nephroureterectomy has remained the standard of care for patients with upper tract urothelial cell cancer (UTUCC) since its inception in the early twentieth century. Experience with the technique was earned largely through procedures related to tuberculosis as clinicians found that the retention of any ipsilateral urinary tract after nephrectomy was prone to recur. Kelly is thought to be the first to perform a nephroureterectomy in 1893 for tubercular disease although the complete excision

J. Bloom · J. L. Phillips (✉)
Department of Urology, Westchester Medical Health Network/New York Medical College, 40 Sunshine Cottage Rd., Skyline 1S-B45A, Valhalla, NY 10595, USA
e-mail: john_phillips@nymc.edu

J. Bloom
Urologic Oncology Branch, National Institute of Health, Bethesda, MD, USA
e-mail: jbbloom@gmail.com

M. Eshghi (ed.), *Urothelial Malignancies of the Upper Urinary Tract*,
https://doi.org/10.1007/978-3-319-51263-1_18

of the ipsilateral bladder cuff was often prevented by dense pelvic inflammation [8]. He later abandoned the transperitoneal approach for an entirely retroperitoneal technique using the so-called 'double incision' maneuver whereby the renal unit was dismembered from its hilar attachments, the organ placed in the pelvis, and then through a Pfannenstiel incision, the specimen, and its distal ureter were removed. Recurrences of urothelial carcinoma were noted in the retained ureteral stump and tumor spillage was of constant concern. Thomas and Regnier in 1924 observed a 9% recurrence rate in the remaining urinary tract in patients who had only a nephrectomy for upper tract tumors. Hunt later wrote that urothelial tumors progressed through the lining of the urothelial system and that the ureter and bladder cuff should be removed as early as possible [8]. Beer published his work on so-called "aseptic nephro-ureterectomies" that addressed his concerns of spillage of urinary contents during the procedure and is credited with espousing the surgical techniques of extraperitoneal bladder cuff resection with the distal ureter which has remained the standard of care for 50 years. Thereafter, many surgeons proposed techniques to remove the distal ureter without performing pelvic surgery, largely through the growing field of endoscopic techniques. An intussusception maneuver was briefly proposed in which a retrograde ureteral catheter is advanced and sutured to the ureteral margin at a level inferior to that of the completed nephrectomy. The ureter is then avulsed from below into the bladder and then unroofed at the bladder cuff endoscopically. Recurrence rates were greater than 15% and these were associated with high mortality. McDonald et al. [9] described the first transurethral resection of the ureteral orifice (TUR-UO) from the bladder prior to performing a nephroureterectomy in 1952 allowing the cystotomy to heal secondarily.

The modern era of nephroureterectomy came with the advent of laparoscopic techniques soon after introduction of the technology required for classic nephrectomy. Clayman et al. performed the first published case of a laparoscopic nephroureterectomy in 1991 in which the bladder cuff underwent transurethral resection (of the ureteral orifice or TUR-UO) with balloon occlusion of the distal ureter [10]. After nephrectomy and distal dissection, the unroofed bladder cuff could be retracted with the surrounding bladder which was then isolated by an EndoGIA™ stapler. Thus, the bladder was never opened to the abdominal cavity and the entirety of the distal ureter and bladder cuff was removed en bloc. As summarized below, a number of alternatives to the Clayman procedure were proposed including the 'clip and pluck' technique, a 'pneumovesicum' and transvesical laparoscopic en bloc bladder cuff mobilization and repair, and hand-assisted, two surgeon maneuvers [11–13]. Robotic surgery has played a role in advancing nephroureterectomy in the facilitation of the bladder cuff and distal ureteral surgery. Its role in surgery of the cephalad upper tract has been subject of debate [14–16].

Purpose of Minimally Invasive Surgery

The goal of minimally invasive surgery in urothelial cancer is to equal the oncology results of open surgery, ensure complete resection of disease, and limit the perioperative morbidity of the procedure. Benefits for the patient can include a shorter hospital stay, decreased narcotic use after surgery, decreased postoperative complications, and a decreased rate of blood transfusion but these short-term gains are vitiated by recurrent disease when minimally invasive surgical approaches are insufficient [14–16]. Still, most series point to the potential standardization of laparoscopy in the surgery of UUT-UC. Patients who undergo laparoscopic versus open nephroureterectomy may have lower mortality (0.3 vs. 0.7%), fewer postoperative complications (9.4 vs. 12.6%) and transfusions (12.9 vs. 20.6%), and shorter lengths of stay. The initial experience of laparoscopic nephroureterectomy, however, has in some studies revealed a longer procedure time (245 vs. 278 min) and cost of hospitalization ($15,691 vs. $12,846) [15]. Robotic-assisted nephroureterectomy is becoming increasingly utilized compared to pure laparoscopic surgery since its inception. In a nationwide study comparing perioperative outcomes of patients undergoing laparoscopic and robotic-assisted nephroureterectomy from 2008 to 2010, overall complications (18.2 vs. 11.9%), mortality (1.4 vs. 0.0%), and length of stay greater than 4 days (49 vs. 39.9%) were lower with the robotic-assisted group when compared to the laparoscopic group although robotic-assisted approaches are associated with hospitalization costs up to 30% higher [15]. The much sought-after metric of the 'learning curve' for robotic nephroureterectomy has been proposed to be 25 procedures, to become proficient with robotic docking positions, suturing, and access techniques that are not used in traditional laparoscopy [17].

Survival and Recurrence After Nephroureterectomy

UTUC is an aggressive cancer with an overall relapse rate of 27% in one large series after surgical intervention [18]. When analyzed by disease stage, freedom of disease at 5 years was Ta/CIS (73%), T1 (76%), T2 (59%), and T3 (40%). The most common sites of relapse are the bladder or remaining urinary tract (68.7%), distant metastases (22.4%), and in the retroperitoneum or lymph nodes (9%). Five-year survivals in these patients by disease stage are Ta/CIS (100%), T1 (92%), T2 (73%), and T3 (41%) with T4 disease having a median survival of only 6 months (Fig. 18.1).

Similar outcomes are seen with minimally invasive surgery. A study of 39 laparoscopic nephroureterectomy patients with various stages of UTUC and a minimum 5-year follow-up had a similar disease recurrence of 69% [19]. Of these patients, 28% went on to die due to their disease at a median time of 31 months after the operation. Another study of patients with pathology comparable to the prior studies and underwent robotic-assisted laparoscopic nephroureterectomy and had recurrence-free survival at 5 years of 57.1% [20]. There is some evidence that not all patients may benefit from a minimally invasive approach. A prospective trial of 80 patients who underwent either laparoscopic nephroureterectomy or open nephroureterectomy was studied and found that overall there was a similar survival between these two groups [21]. However, when analyzing the subgroups with high-grade or stage T3 tumors, there was significantly higher cancer-specific survival in the open group.

The distal ureter and bladder cuff represent a challenge as it often requires repositioning of the patient and increased operative time. However, the importance of completely removing the entire ureter and bladder cuff cannot be understated. Recurrence rates of UCC in the remaining

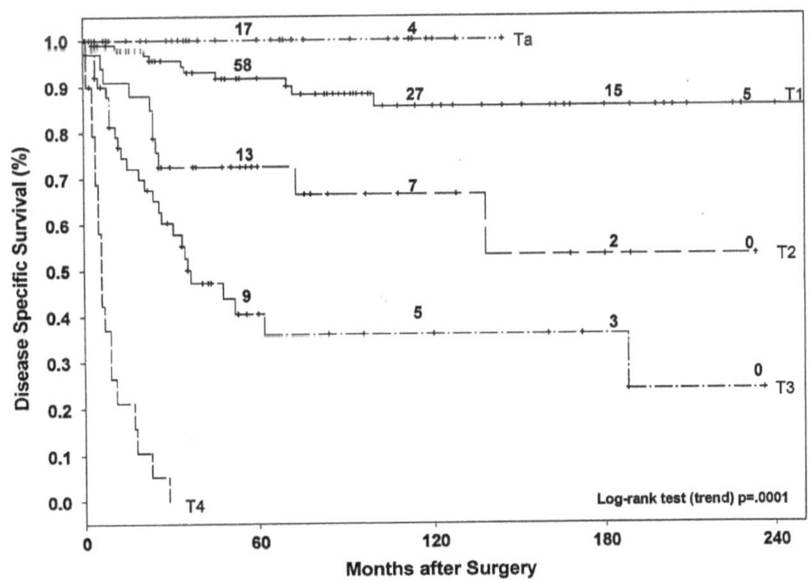

Fig. 18.1 Survival following surgical management of UTUC in 252 patients with a median follow-up of 64 months. Majority of patients (77%) underwent nephroureterectomy. From Hall et al. [18]; used with permission

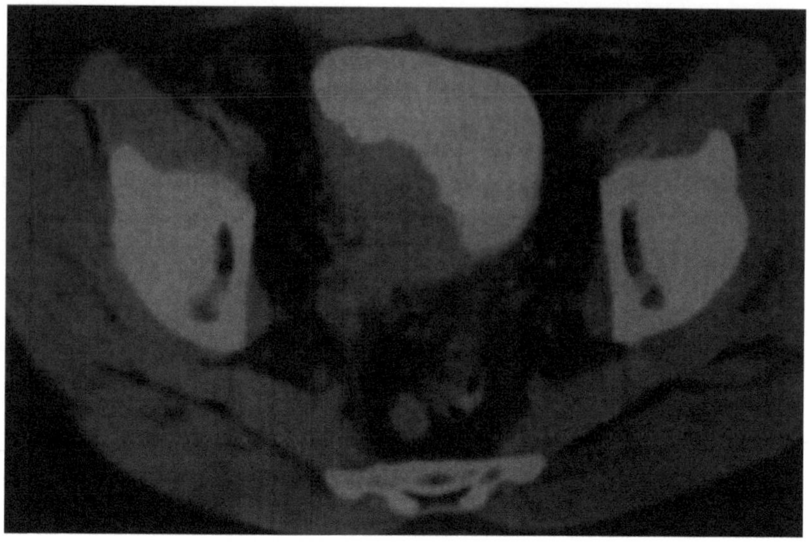

Fig. 18.2 Computed Tomogram scan showing a distal ureteral and bladder cuff recurrence in a patient with upper tract urothelial carcinoma after incomplete right nephroureterectomy. From Arango et al. [16]; used with permission

ureteral stump have been reported to be as high as 14.3–50% [18, 22]. Such patients often present with gross hematuria even years after their original extirpative surgery and will likely require surgical intervention (Fig. 18.2) [23]. Slightly over a third (36%) of patients who have had an incomplete ureteral resection will later present with local recurrence. About 85% of these patients will go on to undergo a distal ureterectomy for their recurrence. However, patients may present with distant metastases and poor survival [24].

Minimally Invasive Techniques

Technical Notes. Laparoscopic nephroureterectomy can be performed transperitoneally or retroperitoneally depending on surgeon preference. Transperitoneal laparoscopic nephroureterectomy is performed by first performing the nephrectomy portion of the procedure with a 10-mm trocar placed supraumbilically, a 5-mm trocar placed in the midclavicular line, and then a 12-mm placed between the first trocar and the xyphoid process [25]. The colon is then mobilized to expose the kidney. The kidney and then the ureter are dissected; a clip can be placed on the ureter to prevent tumor seeding. Two additional 5-mm and 10-mm trocars can then be placed in the pelvis to finish dissecting the distal ureter and bladder cuff if needed [20]. The course of the ureter is often far more sinuous than anticipated and one must be cognizant of the anatomy and neighboring structures along which the ureter courses. The gonadal vessels course anterior to the ureter at a level just above the pelvic brim. Division of the gonadal vessels may compromise blood flow to the testicle especially if the patient has undergone vasectomy or if the vas is divided to obtain pelvic exposure. The ureter courses medial to the iliac vessels but lateral to the medial umbilical ligament which is an important landmark in the male and female. The ureter passes posterior to the superior vesicle pedicle to the bladder (and the uterine artery in the female) deriving the moniker 'water-under-the-bridge' (see Fig. 18.3). The ureter courses inferiorly entering the bladder lateral to the vas deferens in the male and deep to the broad ligament in the female. In the female, the ureter passes just 1.5 cm lateral and slightly anterior to the fornix of the vagina. That proximity was the basis for J. Wesley Bouvee's (1861–1927) original approach to the distal ureter for ureterolithotomy in the female via a lateral incision through the fornix of the vaginal wall. Landmarks in locating the distal ureter, therefore, are the vas deferens in the male and the uterine artery in the female. Adequate exposure of the ureter as it enters the bladder is the only method

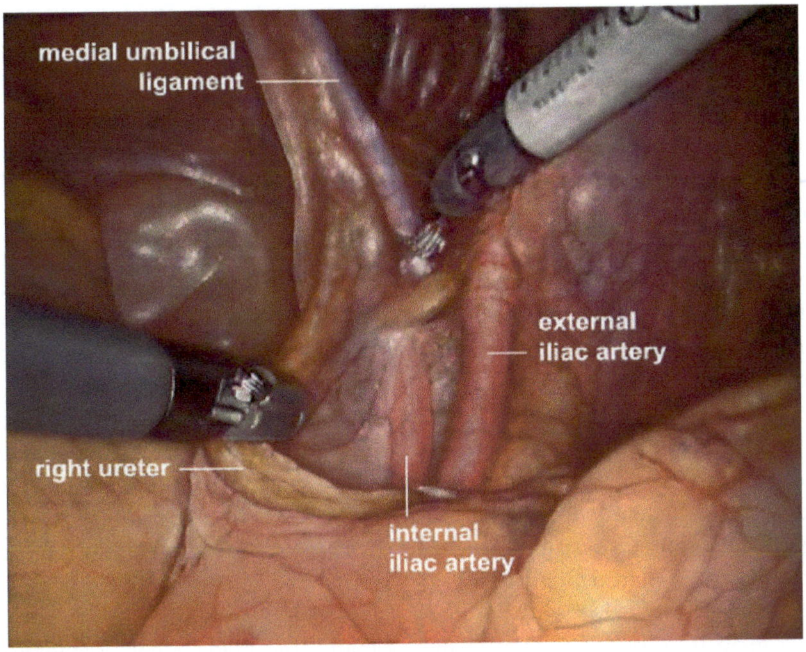

Fig. 18.3 Relationship of Pelvic Landmarks with the ureter. Note the course of the left ureter passing medial to the medial umbilical ligament and then lateral to the left vas deferens (not shown) as it courses along the retrovesical peritoneum toward the prostatic ampulla. The last major structure prior to penetrating the bladder will be the superior vesical artery which courses anterior to the ureter. From Feicke et al. [58]; used with permission

to ensure sufficient resection of the bladder cuff regardless of the approach described below.

A retroperitoneal nephroureterectomy has practical and theoretical advantages. Bowel mobilization, the risk of visceral injury, and ileus may be lessened, intraabdominal pathology is avoided, and tumor spillage may be less catastrophic when confined to the extraperitoneal space. Retroperitoneal surgery requires development of the potential plain between the psoas and the peritoneal cavity. Balloon or manual dissection may be difficult after any pathologic process that causes scarring of the normal tissue plains including prior hematoma, urinoma, fibrosis, or desmoplasia all of which may occur in the setting and potentially the result of multiple endoscopic diagnostic and therapeutic maneuvers. The retroperitoneal approach requires a traditional flank position with the patient flexed to enlarge the space between the 12th rib and the iliac crest. The initial dissection of the space between the renal unit and psoas occurs with blunt, finger dissection through a 1 cm lumbotomy, 2 cm inferior, and medial to the tip of the 12th rib. Often, the kidney can be palpated and mobilized anteriorly. Balloon dissection under direct vision with a 0° lens allows the visualization of the psoas muscle, the ureter, Gerota's fascia, and often genitofemoral nerve. The dissector is replaced by a balloon port that prevents the escape of CO_2 gas from the small space of the retroperitoneum. Laparoscopic ports are typically placed under direct vision one hand breath from the camera port and following the course of the overlying 12th rib. Typically, one port is placed inferior to the tip of the 12th rib, one superior to the superior iliac crest slightly anterior to the mid-axillary line, and the last is placed near the base of the 12th rib near anterior to the erecter spinae muscles [26, 27].

Robotic-assisted nephroureterectomy requires at least 2 more ports that are up to 5 mm larger than required for traditional laparoscopy.

Surgeons who use the patient side cart (PSC) of the DaVinci system for both the kidney and lower ureteral portions of the procedure will need to undock and re-position the PSC. The space for a retroperitoneal robotic nephroureterectomy is the same as traditional laparoscopy but the instrumentation occupies more of it. Robotic arm clashing and limitations of movement will occur unless docking occurs in a standardized manner as follows. The patient is positioned in full flank with the dependent arm either tucked on cushions or raised above the shoulder and flexed. The superior arm must be similarly positioned even lying oblique across the abdomen, thus to allow the docking of the PSC which must come in at a 45° angle over the contralateral shoulder similar to the approach for a robotic-assisted thoracic procedure. The camera is placed first to lock in the PSC. The robotic manipulator arms are then attached so that there is sufficient flexion in the manipulator joint to prevent clashing later in the case. The lens is placed at a 30° 'up' angle and the magnification kept at only 2×. Two assistant ports are required, one, a 10 mm best placed medially and inferior to the medial robotic port, and a 5 mm which courses over the psoas and posterior to the lateral robotic port. The use of the 4th robotic arm can replace the 5-mm assistant port but only if the lateral robotic arm is placed medially to allow one hand breadth between all the robotic ports [28]. The renal hilum is found first using the ureter and the lateral aspect of the vena cava on the right and the ureter and the gonadal vein on the left. Gerota's fascia is entered posteriorly to course parallel with fibers of the psoas until the pulsation of the renal artery is found, its white muscular appearance skeletonized with bipolar and scissors. Weck clips are no longer the primary means of controlling the renal hilum having long been replaced by vascular stapling devices. After the renal hilum is controlled a clip is placed on the ureter to prevent tumor spillage from proximal tumors. The ureter is dissected free distally and this may require division of the vas deferens and division of the superior vesicle artery, the latter of which can be divided with a single Weck clip and Ligasure. Finally, the bladder cuff is addressed surgically herein lies the great variability of the procedure (see below).

The DaVinci Xi may offer 'single docking' for both components of the procedure as the camera can be switched between different arms and trocars (Fig. 18.4) [29]. This feature is especially useful for a nephroureterectomy, where the camera can be shifted caudally to

(a) (b)

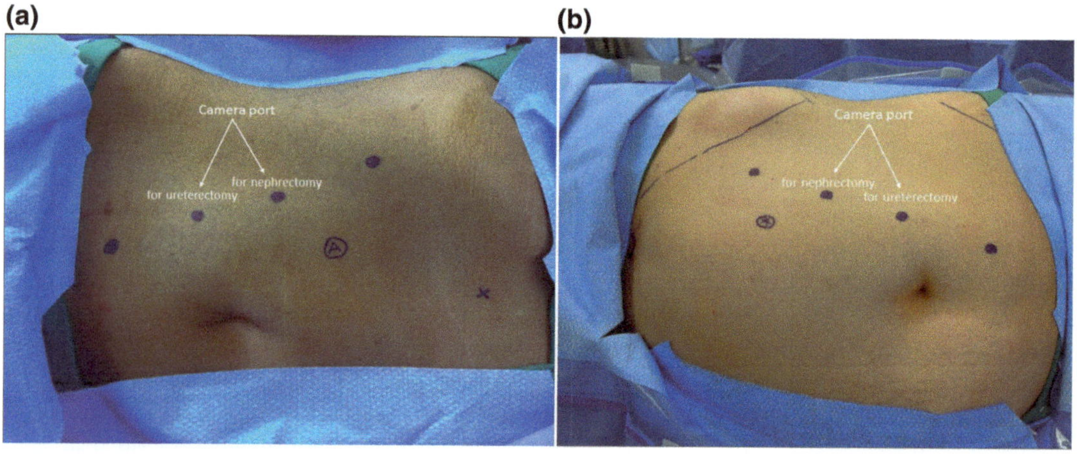

Fig. 18.4 Port placement in robotic-assisted laparoscopic nephroureterectomy (RALNU): the DaVinci Xi. **a** Left-sided transabdominal and **b** Right-sided transabdominal approaches to the kidney and ureter are facilitated by the swivel action of the Xi PSC, allowing for the downward migration of the camera and working robotic instruments for the pelvic portion of the procedure. Note the linear port placement which serves as a useful pattern applicable to most patients. From Darwiche et al. [29]; used with permission

better visualize the approach to the distal ureterectomy after the kidney has been fully mobilized (Fig. 18.4) [30].

Lymphadenectomy. Recently, using retrospective data, the lymph node drainage of UTUC has been mapped to provide a template for surgeons undertaking a lymphadenectomy or for future studies examining the effects of a standard template dissection. Left proximal ureter and renal pelvis tumors drained into the hilar (53%), paraaortic (31%), interaortocaval (4%), suprahilar (1%), common iliac (1%), aortic bifurcation (1%), and other sites (9%) [31]. Right-sided proximal ureteral and renal pelvis tumors drained into the paracaval (44.1%), hilar (22.1%), interaortocaval (20.6%), and retrocaval (10.3%) [32].

The role of lymphadenectomy during nephroureterectomy, however, is debatable. Positive lymph nodes, while providing more accurate staging information, carry a worse prognosis and any potential curative benefit is not known. Retrospective studies evaluating patients who underwent lymphadenectomy compared to those who did not, showed patients with node-positive disease to have decreased overall and recurrence-free survival compared to those who had node-negative disease and those who did not have a node dissection performed [33]. There are currently no randomized controlled trials evaluating the benefit of lymphadenectomy. A meta-analysis examining prior retrospective studies saw a benefit for those with higher stage invasive UTUC who underwent lymph node dissection compared to those who did not [34].

Adrenalectomy. Adrenalectomy during radical nephrectomy is typically reserved for cases of radiographically documented abnormalities, involvement, or feasibility. Management of the adrenal in UUT-UC appears to be similar. A retrospective review of patients who both had adrenalectomy at the time of nephroureterectomy and those who were spared showed no statistical difference in their survival during their median follow-up of 46 months [35]. During this study, the investigators saw none of the 50 patients who underwent adrenalectomy to have spread to the adrenal gland on pathology. In the other group, only one out of 116 patients developed ipsilateral adrenal metastases in those who had adrenal sparing surgery.

Approaches to the Distal Ureter and Bladder Cuff

Open

Multiple approaches have been described for resection of the distal ureter and bladder cuff after mobilization of the kidney and upper ureter laparoscopically or robotically. The classical technique is an open approach with the patient in the supine position through either a low midline, Pfannenstiel, or Gibson incision to provide access to the distal ureter and bladder through which the specimen can be later removed [36–38]. This approach gives greater visualization to ensure complete bladder cuff excision. The bladder cuff can be completely excised extravesically or a cystotomy can be created and the bladder cuff excised transvesically. The transvesical technique ensures direct visualization of a complete bladder cuff and distal ureter excision but should be avoided in patients with concerns of bladder UCC to prevent tumor spillage, patients with a positive urine cytology, and patients who are undergoing treatment for active carcinoma in situ (CIS) of the bladder. Additionally, both the extravesical and transvesical approach may be difficult in obese patients or in those with a history of prior pelvic surgery or radiation [39, 40]. Indeed, there may be some risk to the contralateral ureter in which the orifice is not clearly defined, either with an intubating catheter, or wire, and can be challenging to identify in the thick-walled, heavily trabeculated bladder [41].

TUR-UO

TUR-UO or the "pluck" technique was first described in 1952 by McDonald et al. [9] in a patient with a recurrence in a ureteral stump. Prior to dissection of the kidney and proximal ureter, patients are placed in the dorsal lithotomy position. A resectoscope is then used with a Collins knife to circumscribe the ureteral orifice and then carry this incision through the intramural portion of the ureter into the perivesical fat (Fig. 18.5) [35]. The patient is then repositioned for the nephrectomy portion of the procedure and when dissecting the ureter, the distal ureter can then be "plucked" free and removed along with the entire specimen through a flank incision [36]. The drawback to this technique is the time spent repositioning the patient after the dorsal lithotomy portion. This technique is also contraindicated for patients with multifocal or distal ureteral tumors due to the increased risk of tumor seeding, retroperitoneal recurrence and local recurrence, and positive surgical margins. Multiple case reports exist of local recurrence at the site of the ureteral orifice resection after the 'pluck' technique and may be less than ideal for patients at risk of local recurrence [16, 42]. However, a series of 31 nephroureterectomy patients who all had TUR-UO for high-grade tumor had no resection site or retroperitoneal recurrences at a median follow-up of 20 months [39]. The pluck technique was early incorporated into the laparoscopic nephroureterectomy armamentarium because the procedure would be completed when the ureteral dissection reached the bladder where the previously dissected cuff could be 'plucked' free. The TUR-UO technique, however, may give the appearance that the bladder cuff and UO are completely free from the intramural muscle when they are not. The surgeon will dissect antegrade to the bladder in such cases, find the distal ureter still adequately attached, and require additional dissection into the bladder wall to deliver the specimen. An aide to the dissection is with the combination of hand-assisted (HAL) techniques and transurethral techniques. Some have advocated a combined two-surgeon approach in which the HAL surgeon controls the distal ureter while a second surgeon unroofs the ureteral orifice. The benefit appears to be in the addition of tactical feedback and the confirmation in real time that the UO has been completely resected in toto [43]. Most follow-up studies reported no significant recurrences within the bladder of the 'pluck' technique although would be strongly indicated in cases where there was known CIS or history of high-grade superficial disease [44].

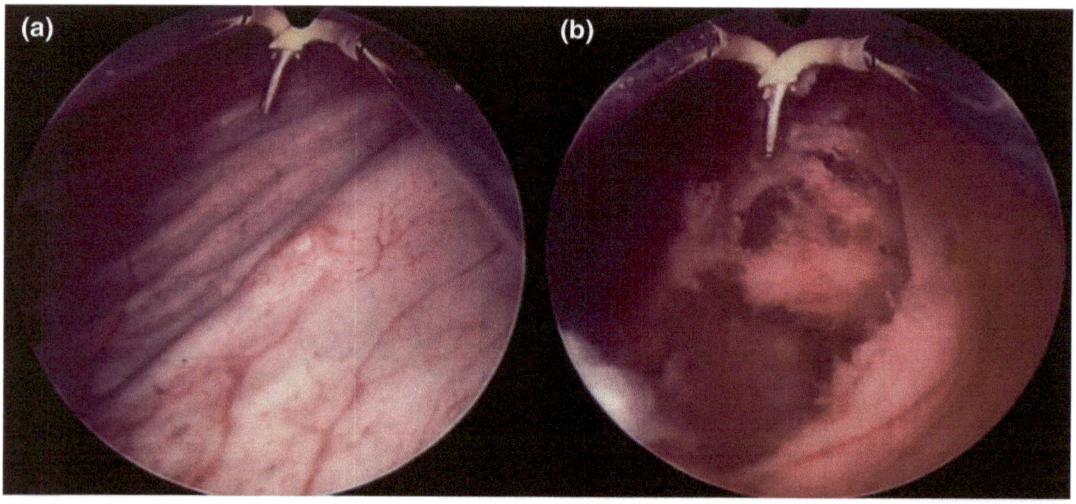

Fig. 18.5 Circumferential incision around the left ureteral orifice in a transurethral approach to the release of the distal ureter and bladder cuff from the intramural detrusor and connective tissue. The technique is often combined with retraction of the bladder cuff into the pelvic portion of the dissection during nephroureterectomy, the so-called 'pluck technique.' From Li et al. [37]; used with permission

Intussusception

A ureteral intussusception technique was originally developed as part of the open approach to aid in delivery of the entire distal ureter without a formal dissection. The technique involves placing a Chevassu catheter, a bulb-tipped ureteral catheter, into the distal ureter at the start of the procedure via cystoscopy (Fig. 18.6) [40, 45, 46]. The nephrectomy and proximal ureteral mobilization are then performed. The ureter is transected and the margin secured to the catheter with ligatures. The patient can then be repositioned into the dorsal lithotomy position for removal of the distal ureter and bladder cuff endoscopically. Traction is placed on the ureteral catheter under direct vision so that the ureter and ureteral orifice are everted. Then, with the resectoscope, TUR-UO can be performed freeing the orifice and distal ureter so that it can be removed through the urethra. A Foley catheter is then placed to allow the bladder to heal. Contraindications to this technique are similar to a TUR-UO, mainly UCC involving the distal ureter as there is a higher likelihood of incomplete resection with a positive margin. Additionally, patients with duplicated ureters, ureteral strictures, prior ureteral surgery, and prior radiation should undergo different techniques to excise the bladder cuff and distal ureter. In a large series of patients undergoing this technique, 6/32 (18.7%) patients failed ureteral intussusception and required an additional incision. These patients were followed for a median time of 35.2 months with 28.1% experiencing local or distant recurrence, similar to published rates of other methods of bladder cuff management. For the majority of low-grade, renal pelvic tumors, ureteral stripping is probably safe and requires a shorter operative time. Its lack of efficacy, violation of the urinary tract, and contraindications for ureteral disease requires caution before its application [45].

Extravesical Resection

Another option for the distal ureter and bladder cuff is an extravesical approach where the distal ureter and its surrounding bladder cuff is dissected

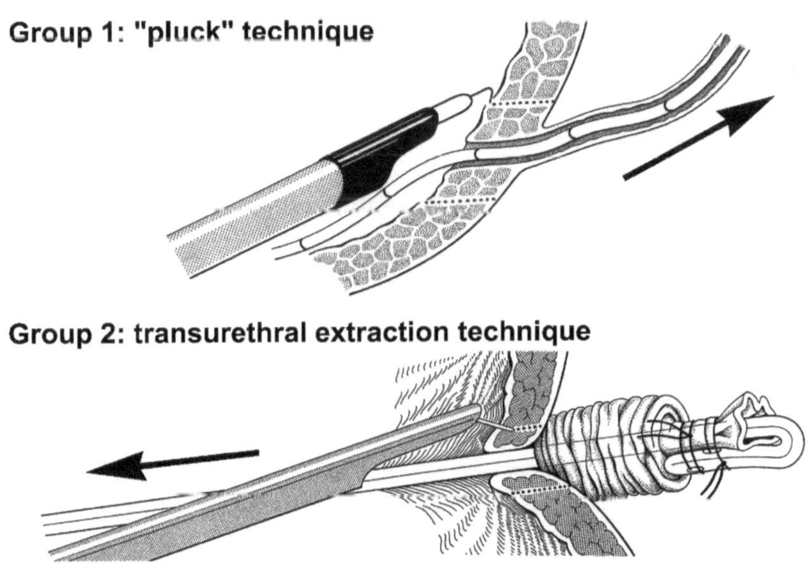

Fig. 18.6 Original approaches to the distal ureter: transurethral incision of ureteral orifice versus the intussusception technique. The kidney is removed after ligation of the proximal ureter. The distal ureter is cannulated with a multi-eye catheter and the ureter is closed in either as a purse-string (*top*) or side cinching (*bottom*) to the catheter. The ureter is then dragged from below as the ureteral orifice is everted and freed by transurethral excision. From Ubrig et al. [46]; Used with Permission

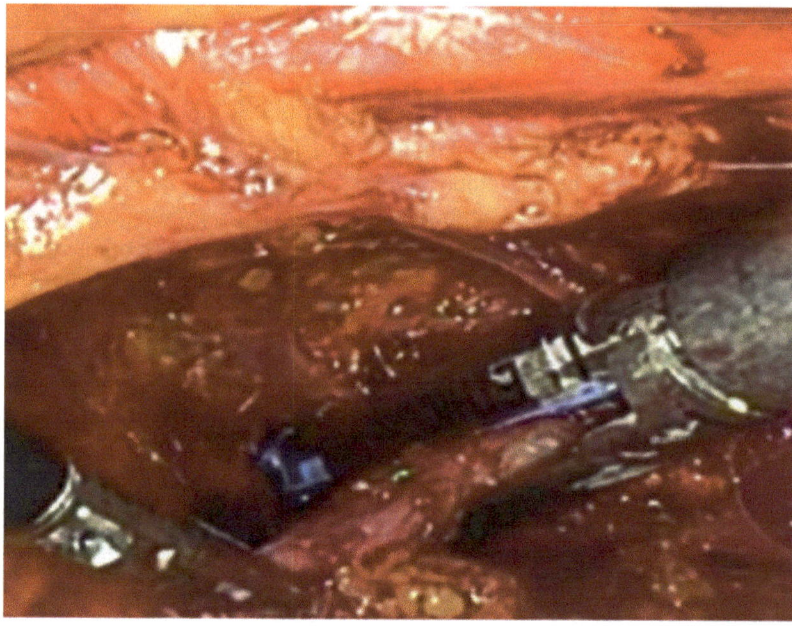

Fig. 18.7 Stapled bladder cuff technique in the management of the left distal ureter in a laparoscopic nephroureterectomy. From Yao et al. [56]; used with permission

free via a lateral low cystotomy. An indwelling open-ended ureteral catheter aids in identification (Fig. 18.7). The bladder defect can then be primarily closed robotically with a running V-Lok suture [35]. Ligasure has been used to replace the older extravesical approach to the bladder cuff using a stapling device. Potential benefits of Ligasure technology use may be the cytolytic effect of tissue sealing of the bladder cuff whereby residual tumor cells are destroyed without opening the bladder to the surgical space [25].

Pneumovesicum, Hydrovesicum, and Lasso Techniques

Guzzo et al. [11] described a 'pneumovesicum' technique of distal ureter management (Fig. 18.8). The patient is placed in dorsal lithotomy position and then two 2-mm needleoscopic ports are placed into the bladder suprapubically under direct vision via a cystoscope. The bladder is insufflated with CO_2. An endoloop is placed through one of the ports and surrounds the ureteral orifice. A guide wire and open-ended ureteral catheter are placed cystoscopically through the loop into the ureter. The resectoscope is used to perform a TUR-UO with the ureteral catheter to guide the resection. A grasper is used through the other port to provide traction during the resection of the intramural ureter. Once the intramural ureter has been sufficiently freed, the ureteral catheter and guidewire are removed and the endoloop is used to retrieve the distal end, preventing tumor spillage, allowing the dissection to occur to the retroperitoneal fat (Fig. 18.9). A Foley catheter is then placed to allow time for bladder healing.

Comparison

When comparing methods of removing the bladder cuff, a study of 301 patients who underwent either transurethral incision, extravesical, or intravesical approach had similar rates of recurrence in the bladder (23.5, 24 and 17.6%), retroperitoneum (7.4, 7.8, 5.5%), and distal metastases (7.4, 10.4, 5.5%) [37]. Another study in which 138 patients underwent TUR-UO or open distal ureterectomy found similar recurrences in the bladder for these two groups (54.4 vs. 47.9%), respectively as well as similar rates of recurrence at the ureteral resection site (3.3 vs. 4.2%), respectively [47]. The main advantage of performing the TUR-UO was a shortening of the

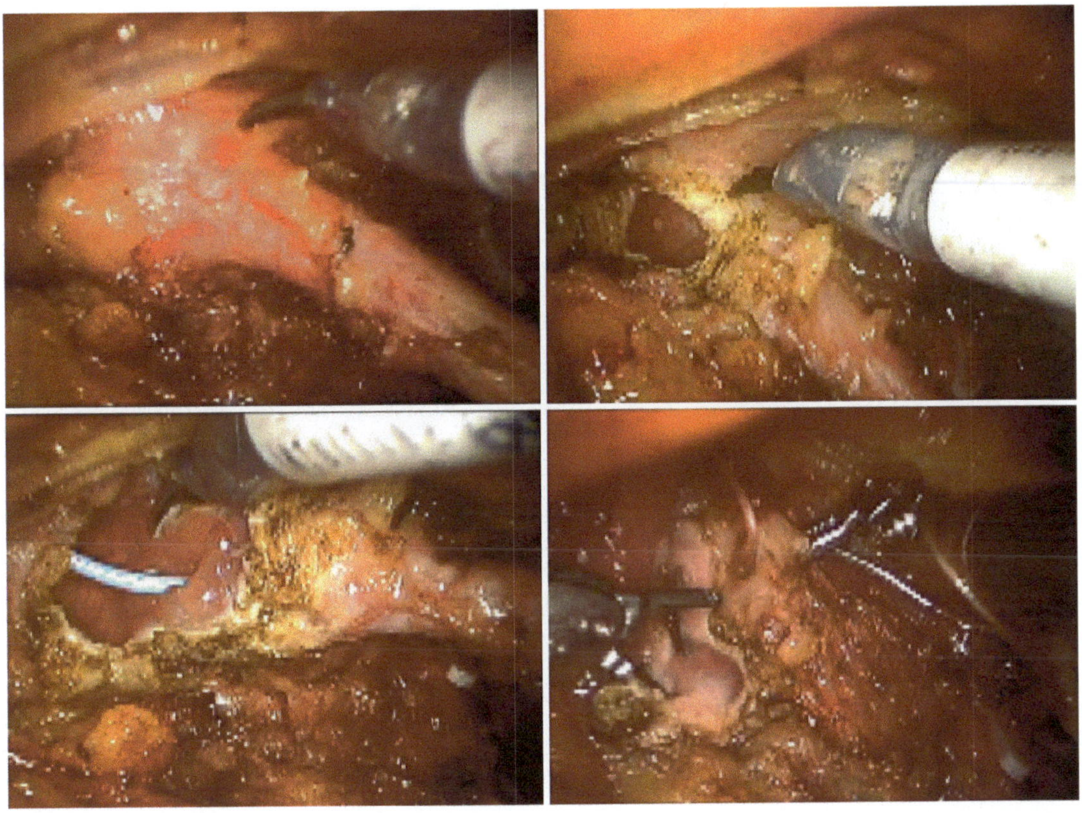

Fig. 18.8 Extravesical excision. Robotic-assisted extravesical excision of ureteral orifice. Note here, the use of a ureteral catheter to assist in dissection. The robotic interface facilitates the two-layer closure of the cystotomy that may decrease Foley catheter drainage. From Khemees et al. [57]; used with permission

operative procedure by an average of 80 min. A contraindication is present of ureteral urothelial disease. In general, the management of the distal ureter and bladder cuff should adhere to the standard of care, namely open bladder cuff resection and en bloc distal ureteral mobilization. Minimally invasive techniques, including the 'pluck,' extravesical excision, ureteral stripping, and stapling, may reach the equivalency of the open technique, especially for low-grade renal pelvis disease, but all may have an increased risk of intravesical recurrence [48]. The surgeon who performs minimally invasive bladder cuff excision as part of a laparoscopic nephroureterectomy may indeed obtain short-term gains. However, vigilant surveillance will be required to ensure that short-term gains do not translate into long-term setbacks and intravesical or intraperitoneal recurrence [16, 49].

Segmental Ureterectomy

Segmental ureterectomy has been considered by some to resection low-grade, isolated ureteral tumors as these may arise as independent neoplasia separate from the renal pelvis (Fig. 18.10). According to Lucca et al. [50] relative indications for segmental ureterectomy and kidney sparing surgery may include feasibility of resected entire tumor burden of a low-grade, non-invasive lesion, absence of hydronephrosis, negative urinary cytology, and patient compliance. Of these, compliance may be the most

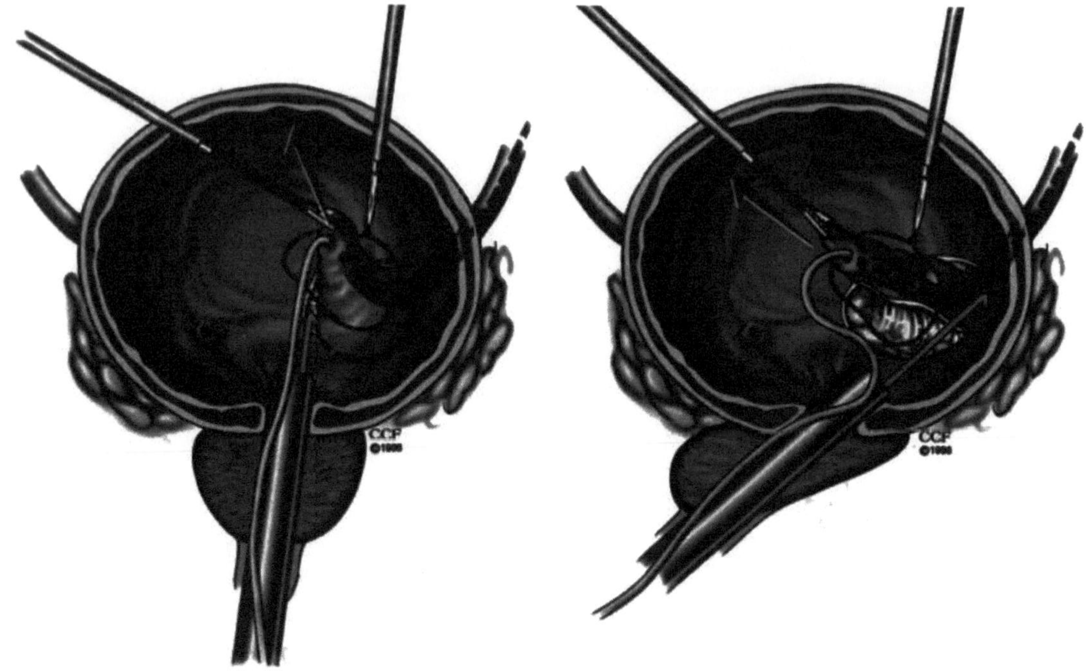

Fig. 18.9 Transvesical approach to the ureteral orifice. Note the use of separate 3- or 5-mm trocars used to place a lasso and graspers that facilitate the transurethral unroofing of the ureteral orifice and its release from the intramural detrusor musculature. From Gill et al. [13]; used with permission

clinically relevant as patients may require follow-up cytologic, imaging, and ureteroscopic evaluation. Small studies of segmental ureterectomy suggest that in properly selected patients, there does not appear to be a negative oncologic consequence of avoiding nephroureterectomy for isolated ureteral lesions [5, 51]. In a retrospective study, there was no perceived difference in recurrence-free or cancer-specific survival comparing 35 subjects who underwent segmental ureterectomy versus 96 who underwent nephroureterectomy [51]. A non-inferiority study confirmed that over a 6-year period, there was no difference in bladder, local/pelvic, or distant recurrences in patients who had undergone nephroureterectomy (n = 77) versus those who underwent segmental ureterectomy (n = 35) for primary ureteral carcinoma including 15 and 11, respectively, who had >T2 disease [5]. Segmental ureterectomy requires the defining of negative margins. Through an open approach, tactical feedback of bulky disease may be helpful combined with intraoperative frozen section analysis of margins. Minimally invasive techniques, however, require different approaches to ensure clear margins. The use of intraoperative ureteroscopy and transmural endoscopic glow can help define a lower ureteral margin, while the upper ureteral margin may require the use of landmarks (e.g., correlation with cross-sectional imaging and the pelvic brim), ultrasound, or antegrade endoscopic techniques (Fig. 18.10). To ensure the lack of spillage, any ureteral tumor should be isolated with ties allowing for the resection of the diseased segment with proximal and distal ties of different colors for pathologic orientation. A gap of 5 cm can ordinarily be closed primarily with proximal and ureteral mobilization. A longer segment may require laparoscopic or robotic-assisted Boari flap creation which may offer longer term patency rates than psoas hitch creation [52].

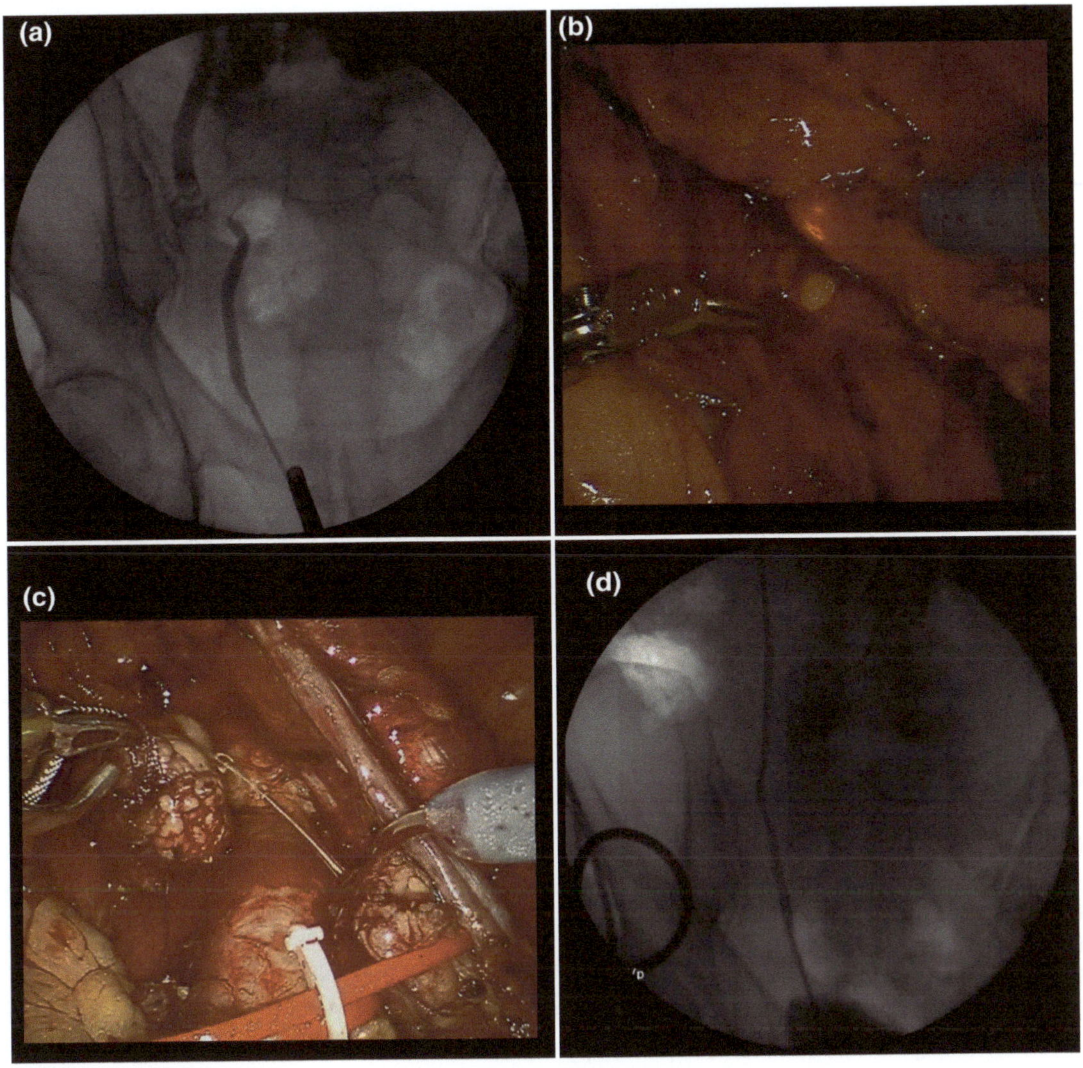

Fig. 18.10 Segmental ureterectomy. Note in **a**, a filling defect consistent with a mid-ureteral high-grade lesion in a 62-year-old smoker undergoing chemotherapy for duodenal carcinoma. In **b**, a flexible ureteroscopic glow allows delineation of the distal margin. In **c**, the proximal margin is resected where a brisk release of obstructed urine is appreciated. A primary spatulated ureteroureterostomy over a 4.8 French ureteral stent is performed. In **d**, a retrograde ureterogram at 6 weeks post-op reveals acceptable patency. Pathology proved to be a pT1N0Mx urothelial carcinoma of the right ureter, 4.6 × 2.8 cm, with negative margins

Neoadjuvant Chemotherapy

Neoadjuvant chemotherapy has become the standard of care for muscle-invasive UCC of the bladder [53, 54]. However, due to a lack of consensus and a paucity of level 1 evidence, neoadjuvant chemotherapy is provided far less often for patients undergoing nephroureterectomy for UUT-UC. Another important consideration is that the loss of kidney function after the procedure may preclude some from being able to receive adjuvant therapy if the pathology warrants. A group of 43 patients receiving different neoadjuvant chemotherapy regimens were compared to a historical group of patients who underwent immediate nephroureterectomy. After receiving neoadjuvant chemotherapy there was significant downgrading in the stage of the disease, as patients were less likely to be T2 or greater 46.5 versus 65.4%, T3 or greater 27.9 versus 47.7%, and 14% of the patients had a complete response with no tumor seen on final pathological evaluation [55]. There is some evidence as well that neoadjuvant chemotherapy improves survival. A comparison between a group receiving neoadjuvant chemotherapy and a historical group that received none showed the chemotherapy group with an overall survival of 80.2 versus 57.65%, respectively. This difference remained statistically significant on multivariate analysis.

While there are currently no prospective trials showing the effectiveness in UUUT-UC, there are some retrospective studies which provide some evidence for its use. Patients with high-grade cancer should be considered for neoadjuvant treatment, especially when considering that after surgery their renal function will decline.

Conclusions

The basis of the nephroureterectomy, to remove the kidney and entirety of the ipsilateral ureter and portion of the bladder cuff, has remained the same since first performed by Kelly in 1893. Surgical advances in this operation have come from innovations in minimally invasive and endoscopic surgeries. Advances in laparoscopy and robotic-assisted surgeries provided tremendous benefits to patients in terms of limiting perioperative complications, less pain postoperatively, and allowing them to stay in the hospital fewer days.

The distal ureter still remains a unique challenge for urologists. Performing this part of the operation requires a great deal of extra time in the operating room. Those where the distal ureter was not resected completely have a high recurrence rate and often poor outcomes. Multiple techniques have been described for the often minimized distal ureteral portion of the surgery including endoscopic, laparoscopic, robotic-assisted, and open all with similar survival and recurrence rates for the patient. Due to the similarities in outcome, surgeon preference, and experience, tumor characteristics and patient characteristics should be the main considerations when planning to perform the nephroureterectomy.

Summary Box

- Nephroureterectomy represents the gold standard in terms of surgical management of upper tract urothelial cancer. Advances in this operation have focused on minimally invasive methods of removal and ease of removal of the distal ureter.
- Minimally invasive surgery has the potential of less morbidity and fewer complications.
- There are multitude approaches to the distal ureter. Options include open surgery, laparoscopic or robotic-assisted, TUR-UO, intussusception, or pneumovesicum. Similar oncologic outcomes are seen with each and should be chosen based on surgeon preference and tumor location.
- Neoadjuvant chemotherapy for upper tract disease has shown potential in preliminary studies but randomized trials are needed before it becomes a standardized recommendation.

References

1. Mitra AP, Alemozaffar M, Harris BN, et al. Outcomes after urothelial recurrence in bladder cancer patients undergoing radical cystectomy. Urology. 2014;84:1420.
2. Raman JD, Messer J, Sielatycki JA, et al. Incidence and survival of patients with carcinoma of the ureter and renal pelvis in the USA, 1973–2005. BJU Int. 2011;107:1059.
3. Makhoul B, De La Taille A, Vordos D, et al. Laparoscopic radical nephrectomy for T1 renal cancer: the gold standard? A comparison of laparoscopic vs open nephrectomy. BJU Int. 2004;93:67.
4. Steinberg JR, Matin SF. Laparoscopic radical nephroureterectomy: dilemma of the distal ureter. Curr Opin Urol. 2004;14:61.

5. Hung SY, Yang WC, Luo HL, et al. Segmental ureterectomy does not compromise the oncologic outcome compared with nephroureterectomy for pure ureter cancer. Int Urol Nephrol. 2014;46:921.
6. Porten S, Siefker-Radtke AO, Xiao L, et al. Neoadjuvant chemotherapy improves survival of patients with upper tract urothelial carcinoma. Cancer. 2014;120:1794.
7. Lin YK, Kaag M, Raman JD. Rationale and timing of perioperative chemotherapy for upper-tract urothelial carcinoma. Expert Rev Anticancer Ther. 2014;14:543.
8. Reservitz GB. A historic review of nephroureterectomy. Surg Gynecol Obstet. 1967;125:853.
9. McDonald HP, Upchurch WE, Sturdevant CE. Nephro-ureterectomy: a new technique. J Urol. 1952;67:804.
10. Clayman RV, Kavoussi LR, Figenshau RS, et al. Laparoscopic nephroureterectomy: initial clinical case report. J Laparoendosc Surg. 1991;1:343.
11. Guzzo TJ, Schaeffer EM, Allaf ME. Laparoscopic radical nephroureterectomy with en-bloc distal ureteral and bladder cuff excision using a single position pneumovesicum method. Urology. 2008;72:850.
12. Kawauchi A, Fujito A, Soh J, et al. Hand-assisted retroperitoneoscopic radical nephrectomy and nephroureterectomy. J Endourol. 2004;18:365.
13. Gill IS, Soble JJ, Miller SD, et al. A novel technique for management of the en bloc bladder cuff and distal ureter during laparoscopic nephroureterectomy. J Urol. 1999;161:430.
14. Trudeau V, Gandaglia G, Shiffmann J, et al. Robot-assisted versus laparoscopic nephroureterectomy for upper-tract urothelial cancer: a population-based assessment of costs and perioperative outcomes. Can Urol Assoc J. 2014;8:E695.
15. Sugihara T, Yasunaga H, Yu C, et al. Perioperative outcome comparisons between open and laparoscopic nephroureterectomy among a population-based Cohort from 2010 to 2012. J Endourol. 2015;29:770.
16. Arango O, Bielsa O, Carles J, et al. Massive tumor implantation in the endoscopic resected area in modified nephroureterectomy. J Urol. 1997;157:1839.
17. Sammon J, Perry A, Beaule L, et al. Robot-assisted radical prostatectomy: learning rate analysis as an objective measure of the acquisition of surgical skill. BJU Int. 2010;106:855.
18. Hall MC, Womack S, Sagalowsky AI, et al. Prognostic factors, recurrence, and survival in transitional cell carcinoma of the upper urinary tract: a 30-year experience in 252 patients. Urology. 1998;52:594.
19. Muntener M, Nielsen ME, Romero FR, et al. Long-term oncologic outcome after laparoscopic radical nephroureterectomy for upper tract transitional cell carcinoma. Eur Urol. 2007;51:1639.
20. Aboumohamed AA, Krane LS, Hemal AK. Oncologic outcomes following robot-assisted laparoscopic nephroureterectomy with bladder cuff excision for upper tract urothelial carcinoma. J Urol. 2015;194:1561.
21. Simone G, Papalia R, Guaglianone S, et al. Laparoscopic versus open nephroureterectomy: perioperative and oncologic outcomes from a randomised prospective study. Eur Urol. 2009;56:520.
22. Roupret M, Babjuk M, Comperat E, et al. European association of urology guidelines on upper urinary tract urothelial cell carcinoma: 2015 update. Eur Urol. 2015;68:868.
23. Bourdoumis A, Syed I, Soosay G, et al. Transitional cell carcinoma of the ureteric stump: a systematic review of the literature. Urol Int. 2013;91:170.
24. Kang M, Jeong CW, Kwak C, et al. The characteristics of recurrent upper tract urothelial carcinoma after radical nephroureterectomy without bladder cuff excision. Yonsei Med J. 2015;56:375.
25. Tsivian A, Benjamin S, Sidi AA. A sealed laparoscopic nephroureterectomy: a new technique. Eur Urol. 2007;52:1015.
26. Fang Z, Li L, Wang X, et al. Total retroperitoneal laparoscopic nephroureterectomy with bladder-cuff resection for upper urinary tract transitional cell carcinoma. J Invest Surg. 2014;27:354.
27. Gill IS, Sung GT, Hobart MG, et al. Laparoscopic radical nephroureterectomy for upper tract transitional cell carcinoma: the Cleveland Clinic experience. J Urol. 2000;164:1513.
28. Zargar H, Krishnan J, Autorino R, et al. Robotic nephroureterectomy: a simplified approach requiring no patient repositioning or robot redocking. Eur Urol. 2014;66:769.
29. Darwiche F, Swain S, Kallingal G, et al. Operative technique and early experience for robotic-assisted laparoscopic nephroureterectomy (RALNU) using da Vinci Xi. Springerplus. 2015;4:298.
30. Patel MN, Aboumohamed A, Hemal A. Does transition from the da Vinci Si to Xi robotic platform impact single-docking technique for robot-assisted laparoscopic nephroureterectomy?. BJU Int. 2015;116:990.
31. Matin SF, Sfakianos JP, Espiritu PN, et al. Patterns of lymphatic metastases in upper tract urothelial carcinoma and proposed dissection templates. J Urol. 2015;194:1567.
32. Kondo T, Nakazawa H, Ito F, et al. Impact of the extent of regional lymphadenectomy on the survival of patients with urothelial carcinoma of the upper urinary tract. J Urol. 2007;178:1212.
33. Mason RJ, Kassouf W, Bell DG, et al. The contemporary role of lymph node dissection during nephroureterectomy in the management of upper urinary tract urothelial carcinoma: the Canadian experience. Urology. 2012;79:840.
34. Yang D, Chen Q, Song X, et al. Effect of lymph node dissection on the outcomes of upper tract urothelial carcinomas: a meta-analysis. Expert Rev Anticancer Ther. 2014;14:667.

35. Huang CY, Chung SD, Wang SM, et al. An audit of nephroureterectomy for upper tract urothelial carcinoma. Eur J Surg Oncol. 2009;35:1333.
36. Stravodimos KG, Komninos C, Kural AR, et al. Distal ureterectomy techniques in laparoscopic and robot-assisted nephroureterectomy: Updated review. Urol Ann. 2015;7:8.
37. Li WM, Shen JT, Li CC, et al. Oncologic outcomes following three different approaches to the distal ureter and bladder cuff in nephroureterectomy for primary upper urinary tract urothelial carcinoma. Eur Urol. 2010;57:963.
38. Macejko AM, Pazona JF, Loeb S, et al. Management of distal ureter in laparoscopic nephroureterectomy—a comprehensive review of techniques. Urology. 2008;72:974.
39. Palou J, Caparros J, Orsola A, et al. Transurethral resection of the intramural ureter as the first step of nephroureterectomy. J Urol. 1995;154:43.
40. Giovansili B, Peyromaure M, Saighi D, et al. Stripping technique for endoscopic management of distal ureter during nephroureterectomy: experience of 32 procedures. Urology. 2004;64:448.
41. Strong DW, Pearse HD, Tank ES Jr, et al. The ureteral stump after nephroureterectomy. J Urol. 1976;115:654.
42. Hetherington JW, Ewing R, Philp NH. Modified nephroureterectomy: a risk of tumour implantation. Br J Urol. 1986;58:368.
43. Brown JA, Strup SE, Chenven E, et al. Hand-assisted laparoscopic nephroureterectomy: analysis of distal ureterectomy technique, margin status, and surgical outcomes. Urology. 2005;66:1192.
44. Kurzer E, Leveillee RJ, Bird VG. Combining hand assisted laparoscopic nephroureterectomy with cystoscopic circumferential excision of the distal ureter without primary closure of the bladder cuff—is it safe? J Urol. 2006;175:63.
45. Saika T, Nishiguchi J, Tsushima T, et al. Comparative study of ureteral stripping versus open ureterectomy for nephroureterectomy in patients with transitional carcinoma of the renal pelvis. Urology. 2004;63:848.
46. Ubrig B, Boenig M, Waldner M, et al. Transurethral approach to the distal ureter in nephroureterectomy: transurethral extraction vs. "Pluck" technique with long-term follow-up; used with permission. Eur Urol. 2004;46:741.
47. Walton TJ, Sherwood BT, Parkinson RJ, et al. Comparative outcomes following endoscopic ureteral detachment and formal bladder cuff excision in open nephroureterectomy for upper urinary tract transitional cell carcinoma. J Urol. 2009;181:532.
48. Srirangam SJ, van Cleynenbreugel B, van Poppel H. Laparoscopic nephroureterectomy: the distal ureteral dilemma. Adv Urol. 2009;2009:1.
49. Otsuka M, Taguchi S, Nakagawa T, et al. Lower ureteral lesion is an independent predictor of intravesical recurrence after radical nephroureterectomy for upper tract urothelial carcinoma. Urol Oncol. 2015;34:e9.
50. Lucca I, Klatte T, Rouppret M, et al. Kidney-sparing surgery for upper tract urothelial cancer. Curr Opin Urol. 2015;25:100.
51. Pedrosa JA, Masterson TA, Rice KR, et al. Oncologic outcomes and prognostic impact of urothelial recurrences in patients undergoing segmental and total ureterectomy for upper tract urothelial carcinoma. Can Urol Assoc J. 2015;9:E187.
52. Fifer GL, Raynor MC, Selph P, et al. Robotic ureteral reconstruction distal to the ureteropelvic junction: a large single institution clinical series with short-term follow up. J Endourol. 2014;28:1424.
53. Rose TL, Deal AM, Basch E, et al. Neoadjuvant chemotherapy administration and time to cystectomy for muscle-invasive bladder cancer: an evaluation of transitions between academic and community settings. Urol Oncol. 2015;33(386):e1.
54. Witjes JA, Comperat E, Cowan NC, et al. EAU guidelines on muscle-invasive and metastatic bladder cancer: summary of the 2013 guidelines. Eur Urol. 2014;65:778.
55. Secin FP, Jiborn T, Bjartell AS, et al. Multi-institutional study of symptomatic deep venous thrombosis and pulmonary embolism in prostate cancer patients undergoing laparoscopic or robot-assisted laparoscopic radical prostatectomy. Eur Urol. 2008;53:134.
56. Yao L, Yang K, Li X. Comparison between completely and traditionally retroperitoneoscopic nephroureterectomy for upper tract urothelial cancer. World J Surg Oncol. 2016;14:171.
57. Khemees TA, Nasser SM, Abaza R. Clinical pathway after robotic nephroureterectomy: omission of pelvic drain with next-day catheter removal and discharge. Urology. 2014;83:818.
58. Feicke A, Baumgartner M, Talimi S. Robotic-assisted laparoscopic extended pelvic lymph node dissection for prostate cancer: surgical technique and experience with the first 99 cases. Eur Urol. 2009;55:876.

Management of Distal Ureter in Nephroureterectomy—Controversies

19

Nariman Ahmadi and Inderbir Gill

Introduction

Management of the distal ureter in radical nephroureterctomy (RNU) for upper tract urothelial tumors has been the topic of controversies in the past. Currently, the practice guidelines recommend excision of the full length of the ureter inclusive of the intramural ureter as well as the ipsilateral periureteric bladder cuff, as gold standard for treatment of the nonmetastatic upper tract urothelial cancers [1].

Radical nephroureterctomy (RNU) is essentially a procedure involving two separate and distinct components: radical nephrectomy and distal ureterectomy. The two main challenges of this operation include resection of the renal hilum and resection of the distal ureter; each located at opposite poles of the abdominopelvic cavity. In order to perform a safe and efficient resection while maintaining good oncological outcomes, surgeons should attempt to either perform them as two separate and distinct procedures via separate incisions or combine the two operations into one. Combining the techniques may vary depending on the surgeon's experience and techniques. Several novel techniques have been described which often utilize a combination of open and laparoscopic approaches with endourological techniques to overcome the challenges in distal ureterectomy and excision of the bladder cuff.

Electronic supplementary material The online version of this chapter (doi:10.1007/978-3-319-51263-1_19) contains supplementary material, which is available to authorized users.

N. Ahmadi (✉) · I. Gill
University of Southern California,
Institute of Urology, 1441 Eastlake Ave,
Suite 7416, Los Angeles, CA 90033, USA
e-mail: nari.ahmadi@gmail.com

I. Gill
e-mail: igill@med.usc.edu

Distal Ureteric Stump—Does It Need to Be Excised?

The first controversy questions the necessity of performing distal ureterectomy for urothelial malignancies of the renal calyces, renal pelvis, or upper ureteric tumors. There is no doubt that the addition of distal ureterectomy, whether performed laparoscopic, open, or endoscopically, increases the operative time, blood loss, post-operative analgesia requirements, length of stay, or even complication rates. A temporary indwelling catheter is almost always required to facilitate healing of the bladder wounds and minimize the risk of urine leak. The urologists have often wondered if excision of the entire distal ureter including intramural ureter or the bladder cuff provides any survival advantage, especially in cases where the tumor is located in the upper

M. Eshghi (ed.), *Urothelial Malignancies of the Upper Urinary Tract*,
https://doi.org/10.1007/978-3-319-51263-1_19

ureter or renal pelvis, or if the tumor is a lower grade urothelial carcinoma. The implication of this question is already evident in a recent multi-institutional review by Capitanio, who reported less than half of all the patients undergoing RNU will have distal ureterectomy and bladder cuff excision [2].

Historically, the first modern (complete) nephroureterctomy was performed in 1898; however, it was not until 1934, that Kimball and Ferris highlighted the high recurrence rate following simple nephroureterctomy for urothelial cancers [3]. In their review of 74 cases, where a ureteral stump was left in situ, 58% developed or had residual malignancies in the ureteric stump. Similarly Kinder and Wallace in their review of 46 cases, found a 45% recurrence rate in the ureteric stump [4]. Other authors reported ureteric stump recurrence rates ranging between 20 and 40% [3, 5, 6]. Ko et al., in his series reported a recurrence rate of 80% (4/5) in patients who had an unplanned incomplete ureterectomy during RNU and 60% (3/5) rate of developing metastatic disease at a median of less than 1 year after RNU, none of which were pre-operatively evident [7]. They attributed the incomplete ureterectomy to higher ASA scores of patients, as well as technical difficulties during the operation, which are the two main factors swaying urologists to electively abandon the completion of distal ureterectomy. Abel et al., examined delayed ureterectomy following incomplete nephroureterctomy for upper tract urothelial carcinoma with a median follow up time of 23 months and found 8 out of 12 (66.7%) patients having recurrent malignancy in the ureteric remnant, and 3 out of 12 (25%) patients developing metastatic disease. Furthermore 9 out of 12 (75%) patients developed bladder recurrences, which is significantly higher than the reported 25–35% recurrence rate with open nephroureterctomy with distal ureterectomy [8].

Does Bladder Cuff Need to Be Excised During Nephroureterctomy?

The second controversy involves the necessity of excision of the bladder cuff. In a large multi-institutional review by Capitanio and colleagues comparing laparoscopic to open RNU, an observation was made that the excision of the bladder cuff on univariate and multivariate analysis did not have an influence on bladder cancer recurrence or cancer-specific mortality [2]. This prompted Lughezzani and colleagues to perform a larger multi-institutional review of tertiary centers of over 4000 patients undergoing RNU focusing on the issue of excision of bladder cuff. The authors observed a 1.25 fold ($p = 0.04$) increased risk of cancer-specific mortality if the bladder cuff excision was omitted. This rate increased to 1.45 fold ($p = 0.02$) for higher stage (T4N0/x) tumors [9]. Consequently, the guidelines currently strongly recommend excision of the full length of ureter as well as the bladder cuff.

What Is the Best Technique for Distal Ureterectomy?

The next topic of controversy is regarding the techniques utilized in the management of the distal ureter in RNU. Several techniques have been described which can be broadly generalized into three major categories: intravesical or transvesical approach, pure extravesical approach, and combination of endoscopic and extravesical. The dissection of the ureter and the nephrectomy component of the procedure can be carried out via an open approach or minimally invasive surgical (MIS) approaches including laparoscopy, hand-assisted, single-port and robotically assisted laparoscopic nephroureterctomy (RALNU). The intravesical/transvesical approach (Fig. 19.1) is traditionally considered the oncological gold standard treatment by many authors. The main advantage of this technique is improved visualization of the contralateral ureter, and the ability to perform a bladder cuff excision under direct vision. The disadvantages include the additional low abdominal incision and the cystotomy and thus the consequent longer recovery time. There are also concerns regarding the potential tumor seeding by not having a “closed” system approach. The extravesical approach does provide the oncological benefit of a “closed” system and avoids the additional

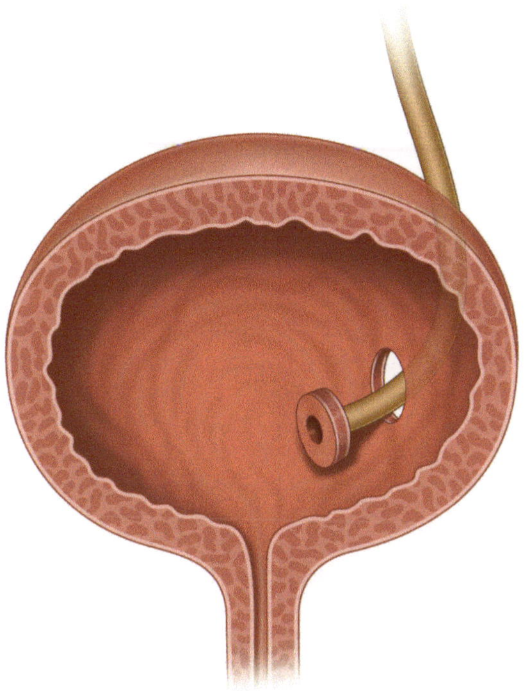

Fig. 19.1 Transvesical left distal ureterectomy with excision of bladder cuff

abdominal incision and cystotomy, hence has a faster recovery time. However, this approach can potentially result in inadvertent damage to the contralateral ureter as well as the potential for incomplete excision of the intramural ureter and the bladder cuff. Several endourological techniques were developed to circumvent the shortcomings of both mentioned approaches; however, their oncological impact has remained the topic of significant controversy. In recent years, more urologists are adopting the extravesical approach due to the increased popularity and utilization of the MIS techniques especially robotic surgery. Consequently, extravesical and endoscopic approaches have been utilized more often with the general objective of improving operative and post-operative parameters.

The Endoscopic Techniques

McDonald in 1952 was the first to describe an endoscopic approach for the management of the distal ureter [10]. Since then, several urologists have described modified techniques to manage the distal ureter endoscopically. The two main pure endoscopic approaches are the transurethral resection of ureteral orifice (TURUO) also known as the "Pluck" technique, and the intussusception technique.

In the TURUO technique, the ureteric orifice and surrounding bladder mucosa are resected with a resectoscope or Collin's knife down to the perivesical fat, facilitating "plucking" of the ureter from above (Fig. 19.2). The two main concerns regarding this technique are potential tumor spillage and seeding into the extravesical space as well as the potential for leaving a segment of intramural ureter behind during "plucking" [11]. Hetherington et al. [12], were the first to report local recurrences in 2 out of 5 patients in whom the "Pluck" technique was utilized. Similarly, Arango et al. [13], reported a case of massive local recurrence following this technique. Both authors subsequently abandoned this technique. However, larger series have advocated the use of this technique, as they observed no difference in recurrence rates. Palou et al. [14], reported 31 cases of RNU utilizing the "pluck" technique, and observed no recurrences with a median follow up of 20 months. Similarly, Geavlete et al. [15], did not observe any local recurrences in their cohort of 72 patients with median follow-up of 44 months.

Modifications of the TURUO technique have been developed with the general aim of reducing tumor spillage and recurrence rates. Their main focus has been on clipping or ligating of the ureter, prior to resection of the intramural ureter. Tan et al. [16], described their technique of clipping the ureter during nephroureterctomy prior to initiation of the endoscopic intervention. Agarwal et al. [17], advocates a novel technique of mobilizing the distal ureter endoscopically with the Collin's followed by endoscopically deployed Endoloop for ligation and occlusion of the distal ureter. No local recurrences were observed in either of these modifications; however, both series had very small sample sizes.

The intussusception technique was initially described by McDonald in 1952 to simplify and eliminate the need for an additional incision [10].

Fig. 19.2 Cross section of bladder and distal ureter before and after resection transurethral resection of the intramural portion of the ureter during 'Pluck' technique

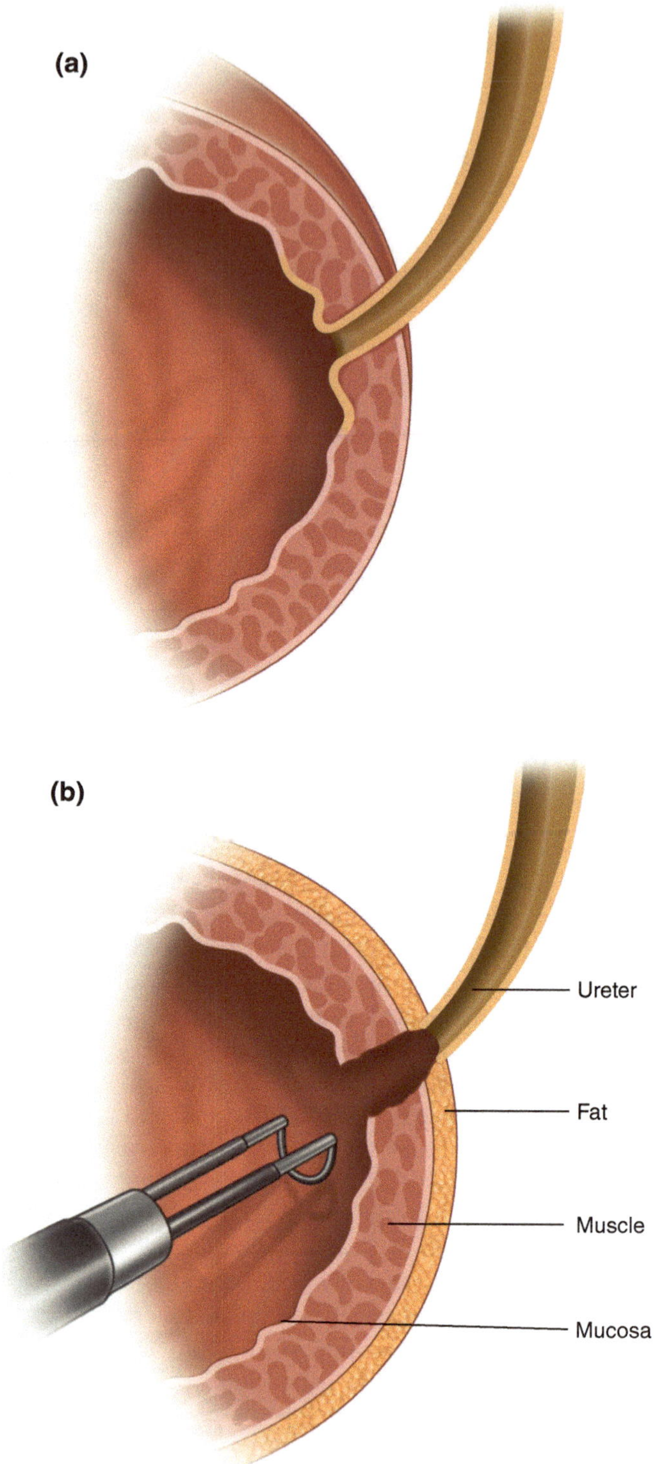

This technique involves tying the distal ureter to a ureteric catheter after completion of the nephrectomy followed by transurethral incision of the bladder mucosa using Collin's knife. This is then followed by traction on the ureteric catheter resulting in intussusception, and retrieval of the distal ureter out of the urethra. So far, limited long-term outcomes have been reported. A literature review by Laguna and de la Rosette [18] compared the intussusception and pluck technique and observed no differences in local recurrence rates. However, the intussusception technique carries approximately a 10% complication rate associated with retrieval of the ureter, and subsequent conversion to open surgery, mainly due to catheter breakage or retained ureter. Generally, both endoscopic techniques are deemed oncologically inappropriate for tumors located in the distal ureter.

The Extravesical Technique

The extravesical laparoscopic stapling technique is often combined with an endoscopic technique for mobilization or resection of the distal ureter. This is followed by laparoscopic extravesical application of a stapling device as the ureter is tented up and away from the bladder. This technique provides the add-on advantage of allowing for a complete minimally invasive approach while maintaining a fully "closed" system. It however carries the disadvantages of potential injury to the contralateral ureter. Furthermore, incorrect application of the stapling device can result in leaving a portion of the distal ureter behind. Histologically, the staple line cannot be accurately assessed and the staple line may be prone to encrustation or formation of stones, years following the operation [11]. Romero et al. [19], compared the stapled extravesical approach with transvesical open excision in 12 patients with median follow up of 4 years and found higher positive margin rates as well as higher local recurrence rates in the laparoscopic approach. Albeit due to small sample size, statistical significance was not established. Similar conclusions have been reported by various authors, indicating higher positive margin rates and local recurrence rates in the stapled extravesical technique [11].

Transvesical Laparoscopic Techniques

Transvesical laparoscopic detachment technique was first introduced by Gill et al. [20]. In this technique, a ureteric catheter is placed initially followed by excision of the bladder cuff and ureteric orifice endoscopically using Collin's knife. Two 2 mm needlescopic ports are inserted suprapubically into the bladder, aiding in the application of an Endoloop to avoid urine leakage from the ureter as well as providing traction to dissect the distal ureter endoscopically using the Collin's knife (Fig. 19.3). The shortcoming of this technique is the potential for extravasation of irrigation fluid and thus potential hyponatremia, which was noted in 1 in 8 cases in their initial series. This approach also carries the potential for port site metastasis, which was not experienced in this series. Gill et al. [20], then went on to perform a comparative review of the described technique with ORNU with mean follow up of almost 2 years, which showed improved positive margin rates, decreased retroperitoneal recurrence rates, and distant metastasis favoring the laparoscopic approach, however statistical significance of this finding could not be determined due to small sample size. Chen et al., described a similar technique using 3 transvesical ports and CO_2 insufflation instead of irrigation fluid for dissection of the distal ureter, aiming to improve vision during dissection and minimizing extravasation of the irrigation fluid to avoid potential of tumor seeding and hyponatremia. The authors later reported their experience in 10 patients with median follow up of 46 months, and observed a systemic recurrence rate of 10%, and bladder recurrence rate of 40%. No cases of port site metastasis were observed [21]. Giannakopoulos et al. [22], using the same technique reported a systemic recurrence rate of 20% and no local pelvic recurrences in their cohort of 10 patients.

Comparison between the three approaches of transvesical, extravesical, and endoscopic has been performed by several authors. Li et al. [23], in

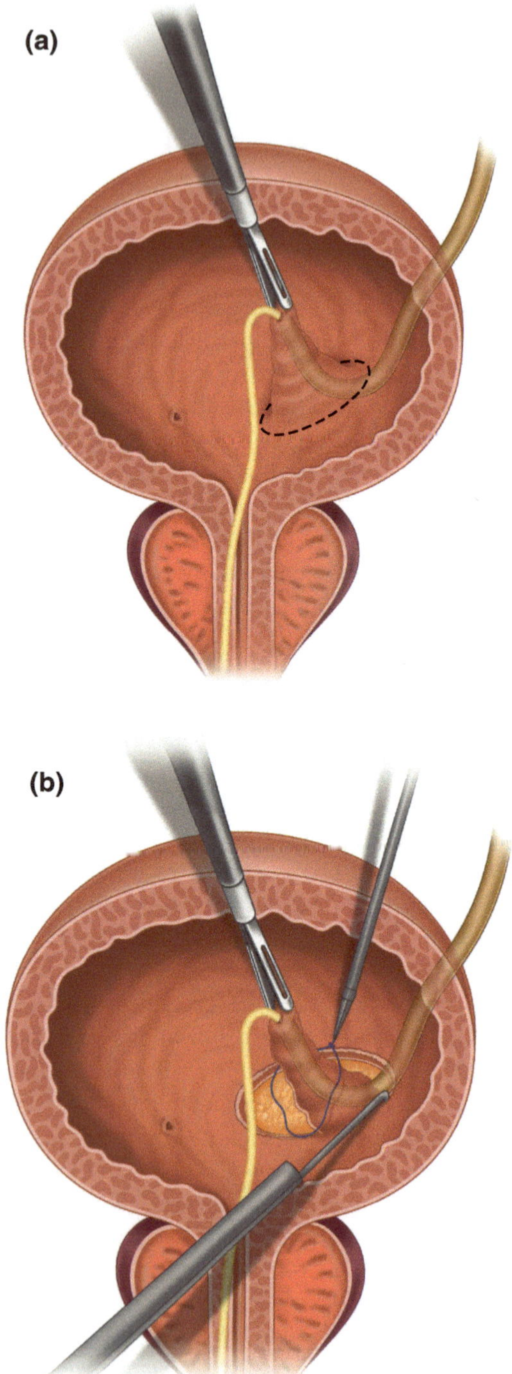

Fig. 19.3 Transvesical laparoscopic distal ureterectomy. **a** The bladder cuff (*dotted line*) is incised by Collins knife. Ureteral orifice is tented by 2 mm. Grasper (*arrow*) and **b** circumferential detachment of bladder cuff and juxtavesical ureter into perivesical fat

a retrospective single center review of 301 patients found no differences between the three groups; however, this study was limited by small sample size, short follow up time as well as low number of events. Krabbe et al. [24], performed a single institution review of 122 patients with median follow up of 32 months and found worse recurrence-free survival (RFS) and cancer-specific survival (CSS) in the nontransvesical approach. Unfortunately, there was no distinction between the extravesical and endoscopic groups in this study. The main limitations of these single institution series include their retrospective nature, variation in operative techniques, inherent bias of assignment of patients to each procedure, and the low number of cases as well as events. To eliminate such biases multi-institutional series can provide a more objective outlook; however, these series are still bound by the same limitations. Kapoor et al. [25], compared intravesical and extravesical techniques at 10 Canadian tertiary centers over a period of 20 years in over 800 patients, assessing RFS and OS. The intravesical group in this review had higher RFS and lower hazard ratios on multivariable analysis. Extravesical and endoscopic approach did not differ on the multivariate analysis. The authors postulated that the incomplete distal ureteric resection in the extravesical approach had accounted for the poor RF rates. In the largest review to date involving 24 international tertiary institutions with a study population of approximately 2500 patients, Xylinas and colleagues assessed the RFS, CSS, and OS of transvesical versus extravesical versus endoscopic management of the distal ureter. The authors did not find any differences between RFS, CSS, and OS between the three approaches of management of the distal ureter. However, the endoscopic groups had a significantly higher rate of intravesical recurrence compared with the other two groups [26].

Laparoscopic versus Open Nephroureterctomy

The next point of controversy is regarding laparoscopic verses open RNU. Since its introduction by

Clayman, laparoscopic nephroureterctomy (LRNU) has gained significant momentum. Multiple initial small series of LRNU have indicated its safety and feasibility; however, these studies were limited by small sample size, short follow-up time, and selection bias in favor of LRNU. The only randomized controlled trial to date comparing LRNU with ORNU favored a better cancer-specific and recurrence-free survival for ORNU; however, the results were not statistically significant [27]. Rassweiler et al. [28], performed a meta-analysis comparing ORNU and LRNU, concluding a longer operative time, lower blood loss, shorter length of stay, and lower analgesia requirement for LRNU. There were no significant differences in intravesical and nonintravesical recurrence, metastasis rates, or disease free survival. More recently Rai et al. [29], confirmed the same findings in a systematic review. Capitanio et al. [2], compared the two modalities in a multi-institutional review of 13 academic centers. On multivariate analysis controlling for the selection biases and confounding variables, there were no differences in RFS or CSS between the LRNU and ORNU.

Laproendoscopic single-site nephroureterctomy and natural orifice transluminal endoscopic surgery are alternative modalities, which have been developed with the aim of minimizing the impact of surgery. Currently, their role in RNU has yet to be fully elucidated with the available data limited to small case series without long-term oncological follow-up.

The Robotic Assisted Laparoscopic Nephroureterctomy

Robotic assisted laparoscopic radical nephroureterctomy (RALNU) has gained considerable momentum in recent years. Due to improved maneuverability in dissection and suturing, RALNU has emerged as an alternative to laparoscopic nephroureterctomy (Fig. 19.4). Nanigian et al. [30], were the first to perform distal ureterectomy and bladder cuff excision with assistance of the robotic system. Since then, several authors have reported their series on safety and feasibility of the RALNU. Trudeau et al. [31], performed a population-based comparison for short term outcomes and costs between LRNU and RALNU of over 1900 patients, demonstrating fewer post-operative complications for patients undergoing RALNU (HR 0.54, CI 0.3–98, $p = 0.04$). There were no differences in length of stay or blood transfusion rates. One of the main challenges of RALNU has been to develop techniques in order to avoid the need for patient repositioning and re-docking of the robot, which subsequently improves operative efficiency and ergonomics. Zargar et al. [32], reported their initial experience in 31 patients undergoing RALNU using a simplified approach to eliminate repositioning and re-docking of the robot. To date, there are few publications on long-term oncological outcomes of RALNU. Aboumohamed et al. [33], reported on the outcomes of 60 patients who underwent RALNU with follow-up of 25 months. This is the largest series to date with intermediate oncological outcomes. The authors reported CSS and RFS rates of RALNU to be comparable to the ORNU series. Larger series with longer follow-ups are indeed required to further assess the oncological outcomes of RALNU.

Use of Intravesical Chemotherapy Post-operatively

One of the main emerging issues is the use of post-operative instillation of intravesical chemotherapy. High quality evidence from randomized controlled trials has recently been published indicating significant reduction in intravesical bladder tumor recurrences. The findings of these trials unfortunately have not yet been assessed in any of the mentioned trials comparing the different approaches and techniques in management of the distal ureter in RNU [34–36].

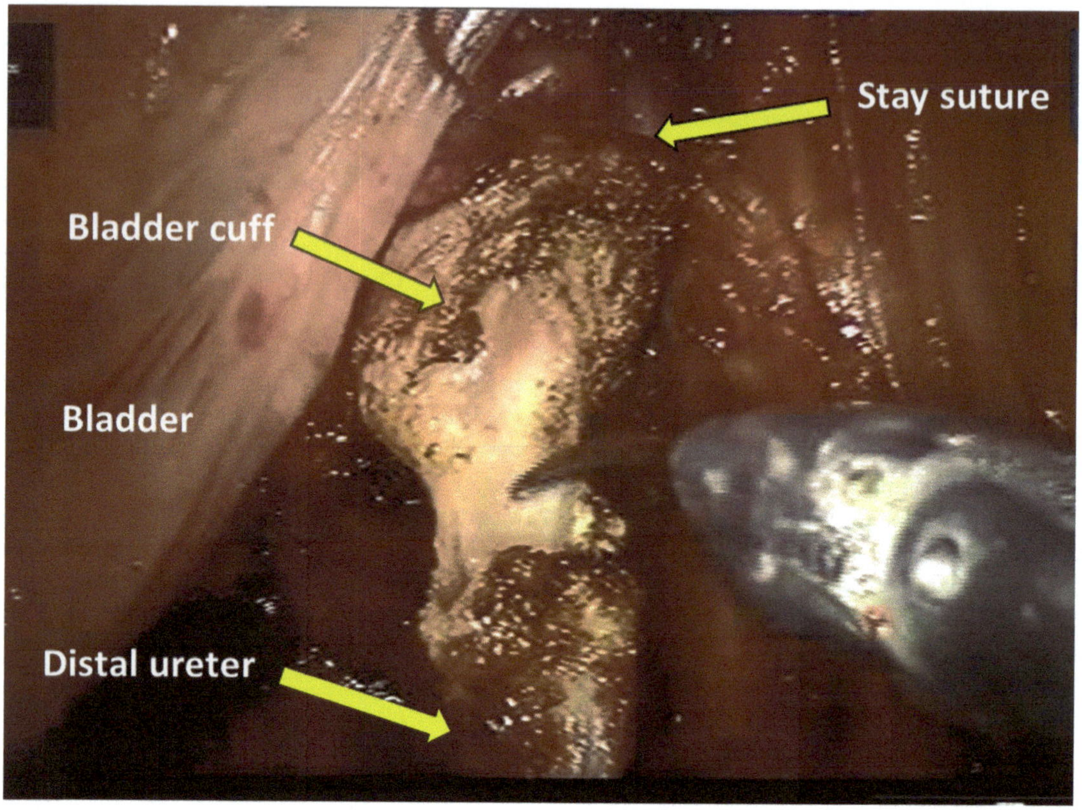

Fig. 19.4 Robotic extravesical distal ureterectomy. A stay suture is placed on bladder mucosa, prior to full detachment of distal ureter, and associated bladder cuff

Conclusion

Management of the distal ureter in upper tract urothelial carcinomas will continue to remain a controversial issue, particularly with the ongoing development of additional novel treatment modalities and operative techniques. The comparison between the techniques in prospective and randomized trials is unlikely due to the rarity of the disease. The current literature supports safety and feasibility of most techniques with each providing their unique advantages and disadvantages. The peri-operative and oncological outcomes highly depends on the appropriateness of the technique applied as well as the surgeon's expertise in that particular technique. Since the oncological outcome remains the most important priority, regardless of the technique utilized, the urologist must adhere to the oncological principles suggested by current literature including but not limited to: achieving a negative margin, excision of full length of the ureter as the bladder cuff, early ligation of the ureter and minimization of urine spillage and potential tumor seeding. Replicating ORNU, which remains to date the gold standard, can be achieved safely with less invasive techniques as long as sound oncological principles are upheld.

Summary Box

- Management of the distal ureter in radical nephroureterctomy remains a controversial topic in urological oncology.
- A variety of techniques including endoscopic, laparoscopic, and open approaches have been described and

shown safety and feasibility; however due to rarity of the disease, comparison of these techniques in high quality study designs is unlikely.
- Current level of evidence supports excision of full length of the ureter at the time of radical nephroureterctomy, including the intramural portion of the distal ureter as well as the bladder cuff.
- Endoscopic techniques such as transurethral resection of the ureteric orifice and the intussusception technique may carry higher risks of local recurrence.
- Extravesical technique provides the advantage of "closed" system, however may carry the risk of inadequate excision of the intramural ureter and bladder cuff as well as the risk of injury to the contralateral ureter.
- Transvesical technique has the advantage of providing better visualization of the contralateral ureter and better bladder cuff excision; however it carries the disadvantage of longer recovery time as well as potential risk of urothelial tumor seeding by not providing a 'closed' system.
- Based on recent systematic reviews, laparoscopic, and open nephroureterctomy have similar oncological outcomes. Data regarding long-term outcomes of single-site and robotic nephroureterctomy is not yet available.
- Post-operative intravesical chemotherapy has been shown to significantly reduce intravesical recurrences in randomized trials.

References

1. Roupret M, Babjuk M, Comperat E, Zigeuner R, Sylvester R, Burger M, et al. European guidelines on upper tract urothelial carcinomas: 2013 update. Eur Urol. 2013;63(6):1059–71.
2. Capitanio U, Shariat SF, Isbarn H, Weizer A, Remzi M, Roscigno M, et al. Comparison of oncologic outcomes for open and laparoscopic nephroureterectomy: a multi-institutional analysis of 1249 cases. Eur Urol. 2009;56(1):1–9.
3. Strong DW, Pearse HD. Recurrent urothelial tumors following surgery for transitional cell carcinoma of the upper urinary tract. Cancer. 1976;38(5):2173–83.
4. Kinder CH, Wallace DM. Recurrent carcinoma in the ureteric stump. Br J Surg. 1962;50:202–5.
5. Bloom NA, Vidone RA, Lytton B. Primary carcinoma of the ureter: a report of 102 new cases. J Urol. 1970;103(5):590–8.
6. Newman DM, Allen LE, Wishard WN Jr, Nourse MH, Mertz JH. Transitional cell carcinoma of the upper urinary tract. J Urol. 1967;98(3):322–7.
7. Ko R, Chew BH, Hickling DR, Razvi H, Luke PP, Chin JL, et al. Transitional-cell carcinoma recurrence rate after nephroureterectomy in patients who undergo open excision of bladder cuff v transurethral incision of the ureteral orifice. J Endourol. 2007;21(7):730–4.
8. Abel EJ, Fisher MB, Matin SF, Kamat AM, Dinney CP, Grossman HB. Delayed ureterectomy after incomplete nephroureterectomy for upper tract urothelial carcinoma: pathologic findings and outcomes. Int Braz J Urol. 2013;39(6):817–22.
9. Lughezzani G, Sun M, Perrotte P, Shariat SF, Jeldres C, Budaus L, et al. Should bladder cuff excision remain the standard of care at nephroureterectomy in patients with urothelial carcinoma of the renal pelvis? A population-based study. Eur Urol. 2010;57(6):956–62.
10. Mc DH, Upchurch WE, Sturdevant CE. Nephro-ureterectomy: a new technique. J Urol. 1952;67(6):804–9.
11. Srirangam SJ, van Cleynenbreugel B, van Poppel H. Laparoscopic nephroureterectomy: the distal ureteral dilemma. Adv Urol. 2009:316807.
12. Hetherington JW, Ewing R, Philp NH. Modified nephroureterectomy: a risk of tumour implantation. Br J Urol. 1986;58(4):368–70.
13. Arango O, Bielsa O, Carles J, Gelabert-Mas A. Massive tumor implantation in the endoscopic resected area in modified nephroureterectomy. J Urol. 1997;157(5):1839.
14. Palou J, Caparros J, Orsola A, Xavier B, Vicente J. Transurethral resection of the intramural ureter as the first step of nephroureterectomy. J Urol. 1995;154(1):43–4.
15. Geavlete P, Georgescu D, Bancu S, Mirciulescu V. Endoscopic ureteral procedures for one-step nephroureterectomy: experience in 100 cases. J Endourol. 2007;21(9):1019–24.
16. Tan BJ, Ost MC, Lee BR. Laparoscopic nephroureterectomy with bladder-cuff resection: techniques and outcomes. J Endourol. 2005;19(6):664–76.
17. Agarwal DK, Khaira HS, Clarke D, Tong R. Modified transurethral technique for the management of distal ureter during laparoscopic assisted nephroureterectomy. Urology. 2008;71(4):740–3.

18. Laguna MP, de la Rosette JJ. The endoscopic approach to the distal ureter in nephroureterectomy for upper urinary tract tumor. J Urol. 2001;166 (6):2017–22.
19. Romero FR, Schaeffer EM, Muntener M, Trock B, Kavoussi LR, Jarrett TW. Oncologic outcomes of extravesical stapling of distal ureter in laparoscopic nephroureterectomy. J Endourol. 2007;21(9):1025–7.
20. Gill IS, Soble JJ, Miller SD, Sung GT. A novel technique for management of the en bloc bladder cuff and distal ureter during laparoscopic nephroureterectomy. J Urol. 1999;161(2):430–4.
21. Mak SK, Ng CF, Chan ES, Yip SK, Cheng CW, Wong WS. Pneumovesicum approach to en-bloc laparoscopic nephroureterectomy with bladder cuff excision for upper tract urothelial cancer: midterm oncological results. J Endourol. 2011;25(4):611–4.
22. Giannakopoulos S, Toufas G, Dimitriadis C, Giannopoulos S, Kalaitzis C, Bantis A, et al. Laparoscopic transvesical resection of an en bloc bladder cuff and distal ureter during nephroureterectomy. ScientificWorldJournal. 2012;2012:658096.
23. Li WM, Shen JT, Li CC, Ke HL, Wei YC, Wu WJ, et al. Oncologic outcomes following three different approaches to the distal ureter and bladder cuff in nephroureterectomy for primary upper urinary tract urothelial carcinoma. Eur Urol. 2010;57(6):963–9.
24. Krabbe LM, Westerman ME, Bagrodia A, Gayed BA, Khalil D, Kapur P, et al. Surgical management of the distal ureter during radical nephroureterectomy is an independent predictor of oncological outcomes: results of a current series and a review of the literature. Urol Oncol. 2014;32(1):54 e19–26.
25. Kapoor A, Dason S, Allard CB, Shayegan B, Lacombe L, Rendon R, et al. The impact of method of distal ureter management during radical nephroureterectomy on tumour recurrence. Can Urol Assoc J. 2014;8(11–12):E845–52.
26. Xylinas E, Rink M, Cha EK, Clozel T, Lee RK, Fajkovic H, et al. Impact of distal ureter management on oncologic outcomes following radical nephroureterectomy for upper tract urothelial carcinoma. Eur Urol. 2014;65(1):210–7.
27. Simone G, Papalia R, Guaglianone S, Ferriero M, Leonardo C, Forastiere E, et al. Laparoscopic versus open nephroureterectomy: perioperative and oncologic outcomes from a randomised prospective study. Eur Urol. 2009;56(3):520–6.
28. Rassweiler JJ, Schulze M, Marrero R, Frede T, Palou Redorta J, Bassi P. Laparoscopic nephroureterectomy for upper urinary tract transitional cell carcinoma: is it better than open surgery? Eur Urol. 2004;46 (6):690–7.
29. Rai BP, Shelley M, Coles B, Somani B, Nabi G. Surgical management for upper urinary tract transitional cell carcinoma (UUT-TCC): a systematic review. BJU Int. 2012;110(10):1426–35.
30. Nanigian DK, Smith W, Ellison LM. Robot-assisted laparoscopic nephroureterectomy. J Endourol. 2006;20(7):463–5; discussion 5–6.
31. Trudeau V, Gandaglia G, Shiffmann J, Popa I, Shariat SF, Montorsi F, et al. Robot-assisted versus laparoscopic nephroureterectomy for upper-tract urothelial cancer: a population-based assessment of costs and perioperative outcomes. Can Urol Assoc J. 2014;8(9–10):E695–701.
32. Zargar H, Krishnan J, Autorino R, Akca O, Brandao LF, Laydner H, et al. Robotic nephroureterectomy: a simplified approach requiring no patient repositioning or robot redocking. Eur Urol. 2014;66 (4):769–77.
33. Aboumohamed AA, Krane LS, Hemal AK. Oncologic outcomes following robot-assisted laparoscopic nephroureterectomy with bladder cuff excision for upper tract urothelial carcinoma. J Urol. 2015;194 (6):1561–6.
34. Ito A, Shintaku I, Satoh M, Ioritani N, Aizawa M, Tochigi T, et al. Prospective randomized phase II trial of a single early intravesical instillation of pirarubicin (THP) in the prevention of bladder recurrence after nephroureterectomy for upper urinary tract urothelial carcinoma: the THP Monotherapy Study Group Trial. J Clin Oncol. 2013;31 (11):1422–7.
35. O'Brien T, Ray E, Singh R, Coker B, Beard R. British Association of Urological Surgeons Section of O. Prevention of bladder tumours after nephroureterectomy for primary upper urinary tract urothelial carcinoma: a prospective, multicentre, randomised clinical trial of a single postoperative intravesical dose of mitomycin C (the ODMIT-C Trial). Eur Urol. 2011;60(4):703–10.
36. Sakamoto N, Naito S, Kumazawa J, Ariyoshi A, Osada Y, Omoto T, et al. Prophylactic intravesical instillation of mitomycin C and cytosine arabinoside for prevention of recurrent bladder tumors following surgery for upper urinary tract tumors: a prospective randomized study. Int J Urol. 2001;8(5):212–6.

Complications of Nephroureterectomy

20

Abhishek Srivastava and Reza Ghavamian

Introduction

Upper tract urothelial cancer (UTUC) comprises 5% of the urothelial cancer [1]. Open radical nephroureterectomy (ONU) and excision of the ipsilateral ureteral orifice with a periureteral cuff of the bladder is the gold standard in the treatment for most patients with UTUC [2]. Clayman et al. [3] first described laparoscopic nephroureterectomy (LNU) in 1991 as an alternative to ONU. Since then, many variations have been described, especially regarding management of the distal ureter and bladder cuff [4–9]. With the advent of robotic surgery in urology, first robotic transperitoneal nephrectomy was described in 2001[10] and retroperitoneoscopic nephroureterectomy was described in 2006 [11], however, the principles of surgical technique and oncologic control remain the same as the open approach. The use of minimally invasive nephroureterectomy (MINU) has increased for the management of UTUC with majority of nephroureterectomies being performed robotically [12, 13]. Several studies have confirmed that MINU can be performed with comparable oncologic outcomes as ONU with the further advantage of decreased length of hospital stay, analgesic requirement, and the need for blood transfusions [14].

In this chapter, we will discuss in detail the identification and management of intraoperative and postoperative complications associated with nephroureterectomy. Generally, renal dissection performed with nephroureterectomy is the same as a nephrectomy except that the ureteral dissection is carried further down into the pelvis past the iliac bifurcation, including the distal ureter. Therefore, many of the complications are similar to those associated with a nephrectomy and are referenced in appropriate sections.

Incidence of Complications

Patients with UTUC are often elderly and comorbid secondary to associated risk factors for developing this malignancy. Significant perioperative complications may occur in this surgical population. Lin et al. [15] reported perioperative complication rates of approximately 40% in patients undergoing radical nephroureterectomy (RNU). One-third of complications were Clavien III or greater. Poor performance status resulted in a fourfold greater risk for perioperative

A. Srivastava
Department of Urology, Montefiore Medical Center, Albert Einstein College of Medicine, 3400 Bainbridge Ave, MAP5, Bronx, NY 10467, USA
e-mail: asrivast@montefiore.org

R. Ghavamian (✉)
Department of Urology, Northwell Health, Northwell Hofstra School of Medicine, Hempsted, NY, USA
e-mail: reza.ghavamian@gmail.com

M. Eshghi (ed.), *Urothelial Malignancies of the Upper Urinary Tract*,
https://doi.org/10.1007/978-3-319-51263-1_20

complications [15]. Similarly, Raman et al. reported complication rates of 26% in 414 patients undergoing RNU from seven academic institutions, of which one-quarter were Clavien grade III or IV [16]. In a recent study, Hanske et al. compared complication rates among patients who underwent MINU or ONU for UTUC within the American College of Surgeons-National Surgical Quality Improvement Program database [14]. 12.7% of patients suffered a complication within 30 days postoperatively, and the rate did not differ among surgical approaches. MINU, however, was associated with a decreased risk of blood transfusions, thromboembolic events, reinterventions, and overall length of stay when compared with ONU [14].

Preoperative Considerations

Patients with substantial cardiovascular or pulmonary disease should be medically optimized and cleared before proceeding with the surgery to avoid life-threatening cardiopulmonary complications. Flank position puts pressure on the great vessels, causing a decrease in preload and an increase in afterload, thereby decreasing cardiac output [17]. Ventilation is also severely impaired by the flank position which could lead to hypoxia. Patients with impaired pulmonary function or cardiac disease are susceptible to carbon dioxide and fluid retention [17]. Close attention to intraoperative end-tidal carbon dioxide monitoring by capnometry is essential [18]. The potential for blood loss and large hemodynamic shifts should prompt preoperative blood typing and crossmatching.

Total and split renal function should be assessed along with the other appropriate imaging to aid in operative planning. Urine culture and sensitivity should be completed to rule out a urinary tract infection. Antibiotic prophylaxis should be administered ≥ 30 min before incision [17]. Subcutaneous heparin can be given preoperatively to decrease the risk of deep vein thrombosis. Compression stockings and sequential compression devices, should be applied to the lower extremities unless contraindicated [17].

The patient must be positioned carefully with pressure points adequately padded to prevent postoperative neurological complications. Vallancien et al. [19] in their experience noted few complications related to patient positioning, but no instances of compartment syndrome were observed. Transient cubital paresis developed in two patients, which resolved within a few days. Trendelenburg position with longer operative times during pelvic operations was responsible for two cases of conjunctivitis secondary to irritation of the cornea. Scapular pain occurred in 11 cases due to prolonged pressure on the shoulder supports [19]. Gill et al. reported brachial palsy of the right arm following an 8.5-h nephrectomy in a morbidly obese patient and a lateral thigh compartment syndrome following a 7.9-h laparoscopic nephrectomy, which rapidly resolved with conservative therapy [18].

Intraoperative Complications

Access Related

The Veress needle puncture, optical trocar access, and the Hasson technique are the three common approaches to obtain pneumoperitoneum for laparoscopic exposure with very low complication rates. In 2001, Schafer et al. reviewed 14,243 laparoscopic procedures where pneumoperitoneum was obtained using the Veress needle, with an overall complication rate of 0.18% [20]. Similarly, Catarci et al. reviewed 12,919 laparoscopic procedures and reported low complication rates of 0.27% with optical trocar access, 0.18% with the Veress needle, and 0.09% with the Hasson technique [21].

Procedure-based surveys of laparoscopic entry access injuries also show a reassuringly low incidence [22]. Claims arising from US and non-US entry access injuries, showed a total of 506 patients had primary access injuries with 65 deaths. 76% of all injuries were incurred to bowel and retroperitoneal vessels in establishing a primary port. Late recognition, along with age ≥ 59 years and major visceral or vascular injuries, were each independent significant predictor of death [22]. To avoid these injuries, midline incisions with the Veress needle (which accounted for nearly one-fifth of all injuries) and trocars must be avoided by the surgeons. Left upper quadrant may be the safest access point. Excessive axial force must also be avoided. To decrease the incidence of unrecognized bowel injuries, the primary trocar site and the bowel beneath it must be visualized from a secondary puncture site before pulling out trocars.

Pareek et al. [23] in a meta-analysis reported less than 0.5% access related complications during laparoscopic renal surgery. The complication rate associated with the access technique (trocar insertion) was only 0.2% in another series [24]. Gill et al. [18] evaluated complications of laparoscopic nephrectomy in 185 patients and described two cases of hernia formation at the trocar site, one abdominal wall hematoma and one trocar injury to a hydronephrotic kidney. Soulie et al. [25] described their complications with 350 laparoscopic procedures and reported two patients with incarcerated hernias through 10 mm port sites whose fascia was not closed. Fascial closure of the port sites 10 mm or greater in size is now encouraged. Bird et al. in their retrospective study noted increased risk of incisional hernia formation with paramedian extraction site in patients with a high BMI [26]. The lower trocar site can be an effective alternative since this site was not associated with incisional hernia development. Other authors have shown reduced complications with specimen removal through a Pfannenstiel incision compared to an expanded port site incision during laparoscopic nephrectomy procedures [27]. Vallancien et al. [19] described their experience after 9 years of practice and complications related to insufflation and placement of trocars were observed only in five patients (0.3%), and required open conversion in 1 patient (0.1%).

Vascular Injury

German Urologic Association reviewed their experience with 482 laparoscopic nephrectomies performed at 14 centers and found complications related to bleeding in 4.6% of patients [28]. The conversion and reintervention rate related to bleeding was 4.3 and 1.4%, respectively [28]. Similarly, Parson et al. in their series of 894 abdominal laparoscopic procedures observed 42 (4.7%) intraoperative complications out of which 23 (2.6%) were related to vascular injuries [29]. Out of 13 emergent conversions to open surgery, 12 (92%) were performed for vascular injury [29].

During radical nephrectomy, the most crucial step is the vascular control of renal hilum. The anatomy can be variable and the proximity to the great vessels requires careful dissection [30, 31]. Siqueira et al. [32] described two intraoperative complications associated with injury to the aberrant right lower pole artery, one required open conversion. They also stressed on the importance of review of preoperative imaging, such as CT or MR angiography when available to identify aberrant renal vessels. The surgeon should avoid clipping at the level of calcification in the artery, if visible on noncontrast CT [32].

The celiac artery, superior mesenteric artery, contralateral renal artery, and lumber vessels may all be mistaken for the renal artery. If an injury occurs to one of these vessels, immediate recognition, and primary repair will minimize subsequent complications. Consultation with a vascular surgeon, if available, is suggested. Siqueira et al. [32] in their initial series of 292 laparoscopic procedures, reported one death, which resulted from the accidental division of SMA. Adrenal arterial branches are also prone to avulsion injury and although they are small, they may bleed profusely [6].

The renal vein must be handled with care because a lumbar vein may drain posteriorly into it, especially on the left. The thinner walls of the vein make avulsion of these small veins a real possibility. Laparoscopic control of renal vein hemorrhage can be particularly difficult. Berger et al. [33] in their series of 100 consecutive LNU at Cleveland Clinic described two emergent open conversions due to excessive renal vein bleeding. Soulie et al. [34] in their series of 1085 laparoscopic procedures noted vascular injury which required open conversion in three cases, one was a vena cava injury close to the renal vein during a right simple nephrectomy.

The renal artery and vein can be safely secured with locking clips or with an endovascular stapler. Kouba et al. analyzed 161 consecutive patients who underwent planned laparoscopic radical nephrectomy or nephroureterectomy, of which 90 had en bloc hilar ligation and 71 underwent individual hilar vessel ligation. The blood loss and open conversion rate were lower in the en bloc group. Postoperatively, no clinical evidence of arteriovenous fistula was found after mean follow-up of 34 months [35].

There have been reports of stapler malfunctions in 1.7–10% of cases [36–38]. Buse et al. described one GIA-stapler failure (1.8%) during laparoscopic nephrectomy in 57 patients, leading to open conversion to recover the stapling device as the device could not be opened after firing the cartridge [36]. Chan et al. reviewed 565 laparoscopic nephrectomies from two institutions and malfunction occurred in 10 cases (1.7%) with two open conversions [37]. Care should be taken not to include clips in the staple line.

Friedman et al. concluded based on survey results from the American Society of Transplant Surgeons members that adverse events tend to be associated more frequently with surgical clips during arterial and venous control [38]. Teleflex Medical subsequently issued a warning against the use of nonabsorbable polymer ligating (NPL) locking clips for the control of the renal hilum during laparoscopic donor nephrectomy. Ponsky et al. reviewed 1695 laparoscopic nephrectomies performed by laparoscopic trained urologists at nine institutions [39] and found no adverse events or failures with the usage of Hem-o-lok ™ clips (Teleflex Medical, Inc., Morrisville, NC) to control the renal artery and the renal vein. They concluded that despite the manufacturer's release of contraindications, Hem-o-lok ™ clips (Teleflex Medical, Inc., Morrisville, NC) are safe for use in laparoscopic nephrectomies when correctly applied by trained urologists [39]. Basic principles for safe Hem-o-lok ™ clip (Teleflex Medical, Inc., Morrisville, NC) placement includes a minimum of two clips placement on the patient side of the renal hilar vessel and complete circumferential dissection of the vessel.

Hsi et al. reviewed U.S. Food and Drug Administration Manufacturer and User Facility Device Experience databases (FDA MAUDE) and discovered 352 reported failures using laparoscopic hemostatic devices, 63% including three deaths with the use of endovascular stapling devices, 33% including one death with the use of nonlocking titanium clips, and 5% including three deaths with the use of locking clips [40]. All three methods used to secure the renal hilum during laparoscopic nephrectomy may result in malfunction, however, based on this study, it was difficult to establish the safety of one device over the other. Meng also performed an extensive search of the FDA MAUDE database, and found 27 adverse events related to the use of locking clips [41]. 48% of the failures occurred during laparoscopic urologic procedures, of these, bleeding was the primary problem in 77%. In all situations, multiple clips were applied to the arterial stump [41].

Bowel Injury

Bowel injury is associated with potentially life-threatening consequences if not promptly recognized and treated. Immediate intraoperative repair is recommended because diagnosis of an unrecognized bowel in the postoperative period is difficult. Early imaging with computerized tomography (CT) of the abdomen and pelvis is vital, and immediate surgical exploration is required when a bowel injury has been identified.

Bishoff et al. [42] performed a retrospective review in 915 patients who underwent laparoscopic urologic procedures between July 1991 and June 1998. Bowel perforation occurred in 0.2% of cases and bowel abrasion occurred in 0.6%. Most bowel abrasion injuries were recognized intraoperatively and repaired immediately. In four cases, perforation injuries were not recognized intraoperatively and patients developed peritonitis and severe sepsis; two patients subsequently died [42]. The authors also reviewed 12 series of laparoscopic bowel complications in the literature and found that the combined incidence of laparoscopic bowel injury was 0.13%, and most injuries (69%) were not recognized at the time of surgery. 50% were related to electrocautery and 32% were access related arising from Veress needle or trocar insertion. The time to identify a bowel injury after surgery was variable and thermal bowel injuries presented later than nonthermal. 80% required laparotomy, and others were treated with total parenteral nutrition, or observation if patients were severely septic. Eight patients died as a direct result of unrecognized bowel injury [42].

Fahlenkamp et al. [24] reported 20 (1.1%) complications associated with injury to adjacent structures, including six bowel injuries. Twelve were associated with the use of monopolar electrocautery and in all 12 cases the injury was not detected during surgery [24]. Use of cold scissors or different energy sources, such as bipolar or ultrasonic energy was recommended. Minor thermal injury may be managed with observation or with superficial suturing but major thermal injury needs a bowel resection with a 6 cm safety margin on either side before completing an end-to-end anastomosis [43]. Nonthermal injuries are typically repaired by direct closure with suturing [23]. Duodenal injuries most commonly occur during anteromedial dissection to the right kidney. Prevention of duodenal injury requires careful dissection and Kocher's maneuver to mobilize the duodenum away from the operative field.

Extensive irrigation with sterile water, drain placement, and postoperative antibiotic prophylaxis should be initiated if unexpected spillage of colonic content occurs [17]. Siqueira et al. [32] described a patient who presented 4 days after an uneventful LNU with lower abdominal pain and was found to have a pelvic abscess on the CT exam. The patient was noted on exploration to have a perforated colonic diverticulum and was treated with a diverting colostomy [32]. Mechanical bowel preparation should be initiated if the probability of tumor extension exists which can complicate resection or require bowel resection. Enterocutaneous fistula has been reported which can be managed with bowel rest and total parenteral nutrition [18, 42]. Other possible complications involving the bowel could be mechanical small bowel obstruction or bowel ischemia resulting from mesenteric vessels compromise, which generally resolves with conservative measures.

Splenic Injury

Higher incidences of splenic injuries were noted during left ONU and ORN (5–10%) compared to left LRN and LNU (1–5%) [43]. These injuries can be managed intraoperatively, with splenectomy or conservative measures [43]. Simon et al. reported four splenic injuries, two splenic lacerations required open conversions for splenectomy and two were managed conservatively with argon beam coagulation or Fibrillar™ (Ethicon, Inc., Somerville, New Jersey) with minimal blood loss [44]. Most splenic injuries occur during mobilization of the splenocolic flexure or dissection of the upper pole of the left kidney [45, 46]. Therefore, the line of Toldt should be incised above the level of the spleen, and the splenorenal and splenocolic ligaments should be divided to allow the spleen to fall medial and retract superior, to prevent any splenic injury. Minimizing splenic retraction prevents inadvertent splenic trauma. Preoperative placement of an oral–gastric tube to empty the stomach facilitates falling of the spleen medially during its mobilization [43]. It is important at the end of a laparoscopic case to inspect the spleen by decreasing pneumoperitoneum to assess adequate hemostasis. Patients undergoing splenic embolization or splenectomy should be provided with appropriate vaccinations postoperatively.

Pancreatic Injury

Pancreatic injuries are relatively uncommon with an incidence rate of <0.5% but can result in significant morbidity mostly from delayed diagnosis. Intraoperative detection and repair can minimize sequelae. Varkarakis et al. [47] reviewed 890 laparoscopic urologic procedures and identified 4 (0.44%) pancreatic injuries, all associated with left-sided procedures. Three patients were treated conservatively and CT-guided drainage of a pancreatic collection was required in 1. Diagnosis of a pancreatic injury is most commonly made in the postoperative period by the patient's symptoms. Measurement of serum and drain amylase can be diagnostic. Prevention of pancreatic injury includes transecting the splenophrenic attachments which will allow the spleen and pancreas to roll medially to minimize the risk of injury [43]. Careful dissection with knowledge of location of the pancreas and complete mobilization of the pancreas and spleen en bloc are key to reducing pancreatic injuries. One should consider placing a drain after a difficult dissection because of the possibility of an unrecognized pancreatic injury.

Recognition of pancreatic lacerations requires immediate repair and it is essential to inspect for pancreatic duct injury. If no injury is noted, simple repair of the pancreatic capsule with nonabsorbable suture and a omental bolster is necessary. If the duct is involved, distal resection of the pancreas is preferable with placement of a surgical drain [17]. General surgical consultation should be obtained if available.

Postoperative management includes bowel rest with the placement of a nasogastric (NG) tube, complete intravenous nutrition, addition of octreotide until serum amylase and/or lipase levels normalize, and percutaneous drainage of the collection.

Liver Injury

Liver injury during nephrectomy is relatively rare with incidences in literature ranging from 0–1.1% [10, 19, 23, 29, 32, 33, 44]. Siqueira et al. [32] reported two cases of liver injury during initial access using the Optiview device. This injury was repaired laparoscopically by packing with hemostatic agents such as Surgicel™ (Ethicon, Inc., Somerville, NJ) and then managed conservatively without the need for reintervention. Liver can be injured by forceful retraction during right nephrectomy. Preventive measures include usage of padded retractors and division of the perihepatic ligaments if necessary to achieve adequate mobilization. On recognition of a liver injury, or during intentional resection of liver extensions of the primary tumor, the liver laceration may be managed with Bovie or argon beam coagulation [17, 30].

Diaphragmatic Injury

Injury to the diaphragm and parietal pleura is an uncommon yet recognized complication during renal surgery regardless of the approach [48, 49]. In a multi-institutional study of 1765 patients, Del Pizzo et al. [48] reported pleural injury in 10 cases (0.6%). Two cases involved inadvertent trocar placement through the pleural cavity, which were managed with chest tube placement. In eight cases, the diaphragm was iatrogenically injured during kidney dissection. A diaphragmatic injury may be identified intraoperatively when the diaphragm is seen billowing down into the surgical field, and is referred to as the *floppy diaphragm* [48]. In all patients, injury was detected intraoperatively and repaired via placement of interrupted sutures laparoscopically. In one patient, residual pneumothorax postoperatively required tube thoracostomy. The authors made several recommendations to avoid diaphragmatic injuries which include (1) Meticulous dissection of the upper pole of the kidney, especially when large masses are present, (2) Minimizing cautery usage when dissecting lesions near the diaphragm, and (3) maintaining a high index of suspicion when a floppy diaphragm is observed intraoperatively [48].

Similarly, Aron et al. also reviewed their series of 1850 laparoscopic procedures in which seven patients (0.4%) sustained iatrogenic diaphragmatic injuries [49]. They described their technique of diaphragmatic repair which mimics the open surgical technique. A running suture is used to close the diaphragmatic defect with the lung deflated. A rubber catheter is introduced through a lateral port into the diaphragmatic tear to enter the pleural space and knot is formed on running suture and held on tension. External end of the catheter is then placed under water seal below the pleural cavity level. The anesthesiologist is then asked to hyperinflate lung to expel all intrapleural CO_2 and abdomen is desufflated. The catheter is then quickly removed and knot is cinched down [49].

Postoperative Complications

Common Complications

RNU may predispose a patient to complications, such as pneumonia, hypertension, and acute renal insufficiency. The risk of pneumonia may be higher after renal surgery compared with other abdominal procedures, as patient's postoperative pain with deep breathing may be substantial, leading to atelectasis, and pneumonia. Early ambulation, incentive spirometry and adequate pain control should be encouraged in the immediate postoperative period [17]. The incidence of postoperative hypertension is <8%, usually mild, and it often resolves. Postoperative acute renal insufficiency may be multifactorial, relating to removal of an affected kidney, direct or indirect manipulation of the contralateral kidney, and rhabdomyolysis related to patient positioning. Postoperative acute renal insufficiency is usually brief but may need dialysis in rare cases. Long-term renal insufficiency is of minimal concern in patients with normal contralateral kidneys [17].

Venous Thromboembolism

Venous thromboembolism (VTE) which includes deep venous thrombosis (DVT) and/or pulmonary embolism (PE) is an important postoperative complication that can be potentially life-threatening after any urologic surgery. Postoperative DVT has been reported in 0.13–1.3% of patients, and PE in 0.08–1% [50, 51]. Prophylaxis with pharmacologic agents such as unfractionated heparin (UFH) and fractionated heparin (FH), and mechanical methods, such as sequential compression devices (SCD) and compression stockings [52] are effective methods for reducing risk of VTE. Montgomery et al. in their retrospective comparison of SCD versus FH found that in both groups the rate of thrombotic complication was 1.2% [50]. Hemorrhagic complication was 9.3% in the FH group, of which 7.0% were major. The hemorrhagic complication rate was 3.5%, with 2.9% being major in the SCD group. The authors recommend some type of prophylaxis to reduce the incidence of DVT and PE after major open and laparoscopic surgery, however, the study was nonrandomized and retrospective in nature [50]. As per the AUA best practice statement, the decision on when and how to start prophylaxis for DVT must be based on the patient's risk stratification, but chemical DVT prophylaxis is strongly recommended in high-risk patients undergoing high-risk procedures, such as RNU [51, 52].

Abscess

Intra-abdominal abscess formation can be a complication of any urologic surgery [28, 29, 45]. Risk factors include preoperative urinary tract infection, entry into the gastrointestinal organs, the kidney parenchyma or the collecting system, and postoperative renal hematoma. Adequate irrigation, prophylactic antibiotics, and surgical drain placement minimize the risk of abscess formation [17]. In the presence of risk factors for infection, unexplained postoperative fever, or leukocytosis should prompt a CT of the abdomen and pelvis to look for an abscess. Treatment involves percutaneous drainage and empiric antibiotics. Antibiotic coverage is adjusted when culture and sensitivity results become available.

Anuria

Complete excision of the ureter with a cuff of bladder is a mandatory part of the procedure. The contralateral ureteral orifice may be damaged by the dissection of bladder cuff. This complication may result in anuria secondary to obstruction of the remaining ureter at the ureteral orifice. Management includes retrograde stent placement if possible or nephrostomy tube placement [17].

Urinary Leakage

Urinary leakage from the bladder is a potential complication after RNU which can be managed with urethral catheter drainage. A cystogram can also be considered at the time of urethral catheter removal. Persistent bladder leak can typically be managed with prolonged urethral catheter drainage. Rarely, persistent urinoma requires urinary diversion either by percutaneous drain or nephrostomy tube placement and allowing the bladder to heal. Urinary fistulas are uncommon but can also be managed in a similar fashion and allowing the fistula to close spontaneously [17].

Tumor Seeding

Low incidence of local recurrence after RNU has been reported in the literature, but it can be a serious complication if the principles of oncologic surgery are not followed. Laparoscopic approach does not result in a clinically significant increased risk of tumor spillage. Local recurrences can be prevented by minimizing tumor handling, using an impermeable bag for specimen retrieval, fixation of trocar to avoid gas leakage, and avoiding laparoscopic surgery in patients with ascites [53].

Conclusions

Complications during RNU vary with the difficulty of the case, patient-related factors and the surgeon's experience. Serious complications can still occur even in competent hands. The incidence and effects of many complications can be minimized with meticulous attention to the anatomic details and proper surgical techniques. Adherence to oncologic principles is imperative to prevent local tumor recurrence.

References

1. Siegel R, Naishadham D, Jemal A. Cancer statistics, 2012. CA Cancer J Clin. 2012;62(1):10–29.
2. Cummings KB, Correa RJ Jr, Gibbons RP, Stoll HM, Wheelis RF, Mason JT. Renal pelvic tumors. J Urol. 1975;113(2):158–62.
3. Clayman RV, Kavoussi LR, Figenshau RS, Chandhoke PS, Albala DM. Laparoscopic nephroureterectomy: initial clinical case report. J Laparoendosc Surg. 1991;1(6):343–9.
4. Steinberg JR, Matin SF. Laparoscopic radical nephroureterectomy: dilemma of the distal ureter. Curr Opin Urol. 2004;14(2):61–5.
5. Gill IS, Soble JJ, Miller SD, Sung GT. A novel technique for management of the en bloc bladder cuff and distal ureter during laparoscopic nephroureterectomy. J Urol. 1999;161(2):430–4.
6. Shalhav AL, Dunn MD, Portis AJ, Elbahnasy AM, McDougall EM, Clayman RV. Laparoscopic nephroureterectomy for upper tract transitional cell cancer: the Washington University experience. J Urol. 2000;163(4):1100–4.
7. McNeill SA, Chrisofos M, Tolley DA. The long-term outcome after laparoscopic nephroureterectomy: a comparison with open nephroureterectomy. BJU Int. 2000;86(6):619–23.
8. Bariol SV, Stewart GD, McNeill SA, Tolley DA. Oncological control following laparoscopic nephroureterectomy: 7-year outcome. J Urol. 2004;172(5 Pt 1):1805–8.
9. Phe V, Cussenot O, Bitker MO, Roupret M. Does the surgical technique for management of the distal ureter influence the outcome after nephroureterectomy? BJU Int. 2011;108(1):130–8.
10. Guillonneau B, Jayet C, Tewari A, Vallancien G. Robot assisted laparoscopic nephrectomy. J Urol. 2001;166(1):200–1.
11. Rose K, Khan S, Godbole H, Olsburgh J, Dasgupta P, Guy S, et al. Robotic assisted retroperitoneoscopic nephroureterectomy—first experience and the hybrid port technique. Int J Clin Pract. 2006;60(1):12–4.
12. Trudeau V, Gandaglia G, Shiffmann J, Popa I, Shariat SF, Montorsi F, et al. Robot-assisted versus laparoscopic nephroureterectomy for upper-tract urothelial cancer: a population-based assessment of costs and perioperative outcomes. Can Urol Assoc J. 2014;8(9–10):E695–701.
13. Yu HY, Hevelone ND, Lipsitz SR, Kowalczyk KJ, Hu JC. Use, costs and comparative effectiveness of robotic assisted, laparoscopic and open urological surgery. J Urol. 2012;187(4):1392–8.
14. Hanske J, Sanchez A, Schmid M, Meyer CP, Abdollah F, Feldman AS, et al. A Comparison of 30-day Perioperative outcomes in open versus minimally invasive nephroureterectomy for upper tract urothelial carcinoma: analysis of 896 patients from the american college of surgeons-national surgical

quality improvement program database. J Endourol. 2015;29(9):1052–8.
15. Lin YK, Deliere A, Lehman K, Harpster LE, Kaag MG, Raman JD. Critical analysis of 30 day complications following radical nephroureterectomy for upper tract urothelial carcinoma. Can J Urol. 2014;21(4):7369–73.
16. Raman JD, Lin YK, Kaag M, Atkinson T, Crispen P, Wille M, et al. High rates of advanced disease, complications, and decline of renal function after radical nephroureterectomy. Urol Oncol. 2014;32 (1):47 e9–14.
17. Nelson EC, Evans CP. Complications of nephrectomy. In: Taneja SS, editor. Complications of urologic surgery: prevention and management. 4th ed. Philadelphia: Saunders, an imprint of Elsevier Inc.; 2009. p. 387–400.
18. Gill IS, Kavoussi LR, Clayman RV, Ehrlich R, Evans R, Fuchs G, et al. Complications of laparoscopic nephrectomy in 185 patients: a multi-institutional review. J Urol. 1995;154(2 Pt 1):479–83.
19. Vallancien G, Cathelineau X, Baumert H, Doublet JD, Guillonneau B. Complications of transperitoneal laparoscopic surgery in urology: review of 1,311 procedures at a single center. J Urol. 2002;168 (1):23–6.
20. Schafer M, Lauper M, Krahenbuhl L. Trocar and Veress needle injuries during laparoscopy. Surg Endosc. 2001;15(3):275–80.
21. Catarci M, Carlini M, Gentileschi P, Santoro E. Major and minor injuries during the creation of pneumoperitoneum. A multicenter study on 12,919 cases. Surg Endosc. 2001;15(6):566–9.
22. Chandler JG, Corson SL, Way LW. Three spectra of laparoscopic entry access injuries. J Am Coll Surg. 2001;192(4):478–90 (discussion 90–1).
23. Pareek G, Hedican SP, Gee JR, Bruskewitz RC, Nakada SY. Meta-analysis of the complications of laparoscopic renal surgery: comparison of procedures and techniques. J Urol. 2006;175(4):1208–13.
24. Fahlenkamp D, Rassweiler J, Fornara P, Frede T, Loening SA. Complications of laparoscopic procedures in urology: experience with 2,407 procedures at 4 German centers. J Urol. 1999;162(3 Pt 1):765–70 (discussion 70–1).
25. Soulie M, Seguin P, Richeux L, Mouly P, Vazzoler N, Pontonnier F, et al. Urological complications of laparoscopic surgery: experience with 350 procedures at a single center. J Urol. 2001;165(6 Pt 1):1960–3.
26. Bird VG, Au JK, Sandman Y, De Los Santos R, Ayyathurai R, Shields JM. Comparison of different extraction sites used during laparoscopic radical nephrectomy. J Urol. 2009;181(4):1565–70.
27. Tisdale BE, Kapoor A, Hussain A, Piercey K, Whelan JP. Intact specimen extraction in laparoscopic nephrectomy procedures: Pfannenstiel versus expanded port site incisions. Urology. 2007;69 (2):241–4.
28. Rassweiler J, Fornara P, Weber M, Janetschek G, Fahlenkamp D, Henkel T, et al. Laparoscopic nephrectomy: the experience of the laparoscopy working group of the German Urologic Association. J Urol. 1998;160(1):18–21.
29. Parsons JK, Varkarakis I, Rha KH, Jarrett TW, Pinto PA, Kavoussi LR. Complications of abdominal urologic laparoscopy: longitudinal five-year analysis. Urology. 2004;63(1):27–32.
30. Green DA, Grasso M. Complications of laparoscopic radical nephrectomy and nephroureterectomy. In: Ghavamian R, editor. Complications of Laparoscopic and Robotic Urologic Surgery. New York: Springer; 2010. p. 113–26.
31. Kaneko N, Kobayashi Y, Okada Y. Anatomic variations of the renal vessels pertinent to transperitoneal vascular control in the management of trauma. Surgery. 2008;143(5):616–22.
32. Siqueira TM Jr, Kuo RL, Gardner TA, Paterson RF, Stevens LH, Lingeman JE, et al. Major complications in 213 laparoscopic nephrectomy cases: the Indianapolis experience. J Urol. 2002;168(4 Pt 1):1361–5.
33. Berger A, Haber GP, Kamoi K, Aron M, Desai MM, Kaouk JH, et al. Laparoscopic radical nephroureterectomy for upper tract transitional cell carcinoma: oncological outcomes at 7 years. J Urol. 2008;180 (3):849–54 (discussion 54).
34. Soulie M, Salomon L, Seguin P, Mervant C, Mouly P, Hoznek A, et al. Multi-institutional study of complications in 1085 laparoscopic urologic procedures. Urology. 2001;58(6):899–903.
35. Kouba E, Smith AM, Derksen JE, Gunn K, Wallen E, Pruthi RS. Efficacy and safety of en bloc ligation of renal hilum during laparoscopic nephrectomy. Urology. 2007;69(2):226–9.
36. Buse S, Gilfrich C, Pfitzenmaier J, Bedke J, Haferkamp A, Hohenfellner M. En bloc stapler ligation of the renal vascular pedicle during laparoscopic nephrectomy. BJU Int. 2008;101(7):878–82.
37. Chan D, Bishoff JT, Ratner L, Kavoussi LR, Jarrett TW. Endovascular gastrointestinal stapler device malfunction during laparoscopic nephrectomy: early recognition and management. J Urol. 2000;164 (2):319–21.
38. Friedman AL, Peters TG, Jones KW, Boulware LE, Ratner LE. Fatal and nonfatal hemorrhagic complications of living kidney donation. Ann Surg. 2006;243(1):126–30.
39. Ponsky L, Cherullo E, Moinzadeh A, Desai M, Kaouk J, Haber GP, et al. The Hem-o-lok clip is safe for laparoscopic nephrectomy: a multi-institutional review. Urology. 2008;71(4):593–6.
40. Hsi RS, Saint-Elie DT, Zimmerman GJ, Baldwin DD. Mechanisms of hemostatic failure during laparoscopic nephrectomy: review of Food and Drug Administration database. Urology. 2007;70(5):888–92.
41. Meng MV. Reported failures of the polymer self-locking (Hem-o-lok) clip: review of data from the Food and Drug Administration. J Endourol. 2006;20(12):1054–7.

42. Bishoff JT, Allaf ME, Kirkels W, Moore RG, Kavoussi LR, Schroder F. Laparoscopic bowel injury: incidence and clinical presentation. J Urol. 1999;161(3):887–90.
43. Breda A, Finelli A, Janetschek G, Porpiglia F, Montorsi F. Complications of laparoscopic surgery for renal masses: prevention, management, and comparison with the open experience. Eur Urol. 2009;55(4):836–50.
44. Simon SD, Castle EP, Ferrigni RG, Lamm DL, Swanson SK, Novicki DE, et al. Complications of laparoscopic nephrectomy: the Mayo clinic experience. J Urol. 2004;171(4):1447–50.
45. Permpongkosol S, Link RE, Su LM, Romero FR, Bagga HS, Pavlovich CP, et al. Complications of 2,775 urological laparoscopic procedures: 1993 to 2005. J Urol. 2007;177(2):580 5.
46. Canby-Hagino ED, Morey AF, Jatoi I, Perahia B, Bishoff JT. Fibrin sealant treatment of splenic injury during open and laparoscopic left radical nephrectomy. J Urol. 2000;164(6):2004–5.
47. Varkarakis IM, Allaf ME, Bhayani SB, Inagaki T, Su LM, Kavoussi LR, et al. Pancreatic injuries during laparoscopic urologic surgery. Urology. 2004;64 (6):1089–93.
48. Del Pizzo JJ, Jacobs SC, Bishoff JT, Kavoussi LR, Jarrett TW. Pleural injury during laparoscopic renal surgery: early recognition and management. J Urol. 2003;169(1):41–4.
49. Aron M, Colombo JR Jr, Turna B, Stein RJ, Haber GP, Gill IS. Diaphragmatic repair and/or reconstruction during upper abdominal urological laparoscopy. J Urol. 2007;178(6):2444–50.
50. Montgomery JS, Wolf JS Jr. Venous thrombosis prophylaxis for urological laparoscopy: fractionated heparin versus sequential compression devices. J Urol. 2005;173(5):1623–6.
51. Rice KR, Brassell SA, McLeod DG. Venous thromboembolism in urologic surgery: prophylaxis, diagnosis, and treatment. Rev Urol. 2010;12(2–3):e111–24.
52. Forrest JB, Clemens JQ, Finamore P, Leveillee R, Lippert M, Pisters L, et al. AUA Best Practice Statement for the prevention of deep vein thrombosis in patients undergoing urologic surgery. J Urol. 2009;181(3):1170–7.
53. Muntener M, Schaeffer EM, Romero FR, Nielsen ME, Allaf ME, Brito FA, et al. Incidence of local recurrence and port site metastasis after laparoscopic radical nephroureterectomy. Urology. 2007;70(5):864–8.

Rigid Uretero-Resectoscopic Management of Ureteral Tumors

21

Joel Hillelsohn and Majid Eshghi

In previous chapters, the management of superficial and small lesions has been described with the use of rigid or flexible ureteroscope. In this chapter, we will outline the evidence for ureteroscopic resection (URS) as well as discuss the management and techniques involved in resection of bulky or deep ureteral tumors. It must be emphasized that the majority of the cases reported in the literature did not involve use of the rigid uretero-resectoscope that will be described in this section. Historically, conservative management of these lesions was indicated in a select subgroup of patients, such as those with bilateral UTUC (upper tract urothelial carcinoma), poor renal function, or a solitary kidney [1]. Now, conservative management of these lesions is guided by patient preference or significant medical morbidities making a patient a poor surgical candidate: imperative case. This chapter will outline the discussion with the patient required prior to initiating conservative treatment of these lesions.

Electronic supplementary material The online version of this chapter (doi:10.1007/978-3-319-51263-1_21) contains supplementary material, which is available to authorized users.

J. Hillelsohn (✉) · M. Eshghi
Department of Urology, Westchester Medical Health Network/New York Medical College, Skyline, 1S-B48, Valhalla, NY 10532, USA
e-mail: jhillelsohn@gmail.com

M. Eshghi
e-mail: majid_eshghi@nymc.edu

Literature Review

Ureteroscopic resection of ureteral tumors was reported in a study by Schmeller et al. [2]. The study reported on 20 patients, 16 of whom were managed by ureteroscopic laser ablation of their upper tract tumor burden. At a median follow up of 13.8 months, three recurrences were noted (19%). A larger study by Martinez-Pineiro et al. [3], examined 185 patients diagnosed with UTUC. Fifty-four of those patients were treated endoscopically, 39 with ureteroscopic resection. Twenty-nine percent of those patients had recurrence at a mean follow up of 30.6 months, while 28% ultimately failed the endourologic management.

However, the low recurrence rate cited above likely reflected a shorter follow up period. In studies with a minimal follow up of 40 months, recurrence rates were between 66 and 90%. In a study by Cutress et al., out of 73 patients selected for conservative endoscopic treatment at a median follow up of 54 months, 66% of patients had a recurrence and 19% required a RNU (radical nephroureterectomy) [4]. The data reveals that recurrences are to be expected and ought to be expressed to the patient prior to initiating treatment.

M. Eshghi (ed.), *Urothelial Malignancies of the Upper Urinary Tract*,
https://doi.org/10.1007/978-3-319-51263-1_21

Factors predicting recurrence have been examined in multiple studies. Tumor size >2 cm, high grade, multi-focality, prior history of bladder UCC (urothelial cell carcinoma), and stage have been reported in multiple studies to be associated with recurrence [5–7]. Other factors such as tumor location have been reported in some studies to be a risk factor for recurrence. However, more recent studies have shown when controlling for grade and stage, the location has no effect on oncological outcomes [7–9]. This disparate data likely reflects the difficulty in adequately staging the disease rather than a higher risk. The most important factor appears to be the grade of the tumor. Rouppret et al. [6] found the five year disease specific survival rate was 82% for low grade tumors and 47% for high grade. In a pooled analysis of existing studies on URS (ureteroscopic) resection Cutress et al. calculated that low-grade disease had a 48% recurrence rate, versus high grade with a 60% recurrence rate [1]. The true recurrence rate for low grade and high grade are likely higher since the studies used in the analysis had variable follow up.

Bladder recurrence although reported in many studies, is likely cofounded by a previous history of bladder UCC. Cutress et al. calculated a bladder recurrence rate of 34% in a pooled analysis, however noted only 15/33 of the studies used reported bladder recurrence and that figure is likely to underestimate the true recurrence rate in studies with longer follow up [1]. Disease-specific survival (DSS) at a follow up of 37 months was reported in the same pooled analysis to be 91%. However, the real DSS is likely to be lower. In larger studies by Krambeck et al. [10] and Thompson et al. [11] tumors were treated as UTUC by visual inspection alone (~50%) in cases where pathological specimens were unable to be processed [11]. Other studies have revealed that visually presumed UTUC may actually be benign in 13–16% of cases [5, 12, 13].

Additionally, most studies did not censor for vital status, significant for a disease that has an OS OF 72–74% [1]. Those that did report DSS showed stratified by grade, had an 81–100% for low grade, and 69–86% for high grade DSS [6, 14, 15]. Renal preservation was also reported to be as high as 81% in pooled analysis [1]. However, like DSS, the numbers are likely to be overestimates, since studies were not censored to vital status. This is likely grade dependent. A study by Cutress et al. showed a 96% renal preservation for grade one and 20% for grade three disease [4].

The greatest concern for endoscopic management especially in non-imperative cases, are the risk of upstaging with a delay to RNU that would impact DSS. Multivariate analysis has shown that more than three previous bladder tumors, high grade, and stage to be significant risk factors for progression and DSS [4, 6, 7]. Ultimately, most studies have close to 20% conversion to RNU. In those patients, it would be important to examine if a delay to RNU changed the DSS. Three small studies examined delay to RNU and DSS. Hendin et al. showed no difference in 5-years DSS and OSS in 48 patients who underwent diagnostic URS prior to RNU [16]. Boorjian et al. compared 12 patients who had conservative treatment for 6 months, followed by RNU, with 34 patients with similar pathology who had immediate RNU. They found no significant difference in DSS (83% vs. 85%) at 39 months [17]. A more recent study by Haddad et al. compared patients with immediate RNU (40) compared to a group with elective conservative treatment, (11) pathologic staging was not significantly different between the two groups [18].

Table 21.1 [19–27] depicts selected studies that had complete follow up data on upper tract recurrence and who examined URS resection alone or distinguished between URS and PCN (percutaneous) resection. These studies are limited by the inability to distinguish between patients selected for conservative treatment for imperative versus elective reasons. Additionally, many of the patients had nonpathological diagnosis of tumors, tumors <2 cm, had significant medical comorbidities and then were not censored for vital status. In our pooled analysis, there was a 55% URS recurrence range (15–90%), 31% bladder recurrence (15–43%), and 22% endoscopic failure (11–47%). However, in studies with follow ups greater than 40 months, (6 studies) UTUC recurrence was 73% (15–90%) however, bladder recurrence was similar 31% (22–43).

Table 21.1 Studies examining ureteroscopic resection for upper tract urothelial carcinoma

Study	*N*	Follow up (mo)	UTCC recurrence (%)	Bladder recurrence *N* (%)	Failed endoscopic management (%)
Schmeller et al. [2]	16	14	3 (19)	ND	2 (13)
Gaboardi et al. [19]	18	15	8 (50)	ND	1 (6)
Engelmyer et al. [20]	10	43	7 (70)	ND	0
Martinez-peneiro et al. [3]	39	31	8 (29)	ND	11 (28)
Daneshmand et al. [21]	30	40	27 (90)	7 (23)	14 (47)
Johnson et al. [22]	35	32	24 (68)	ND	1 (3)
Roupret et al. [6]	27	52	4 (15)	6 (22)	7 (25.9)
Krambeck et al. [10]	37	32	23 (62)	13 (37)	11 (30)
Lucas et al. [14]	39	33	17 (46)	ND	11 (28)
Pak et al. [23]	57	53	51 (90)	ND	11 (19)
Cornu et al. [24]	35	24	21 (60)	14 (40)	4 (11)
Gadzinski et al. [25]	34	58	27 (84)	ND	ND
Raymundo et al. [26]	21	18	4 (31)	2 (15)	ND
Cutress et al. [4]	73	54	50 (69)	31 (43)	22 (30)
Grasso et al. [27]	66	52	51 (66)	18 (27)	15 (23)
Total	537	36.7	325/537 (55)	91/289 (31)	110/482 (22)

Endourologic management failed defined by pathologic progression, undergoing a RNU, or disease-specific mortality

Expert Management

Concomitant disease in the lower tract, are treated in the standard fashion as isolated lower tract urothelial carcinoma. If the tumor invades the ureteral orifice after the bladder resection, the residual tumor in the intraluminal portion of the ureter will be best managed with a rigid uretero-resectoscope. Lesions that are in the lower, mid, and upper ureter also are best managed with a rigid uretero-resectoscope. Additionally, the techniques that will be described in the following pages with the rigid ureteroscope, can be used for resection of benign lesions such as fibroepithelial polyps. These ureteroscopic techniques, are more demanding, require special equipment, which allow for treatment of certain lesions that are rather difficult to manage, with a simple rigid, flexible ureteroscope or if the standard ablation technique is not adequate for the size and the depth of the lesions.

Equipment

The rigid uretero-resectoscope is the main instrument required for the resection of the ureteral tumors. This instrument is a combination of resectoscope and rigid ureteroscope similar to the ones that are used in the bladder, however miniaturized and fitted into ureteroscope. Similar to urethral resectoscopes at the tip of these instruments, there is an insulated portion to allow targeted cutting and fulguration of lesions. The hand portion working elements of the instruments, although smaller have the same function as the urethral resectoscopes with a spring action working element and an outlet for monopolar resection.

At the present time, there are two models of such instruments in the market, however they are not readily available in most institutions. Secondary to the small number of cases, there is a definite learning curve to reach the comfort zone necessary, therefore most urologists are not familiar with nor use it frequently enough to have it as part of their armamentarium in their institutions. As a result, these valuable instruments remain underused. Due to these limitations, there are no large series in the literature dedicated to the management of tumors using these dedicated instruments. The majority of reported cases are managed with semi-rigid and flexible ureteroscopes using either electrocautery/laser or a combination of both.

The Wolf© uretero resectoscope, is approximately 11 French in the outer diameter and it includes an outer sheath with an insulated tip. The working elements that connects to the working sheath of the instrument allows for the insertion of a lens, which is a rod lens similar to cystoscopes. These lenses are very narrow and long, therefore, they are quite fragile and require extremely delicate handling and care. The set that is provided for this instrument also allows for the same lens to be used with a different sheath and placement of a different working element for incision in different areas of the ureter or the UPJ endoureterotome. The lens can also be used with a: 9 French sheath which hosts a different bridge that will allow it to function as a regular rigid ureteroscope (Fig. 21.1).

The energy cord from the working element is connected to the standard electrocautery system used for all transurethral surgeries. The loop that is used is a rather small and extends approximately 1.5 cm past the insulated tip of the scope. The recommended cutting current for the resection and fulguration inside the ureter as well as the renal pelvis is no more than 25–30 W. It can be increased depending on the location of the tumor and surrounding anatomy for example in the distal or pelvic ureter away from major vessels. The knowledge of vascular and paraureteral anatomy is quite essential to avoid inadvertent injuries. In female patient the surgeon must be cognizant of uterine artery in relation to the ureter. One of the concerns with the resection technique is that it requires time and the small loop can build up debris as a result of resection or fulguration. This requires the removal of the bridge and cleaning the loop frequently depending on the size of the lesion and the degree of electrical energy used for resection or fulguration (Video 21.1).

The Storz uretero resectoscope© includes a single sheath, which is approximately 11–12 French. The configuration of the tip creates a larger diameter; however, the loop that is used with this set is larger and allows for a more efficient resection. The other cutting instruments can also be utilized in this same sheath with the use of the working element. The mechanism of action again is similar to the previous instrument and the rest of the instruments that are used in transurethral surgery (Video 21.2).

For centers that perform such surgeries, both of these two instruments together with modern digital flexible video-ureteroscopes, proper biopsy forceps, 3 Fr coagulating electodes, Yag, and Holmium lasers should ideally be available.

In terms of comparison the Storz rigid uretero-resectoscope has a larger outer diameter

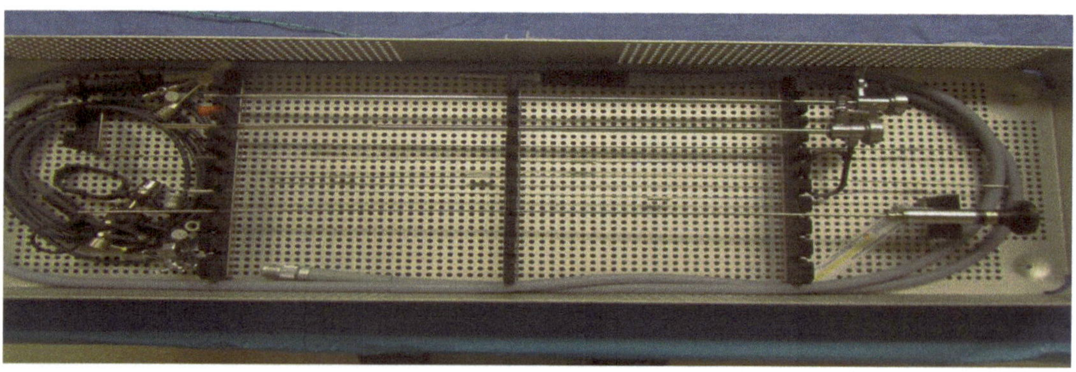

Fig. 21.1 Wolf uretero-resectoscope-complete set

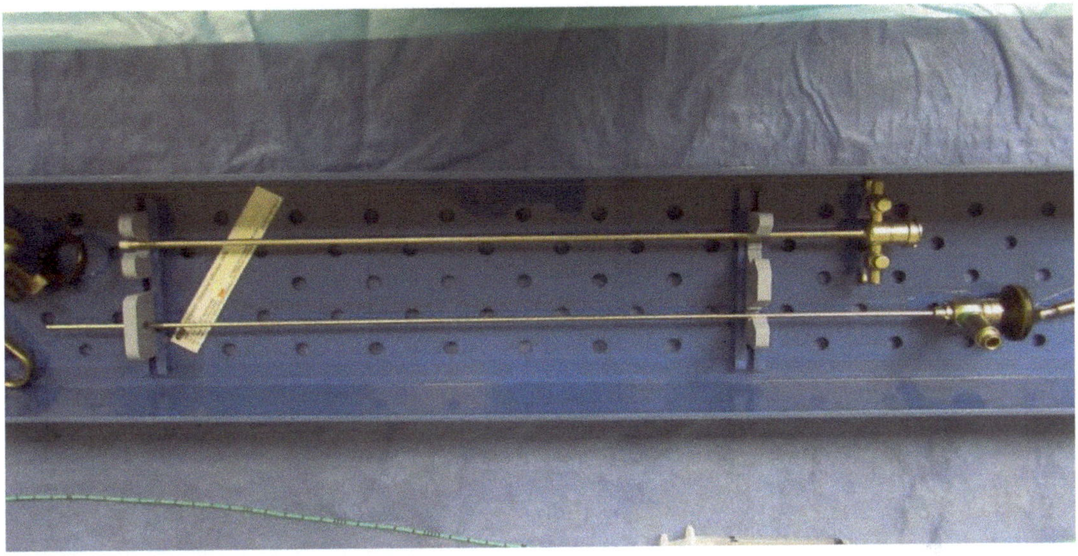

Fig. 21.2 Storz uretero-resectosope-complete set

and is shorter in length, whereas the Wolf instrument has a smaller outer diameter and longer, which allows reaching upper part of the ureter easier. We use the Wolf instrument for more upper tract tumors that are not easy to reach with the Storz resectoscope. Alternatively, we use the Storz resectoscope for bulkier tumors and in lower ureter requiring more extensive resection.

It is critical, when using these instruments, to place a guidewire prior to the start of the resection even if the system is quite dilated. These procedures are typically extensive and can involve resection of the bladder wall and ureteral wall and it is important to maintain access throughout the procedure especially with the high risk of perforation with deep resections. Only an insulated guidewire, such as the Teflon-coated guidewire should be used, to prevent transmission of the electric current throughout the ureteral mucosa. The most common complication from ureteroscopic management of UTC is stricture formation which can be as high as 11% [1]. It is therefore prudent to localize the resection, keep the current as low as possible and place a ureteral stent after complete or incomplete resections. It is not unusual to need to dilate the area of extensive resection several months later during follow up surveillance ureteroscopy. This finding can be compared to areas of scarring seen in the bladder post TURBT. This partially devasculaized area can also serve as landmark for obtaining re-biopsy if indicated clinically or endoscopically (Figs. 21.2 and 21.3).

Resection Technique

The patient's preparation and anesthesia consideration is similar to any other rigid or flexible ureteroscopic techniques. If the patient has previously been diagnosed and the endoscopy is for definitive or palliative resection a significant diagnostic workup does not need to be repeated. In cases where the ureteral lumen is small, it may be difficult in some cases to advance the large 11 French scopes in the ureter. However, if the distal ureter is involved simply by the obstructive effects of the lesion, there can be passive dilatation in the proximal ureter. Additionally, when placing the scope, it passively dilates the ureter. With a hydronephrotic ureter, the resection is simpler, once the scope is advanced past the obstructive lesion, the dilated ureter allows for better visualization and easier resection as the

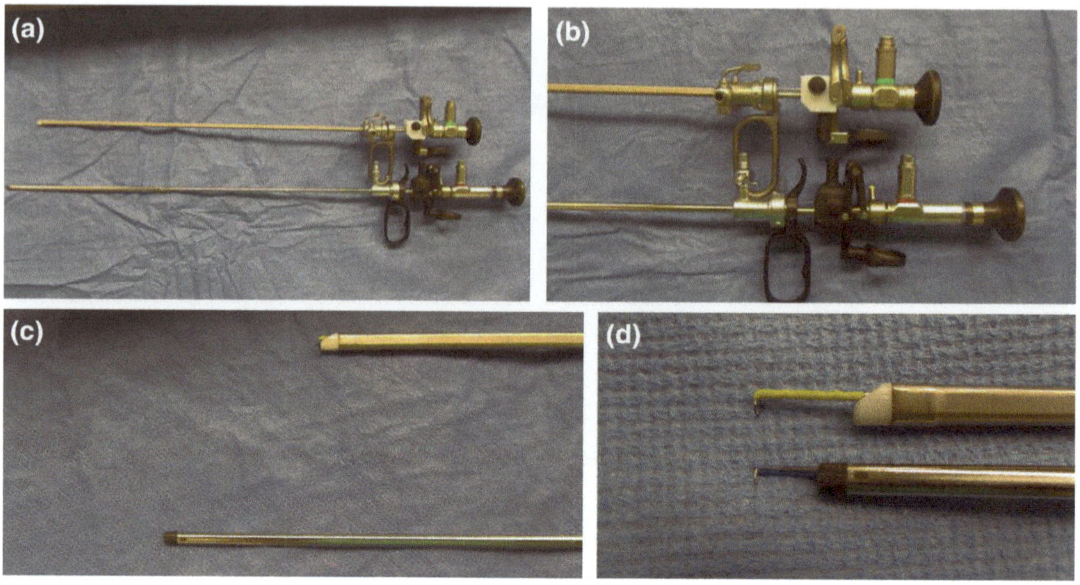

Fig. 21.3 Comparison of Storz and Wolf uretero-resectoscopes **a** assembled uretero-resectoscopes **b** working elements **c** difference in length **d** insulated tip configuration (Storz upper and Wolf lower part of image)

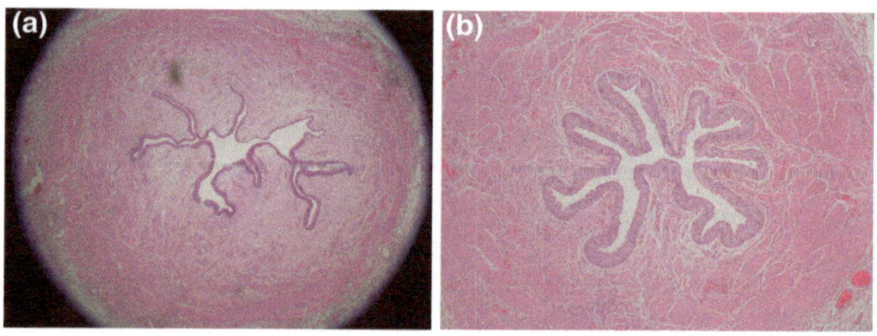

Fig. 21.4 **a** Cross section of uppper ureter showing thin muscular layer. **b** cross section of lower and distal ureter shows 3 distinct muscle layers

instrument is withdrawn leaving the loop extended above the lesion. Undoubtedly, there are cases that are difficult because of the large bulk of the tumor. In some of these cases, the patient may require passive dilation via a stent prior to URS treatment.

One of the fundamental differences of the rigid ureteroscopic resection compared to transurethral resection of bladder tumor is that the ureteral wall is thinner than the bladder, thus resection can be somewhat limited. The thin ureteral wall in general mandates careful and more superficial resection than in the bladder, since the thin-walled ureter can easily perforate. The lower ureter has thicker muscular support as compared to upper ureter which is thinner with usually about two layers limiting resection. None the less this should not eliminate superficial muscle resection is of curative nature. In cases where the bulk of the tumor is intramural, the endophytic Bladder renget part of the lesion can freely be resected until the depth or the base of the lesion is reached. At this point, the resection should be done in thin layers avoiding perforation (Fig. 21.4a and b). In some cases, this leads to inevitable inadequate resection, likely accounting for the high recurrence rates of these lesions. We usually start with 25 W of cutting energy and slightly increase the energy if needed and coagulation should not exceed 25–30 W.

The other technique of superficial biopsy then fulguration is not ideal since it will not reach the deepest part of the tumor. Superficial biopsy technique and fulguration covers the surface of the tumor; however, its coagulation effect will not properly treat of the deep base of the tumor. The recommended laser setting is discussed in the chapter on instruments chapter. This is especially important in cases where the tumor is bulky, high grade, and preoperative imaging clearly indicates that the base of the tumor involves the muscular layer.

In the distal ureter, specifically in the very distal and intramural ureter because of protection from the bladder wall, the operator has the advantage of being able to do deeper resections without causing perforations. In case of distal and bulky ureteral tumors it is usually necessary to extensively resect the intramural ureter. This will allow for free reflux into distal ureter for the purpose of topical chemotherapy or immunotherapy by instillation of agent in the bladder. The operator must be especially careful when resecting in the area of the mid ureter near the iliac vessels. As mentioned earlier one should always be aware of invisible surrounding structures such as uterine vessels, gonadal and iliac vessels, proximity to bowel, as well as ureteral vascular supply. Another critical point is altered anatomy due to previous abdominal and pelvic surgeries, such as colectomy, colostomy, hysterectomy, radical prostatectomy, and renal transplant. History of radiation can additionally pose difficulty due to fixation of the ureter. patient's with excessive vascular variations and aortic aneurysm need careful review of their reconstructed Ct urogram. An assessment of coagulation profile and review of medications with altering coagulation should be done as part of pre op preparation especially if patient requires extensive resection. It needs to be emphasized that this is a laborious process, it is time consuming and the operator needs to be patient to systemically resect the lesion. Considering that these patients usually have multiple co morbidities, it is not prudent to schedule them as a quick case s at the end of the day. Unlike in the bladder the resected fragments and debris have no area to accumulate and one is required to remove the working element and clean the loop multiple times. In some cases, due to the size and the bulk of the tumor, the resection may have to be staged in order to completely resect the lesion. In the first session, the bulk of the tumor is resected, areas of obstruction are removed and stent is placed. In the subsequent session, the remainder of the lesions is resected. Complete resection also improves the outcome when considering topical chemotherapeutic and immunologic adjuvant agents instilled post procedure, such as Mitomycin C and BCG. BCG as we know from lower tract TCC works well only when the lesions is completely resected [1, 28] (Video 21.3).

In the second treatment session, the ureteroscope is readily introduced and the residual tumor and specifically the base of the tumor are completely resected with a much better field of vision and better assessment of demarcation lines and the margins of the tumor (Video 21.4 and Fig. 21.5).

In some of our cases where the lesion appeared to be extensive or high grade, at the completion of the case, we place an open-ended catheter or a single J-catheter in the renal pelvis and then slowly instill Mitomycin C to allow bathing of the collecting system down into the bladder and followed by a stent placement.

Our Preferred Technique. At the completion of the resection a double pigtail stent is placed an additional 5-Fr open-ended catheter is placed parallel to the stent and advanced into the renal pelvis under fluoroscopic control. At this point the bladder is drained and a Foley catheter placed and clamped. Mitomycin C solution can be injected in the 5 Fr catheter to allow for complete bathing of the collecting system as well as the bladder and it is removed under fluoroscopic control after the instillation is completed and the Foley is unclamped after 1 hour. This maneuver will reduce the risk of recurrence as it has been documented after nephroureterectomy Fig. 21.5. The technique of percutaneous intracavitary treatment is discussed in detail in Chap. 28.

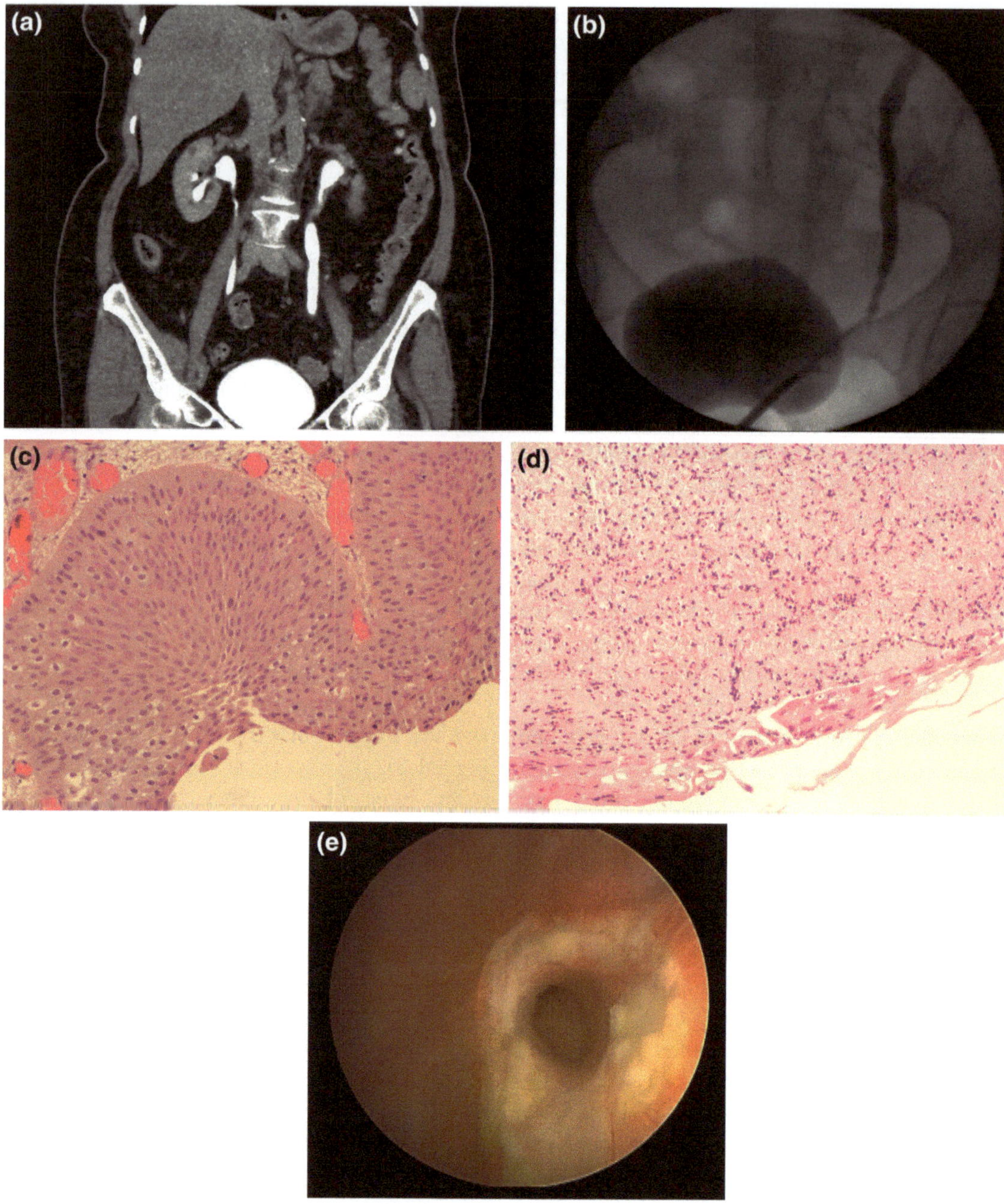

Fig. 21.5 **a**, **b** CT scan and retrograde pyelogram show left hydronephrosis and left distal ureteral lesion **c** pathology reveals low grade urothelial carcinoma **d** follow-up biopsy shows no active tumor **e** appearance of orifice after the completion of treatment

Lastly, the follow up of the patient will include repeat imaging studies, urine cytology, as well as a repeat ureteroscopy and biopsy. It is not unusual for the repeat biopsy samples from the previously resected area to show inflammatory, fibrotic, and granulous tissue suggestive of previous electrocautery effects on the tissues. This will also be discussed in the surveillance Chap. 26 of this book. Virtual ureteroscopy as described in Chap. 5 will clearly play a major

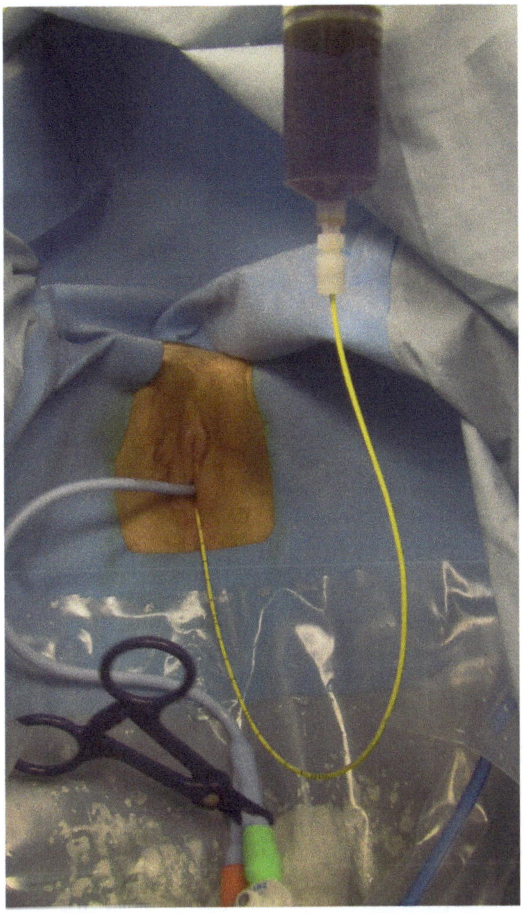

Fig. 21.6 Mitomycin C instilled via 5-Fr ureteral catheters that is placed parallel to the stent. Foley catheter will remain clamped for 1 h to allow complete bathing of the bladder as well. This will reduce the risk of recurrence as it has been documented after nephroureterectomy

role in the future. We perform out patient flexible ureteroscopy in an orifice setting in some of these cases (video 21.5)

Summary Box

- The choice of conservative management for upper tract tumors can be based on patient preference, grade, and comorbidities
- The data on ureteroscopic resection shows that recurrences are common and largely grade dependent
- Studies have shown no impact in disease-specific survival or pathological stage in patients whom had delayed radical nephroureterectomy
- Large ureteral tumors are best treated with uretero-resectoscope since flexible ureteroscopes are not adequate to remove a bulky and deep lesion
- Care must be taken when resecting near the vasculature. As a rule the resection is done in layers rather than scooping deep bites
- Staged resections may be necessary for a complete resection
- Mitomycin C may be used post resection to delay recurrence
- Ureteral orifice should be widely resected to allow reflux into the ureter for topical treatment
- Virtual ureteroscopy and orifice ureteroscopy will play a major role in future as tool of surveillance.

Acknowledgements Author acknowledges the contribution of Sean Fullerton, MD, Westchester Medical Health Network, New YorkMedical College, Valhalla, NY and thanks him for his helpful comments and feedback.

References

1. Cutress ML, Stewart GD, Zakikhani P, et al. Ureteroscopic and percutaneous management of upper tract urothelial carcinoma (UTUC): systematic review. BJU Int. 2012;110:614.
2. Schmeller NT, Hofstetter AG. Laser treatment of ureteral tumors. J Urol. 1989;141:840.
3. Martinez-Pineiro JA, Garcia Matres MJ, Martinez-Pineiro L. Endourological treatment of upper tract urothelial carcinomas: analysis of a series of 59 tumors. J Urol. 1996;156:377.
4. Cutress ML, Stewart GD, Tudor EC, et al. Endoscopic versus laparoscopic management of noninvasive upper tract urothelial carcinoma: 20-year single center experience. J Urol. 2013;189:2054.
5. Deligne E, Colombel M, Badet L, et al. Conservative management of upper urinary tract tumors. Eur Urol. 2002;42:43.
6. Roupret M, Hupertan V, Traxer O, et al. Comparison of open nephroureterectomy and ureteroscopic and

percutaneous management of upper urinary tract transitional cell carcinoma. Urology. 2006;67:1181.
7. Iborra I, Solsona E, Casanova J, et al. Conservative elective treatment of upper urinary tract tumors: a multivariate analysis of prognostic factors for recurrence and progression. J Urol. 2003;169:82.
8. Suh RS, Faerber GJ, Wolf JS Jr. Predictive factors for applicability and success with endoscopic treatment of upper tract urothelial carcinoma. J Urol. 2003;170:2209.
9. Chromecki TF, Bensalah K, Remzi M, et al. Prognostic factors for upper urinary tract urothelial carcinoma. Nat Rev Urol. 2011;8:440.
10. Krambeck AE, Thompson RH, Lohse CM, et al. Endoscopic management of upper tract urothelial carcinoma in patients with a history of bladder urothelial carcinoma. J Urol. 2007;177:1721.
11. Thompson RH, Krambeck AE, Lohse CM, et al. Endoscopic management of upper tract transitional cell carcinoma in patients with normal contralateral kidneys. Urology. 2008;71:713.
12. Lee BR, Jabbour ME, Marshall FF, et al. 13-year survival comparison of percutaneous and open nephroureterectomy approaches for management of transitional cell carcinoma of renal collecting system: equivalent outcomes. J Endourol. 1999;13:289.
13. Fuglsig S, Krarup T. Percutaneous nephroscopic resection of renal pelvic tumors. Scand J Urol Nephrol Suppl. 1995;172:15.
14. Lucas SM, Svatek RS, Olgin G, et al. Conservative management in selected patients with upper tract urothelial carcinoma compares favourably with early radical surgery. BJU Int. 2008;102:172.
15. Gadzinski AJ, Roberts WW, Faerber GJ, et al. Long-term outcomes of immediate versus delayed nephroureterectomy for upper tract urothelial carcinoma. J Endourol. 2012;26:566.
16. Hendin BN, Streem SB, Levin HS, et al. Impact of diagnostic ureteroscopy on long-term survival in patients with upper tract transitional cell carcinoma. J Urol. 1999;161:783.
17. Boorjian S, Ng C, Munver R, et al. Impact of delay to nephroureterectomy for patients undergoing ureteroscopic biopsy and laser tumor ablation of upper tract transitional cell carcinoma. Urology. 2005;66:283.
18. Haddad M, Cloutier J, Cornu JN, et al. Immediate nephroureterectomy or after attempting conservative treatment, on elective indications, for upper urinary tract urothelial carcinoma: comparison of the pathology reports on a retrospective monocentric study. J Endourol. 2015;29:969.
19. Gaboardi F, Bozzola A, Dotti E, et al. Conservative treatment of upper urinary tract tumors with Nd:YAG laser. J Endourol. 1994;8:37.
20. Engelmyer EI, Belis JA. Long-term ureteroscopic management of low-grade transitional cell carcinoma of the upper urinary tract. Tech Urol. 1996;2:113.
21. Daneshmand S, Quek ML, Huffman JL. Endoscopic management of upper urinary tract transitional cell carcinoma: long-term experience. Cancer. 2003;98:55.
22. Johnson GB, Fraiman M, Grasso M, Broadening experience with the retrograde endoscopic management of upper urinary tract urothelial malignancies. BJU Int. 95 Suppl 2; 2005:110.
23. Pak RW, Moskowitz EJ, Bagley DH. What is the cost of maintaining a kidney in upper-tract transitional-cell carcinoma? An objective analysis of cost and survival. J Endourol. 2009;23:341.
24. Cornu JN, Rouprêt M, Carpentier X, et al. Oncologic control obtained after exclusive flexible ureteroscopic management of upper urinary tract urothelial cell carcinoma. World J Urol. 2010;28:151.
25. Gadzinski AJ, Roberts WW, Faerber GJ, et al. Long-term outcomes of nephroureterectomy versus endoscopic management for upper tract urothelial carcinoma. J Urol. 2010;183:2148.
26. Raymundo EM, Lipkin ME, Bañez LB, et al. Third prize: the role of endoscopic nephron-sparing surgery in the management of upper tract urothelial carcinoma. J Endourol. 2011;25:377.
27. Grasso M, Fishman AI, Cohen J, et al. Ureteroscopic and extirpative treatment of upper urinary tract urothelial carcinoma: a 15-year comprehensive review of 160 consecutive patients. BJU Int. 2012;110:1618.
28. Yokogi H, Wada Y, Mizutani M, et al. Bacillus Calmette-Guérin perfusion therapy for carcinoma in situ of the upper urinary tract. Br J Urol. 1996;77:676.

Percutaneous Resection of Renal Pelvis and Calyceal Tumors

22

Majid Eshghi, Joel Hillelsohn and Roger Yau

The percutaneous approach is reserved for cases that cannot be managed with more minimally invasive techniques utilizing either rigid or flexible ureteroscopy with biopsy, resection or laser/Bugbee ablation. With the advent of new ureteroscopes with flexible distal tips and digital optics, the percutaneous (PCN) approach is limited to large renal pelvic or calyceal tumors extending into the infundibulum in the same way that ureteroscopy is not an adequate approach for management of staghorn calculus. Percutaneous resection though has significant advantages over ureteroscopic (URS) resection for better and more adequate resection. There is better visualization and larger instruments can be used, thereby improving staging, decrease understaging and allowing for more reliable resection capabilities thus eliminating one of the major drawbacks of ureteroscopy: inability to obtain deep biopsies in all areas of the upper tract. Large cold cup biopsies will rarely understage surface tumor carpeting with infiltrating and invasive nature. One of the poor prognostic factors of UTUC is hydronephrosis but this, at times, could be secondary to the large volume of the disease located near ureteropelvic or calycioinfundibular junctions and simply create a mechanical intraluminal obstruction similar to the cases of large fibroepithelial tumors in the ureter. Percutaneous access also allows easy instillation of adjuvant topical therapy in an outpatient setting. Lastly PCN access facilitates second look surveillance nephroscopy that can reliably gain access to areas that are difficult to reach, after urinary diversion, cystectomy, orthotopic urinary reservoir or for adequate survey with a larger flexible cystoscope in difficult areas of upper urinary tract such as the lower pole calyx [1]. The percutaneous approach will therefore provide a more reliable method for risk assessment, staging and help prognosticating patient's treatment outcome specially for the reason that these patients have a tendency to have an initial presentation with invasive disease. The risks of ureteroscopic understaging and under treatment are similarly higher.

Similar to ureteral lesions that are managed endoscopically or using uretero-resectoscope, the

Electronic supplementary material **The online version of this chapter (doi:10.1007/978-3-319-51263-1_22) contains supplementary material, which is available to authorized users.**

M. Eshghi (✉)
Chief Section of Endourology and Minimally Invasive Urology, Department of Urology, New York Medical College, Westchester Medical Health Network, Valhalla, NY, USA
e-mail: majid_eshghi@nymc.edu

J. Hillelsohn · R. Yau
Department of Urology, Westchester Medical Health Network/New York Medical College, Valhalla, NY, USA
e-mail: jhillelsohn@gmail.com

R. Yau
e-mail: Roger.yau@wmchealth.org

M. Eshghi (ed.), *Urothelial Malignancies of the Upper Urinary Tract*,
https://doi.org/10.1007/978-3-319-51263-1_22

percutaneous technique for the resection of renal pelvic tumors has similar indications. The patients are typically older with multiple comorbidities or imperative conditions such as physically or functionally solitary kidneys, poor renal function which is associated with lower life expectancy, a varied combination of bilateral ureteral and or renal pelvic tumors as well as other contraindications for radical surgeries such as nephroureterectomy. Additional indications include low grade, unifocal upper tract urothelial carcinoma (UTUC) of the renal pelvis, per European Urology 2015 guidelines [2]. Percutaneous tumor resection can be curative with small low-grade lesions versus palliative in patients who have had multiple procedures such as previous nephrectomy, cystectomy, or have single functioning renal unit with recurrence of tumor [3]. Another indication is preservation of renal function to allow the patient undergo nephrotoxic chemotherapy such as cisplatinum. The chemotherapy could be for urologic or other non urologic malignancies. Such an example is a patient whose nephrostogram is shown in Fig. 22.1. This patient had a very high recurrence of urothelial carcinoma. He was status post right nephroureterctomy, cystectomy, Left ureterectomy and a solitary left renal unit which was drained through a jejunal conduit. He eventually developed recurrence in this solitary renal pelvis which was resected percutaneously. This was purely a palliative procedure according to the patient's choice to avoid hemodialysis.

The studies examining percutaneous resection are similar to the ones examined for ureteroscopic resection in the previous chapter. Most are limited by short follow up time, did not censor for vital status and had small retrospective cohorts consisting of many patients with low grade and low volume disease. Recurrence has ranged in studies between 13 and 65%, and as in URS resection it is grade and stage dependent [4–13]. The largest study was reported by Motamedinia, et al. They reported on a 141 patients treated with PCN resection followed for 66 months. Recurrence rates were 33% for low grade and 44% for high grade patients. Significantly, 87% of the patients avoided a radical nephroureterectomy (RNU) [14]. These recurrence rates are similar to what is seen in the

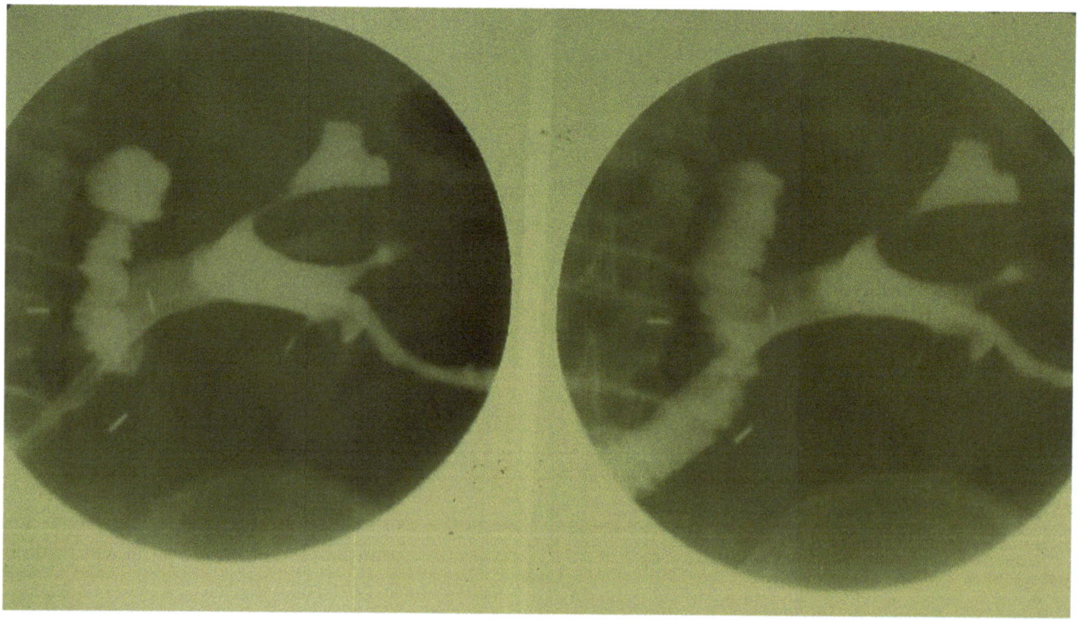

Fig. 22.1 This image shows a percutaneous nephrostomy tube in a solitary left kidney, draining via a jejunal conduit with recurrent upper tract urothelial carcinoma which was resected percutaneously

literature. Cutress et al. did a pooled analysis of PCN resection studies and showed a recurrence rate of 35% for low grade disease and a 42% for high grade disease [15]. The complication rate for PCN resection though is higher than URS resection. Cutress et al. showed a pooled complication rate of 27% for PCN resection versus 14% for URS resection. The most common complication was blood transfusion at 17% (Table 22.1) [4–11, 14, 16, 17]. A rare but serious concern when performing PCN resection is the possibility of tract seeding. However, this is an extremely rarely seen complication. In one of the largest studies evaluation PCN resection by Rastinehad et al., tract seeding was seen in only 0.75% of cases (1/133) [13].

An essential part of our practice protocol is to have a frank discussion with the patient and relatives who are intimately involved with the patient peri-operatively regarding the risk and benefits of conservative treatment. An outline for that discussion will be summarized in Chaps. 26 and 28 on intracavitary treatment and surveillance. The following is our protocol for PCN resection.

Preoperative Assessment

The preoperative assessment of the patients for percutaneous resection of UTUC is similar to percutaneous stone cases. The routine preoperative assessments include cardiopulmonary, preoperative diagnostic imaging studies, retrograde pyelograms, selective urinary cytology from upper tracts and/or flexible ureteroscopic biopsy. Particular attention should be paid to the patient's coagulation profile and an active blood type and cross should be in the system. Bleeding blood is the most common complication of PCN and blood transfusion has been reported in as many as 17% of cases. We recommend to have 2 units available prior to the start of the procedure. If indicated, the patient will be started on preoperative oral antibiotic. Otherwise, if the patient has

Table 22.1 Recurrence and complication rates after percutaneous tumor resection

Study	*N*	Follow Up (mo)	Upper tract recurrence *N* (%)	Bladder recurrence *N* (%)	RNU *n* (%)	Complications *N* (%)
Tasca et al. [16]	10	19	5 (50)	ND	3 (30)	ND
Fuglsig et al. [4]	26	21	8 (31)	ND	9 (35)	2 (8) tranfusion 1 (4) tumor seeding
Plancke et al. [5]	10	28	1 (10)	1 (10)	1 (10)	0/10
Patel et al. [6]	26	45	9 (35)	11 (42)	5 (19)	7 (27) overall, 3 (12) transfusion
Martinez-Pinerio et al. [7]	18	31	2 (11)	ND	1 (6)	7 (33) overall
Clarke et al. [8]	17	24	6 (33)	ND	2 (12)	2 (12) transfusion 1 (6) UTI
Goel et al. [9]	20	64	13 (65)	3 (15)	10 (50)	4 (20)
Suh et al. [10]	14	21	14 (100)	ND	5 (14)	ND
Palou et al. [11]	34	51	15 (44)	ND	9 (26)	2 (6)
Roupret et al. [17]	24	62	3 (13)	4 (17)	5 (21)	7 (29) overall, 3 (13) transfusion
Motamedinia et al. [14]	141	66	50 (35)	ND	19 (13)	ND
Overall	340	39.27	126/340 (37)	19/80 (24)	69/340 (20)	64/236 (27) overall 37/218 (17) transfusion 5/256 (2) renal failure 1/236 (seeding of tract)

a negative urine culture, antibiotics will be administered intravenously prior to the start of the case. Patients must also be informed and prepared for having nephrostomy tubes that will be draining to a leg-bag and be instructed on its care prior to the procedure.

Instrumentation

The following equipments are needed for percutaneous renal pelvic tumor resection.

We use standard percutaneous entry system for puncture and dilation, a standard nephroscope, a urethro-resectoscope, a flexible cystoscope and flexible ureteroscope (Fig. 22.2). An essential component for obtaining adequate biopsies is a cold-cup nephroscopic biopsy forceps. It is used for de-bulking tumor as well as deep biopsies of the tumor base (Fig. 22.3). The cup-shaped uni-action forceps helps obtain adequate tissue for pathology. Moderate size tumors can sometimes be completely removed this way and the base can be further lasered or coagulated. If the tumor is resected using hot loop, this cold cup will allow for biopsy of the base and margins (Video 22.1). It is important to maintain an open communication with the pathology department to ensure adequate tissue is obtained for diagnosis.

For initial evaluation and inspection of the renal calyces a nephroscope or if needed a flexible cystoscope is used (Video 22.2). A urethro-resectoscope that is used for transurethral resection of bladder tumors (TURBT), or prostate (TURP) is the main instrument. We usually use a 24 Fr urethro-resectoscope utilizing slender bipolar as opposed to monopolar electrocautery which was used earlier. This is essential for resection of bulky tumors. A flexible cystoscope with proper forceps is also essential to reach adjacent calyces not easily reachable with rigid scopes. For follow up, surveillance procedures or with a small disease burden a #12 French mini-scope can be used. (MIP-Minature nephroscope sizes 9.5, 12, 17.5) (Karl Storz Endourolgy) Adequate inspection, sampling and use of a laser or electrocautery for ablation can be performed with the mini-scope without the need for over dilation of the tract. The mini-scope has its own reusable metallic sheaths and dilators. The metal dilator is passed over the guidewire, over which the sheath is advanced. The metal dilator is then removed and the mini nephroscope is inserted through the sheath (Fig. 22.4). This mini-scope can be used without a working sheath for surveillance through mature tracts, follow up biopsy and for removal of small volume disease (Fig. 22.5) (Video 22.3). There is also a 17 Fr pediatric nephroscope which can be used, with a 5 Fr working channel. The working port utilizes the same biopsy forceps as the 12 Fr scope. Both instruments can accommodate laser fibers and small Bugbee for coagulation (Fig. 22.6). The mini-scope is a single unit whereas the pediatric nephroscope is a two piece system similar to the adult scope. These two instruments are not adequate for initial phase of resecting a large lesion because of lacking a loop, on the other hand they are ideal for follow-up and for small lesions. In cases where the small scopes are used, a dedicated 18 Fr balloon dilator with sheath can be utilized to dilate the tract instead of the mini-scope dilators (Fig. 22.7). In cases of bulky lesions we recommend a clear working sheath that allows visualization in the periphery through the sheath, thereby ensuring small peripheral lesions are not missed. Holmium or Neodymium YAG laser should be available for ablation of the base of the lesion after the tumor is completely resected (Fig. 22.8; Video 22.4). A flexible ureteroscope should also be available if the operator needs to inspect the ureter in an antegrade fashion.

Post procedure nephrostomy tube configurations will depend on the need for possible second stage procedure or if the patient is being considered for intracavitary treatment. It is recommended to have multiple types of nephrostomy tubes available based on the extent, the location of the lesion, anatomy of the collecting system, involvement of the UPJ area and consideration of intracavitary treatment. We will review the exit strategy later in the chapter.

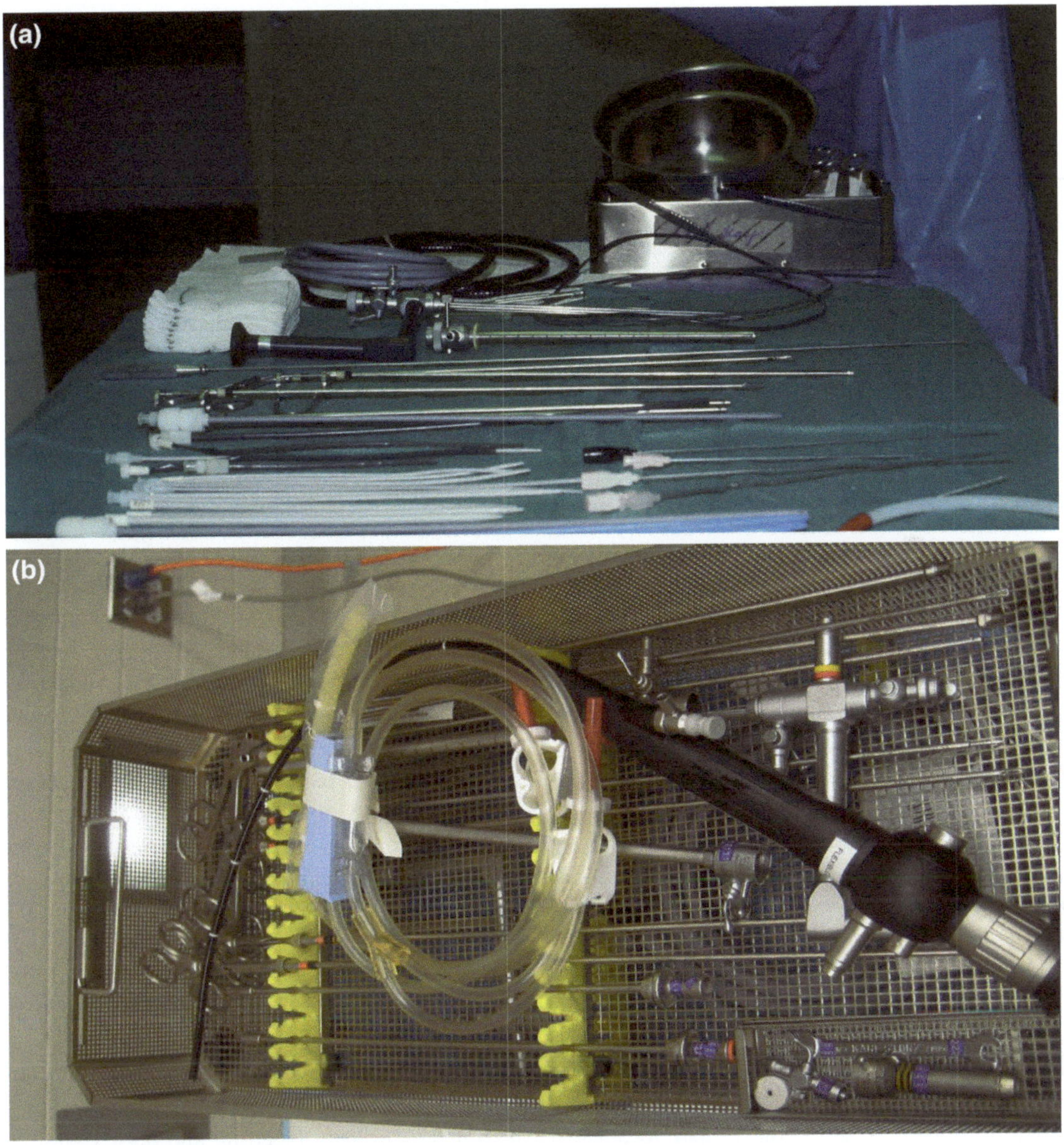

Fig. 22.2a, b Standard percutaneous nephrostomy table set up

Procedure

Operating Room Set Up

After the patient is brought to the room, the anesthesized on the stretcher and draped and prepped for a simple cystoscopy. A standard patient identification and time out is performed.

A flexible cystoscope (15–16 FR) is used to evaluate the bladder. Typically, the bladder is evaluated in the office preoperatively, so the primary goal of the cystoscopy is for the placement of a ureteral catheter. An unexpected small low grade appearing lesion can be simply biopsied and fulgurated with a Bugbee electrode or lased through the flexible cystoscope.

The ureteral orifice on the affected side is intubated with a 5–6 Fr open ended catheter and

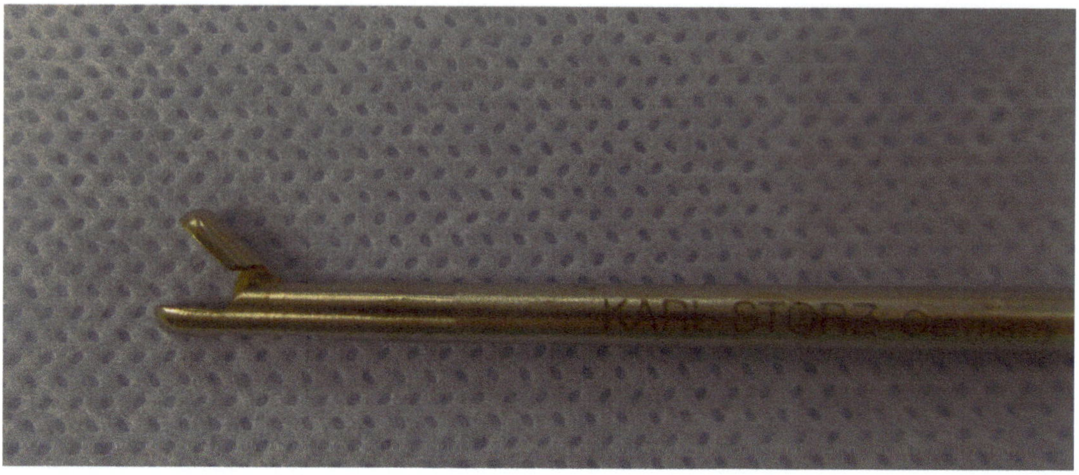

Fig. 22.3 Cold Cup biopsy allows for obtaining large deep biopsies for pathological diagnosis without cautery artifact

an 0.038 Sensor Guide Wire is advanced through the open ended catheter. Care must be taken not to advance the open ended catheter forcibly and too far blindly specially if there is preexisting ureteral or UPJ obstruction as it can cause perforation or renal injury. The open ended catheter is then secured to a Foley catheter using anesthesia pink tape with a butterfly configuration (Fig. 22.9).

The patient is placed in the prone position. Positioning, prepping and draping are done similar to percutaneous stone surgery cases. One should be sure to pad all pressure points.

The Puncture Technique

After the C-arm is set in the proper location a retrograde pyelogram is performed to outline the collecting system. The preoperative CT scan is reviewed prior to the procedure and is brought up on the screen in the operating room for easy review. A 3 dimensional reconstructed CT urogram is helpful for proper mapping of collecting system and tumor volume and orientation. Based on the preoperative imaging and intraoperative retrograde pyelogram a calyx is chosen for access (Fig. 22.10). The general recommendation is to perform the puncture using an 18 g needle into a calyx that is not directly on the lesion, but should easily be accessible the lesion. Accessing the diseased calyx may lead to crushing of the tumor against the wall when dilating the tract, leading to missed lesions and bleeding from avulsion of the tumor. There are cases where it is necessary to access the diseased calyx directly. The dilation and sheath placement should be limited to the parenchyma not to violate the tumor architecture. Tumors extending to the upper pole calyxes are difficult to access through a lower calyx. In such a case, it is recommended to directly access the upper pole calyx (Fig. 22.11). The access is thus decided on by considering all of the above factors and the experience of the operating surgeon. A short tract is obviously always preferred and direct puncture into the renal pelvis or calyceal infundibulum must be avoided at all times. Since it causes significant bleeding and poor visibility. The interlobar vessels travel along the infundibulum and additionally there is very little underlying muscular support in this area similar to renal sinus.

Once access is obtained with the needle and confirmed with aspiration urine cytology can be sent if it is helpful for diagnostic and staging. The subsequent steps in obtaining access are similar to stone extraction procedures. An 0.038 guide wire is placed through the needle and is manipulated down to the ureter and into the bladder. Typically, an angled tip guide wire is

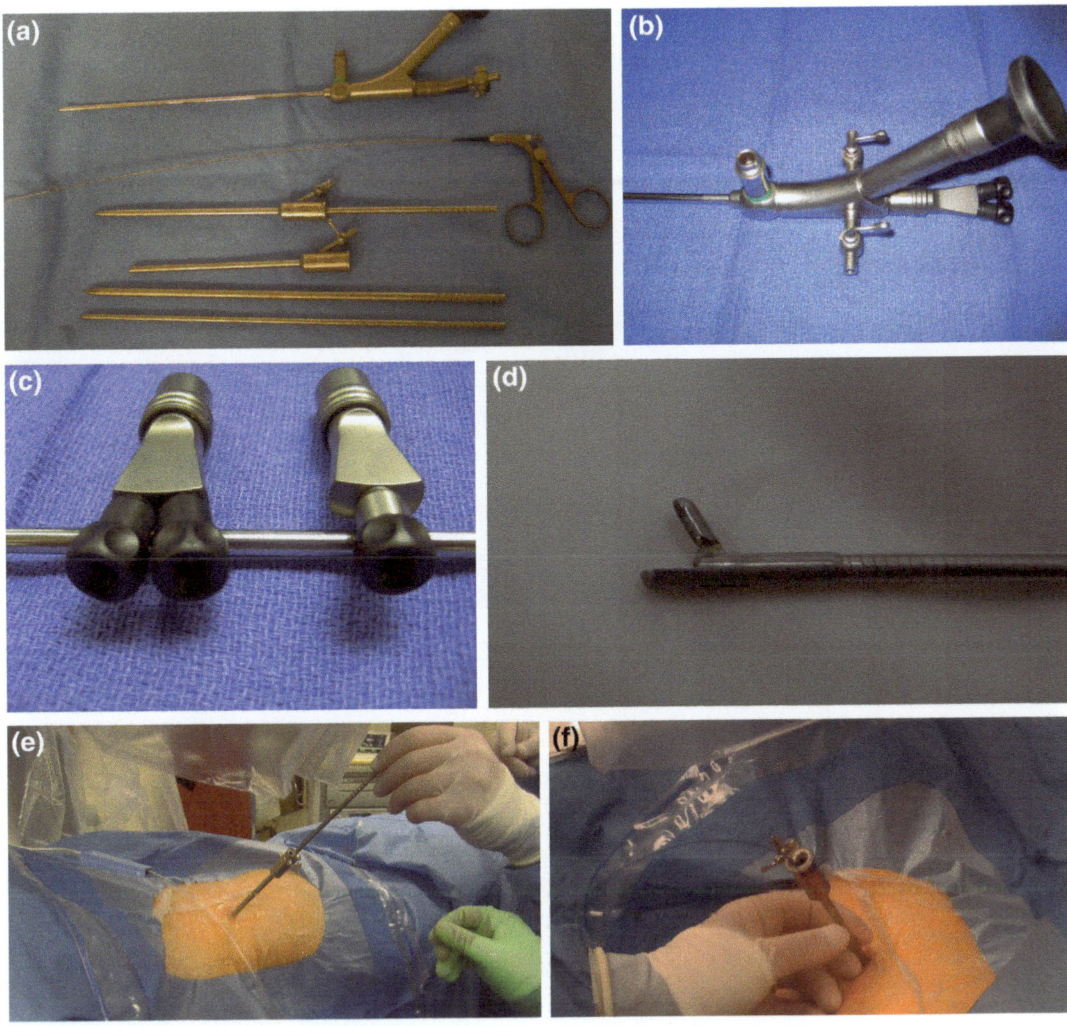

Fig. 22.4 **a** A mini-nephroscope with sheath and dilator **b** angled optic allows for use of rigid straight instrument, **c** double or single channel options, **d** cold cup biopsy, **e** dilation of tract, **f** work sheath in place, (22-V-2-Dilation prior to the use of miniscope)

required to avoid perforation of the collecting system. The wire can be angulated and directed down with use of a Cook Kumpe or similar angiographic catheters (Fig. 22.12). Once an angled tip catheter is in the renal pelvic with a straight tip wire can be used with angiographic catheter if needed. In some cases a glide wire is needed to manipulate past any lesions and down into the ureter yet there are times in which despite much effort, a wire cannot be passed down to the ureter. In such circumstance a guide wire is typically curled into the renal pelvis and the tract is dilated over the wire and once nephroscopy is performed usually a retrograde guide wire placed through the ureteral catheter can be retrieved to provide a safe through and through access.

Dilation

Dilation of the tract largely depends on the type of instrumentations that will be utilized. For large lesions and initial resections, a 24 Fr

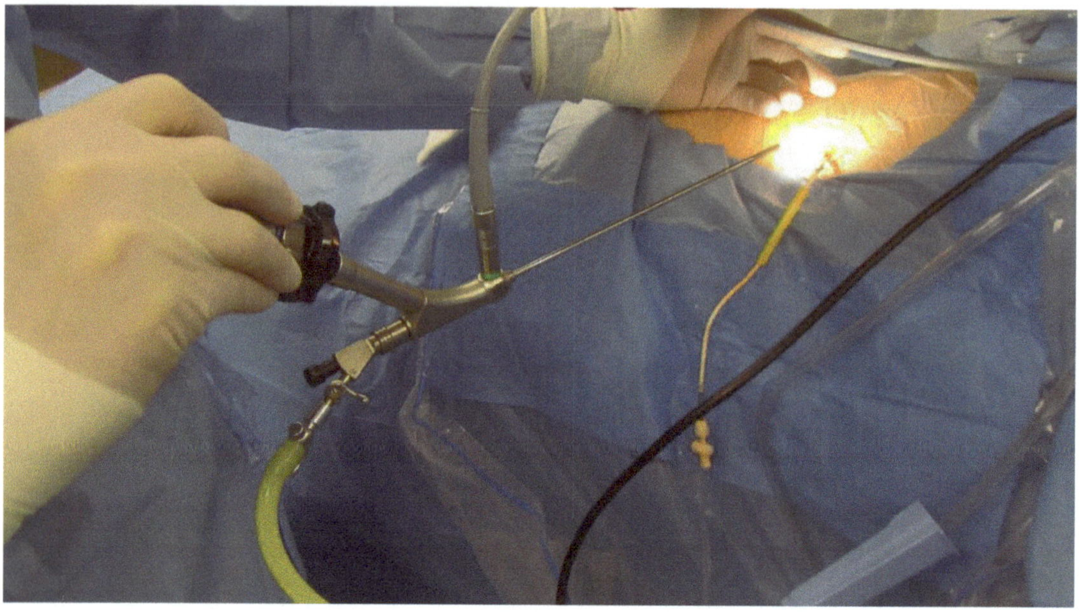

Fig. 22.5 In mature tracts the miniscope can be used for follow up surveillance without dilation or sheath

Fig. 22.6 Pediatric nephroscope

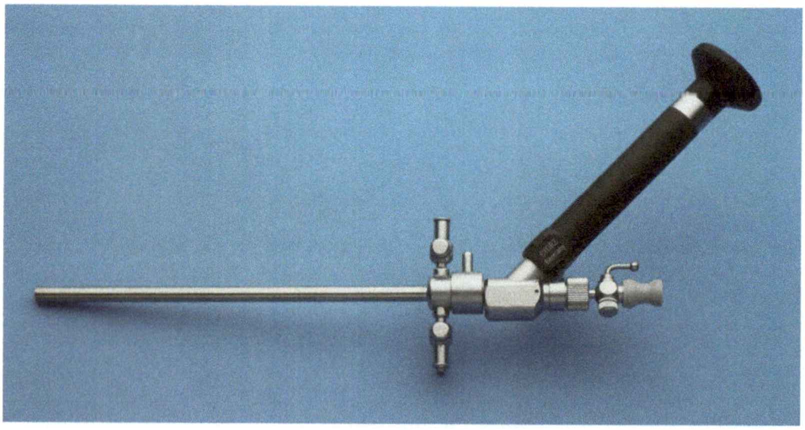

urethro-resectoscope or nephroscope is used and the tract is dilated as per standard percutaneous stone cases up to 30 Fr. However, for surveillance or low volume lesions we suggest using either a 12 Fr mini nephroscope, a 17.5 Fr pediatric nephroscope or a flexible cystoscope. If the operator decides to use a flexible cystoscope and to obtain large biopsies and perform electrocoagulation or laser ablation, an 18 Fr sheath with a balloon dilator can be used for this purpose (Cook Medical). If this equipment is not available, one can use sequential Teflon dilators up to 15 or 16 Fr and then use a 10 cm long balloon with a 6 Fr outer diameter to dilate up to 18 Fr and a backloaded 18 Fr sheath can be advanced over this to allow for nephroscopy using either pediatric nephroscope or flexible cystoscope. Individual clear sheath and small caliber sheaths are commercially available (Boston Scientific).

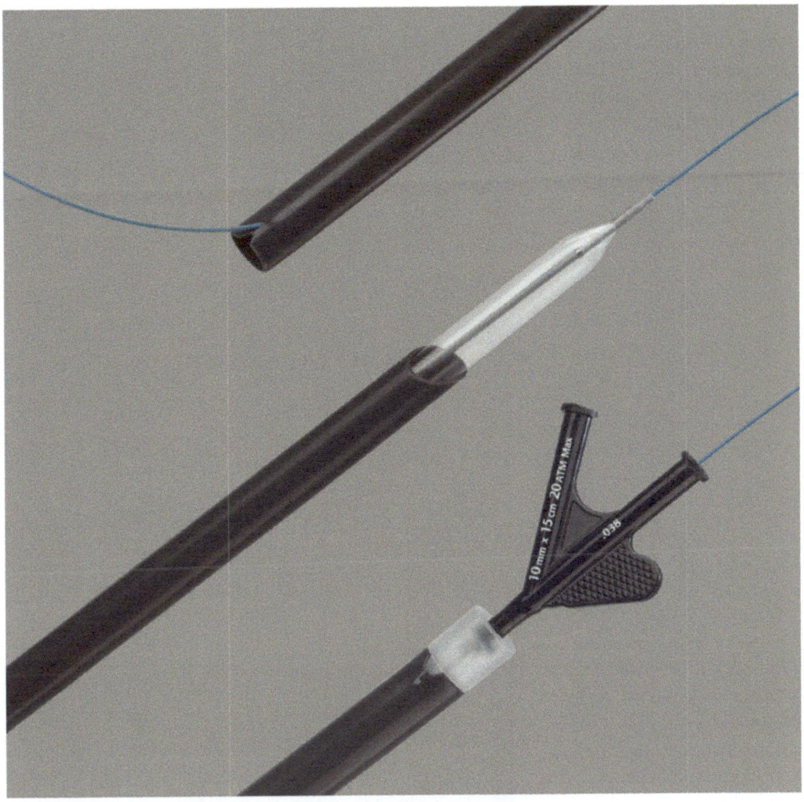

Fig. 22.7 18 Fr balloon and working sheath-Cook Medical

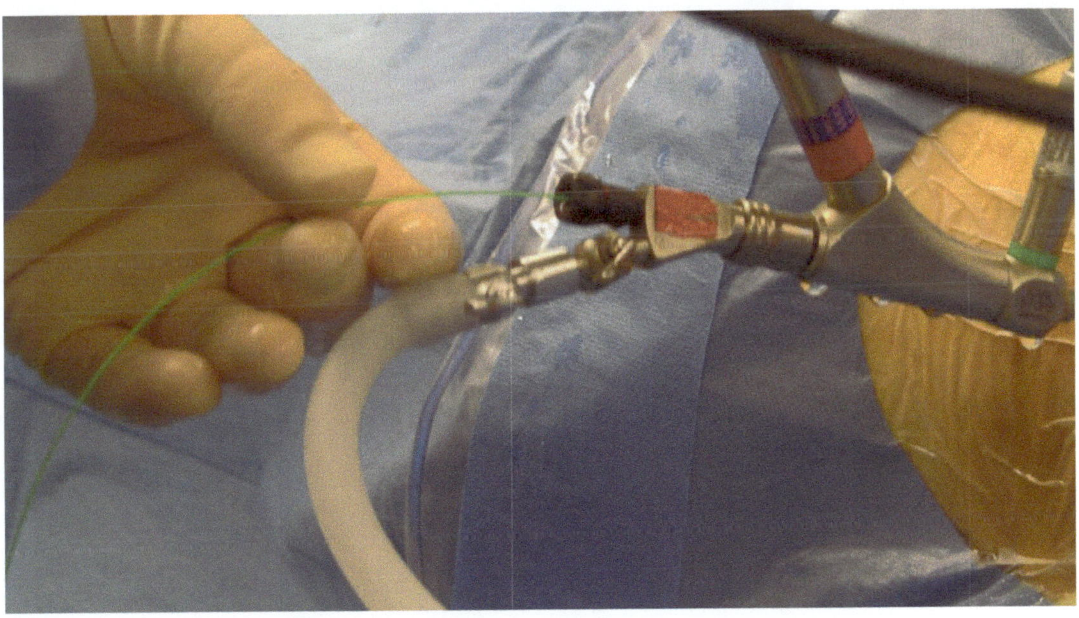

Fig. 22.8 Application of laser through a miniscope

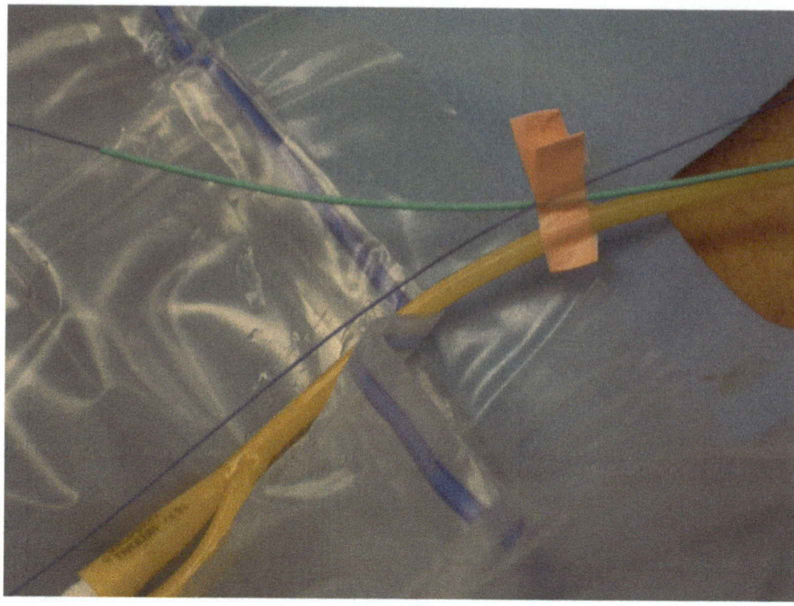

Fig. 22.9 Open ended catheter in sterile field for retrograde injection. Butterfly configuration allows for easy removal of tape

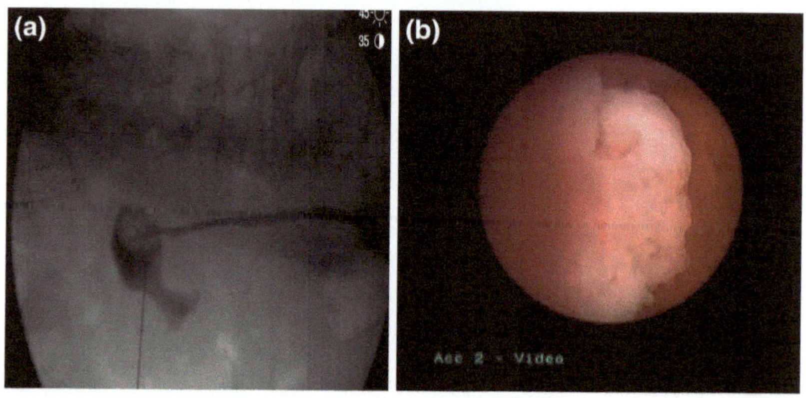

Fig. 22.10 **a** A mid calyceal puncture will allow perfect angle and view if a tumor involving renal pelvis and UPJ area **b** Endoscopic view of tumor

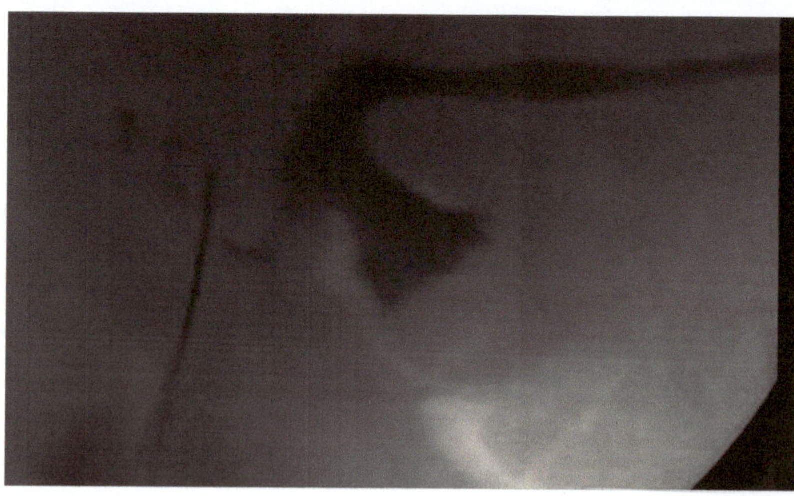

Fig. 22.11 A direct upper pole access for resection of upper pole calyx and infundibular tumor

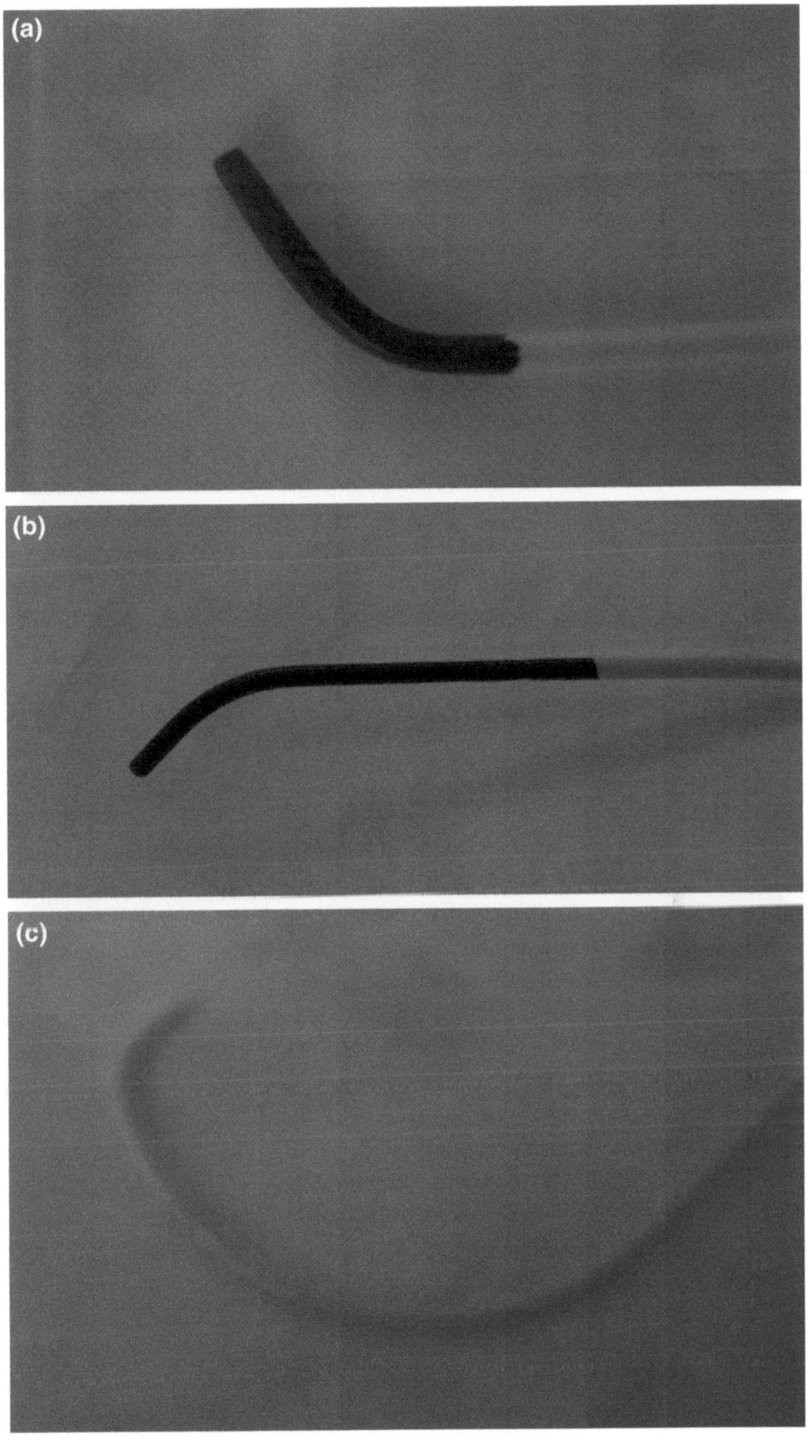

Fig. 22.12 **a–c** A variety angiographic type catheters for manipulation of wire in collecting system (Cook Urological©, Spencer, Indiana)

Initial Inspection

It is advisable to initially inspect all the calyces, the renal pelvis and the UPJ area thoroughly to assess the extent of the tumor prior to resection. Obviously, after extensive resection, it may be harder to use a flexible scope to access some of the peripheral calyces. So if there are small lesions in peripheral calyces, it may be advisable to use a flexible scope and ablate or remove these smaller lesions prior to resecting the larger central pelvic lesion. We use the large cold cup biopsy forceps to obtain several samples of tissue before any electrical resection. To avoid any electrocautery artifact that can affect pathologic assessment. At the completion of the resection one can take a deep biopsy of the base of the tumor for pathologic staging. In low volume disease, several large bite biopsies with the cold cup forceps will completely remove the tumor. One can then simply ablate the base with laser or electro cauterization.

Resection

As stated above with large volume disease, it is suggested to use a slender or standard resectoscope. Either a standard urethro-resectoscope with glycine or preferably a bipolar resectoscope with saline. It is recommended to use much lower energy settings than are used for TURBT or TURPS. In the kidney there is risk of transmission of electrical energy causing injury to the UPJ or vessels beyond the renal pelvis. One should use the minimal amount of energy that will allow for effective resection and fulguration, this also helps to avoid cautery artifact on the pathological specimens. The technique of resection is similar to resection for bladder tumors. Our practice is to resect the lesion starting from the periphery from one end of the lesion to the other. Careful resection must be performed near UPJ, the medial and ventral aspects of the renal pelvis to avoid resecting into the vasculature and causing strictures. If extensive tumor volume near the UPJ can prevent safe excursion of the resectoscope loop, we recommend using cold cup biopsy forceps to debulk the area allowing needed space and improved visibility for safe resection. Another area requiring careful and cautious resection is the infundibular conduit due to the vicinity of vessels and poor subepithelial musculature as was mentioned earlier. In cases where tumor has originated in a calyx and extended into the infundibular area the resection of calyceal area can be deep and cautiously advanced across the infundibulm and into the pelvis depending on the extent of the pathology. In the calyceal area urothelial muscureal layer is thin and directly over the parenchyma without submucosal or muscular layers (Fig 22.13a). In the infudibular area there is a very thin submucosal area and no significant muscle layers and as it merges with renal pelvis muscular layers become evident (Fig. 22.13b). Therefore an infiltrative high grade lesion in the calyx has different pathologic significance compared to renal pelvic lesion. Once the resection is complete a thorough inspection of the renal pelvis and calyces is performed before the resectoscope is removed. If adequate deep biopsies and tumor base samples are not obtained earlier, it is recommended to obtain deep cold cup biopsies of the base and the margins of the tumor at this time. In case resection is not adequate or as per surgeon's preference laser ablation of the base and margins can be performed at this stage. For review of Laser safety and settings refer to Chap. 14 (Video 22.5).

Unless the patient has previously undergone ureteroscopy we perform and antegrade flexible ureteroscopy at this time. In cases of intact ureteropelvic junction area antegrade ureteroscopy can be performed prior to resection of the tumor. To avoid egress of resected tissue and cells down the ureter a UPJ occlusion balloon can be placed over the through and through guide wire prior to the start of the resection. This maneuver can theoretically allow for holding a small amount of Mitomycin C in the renal pelvis before removal of occluding catheter. The post resection treatment with Mitomycin can then be completed as described later in this chapter.

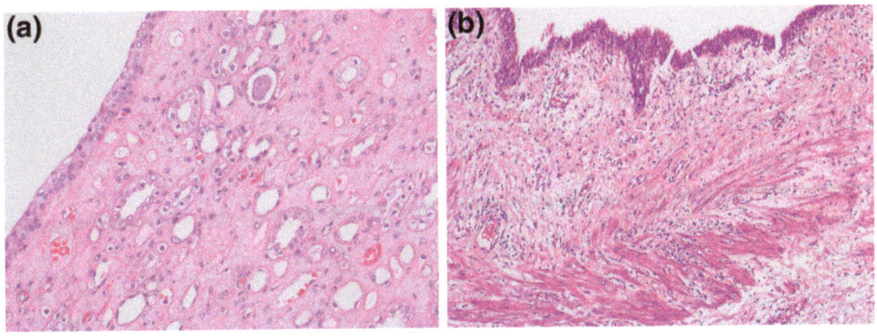

Fig. 22.13 **a** pathology slide showing calyceal resection showing no muscular layer **b** pathology slide showing resection closer to the pelvis showing muscular layer

Exit Strategy

The exit strategy for percutaneous resection of the renal pelvis depends on the following factors:

Location of the tumor.
Size of the tumor.
Invasive stage of the tumor that may dictate further treatment.
Consideration of postop intracavitary treatment.

At the completion of the procedure in the absence of obvious bleeding from the collective system, the following options are used.

If dilation is minimal and the mini nephroscope was used, a 10–12 Fr pigtail nephrostomy (Fig. 22.14) is placed.

If the dilation has been to #18 French, with resection, usually a 14 Fr pigtail or 16 Fr Foley type universal nephrostomy (Cook Urological) is a good option (Fig. 22.15).

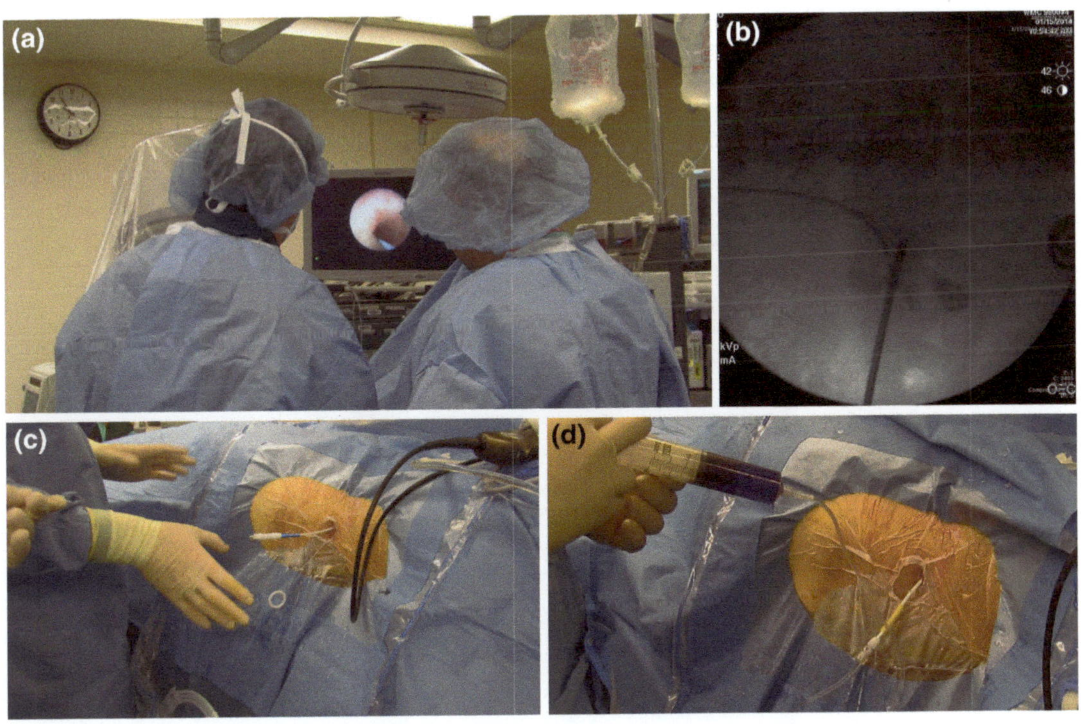

Fig. 22.14 **a** Mini nephroscope evaluation, **b** radiographic appearance of mini scope in collecting system, **c** placement of a 10.2 Fr single pigtail nephrostomy for postop intracavitary treatment and **d** immediate post nephroscopy mitomycin treatment

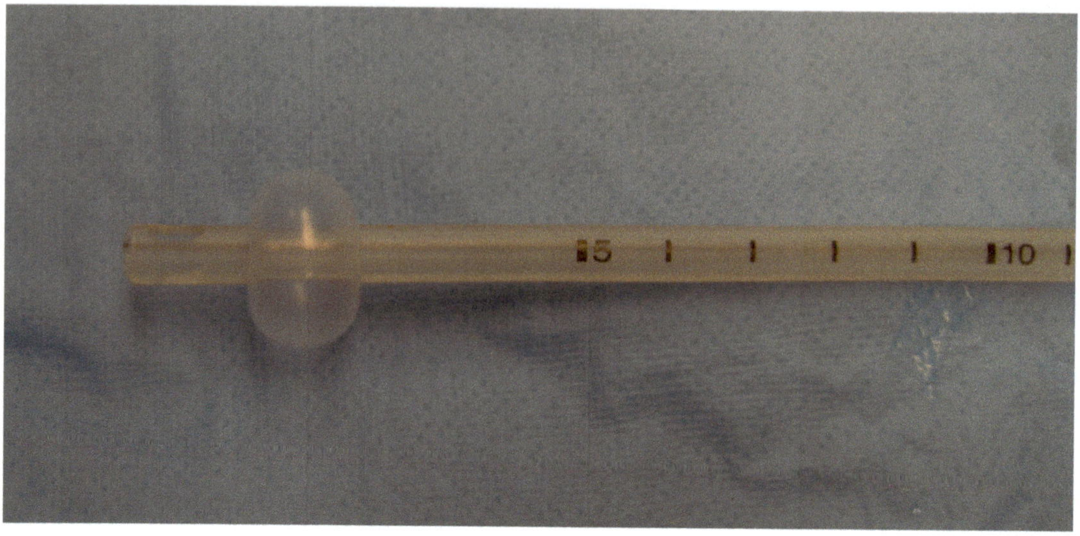

Fig. 22.15 Universa Foley Type nephrostomy tube (Cook Medical) with a rather short tip is ideal for a large renal pelvis post resection

After resection of large volume tumors, one can place a Malecot, a larger pigtail nephrostomy or a large Foley that can later on be exchanged to a smaller pigtail nephrostomy in anticipation of intracavitary treatment. In cases where hemostasis is an issue, it is always recommended to use larger nephrostomy tubes for initial control of the postoperative bleeding. This tube can later be modified to a smaller nephrostomy tube for postoperative intracavitary treatment.

For tumors resected near the UPJ, one can initially use a Malecot re-entry nephrostomy tube (Fig. 22.16), or a modified nephrostent (the distal end is custom cut) that goes halfway down the

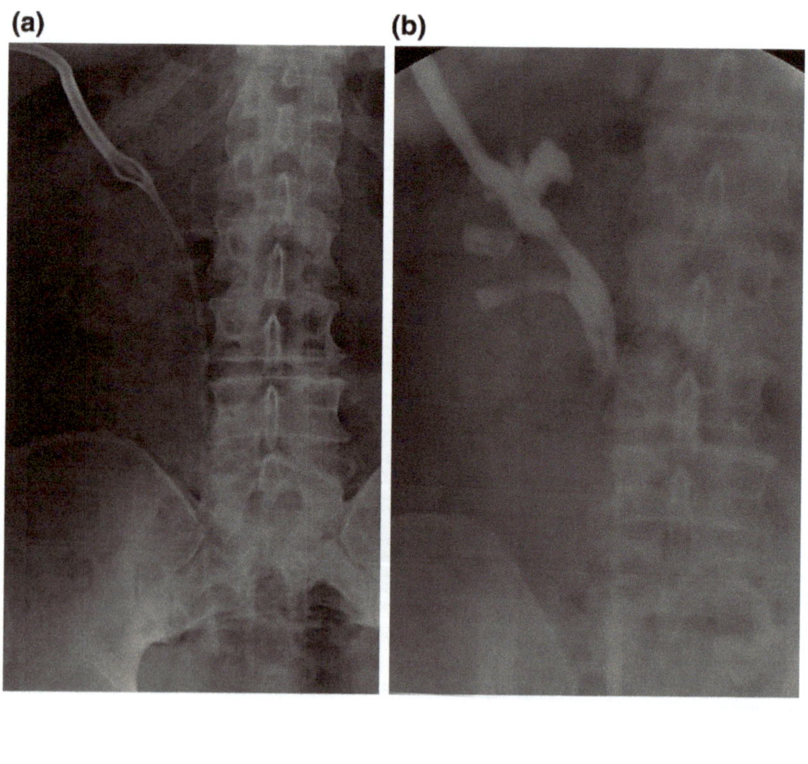

Fig. 22.16 **a** A Malecot re-entry nephrostomy tube used after resection of tumor in the renal pelvis and UPJ area **b** nephrostogram in a patient after resectio of upper calyceal tumor

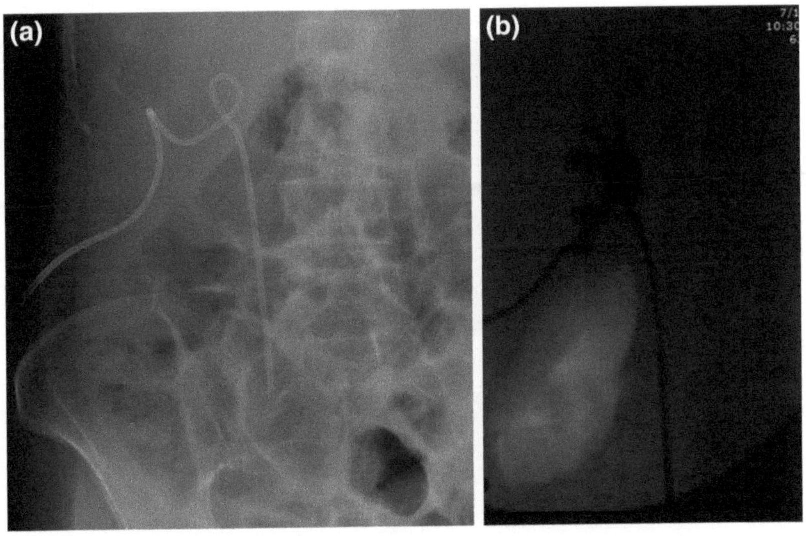

Fig. 22.17 **a** A modified distal end of nephrostent: custom cut to end in proxiamal to mid ureter after resection of pelvic tumor near UPJ **b** nephrostogram in the same patient

ureter to the level of iliac vessels (Fig. 22.17). They allow for drainage and stenting of the UPJ and upper ureter and eliminate the irritative effects of stent in the bladder. Another option is placement of a pigtail nephrostomy tube and placement of an open-ended ureteral catheter down the ureter. This is a temporary tube to allow initial healing of the UPJ and proximal ureter. If the surgeon deems long term stenting is needed, antegrade double pigtail stent can be placed with an additional nephrostomy for postop treatment. After adequate nephrostograms, one week later, it can be removed, smaller tubes placed and proceed with the intracavitary treatment. A modified nephrostent does not need to be changed, capping this tube turns into internal drainage system.

After the resection of tumor involving the calyces and infundibulum, a modified catheter is recommended. We use a sharp pair of scissors and create additional fenestration in the shaft of the pigtail nephrostomy or a regular nephrostomy tube. This allows drainage of the infundibular area where it is traversing. This is also helpful during the postoperative period for bathing the area during intracavitary treatment (Fig. 22.18).

Nephrostogram

After the nephrostomy tube is placed, a nephrostogram is performed under fluoroscopic control to confirm the location of the tube and make adjustment as needed with an eye for assessment of adequate drainage, bathing and surface contact anticipating postop intracavitary treatment.

Postop Intracavitary Treatment

Similar to treatment of bladder tumors at the completion of the procedure, 40 mg of mitomycin diluted in 60 cc of normal saline is slowly instilled through the nephrostomy tube over approximately 10–15 min to destroy possible floating cells. A full discussion of the indications and technique of intracavitary therapy is provided in Chap. 28.

Postop Management

During the initial postoperative phase, the nephrostomy tube is left open to allow for the

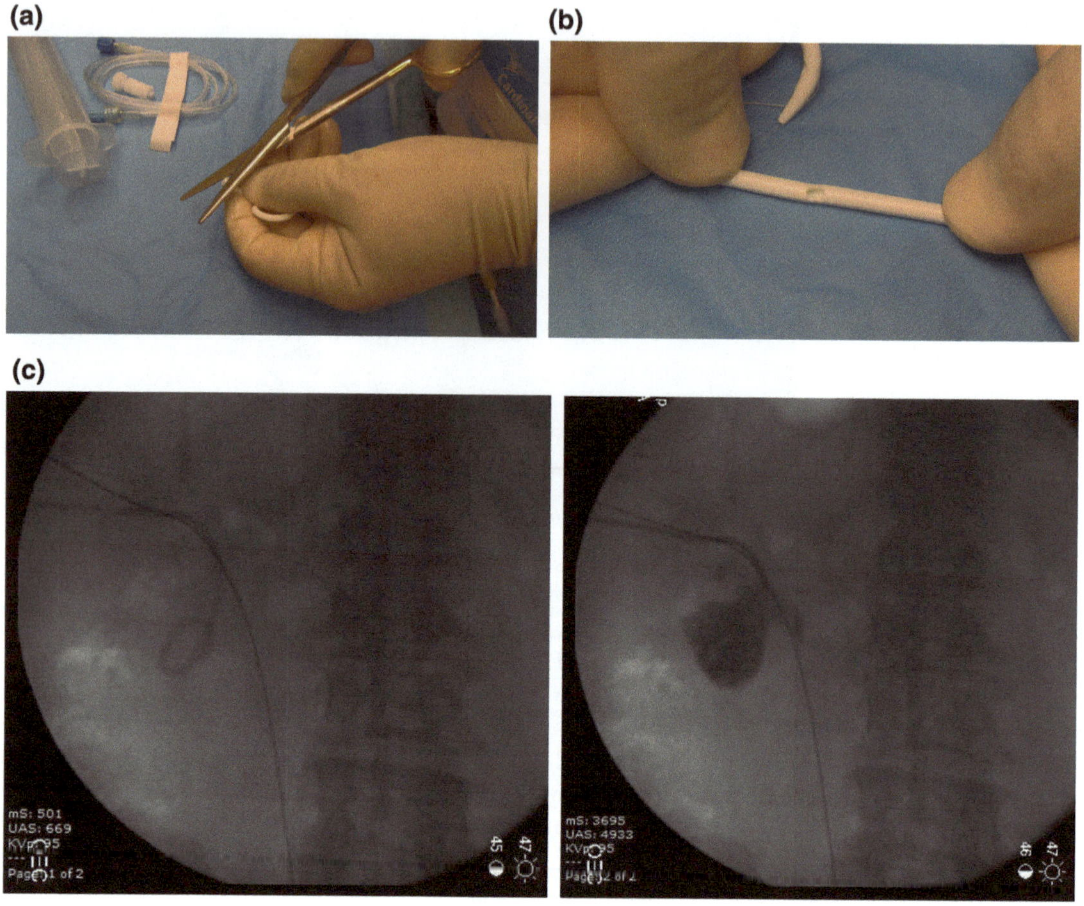

Fig. 22.18 **a** Creating a proximal fenestration, **b** appearance of proximal fenestration, and **c** radiologic appearance of tube in patient

healing of the resected area and sealing around the nephrostomy tube since the size of the tract is usually larger than the nephrostomy tube. After one week a nephrostogram is performed. If it shows satisfactory position of the nephrostomy tube for intracavitary treatment and no obvious extravasation, the nephrostomy tube can be capped with a three-way stopcock or preferably an autoseal Hep-Lock. This then can be accessed for outpatient intracavitary therapy.

If the final pathologic diagnosis suggests probable residual disease based on pathologic margins or intraoperative observation a second look procedure is performed within two to three days. In cases of large and bulky tumors we often plan a two stage procedure two to three days apart.

Electrocautery and Laser Ablation

Electrical ablation using Bugbee-type electrodes or laser ablation is safe inside the renal system. In cases where the surgeon does not feel comfortable with a resectoscope, they can be an alternative to resection. The Holmium laser is a pulsed laser familiar to most urologist due to its use for nephrolithiasis. It has a tissue penetration of only 0.5 mm, so it can be observed endoscopically. Typical settings for ablation is an energy of 0.8–1.2 J and frequency of 5–10 Hz. In contrast, the ND-YAG laser penetrates the tissue at least 5–10 mm, and unlike the Bugbee or the holmium laser it does not need to be in contact with the tissue for coagulation. However, its effect cannot be easily seen endoscopically, so care must be taken not to use higher settings than 25–30 W to avoid necrosing the renal pelvis and developing infundibular stenosis. Typically, the protocol is to ablate the surface lesion with holmium or Bugbee, or use the ND YAG to coagulate the bulk stalk and the base of the tumor. Finally, the periphery is coagulated to ensure hemostasis. Special care should be taken when using any of these instruments around the UPJ and ureter, as stricture formation is the most common complication of the treatment [18]. It also important to note if utilizing ablation therapy as a sole mode of tumor removal to obtain cold cup biopsies prior to ablation for grading and after ablation for assessment of pathologic margins. One of the limitations of the ablation technique is often the deep cold cup biopsy specimen is hard to process secondary to necrotic artifact from the Bugbee or laser [15]. In summary a variety of *combination techniques* can be used with variety of electrodes and laser fibers with precaution according to the preference of the surgeon. Deep lasering should be avoided in the medial, ventral aspects of renal pelvis, hilar and UPJ areas.

Summary Box

- Bulky tumors are best managed percutaneously.
- Percutaneous resection has the best outcome in low-grade disease.
- Follow up should include biopsy of resection site.
- Large cold cup biopsy provides accurate grade and stage.
- The shape of nephrostomy should allow for intracavitary treatment.
- Yag laser ablation allows for deep destruction of tumor.
- Primary resection of bulky tumor is best achieved with a resectoscope.
- UPJ and medial pelvic resection should be done cautiously.
- Intracavitary treatment is done as an outpatient.
- Antegrade or retrograde ureteroscopy should be part of surveillance nephroscopy.

References

1. Iwaszko MR, Krambeck AE. Conservative management of upper tract transitional cell carcinoma. Indian J Urol. 2008;24:159.
2. Rouprêt M, Babjuk M, Compérat E, et al. European association of urology guidelines on upper urinary tract urothelial cell carcinoma: 2015 update. Eur Urol. 2015;68:868.
3. Adamis S, Varkarakis J. Minimally invasive approach in the management of upper- urinary-tract tumours. Scand J Urol Nephrol. 2011;45:381.
4. Fuglsig S, Krarup T. Percutaneous nephroscopic resection of renal pelvic tumors. Scand J Urol Nephrol Suppl. 1995;172:15.
5. Plancke HR, Strijbos WE, Delaere KP. Percutaneous endoscopic treatment of urothelial tumours of the renal pelvis. Br J Urol. 1995;75:736.
6. Patel A, Soonawalla P, Shepherd SF, et al. Long-term outcome after percutaneous treatment of transitional cell carcinoma of the renal pelvis. J Urol. 1996;155:868.
7. Martínez-Piñeiro JA, García Matres MJ, Martínez--Piñeiro L. Endourological treatment of upper tract urothelial carcinomas: analysis of a series of 59 tumors. J Urol. 1996;156:377.
8. Clark PE, Streem SB, Geisinger MA. 13-year experience with percutaneous management of upper tract transitional cell carcinoma. J Urol. 1999;161:772.
9. Goel MC, Mahendra V, Roberts JG. Percutaneous management of renal pelvic urothelial tumors: long-term followup. J Urol. 2003;169:925.
10. Suh RS, Faerber GJ, Wolf JS. Predictive factors for applicability and success with endoscopic treatment of upper tract urothelial carcinoma. J Urol. 2003;170:2209.
11. Palou J, Piovesan LF, Huguet J, et al. Percutaneous nephroscopic management of upper urinary tract transitional cell carcinoma: recurrence and long-term followup. J Urol. 2004;172:66.
12. Cornu JN, Rouprêt M, Carpentier X, et al. Oncologic control obtained after exclusive flexible ureteroscopic management of upper urinary tract urothelial cell carcinoma. World J Urol. 2010;28:151.
13. Rastinehad AR, Ost MC, Vanderbrink BA, et al. A 20-year experience with percutaneous resection of upper tract transitional carcinoma: is there an oncologic benefit with adjuvant bacillus Calmette Guérin therapy? Urology. 2009;73:27.

14. Motamedinia P, Keheila M, Leavitt DA, et al. The expanded use of percutaneous resection for upper tract urothelial carcinoma: a 30-year comprehensive experience. J Endourol. 2015.
15. Cutress ML, Stewart GD, Zakikhani P, et al. Ureteroscopic and percutaneous management of upper tract urothelial carcinoma (UTUC): systematic review. BJU Int. 2012;110:614.
16. Tasca A, Zattoni F. The case for a percutaneous approach to transitional cell carcinoma of the renal pelvis. J Urol. 1990;143:902.
17. Rouprêt M, Traxer O, Tligui M, et al. Upper urinary tract transitional cell carcinoma: recurrence rate after percutaneous endoscopic resection. Eur Urol. 2007;51:709.
18. Johnson GB, Fraiman M, Grasso M. Broadening experience with the retrograde endoscopic management of upper urinary tract urothelial malignancies. BJU Int. 2005;95 Suppl 2:110.

Urothelial Carcinoma in Transplanted, Pelvic, and End Stage Kidneys

23

Roger Yau and Majid Eshghi

Historically, the pelvic kidneys are either congenital in the form of a single pelvic kidney or transplanted kidneys in the lower quadrant. Additionally, the end stage renal kidneys in hemodialysis dependent and transplanted patients also have the potential of forming urothelial cell carcinoma. Overall, the incidence of urothelial cell carcinoma in congenital pelvic kidneys is not different or higher than normally positioned native kidneys, and there are a very few reports of urothelial cell carcinoma in such kidneys. The end stage renal kidneys have generally a higher incidence of developing transformations into malignancy and urothelial cell carcinoma will be one of those. Patients with end stage renal disease who undergo renal transplant and have a history of smoking and bladder cancer and who are generally immunocompromised, carry a higher risk of developing urothelial cell carcinoma as well. The more common pathology in these patients is the classical renal cell carcinoma, unless the patient has had significant exposures to possible risk factors for urothelial cell carcinoma.

The urothelial cell carcinoma in transplanted kidneys is not a very common entity, and if the patient is the recipient and has had strong history of urothelial cell carcinoma of the bladder or previous nephroureterectomy, they can be at a higher risk of developing this disease, but again based on the reported cases in the literature, these cases are very few and far between.

The only exception to this is the region of Southeast Asia where when compared to the rest of the world, a relatively large number of cases are reported. There are several factors that can be accounted for and contributory to this entity of higher incidence of urothelial cell carcinoma in Southeast Asia in patients with transplanted kidney. Environmental factors are considered to be the most obvious of them all. Obviously, because of the low incidence of this disease, the literature of this subject is very sparse. In this chapter, we will address available data on upper tract urothelial cell carcinoma (UTUC) in patients with end stage renal disease as well as pelvic kidneys.

Congenital Pelvic Kidney

Congenital pelvic kidneys are due to an embryologic anomaly of ascent. In autopsy studies, the incidence averages 1 in 900 [1]. It is usually unilateral and more common on the left side. Due to the ectopia, pelvic kidneys are malrotated.

R. Yau · M. Eshghi (✉)
Department of Urology, Westchester Medical Health Network/New York Medical College, Valhalla, NY, USA
e-mail: majid_eshghi@nymc.edu

R. Yau
e-mail: Roger.yau@wmchealth.org

M. Eshghi (ed.), *Urothelial Malignancies of the Upper Urinary Tract*,
https://doi.org/10.1007/978-3-319-51263-1_23

Hydronephrosis, ureteropelvic obstruction, and reflux are common. Furthermore, pelvic kidneys are prone to developing urolithiasis. There have been no studies or case reports in the literature associating pelvic kidneys to increased UTUC. Urinary stasis and ectopic location is not associated with UTUC.

Autotransplantation and UTUC

Autotransplantation of the kidney is primarily used for ureteral injuries, obstruction, bench surgery for tumor, pain, or vascular anomalies. Patients do not need to be on immunosuppressants afterwards. In a 27 year retrospective review at two institutions at University of Oregon and Washington, they reviewed 51 patient who underwent renal autograft transplantation. With a median follow up of almost 2 years, none of their patients developed urothelial cell carcinoma [2]. The surgical action of moving the kidney and reanastomosis does not increase the risks of developing cancer unlike renal transplants.

Transplant Kidney and UTUC

The incidence of UTUC in the United States from 1985 to 1994 is 0.73 to 1.0 per 100,000 people per year from SEER database [3]. They only account for 6% of all renal tumors. The mean age of presentation is 65 years old. It is two times more likely in Caucasians and men, three times more likely in smokers, and up to 100–200 times more likely in the Balkan region due to diet and environmental influences. Southwestern Taiwan is another region afflicted by increased UTUC which is endemic due to high levels of arsenic in the soil which cause Blackfoot Disease [4].

During a renal transplant, the graft kidney is usually placed in the pelvis and the native kidneys are left in situ. There are some scenarios where the native kidneys are removed during transplantation which include: solid tumor, symptomatic kidney stones, chronic infections, unresponsive proteinuria mass effect from polycystic kidney disease, unresponsive hypertension, and persistent anti-GBM antibodies. Malignancies can occur both in the native kidneys and in the graft kidney. New cancers which develop after transplantation are called de novo malignancies.

Historically, in 1954, the first kidney transplant was successfully performed in identical twins. By the early 1960s there were 30 worldwide transplant centers. Immunosuppression is the mainstay medical therapy to prevent rejection of the graft. Throughout history there have been three main families of immunosuppressants used: azathioprine, cyclosporine (CYA), and mTOR inhibitors. Even in the early days of transplantation it was known that de novo malignancies were more common in transplant recipients due to immunosuppression. The most common types of cancer were skin, lymphoma, Kaposi sarcoma, and renal tumors in that order. It was estimated that the incidence of lymphoma was 40 times greater than the general population. The most common solid organ tumor was from the genitourinary tract. From review papers, the percentage of GU de novo malignancies ranges from 9.7 to 17% [5]. Many studies have also shown an association in de novo malignancies with male gender, increased age, and diabetes mellitus. There has even been one case study that reported complete regression of hepatocellular carcinoma after immunosuppressive therapy was decreased [6]. There have also been studies that have shown a direct cellular effect for cancer promotion by CYA. The newest family of immunosuppression, mTOR inhibitors, have been linked with up to 60% lower risk of de novo malignancies in post-transplant patients [5].

Urothelial carcinoma is an uncommon malignancy and most studies are retrospective. Most of the staging, grading, and treatment is borrowed from what is known about bladder cancer. However, studies have shown an increased association with UC and renal transplant recipients. Urothelial cell carcinoma in renal transplant recipients is endemic in some Asian countries and associated with Chinese herbal medicine use [7].

Aristolochic acid in Chinese herbal medicine leads to UC. It is known that Balkan nephropathy leads to increased UC due to diet which is high in Aristolochic acid. It is also found in Chinese herbal medicine used for weight loss and as a digestion aid. The use of the Chinese herb is associated with increased UC especially in Taiwan [8]. Other areas of Taiwan also have naturally high arsenic content in the soil that leads to Blackfoot disease and UTUC. Female predominance in Taiwan has been shown across many studies in acquired UTUC.

A single center in Taiwan analyzed their data of 52 renal transplant recipients and found 24 cases of UC which represented 43.6% of all de novo cancers [9]. Mean time to diagnosis was 46 months. The most common clinical signs were painless hematuria and pyuria. 9 patients (41%) had synchronous bilateral UTUC. 6 patients had widespread metastasis that resulted in death. In the literature this is one of the highest percentage of de novo UTUC. To note, these cases were often multifocal and invasive. Due to their findings they recommended prophylactic bilateral native nephroureterectomies in their patient population at the time of renal transplant.

A large single center in Beijing, China published their data on de novo UC in renal transplant recipients to add to the little known literature outside of Taiwan [9, 10]. They looked at a total of 1429 transplant recipients and found 27 to have developed de novo upper tract UC on average of 44 months later. 59.3% of the UTUC patients had taken Chinese herbs containing aristolochic acid. The incidence of UTUC was 5.42% compared to 0.97% in the group that took aristolochic acid and those that did not respectively. They found that female gender, the Chinese herb, and persistent immunosuppression were risk factors for developing post transplant UTUC. This is contrary to previous findings that males were more susceptible to genitourinary cancers. The most common clinical presentations were gross and microscopic hematuria. One patient had asymptomatic hydronephrosis (Fig. 23.1).

A US study by Engels et al. of all solid organ transplant recipient registries, found the incidence of de novo cancers, and compared them to the expected incidence from cancer registries [11]. They found men at increased risk. Renal transplant recipients were 6.6 times likely to have kidney cancer. These commonly presented in a bimodal fashion; at 1 year and 4–15 years post transplant. They did not distinguish between RCC and UTUC. Bladder cancer was 1.52 times more likely to occur in transplant recipients.

As mentioned earlier, malignancies can also occur in the graft. There have been case reports of UC developing in the kidney graft. In a retrospectively reviewed study of 1365 renal transplant recipients and found 2 that developed UC of the graft [12]. Both patients were women and presented with hydronephrosis. They were found to have high grade UC invading into the fat. Cytogenetics was performed on one female patient's pathology sample and the cells were found to be male which corresponded with her donor's gender. Both patients were successfully treated with transplant nephrectomies. When a living donor develops UTUC in the ureteral remnant of the donated kidney, the recipient must be evaluated and followed closely for developing the same cancer.

Urothelial Cell Carcinoma in End Stage Renal Disease (ESRD)

Sadly, the majority of people with ESRD do not receive a kidney transplant and remain on dialysis due to the lack of available donor grafts. There have been studies comparing the cancer risk in dialysis versus post-transplant that showed the risk only increased after transplantation [13] however others have found ESRD on dialysis have their independent association with increased risk of de novo cancers. In an international collaborative study by Maisonneuve et al. more than 800,000 patients were reviewed from 3 continents [14]. They found 3–7% de novo cancer rate among ESRD patients on dialysis. Genitourinary cancers were the most common type of cancer. Bladder cancer was one and a half times more likely and kidney cancer was 3.6 times more likely. Kidney cancer was also found to be associated with longer time on

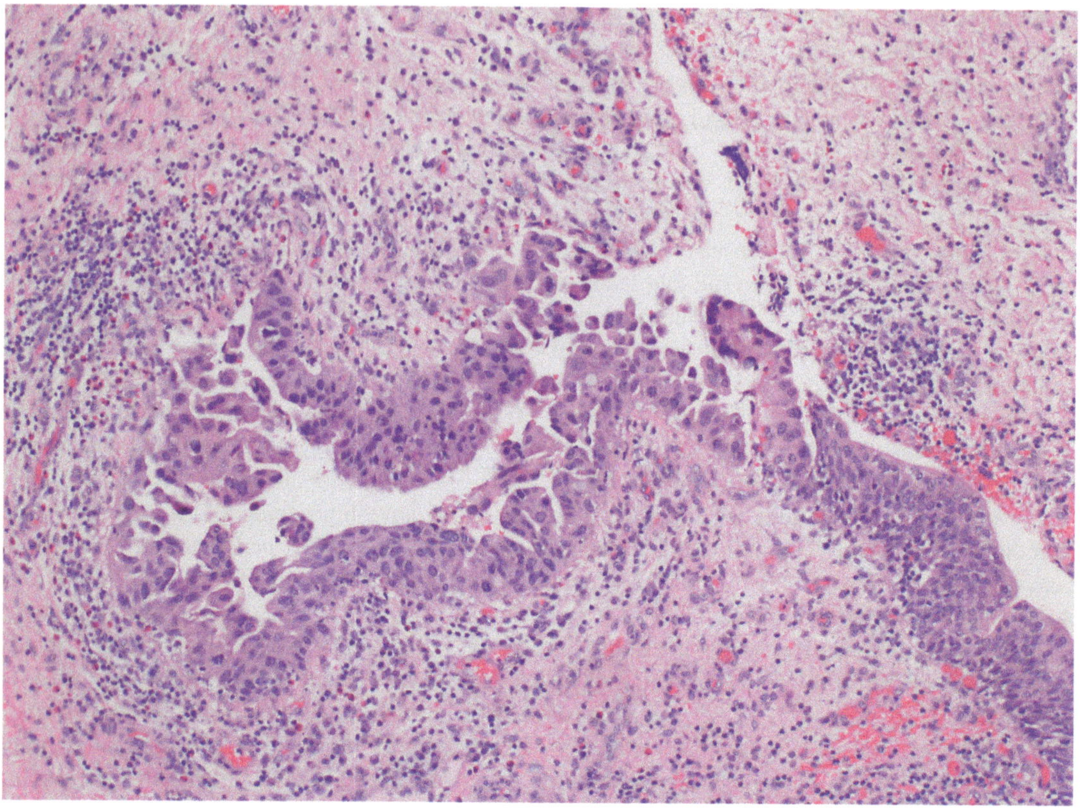

Fig. 23.1 High power histologic evaluation in a collecting system in transplant kidney with UC

dialysis. Interestingly, younger patients in the 35–64 year old age group were at a higher risk. Genitourinary cancers were most highly associated with infectious or toxic renal disease. The type of dialysis was not significant for the risk of de novo malignancies. However, this study did not distinguish kidney cancers into renal or urothelial cell carcinoma.

Bladder Cancer in Renal Transplant Recipients

Bladder cancer is much more common than UTUC and therefore has many NCCN guidelines for management and treatment. Renal transplant recipients have a higher incidence of developing bladder cancer, however, treatment remains the same. A study from Sloan Kettering Cancer Center reported on 17 patients in an 11 year span who developed bladder cancer after renal transplantation [15]. BCG was seen to be a viable option for non-muscle invasive bladder cancer even though the patients continued on their immunosuppressive regimen [16]. The use of BCG immunotherapy in post organ transplant and other immunosuppressed or compromised conditions should be exercised with extreme caution. It requires survey of all potential organs at danger (lungs, endstage kidneys, etc.) and close follow up of patients.

Summary Box

- There is no increase incidence of UTUC in congenital pelvic kidneys or autotransplanted kidneys.
- Renal transplant recipients are at a higher risk of de novo malignancies due to immunosuppression. They have substantially elevated rates of skin

cancer, Kaposi sarcoma, and genitourinary malignancies such as UTUC, kidney cancer, and bladder cancer.

- Chinese herb nephropathy is caused by aristolochic acid.
- There is a male predominance in post transplant recipient de novo UTUC except in Chinese herb nephropathy.
- Renal cancer and UC in ESRD patients on dialysis is increased. It is associated with a younger age group, length of time on dialysis, and toxic renal disease.
- Bladder cancer can be treated safely with BCG in renal transplant recipients on immunosuppression.
- Radical cystectomy and urinary diversion is possible but challenging in renal transplant recipients.

References

1. Abeshouse BS, Bhisitkul I. Crossed renal ectopia with and without fusion. Urol Int. 1959;9:63–91.
2. Cowan NG, et al. Renal autotransplantation: 27-year experience at 2 institutions. J Urol. 2015; 194(5):1357–61.
3. Munoz JJ, Ellison LM. Upper tract urothelial neoplasms: incidence and survival during the last 2 decades (0022–5347 (Print)).
4. Wein AJ, et al. Campbell-Walsh urology. Elsevier Health Sciences; 2015.
5. Kauffman HM, et al. Post-transplant de novo malignancies in renal transplant recipients: the past and present. Transpl Int. 2006;19(8):607–20.
6. Chuang FR, et al. Increasing transplant cancer patient survival by conversion of immunosuppressive agents (0041–1345 (Print)).
7. Zhang A, et al. A retrospective review of patients with urothelial cancer in 3370 recipients after renal transplantation: a single-center experience. World J Urol. 2015;33(5):713–7.
8. Lai MK, Tai HC, Wang SM. Urothelial carcinoma in renal transplant recipients. In: Trzcinska M, editor. Kidney transplantation—new perspectives. InTech; 2011.
9. Kao Y-L, et al. Transitional cell carcinoma in renal transplant recipients. World J Surg. 2003;27(8):912–6.
10. Li XB, et al. Transitional cell carcinoma in renal transplant recipients: a single center experience. Int J Urol. 2008;15(1):53–7.
11. Engels EA, et al. Spectrum of cancer risk among US solid organ transplant recipients. JAMA. 2011;306 (17):1891–901.
12. Hevia V, et al. Transitional cell carcinoma of the kidney graft: an extremely uncommon presentation of tumor in renal transplant recipients. Case Rep Transplant. 2013;2013:196528.
13. Birkeland SA, Lokkegaard H, Storm HH. Cancer risk in patients on dialysis and after renal transplantation. Lancet. 2000;355(9218):1886–7.
14. Stewart JH, et al. Cancers of the kidney and urinary tract in patients on dialysis for end-stage renal disease: analysis of data from the United States, Europe, and Australia and New Zealand. J Am Soc Nephrol. 2003;14(1):197–207.
15. Prabharasuth D, et al. Management of bladder cancer after renal transplantation. Urology. 2013;81(4):813–9.
16. Master VA, et al. Treatment and outcome of invasive bladder cancer in patients after renal transplantation. J Urol. 2004;171(3):1085–8.

24 Metastatic Nodal Pattern: Is There a Role for Paraaortic Lymph Node Dissection

David M. Golombos, Patrick Lewicki, Jullet Han and Douglas S. Scherr

Introduction

Upper tract urothelial carcinoma (UTUC) represents only 5% of urothelial carcinomas [1, 2], but the overall incidence has slowly risen from 1.88 to 2.06 cases per 100,000 person-years from 1973 to 2005 [3]. Over that period, there has been an increased detection of in situ lesions, which may be a result of increased use of bladder cancer surveillance regimens and improved cross-sectional imaging. However, in those treated surgically with either radical nephroureterctomy (RNU) or segmental ureterectomy (SU) there has been a stage and grade migration toward more aggressive disease, with more extensive and aggressive surgery used in individuals with more advanced disease stages in the most contemporary years [4]. Overall, up to about 30% of UTUC cases have lymph node (LN) involvement, the most common site of metastasis [5–7]. Nodal involvement is a poor prognostic indicator. It represents the strongest adverse pathological feature in regard to prognosis in patients treated with RNU, and chemotherapy or radiotherapy rarely results in improvement in patient survival [8, 9]. Novara et al. [10], in one of the largest published series of RNU for UTUC, found LN involvement to be an independent predictor of cancer-specific mortality (CSM), with a threefold increased risk compared to node-negative patients. Evidence suggests lymphadenectomy plays at least a staging role in renal cell carcinoma [11] and prostate cancer [12]. Pelvic LN dissection is widely accepted as a crucial component of surgical management of urothelial carcinoma of the bladder (UCB), with retrospective evidence demonstrating possible improvement in cancer-specific survival (CSS) and overall survival (OS) [13–15]. However, at least in part due to the relative rarity of UTUC, practice patterns regarding nodal management widely vary and questions remain about the role of lymph node dissection (LND) in this disease. This chapter hopes to address some of these outstanding questions as we examine the role of LND in the surgical management of patients with UTUC.

D. M. Golombos · D. S. Scherr (✉)
Department of Urology, New York Presbyterian Hospital—Weill Cornell Medical Center, 525 East 68th Street, Starr Pavilion, 9th floor, New York, NY 10065, USA
e-mail: dss2001@med.cornell.edu

D. M. Golombos
e-mail: dag2042@med.cornell.edu

P. Lewicki · J. Han
Department of Urology, Weill Cornell Medical College, New York, NY 10021, USA
e-mail: pjl2002@med.cornell.edu

J. Han
e-mail: jh2383@gmail.com

M. Eshghi (ed.), *Urothelial Malignancies of the Upper Urinary Tract*,
https://doi.org/10.1007/978-3-319-51263-1_24

Incidence of Lymph Node Invasion

The incidence of LN involvement has been shown to be influenced various by factors, including tumor location, stage, and grade. Kondo et al. [16] showed tumors involving the renal pelvis, upper ureter, and middle ureter had a higher incidence of LN metastasis (20–43%) while tumors involving the distal ureter had a lower incidence (8–13%). In this same analysis, incidence of positive LNs increased in a step-wise fashion with increasing stage, with 0, 5, 24, and 84% in patients with Tis/Ta/T1, T2, T3, and T4 respectively. High-tumor grade was associated with increased nodal involvement, as LN invasion was present in 0, 11, and 35% of patients with G1, G2, and G3 tumors, respectively. In 2009, a multi-institution collaboration, the Upper Tract Urothelial Carcinoma Collaboration (UTUCC) was created to collect data on RNUs performed across 13 tertiary care institutions. Evidence from these studies also demonstrates the impact of stage and grade, with 6, 16, and 35% of patients with positive LNs in pT1, pT2, and pT3–4 disease. With the now standard two tiered grading system, they found only 6% of patients with LN involvement to have low-grade (LG) disease, with the remaining having high-grade (HG) tumors [8, 17].

Regional Lymph Nodes

Multiple studies have demonstrated that patterns of UTUC nodal metastasis are highly dependent on tumor location and laterality. Early studies conducted from the 1980s showed that tumors of the renal pelvis and upper ureter primarily spread to the paraaortic and paracaval nodes, and those of the distal ureter spread to the pelvic nodes [18–20].

Compared with bladder cancer, LND for UTUC has the additional consideration of laterality and asymmetry of great vessels and renal vasculature, which more recently has been the subject of further investigation. In 2006, Assouad et al. [21] injected dye into cadavers in an attempt to understand renal lymphatic drainage patterns, highlighting this asymmetry by demonstrating para- and retrocaval drainage from the right kidney and predominantly hilar and paraaortic drainage from the left kidney. Kondo and colleagues have done extensive work to try to provide a better understanding of the influence of laterality and the location of the primary tumor in regards to patterns of lymphatic metastasis. Starting in 2007, they have performed mapping studies to analyze the primary sites of lymphatic metastases of UTUC according to the location of the primary tumor using surgically excised specimens and/or imaging analysis [6]. Their initial work supported that of Assouad, noting again that the primary sites of lymphatic metastasis encompassed a relatively wide area, especially on the right side. The mapping studies will be discussed in greater detail later in this chapter in regards to surgical templates. However, largely they have reported primary tumors originating from the right renal pelvis and upper two-thirds of the ureter to metastasize to the hilar, paracaval, retrocaval, and interaortocaval nodes. Tumors involving the left renal pelvis and upper two-thirds of the ureter metastasize to the renal hilum, interaortocaval, and paraaortic nodes. Tumors involving the distal ureter commonly spread to the ipsilateral pelvic lymph nodes beyond the aortic bifurcation (Fig. 24.1) [6, 22].

In the 2009 TNM classification of upper urinary tract urothelial cell carcinoma [23], the regional lymph nodes are considered to be the hilar, abdominal paraaortic, and paracaval nodes, and for the ureter the intrapelvic nodes. Laterality currently does not affect the *N* classification.

Role of Lymphadenectomy

LND has been shown to offer staging benefits for many malignancies, including UCB, as it assesses for microscopic metastasis and often guides postoperative management regarding systemic adjuvant chemotherapy. Furthermore, it offers a therapeutic benefit by reducing the overall tumor burden if micro-metastatic disease is present. LND for UCB has been shown to offer both staging and therapeutic benefits and is highly

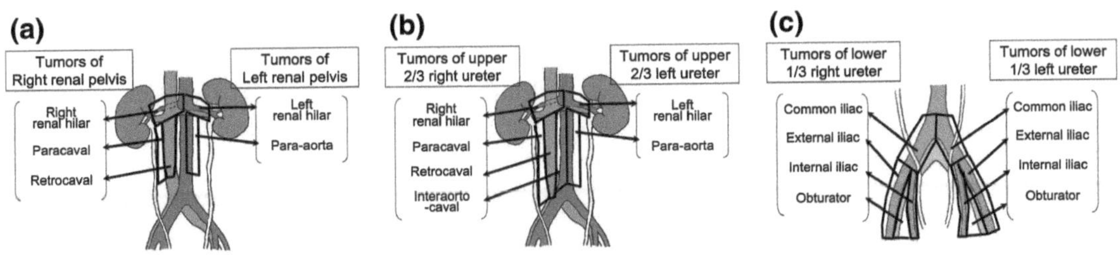

Fig. 24.1 Regional lymph node schema according to primary tumor locations **a** renal pelvis; **b** upper two-thirds of ureter; **c** lower third of ureter. From Kondo et al. [16]; used with permission

recommended for those undergoing a cystectomy [24–26]. However, given the low incidence of UTUC, most studies are retrospective and underpowered, resulting in an increase in combined multi-institutional data. Inconsistencies in practice patterns regarding the performance, location, and extent of LND also make it more difficult to extrapolate tangible benefits of performing LND for UTUC. Secin et al. [27] found that the individual surgeon was a significant predictor of whether LND was performed, even after controlling for tumor and patient characteristics. Consequently, up to 60% of patients undergoing RNU for UTUC do not undergo LND at the time of surgery [17].

Staging Role

There is a growing body of evidence to support that LND performed at the time of RNU is the best way to completely and accurately stage UTUC. This is especially important considering our lack of ability to accurately stage patients preoperatively. Urine cytology has limited diagnostic accuracy in the detection of UTUC, with sensitivity and positive predictive values (PPV) at 56 and 54% for HG and 62 and 44% for muscle-invasive UTUC [28]. Ureteroscopic biopsy is the gold standard for visualizing and establishing the definitive diagnosis of UTUC. However, while grade specification for biopsies are highly correlative with pathological grade [29], studies have shown as low as 60% concordance rates between pT stage from initial biopsy to follow up biopsy or surgical resection [30].

Computed tomography (CT) imaging has also demonstrated limited utility in the staging of upper tract disease. Scoleri et al. [31] reported the overall accuracy of CT in predicting the pathologic TNM stage was 59.5%, with understaging in 16.2% of patients, and failure to detect metastatic disease in 24.3% of scans. Secin et al. [27] found 40% of pN+ patients had no sign of LN enlargement on previous CT scan.

Several papers have investigated the role of LND and nodal status, including two large multi-institutional studies. In the first, Roscigno et al. [32] looked at 132 consecutive patients with muscle-invasive UTUC who underwent radical surgery and found that 5 year CSS in pNx patients was significantly worse than in pN0 patients (48% vs. 73%, $p = 0.001$). Interestingly, both disease-free survival (DFS) and CSS of pNx patients was comparable to those of pN+ patients, which was confirmed on multivariable Cox regression analysis, where LN status was a significant predictor of DFS and CSS. Based on their findings, authors strongly supported the need for LND in patients with muscle-invasive disease.

In a second large multi-institutional study, the UTUCC collected data on 1130 consecutive patients with pT1–4 UTUC treated with RNU [8]. 522 (49%) underwent LND, which was performed based on surgeon decision. The 5 year CSS was lower in patients with pNx disease, which in turn was lower than those with pN0 disease. In pT1 patients, CSS was not different in patients with pN0 and pNx disease, although this may be reflective of the low probability of LN involvement ($n = 7$) in this subset of patients. In pT2–4 cases, CSS estimates were lowest in pN+

patients, intermediate in pNx, and highest in pN0 (33% vs. 58% vs. 70% $p = 0.017$). These findings once again indicate improved disease staging with LND, especially in those with muscle-invasive disease, and show LAD may aid in identifying the patients with worse prognosis who should be considered for adjuvant chemotherapy.

While up to 30% of patients with muscle-invasive UTUC have metastasis to regional LNs [33, 34], patients with lower stage disease have lower incidence of LN metastasis and the staging role of LND becomes less clear. In their examination of 184 patients who underwent RNU for UTUC, Brown et al. [35] failed to demonstrate a survival advantage in pNx versus pN0 patients. This series examined all tumors, and nearly 50% were noninvasive. Lughezzani et al. [36] also found no statistically different difference in CSM rates examining >2800 patients using Surveillance, Epidemiology and End Results (SEER) registries. Authors offer several explanations for the observed discrepancy between their findings and previous findings supporting benefit to LND. These include the possibility that low-risk patients were identified by their surgeons as such and thus were spared from LND.

Recently, Xylinas et al. [37] analyzed 814 patients treated by RNU with LND and estimated the sensitivity of pathological nodal stating using a beta-binomial model. They determined that the probability of missing lymph node metastasis decreased as the number of LN examined increased, and if only a single node was examined, 44% of patients would have been misclassified at having pN0 disease while harboring LN metastasis. They used their analysis to create a pathological nodal staging score (pNSS) which predicts the probability that a patient with pathologically confirmed negative LNs is free of occult LN metastasis based on pT stage, lymphovascular invasion (LVI), and the number of LN analyzed. They concluded that each patient who undergoes RNU for UTUC needs LND, and believe the pNSS may help refine clinical decision-making regarding the administration of adjuvant chemotherapy.

Therapeutic Role

While LND performed at the time of RNU remains the most accurate means to completely and accurately stage patients with UTUC, several reports have also offered persuasive rationale for the therapeutic benefits of comprehensive LND in urothelial cancer.

Skinner [38] was one of the first to report on the possibility of curative pelvic LND during radical cystectomy (RC) in patients with advanced UCB. Poulsen et al. [39] reported on improved recurrence-free survival (RFS) rates for patients undergoing RC when extending the limits of pelvic LND from the bifurcation of the common iliac vessels to the bifurcation of the aorta. A large retrospective series by Stein et al. [40] reported a durable 34% 10-year RFS in patients with LN metastasis identified from LND at the time of RC, and later reported a survival advantage associated with greater than 15 nodes. Herr et al. [41] demonstrated improved survival for patients with >10 LN versus <10 LN removed at the time of RC. Furthermore, a report from Koppie et al. [13] showed the probably of survival did not plateau but instead continued to rise as the number of LNs removed increased. These studies highlight the importance of LND in the surgical management of urothelial cancer, and led the Bladder Cancer Collaborative Group to suggest surgical standards for RC, including at least 10–14 LN retrieval [42]. However, although there is general agreement on the need for optimizing the quality of LN dissection, this is hindered by the lack of a defined template of LN dissection and a standardized method of evaluating and reporting LN specimens.

The therapeutic benefit of LND for UTUC is less well established due to its relative rarity. Rational is supported by repots as previously noted, and several studies have investigated its potential therapeutic role. In 1998, Miyake et al. [43] reported on 72 patients and demonstrated a survival advantage in patients undergoing LND who did not have LVI. Brausi et al. [44] described the possible curative role of LND in patients with infiltrative UTUC. Retrospective review of 82 patients with invasive UTUC revealed advantage in both DFS and CSS in those who received LND versus those who did not. Margulis et al. [34] also provided evidence for possible curative role of LND in a subset of patients, where they looked at over 1300 patients treated with RNU, they noted despite LN involvement, 35% of patients were alive at 5 years, and 32% alive at 10 years. In a prospective, nonrandomized, multi-institutional trial of template-based LND, Kondo et al. [45] showed a significant benefit of LND on CSS and OS in patients with invasive cancer of the renal pelvis.

Roscigno et al. [32] also reported LND as a strong independent predictor of DFS and CSS in patients surgically managed for muscle-invasive UTUC. They were also one of the first to suggest that the number of LNs removed and examined may play a significant role in predicting clinical outcome after radical surgery for UTUC, as they noted that the higher number of LNs removed and examined was associated with significant improvement in both DFS and CSS.

However, conflicting evidence exists as to whether the number of nodes affects the therapeutic value of LND. In a large multicenter study from the UTUCC, the number of LNs removed was an independent predictor of CSM in node-negative patients. They observed longer survival in patients in whom at least eight LNs had been removed, essentially demonstrating that at least eight LN must be removed to ensure a higher likelihood of true pN0 status [17]. On the contrary, when reviewing 312 patients with UTUC treated predominately with RNU, Abe et al. [46] did note a difference in survival between pN0 and pNx groups. However, in those who did undergo LND, the median number of LN removed was six, and they were unable to show a significant difference in CSS between the patients who had more or less than six LN removed. Similarly, in patients with muscle-invasive clinical node-negative patients, Kondo et al. [47] found that the total number of LN removed had no significant influence on survival. Rather, authors suggested the total number of LN removed may be used only for assessing the quality of the LND.

Lymph node density (the percentage of the number of LNs involved with tumor divided by the total number of LNs examined) has been examined in UCB [14]. Stein et al. [48] found lymph node density lower than 20% is likely to predict better survival of patients with UCB who had LN involvement. Several studies in various malignancies have also suggested that lymph node density may have greater prognostic value than absolute numbers of LNs [49, 50]. This concept was examined in UTUC by Bolenz et al. [51] in a multi-institutional retrospective cohort of patients undergoing RNU with regional LND. They found patients with a lymph node density of lower than 30% were at less risk of disease recurrence and had improved CSM. However, this represents the only study of its kind, and more results are required to validate the lymph node density concept in the setting of UTUC.

Templates

One important surgical consideration and an area of recent investigation is the anatomical template upon which LND at the time of RNU should be based. There exists little in the way of consensus regarding anatomical boundaries for dissection and the extent of dissection (i.e., number of LN) that is most appropriate in the surgical management of UTUC. This fact complicates many of the studies looking at survival and prognostic data, which have not been able to account for the anatomical extent of the dissection that was employed.

In contrast to the situation in UTUC, the specifics of LND are much better understood and more universally accepted in the operative management of UCB. In 2009, Karl et al. [52] published a systematic review of the literature on LND at the time of RC, focusing mainly on randomized trials with some control and comparative studies. They concluded that evidence advocates for a pelvic LND that minimally includes regions of the internal and external iliac vessels, the obturator fossa, and the distal part of the common iliac vessels including their bifurcation. More recently, Bi et al. [53] published their own systematic review and meta-analysis investigating the therapeutic efficacy of extended pelvic LND for UCB. This dissection includes LN between the bifurcation of common iliac and the aortic bifurcation, as well as a distal extension to the circumflex iliac vein and nodes of Cloquet, in addition to those nodes described by Karl et al. [52]. Extended pelvic LND was found to be associated with better RFS than the non-extended dissection, with a hazard ratio of 0.65 ($p < 0.001$). Due to a lack of prospective randomized controlled trials, the EAU currently gives a Grade B recommendation to this extended template as an *option* beyond standard bilateral LND [54].

In regards to UTUC, the relative rarity of disease, wide anatomic variation of possible tumor involvement, and the vast arcades of vascular and lymphatic channels have all hindered the ability to establish a universally accepted anatomic template for LND at the time of RNU.

In 2007, Kondo et al. [6] performed retrospective mapping studies on the primary site of LN metastasis representing the most detailed description at the time. Their study characterized the location of primary tumor as either left or right; and either belonging to renal pelvis, or upper [superior to the level of the inferior mesenteric artery (IMA)], middle (between IMA and where the ureter crosses the common iliac artery), or lower ureter (below this crossing). Imaging studies and pathology results were used to retrospectively determine the site of primary nodal metastasis for 181 patients with UTUC. 42 patients were found to have LN involvement. They found LN involvement to be highly dependent upon location of primary tumor, and that nodal spread was much wider than previously thought, especially for cancers of the right ureter. Nodal sites where the incidence of metastasis was 30% or more were then classified as regional lymph nodes. For tumors of the right renal pelvis, upper and middle ureter, paracaval and retrocaval nodes (and interaortocaval nodes for the ureteral tumor) were considered to be regional lymph nodes. For tumors of the left renal pelvis, upper and middle ureter, the renal hilar and paraaortic nodes were regional nodes. For tumors of the lower ureter, the ipsilateral common iliac, external iliac, obturator, and internal iliac nodes were included as regional lymph nodes, as for UCB.

To follow this, Kondo et al. [47] published in 2010 on the impact of template-based LND on survival. They retrospectively compared 109 patients with UTUC in two groups receiving RNU with simultaneous LND; one group ($n = 41$) received a "complete" dissection of all regional nodes, while the other group ($n = 78$) received an "incomplete" dissection that did not include all regional nodes. The group also investigated the impact on survival of number of LNs removed. Their analysis indicated an association between complete LND and increased survival, while they found no survival association with number of LNs removed. It is worth noting that some of the patients receiving incomplete LND did so on the basis of significant comorbidity, and that the complete LND group received more adjuvant chemotherapy (although when the hazard ratio adjusted for adjuvant chemotherapy was obtained, complete LND remained a significant prognostic factor). The implication that a complete dissection has survival benefit beyond simply including more LNs strongly argues for standardization of this aspect of surgical management.

In 2012, Kondo and Tanabe [22] reanalyzed their 2007 mapping studies to now include 75 patients with LN positive for metastases. The results were largely confirmatory of their initial study, but also showed the spread of metastases to the interaortocaval nodes from the tumor of the right renal pelvis and the pre-sacral nodes from those of the lower ureters, which are now included in their template recommendation as regional LN.

More recent data from Matin et al. [55] serves to further modify the existing framework for template-based dissection. In a similar approach to that of Kondo [6], Matin et al. looked retrospectively at LN involvement in patients with UTUC undergoing RNU with LND, and characterized anatomic sites of LN metastasis based on final pathology reports. Their findings were similar to those previously published, with some differences and additional insights. For right renal pelvis and proximal ureteral tumors, authors found that dissection of the hilum, paracaval, retrocaval, and interaortocaval regions would capture nearly all LN metastasis. For the left, the same was found for a hilar and paraaortic dissection. For mid ureteral tumors, a significant proportion of LN metastasis were identified in the interaortocaval and paracaval/retrocaval (right) and paraaortic (left) regions, suggesting a cranial lymphatic drainage pattern. For distal tumors, typical pelvic templates would remove majority of LN metastasis, but again found a proportion could remain adjacent to the ipsilateral great vessel in a pattern not previously described. Interestingly, interaortocaval involvement from both sides as well as other "out-of-field" LN metastasis appeared to occur secondarily. For example, in right-sided proximal tumors, only one of the five patients with interaortocaval LN metastasis had no other sites of LN metastasis, suggesting that patients without any disease in the paracaval or retrocaval areas may be able to have this region omitted, or possibly guided by frozen section at the time of surgery. Even with these new insights, large prospective studies evaluating standardized LND templates are still lacking.

Open Versus Laparoscopic/Robotic

An additional consideration that has been the recent subject of investigation is the surgical approach employed in LND; open versus laparoscopic or robotic. In RC with LND for UCB, open and robotic approaches have demonstrated similar yield regarding number of LNs, although the impact of number of LN removed on survival is better understood in that disease [56]. That considered, the majority of the literature comparing surgical approaches focuses on number of LN retrieved. Busby et al. [57] demonstrated the feasibility of laparoscopic LND during RNU, showing median number of LNs retrieved to be six and three for laparoscopic and open dissections, respectively. Abe et al. [58] showed similar findings in reporting on a prospective cohort undergoing laparoscopic RNU. In this series, the median number of LNs removed was 14 (range 1–33), which was comparable to another recent prospective series by Kondo and Tanabe [22], where a mean of 13 LN were removed during open RNU using similar dissection templates.

A comparison of surgical approach in LND for UTUC is limited by the fact that a complete understanding of the most important aspects of LND has not been established. It is difficult to say that one approach is truly inferior to the other on the basis of, say, a marginal decrease in number of LN retrieved, when the impact on survival of number of nodes dissected is still uncertain. In one of the largest studies Capitanio et al. [59] retrospectively compared the two approaches, open RNU ($n = 979$) versus laparoscopic RNU ($n = 270$) with non-metastatic UTUC and compared RFS and CSS between groups. Short-term oncologic data between the two groups was comparable when adjusting for the fact that laparoscopic surgery was selectively performed in patients with less advanced disease. As in the aforementioned studies, there was no significant difference in median number of LN removed.

Complications

The disadvantage of performing LND at the time of RNU, or the potential adverse effects from extending the limits of LND have not been well studied.

In their prospective series of laparoscopic RNU, Abe et al. [58] reported LND usually added about 0.5 to 1 h to total operative time, although this was not recorded separately. In their series, Kondo and Tanabe [22] compared those who underwent "complete" LND versus "incomplete" LND providing some insight into the influence of the extent of dissection. Complete LND resulted in an increase in minor complications, but operative time, intraoperative bleeding, and length of stay did not differ.

In a phase III randomized trial of over 700 patients, the European Organization for Research and Treatment of Cancer (EORTC) 30881 trial [60] found that LND did not affect the surgical complication rate, but that trial compared radical nephrectomy (RN) with modified retroperitoneal lymph node dissection (RPLND) with RN alone.

In the only study of its kind, Rao et al. [61] looked to prospectively validate the safety and feasibility of LND at the time of RNU for UTUC in a phase II clinical trial. 20 patients with suspected UTUC underwent open ($n = 10$), laparoscopic ($n = 4$) or robot-assisted ($n = 6$) RNU with a modified RPLND. The modified template consisted of a perihilar, paracaval, and pelvic LND for right-sided tumors, and perihilar, paraaortic, and pelvic LND for left-sided tumors, with removal of interaortocaval LN at the discretion of the surgeon. The overall post-op complication rate was 9/19 patients, with eight minor complications (Clavien Grade I–II) [62] and just one major complication (Calvien grade III or more), a patient who developed chylous ascites requiring surgical reexploration. These complication rates are similar to previous open and laparoscopic RNU series conducted without LND [55, 61, 63]. There were no statistical differences in complication rate with regard to surgical approach or length of stay, and authors concluded that modified RPLND during RNU is a feasible procedure with acceptable morbidity.

Current 2015 Guidelines

Campbell-Walsh Urology 10th edition [64] endorses regional LND for all RNUs, except in rare occasions such as severe atherosclerosis of the aorta or grossly positive, fixed LN, where it may be limited or omitted. Otherwise, for renal pelvis and proximal/middle ureteral tumors, the ipsilateral renal hilar nodes and adjacent paraaortic or paracaval nodes should be resected, noting this dissection adds little time or morbidity to the surgery.

According to the National Cancer Institute (NCI)—Physician Data Query (PDQ) [65], LND at the time of nephrectomy may offer prognostic information, but little, if any, therapeutic benefit.

The EAU Guidelines [66] note that anatomic sites for LND have not been clearly defined, and the LND template is likely to have a greater impact on survival than number of LN removed. Guidelines suggest that LND appears to be unnecessary in cases of Ta or T1 UTUC due to low yield of LNs in this setting, as there is an increase in the probability of LN positive disease with pT classification [36]. With the caveat that it currently is not possible to standardize the indication or extent of LND, suggestion is made that LND can be achieved following lymphatic drainage as follows: LND medial to the ureter in ureteropelvic tumors, retroperitoneal LND for higher ureteral tumors and/or tumors of the renal pelvis (i.e., right side: border of the venal cava or right side of the aorta: and left side: border of the aorta).

The National Comprehensive Cancer Network (NCCN 2.2015) [67] guidelines for LND vary depending on the location of the primary tumor. For tumors originating in the renal pelvis, regional LND is recommended for HG or large tumors, or those that invade the parenchyma. LND is recommended for all HG ureteral tumors regardless of location, with consideration for LG tumors of the mid-ureter if RNU is performed.

Conclusions

A precise understanding of the benefit of LND at the time of RNU is still lacking, and it is currently impossible to standardize the indications or extent of dissection. However, current evidence suggests at minimum a staging benefit, and potentially a survival advantage to performing LND, especially in those with invasive or high-grade disease. Standard dissection templates based on tumor location require large-scale prospective evaluation in order to fully understand the clinical utility of LND in patients with UTUC.

Summary Box

- The overall incidence of UTUC is slowly rising, with a stage and grade migration toward more aggressive disease in patients undergoing surgical management.
- Nodal involvement, present in up to 30% of cases, represents the strongest adverse pathologic feature in patients treated with RNU.
- Multiple studies have demonstrated that patterns of UTUC nodal metastasis are highly dependent on tumor location and laterality. Tumors originating from the right renal pelvis and upper two-thirds of the ureter generally metastasize to the hilar, paracaval, retrocaval, and interaortocaval nodes, while tumors in the left renal pelvis and upper two-thirds of the ureter metastasize to the renal hilum, interaortocaval, and paraaortic nodes. Tumors involving the distal ureter commonly spread to the ipsilateral pelvic nodes beyond the aortic bifurcation.
- LND performed at the time of RNU is the best way to completely and accurately stage UTUC. The therapeutic benefit is less well established.
- No universally accepted anatomic template for LND at the time of RNU exists due to the relative rarity of disease, wide anatomic variation of possible tumor involvement, and the vast arcades of vascular and lymphatic channels.
- Current guidelines generally recommend that LND be performed for all large, invasive, or high-grade tumors.
- Large, prospective studies are needed to create defined templates and more clearly define the role of LND in surgical management of UTUC.

References

1. Munoz JJ, Ellison LM. Upper tract urothelial neoplasms: incidence and survival during the last 2 decades. J Urol. 2000;164(5):1523–5.
2. Oosterlinck W, Solsona E, van der Meijden AP, Sylvester R, Bohle A, Rintala E, et al. EAU guidelines on diagnosis and treatment of upper urinary tract transitional cell carcinoma. Eur Urol. 2004;46(2):147–54.
3. Raman JD, Messer J, Sielatycki JA, Hollenbeak CS. Incidence and survival of patients with carcinoma of the ureter and renal pelvis in the USA, 1973–2005. BJU Int. 2011;107(7):1059–64.
4. Lughezzani G, Jeldres C, Isbarn H, Sun M, Shariat SF, Widmer H, et al. Temporal stage and grade migration in surgically treated patients with upper tract urothelial carcinoma. BJU Int. 2010;105 (6):799–804.
5. Komatsu H, Tanabe N, Kubodera S, Maezawa H, Ueno A. The role of lymphadenectomy in the treatment of transitional cell carcinoma of the upper urinary tract. J Urol. 1997;157(5):1622–4.
6. Kondo T, Nakazawa H, Ito F, Hashimoto Y, Toma H, Tanabe K. Primary site and incidence of lymph node metastases in urothelial carcinoma of upper urinary tract. Urology. 2007;69(2):265–9.
7. Zigeuner R, Pummer K. Urothelial carcinoma of the upper urinary tract: surgical approach and prognostic factors. Eur Urol. 2008;53(4):720–31.
8. Roscigno M, Shariat SF, Margulis V, Karakiewicz P, Remzi M, Kikuchi E, et al. Impact of lymph node dissection on cancer specific survival in patients with upper tract urothelial carcinoma treated with radical nephroureterectomy. J Urol. 2009;181(6):2482–9.
9. Ozsahin M, Zouhair A, Villa S, Storme G, Chauvet B, Taussky D, et al. Prognostic factors in urothelial renal pelvis and ureter tumours: a multicentre Rare Cancer Network study. Eur J Cancer (Oxford, England: 1990). 1999;35(5):738–43.
10. Novara G, De Marco V, Gottardo F, Dalpiaz O, Bouygues V, Galfano A, et al. Independent predictors of cancer-specific survival in transitional cell carcinoma of the upper urinary tract: multi-institutional dataset from 3 European centers. Cancer. 2007;110(8):1715–22.
11. Capitanio U, Becker F, Blute ML, Mulders P, Patard JJ, Russo P, et al. Lymph node dissection in renal cell carcinoma. Eur Urol. 2011;60(6):1212–20.
12. Miki J, Egawa S. The role of lymph node dissection in the management of prostate cancer. Int J Clin Oncol. 2011;16(3):195–202.
13. Koppie TM, Vickers AJ, Vora K, Dalbagni G, Bochner BH. Standardization of pelvic lymphadenectomy performed at radical cystectomy: can

we establish a minimum number of lymph nodes that should be removed? Cancer. 2006;107(10):2368–74.
14. Konety BR, Joslyn SA, O'Donnell MA. Extent of pelvic lymphadenectomy and its impact on outcome in patients diagnosed with bladder cancer: analysis of data from the surveillance, epidemiology and end results program data base. J Urol. 2003;169(3):946–50.
15. Leissner J, Hohenfellner R, Thuroff JW, Wolf HK. Lymphadenectomy in patients with transitional cell carcinoma of the urinary bladder; significance for staging and prognosis. BJU Int. 2000;85(7):817–23.
16. Kondo T, Nakazawa H, Ito F, Hashimoto Y, Toma H, Tanabe K. Impact of the extent of regional lymphadenectomy on the survival of patients with urothelial carcinoma of the upper urinary tract. J Urol. 2007;178(4 Pt 1):1212–7; discussion 7.
17. Roscigno M, Shariat SF, Margulis V, Karakiewicz P, Remzi M, Kikuchi E, et al. The extent of lymphadenectomy seems to be associated with better survival in patients with nonmetastatic upper-tract urothelial carcinoma: how many lymph nodes should be removed? Eur Urol. 2009;56(3):512–8.
18. Batata MA, Whitmore WF, Hilaris BS, et al. Primary carcinoma of the ureter: a prognostic study. Cancer. 1975;35:1626–32.
19. McCarron JP Jr, Chasko SB, Gray GF Jr. Systematic mapping of nephroureterectomy specimens removed for urothelial cancer: pathological findings and clinical correlations. J Urol. 1982;128:243–6.
20. Akaza H, Koiso K, Niijima T. Clinical evaluation of urothelial tumors of the renal pelvis and ureter based on a new classification system. Cancer. 1987;59:1369–75.
21. Assouad J, Riquet M, Foucault C, Hidden G, Delmas V. Renal lymphatic drainage and thoracic duct connections: implications for cancer spread. Lymphology. 2006;39:26–32.
22. Kondo T, Tanabe K. Role of lymphadenectomy in the management of urothelial carcinoma of the bladder and the upper urinary tract. Int J Urol. 2012;19(8):710–21.
23. Sobin L, Gospodarowicz M, Wittekind C. TNM classification of malignant tumours. Urological tumours. Renal pelvis and ureter. 7th revised edn. New York: Wiley-Blackwell, UICC; 2009, p. 258–61.
24. Stenzl A, Cowan NC, De Santis M, Kuczyk MA, Merseburger AS, Ribal MJ, et al. Treatment of muscle-invasive and metastatic bladder cancer: update of the EAU guidelines. Eur Urol. 2011;59(6):1009–18.
25. Dretler SP, Ragsdale BD, Leadbetter WF. The value of pelvic lymphadenectomy in the surgical treatment of bladder cancer. J Urol. 1973;109(3):414–6.
26. Skinner DG. Management of invasive bladder cancer: a meticulous pelvic node dissection can make a difference. J Urol. 1982;128(1):34–6.
27. Secin FP, Koppie TM, Salamanca JI, Bokhari S, Raj GV, Olgac S, et al. Evaluation of regional lymph node dissection in patients with upper urinary tract urothelial cancer. Int J Urol Official J Jpn Urol Assoc. 2007;14(1):26–32.
28. Messer J, Shariat SF, Brien JC, Herman MP, Ng CK, Scherr DS, et al. Urinary cytology has a poor performance for predicting invasive or high-grade upper-tract urothelial carcinoma. BJU Int. 2011;108(5):701–5.
29. Keeley FX, Kulp DA, Bibbo M, McCue PA, Bagley DH. Diagnostic accuracy of ureteroscopic biopsy in upper tract transitional cell carcinoma. J Urol. 1997;157(1):33–7.
30. Vashistha V, Shabsigh A, Zynger DL. Utility and diagnostic accuracy of ureteroscopic biopsy in upper tract urothelial carcinoma. Arch Pathol Lab Med. 2013;137(3):400.
31. Remzi M, Shariat S, Huebner W, Fajkovic H, Seitz C. Upper urinary tract urothelial carcinoma: what have we learned in the last 4 years? Ther Adv Urol. 2011;3(2):69–80.
32. Roscigno M, Cozzarini C, Bertini R, Scattoni V, Freschi M, Da Pozzo LF, et al. Prognostic value of lymph node dissection in patients with muscle-invasive transitional cell carcinoma of the upper urinary tract. Eur Urol. 2008;53(4):794–802.
33. Roscigno M, Brausi M, Heidenreich A, Lotan Y, Margulis V, Shariat SF, et al. Lymphadenectomy at the time of nephroureterectomy for upper tract urothelial cancer. Eur Urol. 2011;60(4):776–83.
34. Margulis V, Shariat SF, Matin SF, Kamat AM, Zigeuner R, Kikuchi E, et al. Outcomes of radical nephroureterectomy: a series from the upper tract urothelial carcinoma collaboration. Cancer. 2009;115(6):1224–33.
35. Brown GA, Busby JE, Wood CG, Pisters LL, Dinney CP, Swanson DA, et al. Nephroureterectomy for treating upper urinary tract transitional cell carcinoma: time to change the treatment paradigm? BJU Int. 2006;98(6):1176–80.
36. Lughezzani G, Jeldres C, Isbarn H, Shariat SF, Sun M, Pharand D, et al. A critical appraisal of the value of lymph node dissection at nephroureterectomy for upper tract urothelial carcinoma. Urology. 2010;75(1):118–24.
37. Xylinas E, Rink M, Margulis V, Faison T, Comploj E, Novara G, et al. Prediction of true nodal status in patients with pathological lymph node negative upper tract urothelial carcinoma at radical nephroureterectomy. J Urol. 2013;189(2):468–73.
38. Skinner DG. Management of invasive bladder cancer: a meticulous pelvic node dissection can make a difference. J Urol. 1982;128:34–6.
39. Poulsen AL, Horn T, Steven K. Radical cystectomy: extending the limits of pelvic lymph node dissection improves survival for patients with bladder cancer confined to the bladder wall. J Urol. 1998;160:2015–9.
40. Stein JP, Lieskovsky G, Cote R, Groshen S, Feng AC, Boyd S, et al. Radical cystectomy in the treatment of invasive bladder cancer: long-term

results in 1,054 patients. J Clin Oncol Official J Am Soc Clin Oncol. 2001;19(3):666–75.
41. Herr HW, Faulkner JR, Grossman HB, Natale RB, deVere White R, Sarosdy MF, et al. Surgical factors influence bladder cancer outcomes: a cooperative group report. J Clin Oncol Official J Am Soc Clin Oncol. 2004;22(14):2781–9.
42. Herr H, Lee C, Chang S, Lerner S, Bladder Cancer Collaborative G. Standardization of radical cystectomy and pelvic lymph node dissection for bladder cancer: a collaborative group report. J Urol. 2004; 171(5):1823–8; discussion 7–8.
43. Miyake H, Hara I, Gohji K, Arakawa S, Kamidono S. The significance of lymphadenectomy in transitional cell carcinoma of the upper urinary tract. Br J Urol. 1998;82:494–8.
44. Brausi MA, Gavioli M, De Luca G, Verrini G, Peracchia G, Simonini G, et al. Retroperitoneal lymph node dissection (RPLD) in conjunction with nephroureterectomy in the treatment of infiltrative transitional cell carcinoma (TCC) of the upper urinary tract: impact on survival. Eur Urol. 2007; 52(5):1414–8.
45. Kondo T, Hara I, Takagi T, Kodama Y, Hashimoto Y, Kobayashi H, et al. Template-based lymphadenectomy in urothelial carcinoma of the renal pelvis: a prospective study. Int J Urol. 2014;21 (5):453–9.
46. Abe T, Shinohara N, Muranaka M, Sazawa A, Maruyama S, Osawa T, et al. Role of lymph node dissection in the treatment of urothelial carcinoma of the upper urinary tract: multi-institutional relapse analysis and immunohistochemical re-evaluation of negative lymph nodes. Eur J Surg Oncol J Eur Soc Surg Oncol Br Assoc Surg Oncol. 2010; 36(11):1085–91.
47. Kondo T, Hashimoto Y, Kobayashi H, Iizuka J, Nakazawa H, Ito F, et al. Template-based lymphadenectomy in urothelial carcinoma of the upper urinary tract: impact on patient survival. Int J Urol Official J Jpn Urol Assoc. 2010;17(10):848–54.
48. Stein JP, Cai J, Groshen S, Skinner DG. Risk factors for patients with pelvic lymph node metastases following radical cystectomy with en bloc pelvic lymphadenectomy: concept of lymph node density. J Urol. 2003;170(1):35–41.
49. Ooki A, Yamashita K, Kobayashi N, Katada N, Sakuramoto S, Kikuchi S, et al. Lymph node metastasis density and growth pattern as independent prognostic factors in advanced esophageal squamous cell carcinoma. World J Surg. 2007;31(11):2184–91.
50. Daneshmand S, Quek ML, Stein JP, et al. Prognosis of patients with lymph node positive prostate cancer following radical prostatectomy: long-term results. J Urol. 2004;172:2252–5.
51. Bolenz C, Shariat SF, Fernandez MI, Margulis V, Lotan Y, Karakiewicz P, et al. Risk stratification of patients with nodal involvement in upper tract urothelial carcinoma: value of lymph-node density. BJU Int. 2009;103(3):302–6.
52. Karl A, Carroll PR, Gschwend JE, Knuchel R, Montorsi F, Stief CG, et al. The impact of lymphadenectomy and lymph node metastasis on the outcomes of radical cystectomy for bladder cancer. Eur Urol. 2009;55(4):826–35.
53. Bi L, Huang H, Fan X, Li K, Xu K, Jiang C, et al. Extended vs non-extended pelvic lymph node dissection and their influence on recurrence-free survival in patients undergoing radical cystectomy for bladder cancer: a systematic review and meta-analysis of comparative studies. BJU Int. 2014;113(5b):E39–48.
54. Witjes JA, Comperat E, Cowan NC, De Santis M, Gakis G, Lebret T, et al. EAU guidelines on muscle-invasive and metastatic bladder cancer: summary of the 2013 guidelines. Eur Urol. 2014; 65(4):778–92.
55. Matin SF, Sfakianos JP, Espiritu PN, Coleman JA, Spiess PE. Patterns of lymphatic metastases in upper tract urothelial carcinoma and proposed dissection templates. J Urol. 2015.
56. Yuh B, Wilson T, Bochner B, Chan K, Palou J, Stenzl A, et al. Systematic review and cumulative analysis of oncologic and functional outcomes after robot-assisted radical cystectomy. Eur Urol. 2015;67 (3):402–22.
57. Busby JE, Brown GA, Matin SF. Comparing lymphadenectomy during radical nephroureterectomy: open versus laparoscopic. Urology. 2008;71(3): 413–6.
58. Abe T, Takada N, Matsumoto R, Osawa T, Sazawa A, Maruyama S, et al. Outcome of regional lymphadenectomy in accordance with primary tumor location on laparoscopic nephroureterectomy for urothelial carcinoma of the upper urinary tract: a prospective study. J Endourol. 2015;29(3):304–9.
59. Capitanio U, Shariat SF, Isbarn H, Weizer A, Remzi M, Roscigno M, et al. Comparison of oncologic outcomes for open and laparoscopic nephroureterectomy: a multi-institutional analysis of 1249 cases. Eur Urol. 2009;56(1):1–9.
60. Blom JH, van Poppel H, Marechal JM, Jacqmin D, Schroder FH, de Prijck L, et al. Radical nephrectomy with and without lymph-node dissection: final results of European Organization for Research and Treatment of Cancer (EORTC) randomized phase 3 trial 30881. Eur Urol. 2009;55(1):28–34.
61. Rao SR, Correa JJ, Sexton WJ, Pow-Sang JM, Dickinson SI, Lin HY, et al. Prospective clinical trial of the feasibility and safety of modified retroperitoneal lymph node dissection at time of nephroureterectomy for upper tract urothelial carcinoma. BJU Int. 2012;110(11 Pt B):E475–80.
62. Dindo D, Demartines N, Clavien P-A. Classification of surgical complications. Ann Surg. 2004; 240(2):205–13.
63. Rajput MZ, Kamat AM, Clavell-Hernandez J, Siefker-Radtke AO, Grossman HB, Dinney CP, et al. Perioperative outcomes of laparoscopic radical nephroureterectomy and regional lymphadenectomy

in patients with upper urinary tract urothelial carcinoma after neoadjuvant chemotherapy. Urology. 2011;78(1):61–7.

64. Wein AJ, Kavoussi LR, Novick AC, Partin AW, Peters CA. Campbell-Walsh urology: expert consult premium edition: enhanced online features and print, 4-Volume Set:Amsterdam: Elsevier Health Sciences; 2011.
65. Transitional Cell Cancer of the Renal Pelvis and Ureter Treatment (PDQ″) (database on the Internet) (2015). National Cancer Institute. Available from: http://www.cancer.gov/types/kidney/hp/transitional-cell-treatment-pdq.
66. Roupret M, Babjuk M, Comperat E, Zigeuner R, Sylvester RJ, Burger M, et al. European association of urology guidelines on upper urinary tract urothelial cell carcinoma: 2015 update. Eur Urol. 2015.
67. National Comprehensive Cancer Network. NCCN clinical practice guidelines in oncology—bladder cancer. Version 2.2015 http://www.nccn.org/professionals/physician_gls/pdf/bladder.pdf.

Diagnosis and Management of Upper Urinary Tract Recurrences After Radical Cystectomy

25

Mark Ferretti, Jonathan Bloom and John L. Phillips

Introduction

The diagnosis and management of upper urinary tract (UUT) urothelial carcinoma (UC) recurrences after urinary diversion represents a challenge from both an oncologic and endoscopic perspective. Patients who undergo radical cystectomy and survive their disease have a long-life risk of recurrence of UC in the upper urinary tract [1]. Current surveillance techniques, however, may miss nearly half of those who present with recurrent UUT after radical cystectomy [2]. Upper Urinary Tract Urothelial Carcinoma (UUT-UC) after radical cystectomy may have a significant delay in diagnosis in an elderly population with significant comorbidities [3, 4]. The current chapter will summarize the epidemiology, pathophysiology, diagnosis, and treatment options of UUT-UC after radical cystectomy.

M. Ferretti · J. Bloom · J. L. Phillips (✉)
Department of Urology, Westchester Medical Health Network/New York Medical College, 40 Sunshine Cottage Rd, Skyline 1S-B45A, Valhalla, NY 10595, USA
e-mail: john_phillips@nymc.edu

M. Ferretti
e-mail: mark.ferretti@gmail.com

J. Bloom
Urologic Oncology Branch, National Institute of Health, Bethesda, MD, USA
e-mail: jbbloom@gmail.com

UC represents a 'field defect' in that all cells of the urinary tract are exposed to the same concentration of urinary mutagens and thus share some increased clonal and non-clonal propensity towards carcinogenesis. In classic studies, UUT-UC is said to occur in about 5% of those with bladder cancer but with modern surveillance strategies, the true incidence may be 20% and rise as high as 35% in those with a history of non-muscle-invasive bladder cancer (NMIBC) and carcinoma in situ (CIS) where prolonged survival may increase upper tract recurrences [5–8]. More than a third of patients who have primary UUT-UC of the renal pelvis or ureter and undergo nephro-ureterectomy (NU) may experience a bladder recurrence at a median of 25.9 months and 60% of such patients recur >2 years after NU [9]. The incidence, location, and disease course of UC in the UUT is influenced by exposure time to urinary mutagens (i.e., 'dwell' time), rates of spontaneous somatic mutagenesis and DNA mismatch repair defects, and organ susceptibility to the establishment of invasive, i.e., ≥ T2 disease [10–14]. Upper urinary tract UC (UUT-UC) is far less common than bladder UC occurring at a rate in UK males of 1.7–2.0/100,000 compared to 15.2–19.4/100,000 for bladder UC (National Cancer Intelligence Network, 2013). SEER data indicate that the incidence of UUT-UC increased from 1.88 to 2.06 cases per 100,000 person-years from 1973 to 2005 largely due to the identification of in situ tumors [15]. However, over 40% of

M. Eshghi (ed.), *Urothelial Malignancies of the Upper Urinary Tract*,
https://doi.org/10.1007/978-3-319-51263-1_25

patients still present with >T2 disease, continues to have poor 5-year overall survival rates, and has kept the prognosis of UUT-UC from improving demonstrably over the past few decades. Overall mortality rates vary with gender (11% increased risk of death in males), race (African-Americans have a 29% increased risk of death over non-hispanic whites), and age with the elderly over 80 years of age have double the risk of death as stage-matched patients <70 years of age. These differences are similar to bladder cancer itself in that overall 1- and 5-year survival rates for both UUT-UC and BC are 75 and 50%, respectively. These data reflect the behavior of UUT-UC in subjects with an intact bladder. Information regarding UUT-UC after radical cystectomy (RC) requires an evaluation of data concerning UUT-UC 'relapses'.

Relapses of UUT-UC after radical cystectomy may be viewed in two groups: *de novo* occurrences of new-onset UUT tumors clonally unrelated to a treated bladder cancer or recurrences of previously treated or unrecognized upper tract tumors (Fig. 25.1). Of 2029 patients who underwent RC over a 40 year period, 25 or 1.2% developed UC in the UUT requiring NU. Similarly, 2.5% of 1069 patients status post radical cystectomy from 1985–2001 required NU for UUT-UC [2, 4]. A meta-analysis of 13,185 subjects from 22 studies found that between 0.75 and 6.40% of patients undergoing radical cystectomy may experience a UUT recurrence between 0.4 and 349.2 months post-operatively, a third of whom may present with metastatic disease, and half of whom will ultimately die of their original bladder cancer [1]. The incidence of UUT-UC in patients' status post radical cystectomy may appear to be 2–3 times lower than the UUT-UC rate in patients with an intact bladder but may more likely reflect the decreased life-span and follow up for patients undergoing RC for muscle-invasive bladder cancer in the first place [5].

Still, patients who undergo NU after radical cystectomy have higher rates of T3 and T4 disease compared to those who undergo NU with an intact bladder, whether or not they have had a history of bladder cancer (Table 25.1). Such tumors are also of higher grade and are associated with increased positive lymph node yields than patients without bladder cancer [16].

NU induces some degree of renal insufficiency. Organ-sparing or conservative therapy (CT) to maintain a renal unit in the setting of UUT-UC may offer a maintained level of renal function and does not appear to convey a worse prognosis in patients who ultimately undergo NU [17, 18]. Early identification of UUT-UC after radical cystectomy, therefore, may help identify patients with lower stage disease who would be amenable to CT. Despite standardized surveillance regimens using cross-sectional imaging and urinary cytology, 75% of patients with UUT-UC after radical cystectomy present with symptoms including gross hematuria or hydronephrosis-related pain [2, 16].

UUT-UC represents true challenges, therefore, to the practicing urologist. UUT-UC, once diagnosed, has few therapeutic options other than radical extirpative surgery even for non-invasive disease compared to the multiple options over a long duration for both therapy and surveillance seen in non-muscle-invasive bladder cancers (NMIBC). The ability to diagnose, and, in some cases, monitor for recurrent UUT-UC, is aided by endoscopic access to the UUT through the predictable location and anatomy of the ureteral orifices. For patients who have undergone radical cystectomy and urinary diversion for lower UC, the surveillance of the UUT for de novo, recurrent, or occult UC, represents a diagnostic and therapeutic challenge. This chapter will focus on the diagnosis and management of UUT-UC in those patients who have undergone radical cystectomy and some form of permanent urinary diversion.

Epidemiology, Pathologic, and Molecular Features

Risk factors for bladder and UUT cancer may be different than in those who sustain a relapse of UUT after cystectomy. Smoking, which is the strongest risk factor for UC, and is associated with half of all cases, does not appear related to the risk of relapse [19]. The roles of arsenic, hair

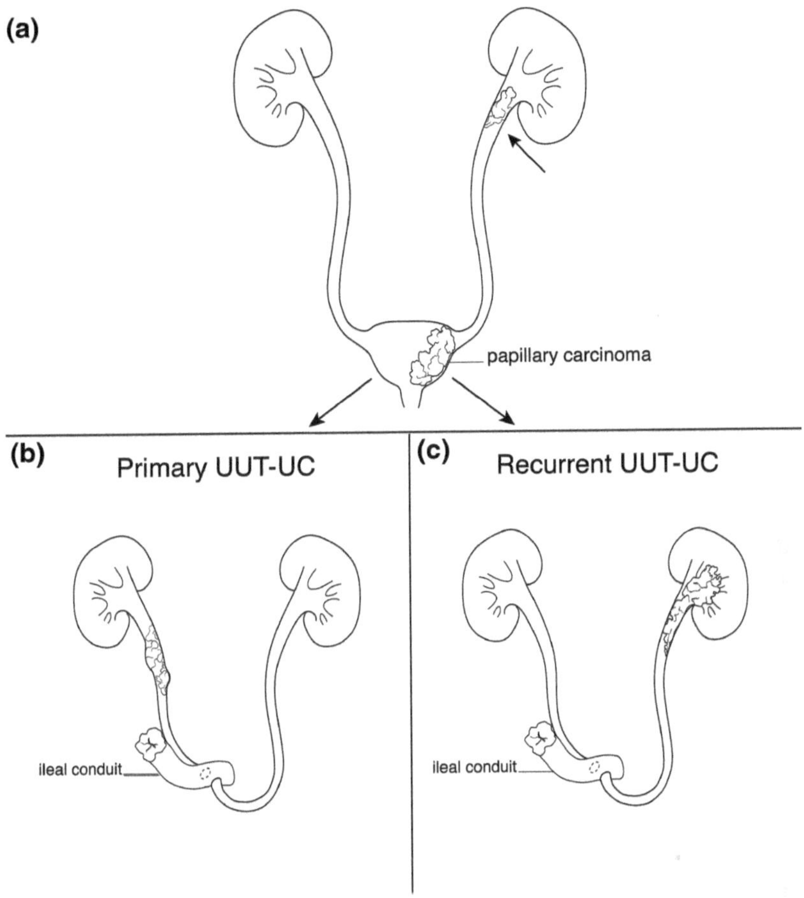

Fig. 25.1 Upper urinary tract urothelial carcinoma (UUT-UC) after cystectomy may occur as 'primary' or 'recurrent' disease. For example, a patient **a** has a large, invasive bladder tumor and, in this example, a small left sided non-invasive UUT-UC of the proximal ureter (*arrow*) which may or may not have been detected or treated. The patient undergoes cystectomy and urinary diversion. In one scenario, the patient presents with a new unrelated primary tumor of the right ureter (**b**). Alternatively, the patient presents with a recurrence of the missed or undertreated UUT-UC of the left ureter and pelvis (**c**). ClarityArt, sdphillips94@gmail.com, New York

Table 25.1 Pathologic findings of nephroureterectomy specimens in patients with and without a history of bladder cancer (BC) and those status post radical cystectomy (RC) [1, 2]

p Stage	No h/o BC [1]	History of BC, no RC [1]	Relapse after RC [2]
CIS	1.6	2.7	
Ta	26.7	28.7	
T1	23	21.8	54.2
T2	9.3	12.3	0
T3	31	32.7	45.8
T4	8.4	1.8	
Nx	60.4	61.3	0
N+	6.4	8.6	32
N0	33.2	30.1	68
Low grade	49.1	44.1	8.3
High grade	50.9	55.9	91.7

dye, phenacetin abuse, and aromatic amine exposure are suspected to contribute to the incidence of lower and UUT-UC but there is no data suggesting they play a role in UUT relapses.

The role of gender and race in the incidence and mortality of bladder cancer and UUT-UC is well established [15]. For example, US bladder cancer related death rates from 2008 to 2012 were 8.1, 2.2, 5.3, and 2.5 per 100,000 person-years in white men and women, and black men and women, respectively (SEER). For UUT-UC, male gender was still associated with a worse overall survival with a risk of death of 7 and 5% greater than women at 3 and 5 years and for ureteral carcinoma, the mortality rate was 16% higher [15]. However, non-hispanic blacks appear to have worse 5 and 10 year survival rates than white non-hispanics and have a 30% increased risk of death from either renal pelvic or ureteral UUT-UC. Gender and racial differences after radical cystectomy are less clear and may reflect the biologic behavior of the original bladder cancer. No gender or racial differences in either the rate, location, or survival have been reported suggesting that once the prognosis and outcome of the lower urinary tract has been defined, there exist fewer differences that separate the patterns of UUT-UC among men and women of different races [4].

There are some pathologic parameters that appear to predict for recurrences in the upper tract in those with bladder cancer who ultimately undergo radical cystectomy. Urethral involvement in women, prostatic stromal involvement in men, CIS of the bladder, intramural ureteral carcinoma, recurrent superficial disease, and positive ureteral margins all appear to predict relapses of UUT UC after RC [2, 20–23]. As discussed, patients who undergo RC for muscle-invasive bladder cancer (MIBC) have 5-year survival rates that may be as low as 40%. Many patients with MIBC may not survive long enough to develop UUT-UC that can be found on surveillance or which presents with symptoms. In contrast, patients who undergo cystectomy for recurrent Ta, T1, or CIS disease may have been managed for long intervals and who may therefore be at increased risk for development of the UUT either at the time of cystectomy or at a later date.

Molecular studies of UUT in patients with and without bladder cancer may suggest which patients are at risk for relapse after radical cystectomy. BC is thought to derive from mutations in one of two pathways—those of the positive oncogene p53 and those of the stroma-modifying modeling gene FGFR3. Mutations of p53 are associated with CIS and MIBC while tumors derived from mutant FGFR3 tend to be of lower grade, superficial, and, thus, carry a better prognosis. As NMIBC is far more common than MIBC, it follows that the prevalence of FGFR3-positive tumors is higher in TURBT but not in RC specimens. The proportion of p53 and FGFR3-positive tumors in renal pelvis cancer is similar to that found in bladder cancer specimens although genetic studies are limited to whole organ NU analysis and not endoscopically derived biopsies which poorly correlate with tumor histology [14, 24].

Chinese herbal nephropathy may cause increased exposure of the upper tracts to aristolochic acid (AA) which ultimately lead to p53 mutations and an increased rate of UUT-UC [14]. Balkan endemic nephropathy (BEN) has been long shown to increase the rate of UUT-UC nearly 100-fold in endemic areas and potentially through an AA-like p53 mutation pathway associated with proteinuria, renal failure, and mutations of the oncogene c-myb [25]. BEN patients with end-stage renal failure have undergone preventative nephroureterectomy. It follows, then, that patients with BEN who undergo RC are at particularly increased risk for relapse of the upper urinary tract. Other familial conditions with genetic predispositions towards UUT-UC would include Lynch Syndrome or Hereditary Non-Polyposis Colorectal Cancer (HNPCC). Patients with HNPCC have germline mutations in the DNA mismatch repair (MMR) genes, most commonly MSH2 and MLH1, and are at nearly a 22-fold risk of UUT-UC, occur at an earlier age, and have a higher rate of bilaterality [26]. MMR mutations are thought to lead to microsatellite instability (MSI) and chromosomal breakage, the hallmark of carcinogenesis. MSI mutations pathways may be important in non-familial cases of UUT-UC as well and point to a distinct pathway for carcinogenesis that is different than for BC. MSI mutations are thought to be the driver of other mutations, such as p53 or FGFR3, and may be a distinct feature of UUT-UC. Mismatch repair mutations, for example, were found in nearly 15% of potentially sporadic UUT tumors compared to only 1% of bladder cancers [27]. It would follow, then, that the absence of MSI mutations in a cystectomy patient would not guard against relapse of disease in the upper tract.

Molecular profiling may identify driver mutations but, more importantly, networks of a larger number of normal and/or abnormal genes that drive the carcinomatous phenotype. Molecular profiling of bladder cancers that could predict recurrence in the upper tract would be particularly useful. Affymetrix gene array analysis has revealed that expression of FXDY3 appears prevalent in both UUT- and bladder UC and suggests a potentially prognostic role [28]. In a study of 10 bladder carcinomas and 14 unrelated UUT-UCs, 21 genes could be used to differentiate BC from UUT including increased expression of CLCA2 and GABRA [29]. Thus, genomic profiling of tumor from a radical cystectomy specimen may help predict which patients have occult synchronous UUT disease or who are destined to relapse in the UUT.

Imaging

Imaging is a mainstay in the diagnosis and surveillance of patients with UC. NCCN guidelines suggest that in patients who have undergone RC for bladder cancer, imaging of the "chest, upper tracts, abdomen, and pelvis every 3–6 months for 2 years based on risk of recurrence and then as clinically indicated" is suggested. More than half of patients who sustain a relapse in the UUT after RC do so beyond the 2 year limit suggested by the NCCN guidelines. Clinically indicated therefore must be applied broadly to RC patients in order to ensure timely follow up and early detection of relapsed disease. The application of NCCN guidelines after radical cystectomy is known to be low [30, 31]. The number needed to image, however, would be low itself, as larger series suggest that only 1 of 50 patients' status radical cystectomy live to develop upper tract recurrences and more than half of those presented with disease that eluded regular upper tract imaging [2].

In general, however, GU imaging is still dependent on the use of a urinary contrast agent that allows for the detection of filling defects, urothelial masses, and tumor formation before the onset of a mass effect. Up to half of all patients' status post RC have renal insufficiency and are not candidates for traditional intravenously delivered iodinated contrast agents. CT is the most widely used modality in the work up and surveillance of patients with UUT-UC, although this modality may have difficulty in detecting small, superficial lesions in the absence of a mass >5 mm or a positive cytology [32, 33]. CT urography has replaced intravenous or excretory urography in the initial and prospective work up of patients with gross hematuria or known UUT-UC [34]. The performance of CT urography is best with so-called 4-phase or 'multidetector' CT (MDCTU) especially when radiologists work with the ordering physician and have access to pertinent clinical information [35]. The sensitivity, specificity, and accuracy of excretory urography is 75, 86, and 85%, respectively, which increases on MDCTU to 96, 98, and 98% on MDCTU, respectively [35]. Still, CT may have some limitations even in those with normal renal function. In one study, biopsy-proven UUT-UC was found in only 40 of 76 patients with a 'positive' CT urogram (positive predictive value of 53%) [33]. MDCTU detection rates for ureteral UUT-UC are decidedly lower than for renal pelvic disease with areas under the curve (AUCs) of 0.84 and 0.98, respectively, by radiologists blinded to clinical data [35]. Limitations of CT urography would include the reliance of intravenous contrast agents, reactions to contrast material, and radiation exposure. Traditional radiation exposure after CT urography is well-tolerated, especially in the older population in whom an evaluation of UUT-UC is warranted, but newer maneuvers, such as iterative reconstruction, can help halve dose rates to as low as 6.1 mSv [36]. Contrast reactions in the low ionic era are rare and are quoted as occurring in as few as

1 event in 500 studies [37]. Patients in whom contrast-associated opacification is important, which would include nearly all patients under surveillance for UUT-UC, will need to consider alternatives, namely magnetic resonance imaging (MRI).

Upper tract MRI has evolved to become highly accurate, in some cases more so than CT urography, without the use of radiation or iodinated contrast agents. Rates of nephrogenic systemic fibrosis (NSF) are unreported in those with normal renal function and rare in the modern era of MRI imaging in those with renal insufficiency. Gadodiamide (Omniscan™), gadopentetate dimeglumine (Magnevist™), and gadoversetamide (Optimark™) are associated with NSF in stage 4 and 5 renal disease suggesting that immediate post-MRI dialysis may be a useful rule to limit toxicity. For those patients who can tolerate gadolinium, diffusion weighted MRI appears slightly superior to CT urography in terms of detection rates, especially in cases where the collecting system has little structural abnormality and tumor burden may be subtle (Fig. 25.2). MRI can be performed using urine itself as the 'contrast' agent, so-called 'static fluid MRI', or with traditional contrast enhanced studies. Diffusion weighted MRI has increased accuracy over static fluid MRI because malignant tissue has higher signal intensity than normal tissue but the detection rate is less than seen in conventional MDCTU [38, 39]. Quoted rates of performance for static MRI urography are a sensitivity, specificity, and accuracy of 76, 91, and 83% which improves to 84, 89, and 87%, respectively, with diffusion weight imaging (compared to 95, 89, and 92% on CTU by the same radiologist on the same patients) [38]. For patients who are status post cystectomy, however, who may have renal insufficiency, CT urography may not be applicable. The next best choice would be, therefore, MR urography especially in patients in whom lesions are superficial or <5 mm [42]. Gadolinium-enhanced MRI is quoted to detect renal pelvic lesions as small as 2 mm, can differentiate from benign disease seen in some chronic kidney disease (e.g., papillary necrosis), and can help discriminate central renal cell carcinomas from urothelial carcinomas in patients who cannot tolerate MDCTU [40–42].

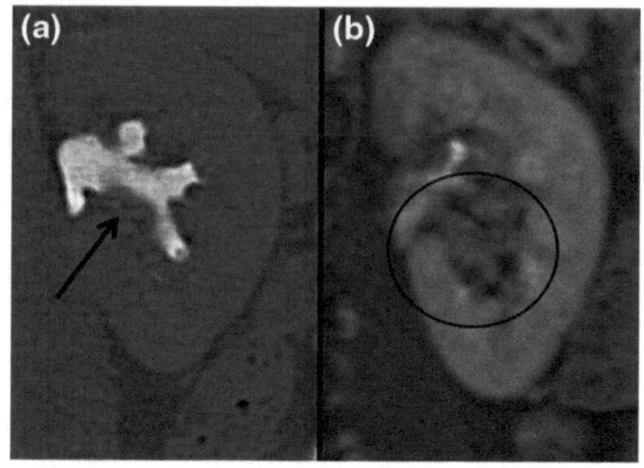

Fig. 25.2 Diagnosis of upper urinary tract urothelial carcinoma: CTU versus static DWMRI. **a** Delayed contrast phase of MDCTU showing <2 mm filling defect (*black arrow*) missed by prospective radiologist. **b** Static DWMRI of same patient 2 weeks later demonstrating poorly demarcated, larger lesion with parenchymal involvement (*black circle*) that proved to be T2 UUT-UC

An intriguing alternative in development for upper tract imaging would be bubble contrast-associated ultrasound technology. Microbubbles of perfluorocarbon or nitrogen gas appear to be well-tolerated after intravenous injection when contained by a lipid or protein macromolecular coating. Contrast ultrasound would in theory therefore allow for dynamic, real-time imaging of the renal unit without concern for renal function, radiation, or the cost of MRI [43]. Current ultrasound technology allows for the discrimination of renal cell carcinoma from columns of Bertin or pseudotumor, angioma, oncocytoma, and inflammatory masses but there are no current indications that ultrasound can detect urothelial carcinomas with the level of accuracy of either MRU or MDCTU.

The toxicity and immunogenicity of iodinated contrast reagents is related to their intravenous administration. The classic work up of hematuria included cystoscopy and retrograde pyelography with Urografin™ or Cystografin™ contrast reagents. The technique is still ideal for patients with renal insufficiency, severe contrast allergies (who may react to venous extravasation), or who cannot tolerate MRI but most typically requires the cost, burden, and time of general anesthesia. For those with a urinary diversion to an ileal conduit, retrograde pyelography is nearly precluded but may be possible by utilizing the reflux often associated with Bricker type ureterointestinal anastomoses. So-called 'loopograms' should be considered in the work up and or surveillance of patients after radical cystectomy where MDCTU, MRU, or ultrasound is inaccurate or infeasible or fails to opacify the collecting system. 'Pouchography' has less accuracy in that many ureterointestinal anastomoses are designed to be non-refluxing and reflux via a Studer type afferent limb or Indiana pouch is not predictable. No recent study has evaluated loopography in the detection of urothelial cancers but may help to lateralize abnormalities through a safe, often in-office procedure that has fluoroscopic capabilities. Still, loopographic detection may occur in <25% of patients with recurrences and likely only in patients who present with symptoms or hematuria [44].

In summary, the use of imaging is critical in the long-term surveillance of patients' status post cystectomy for the detection or recurrent UUT-UC. For those who can tolerate intravenous contrast, CTU appears to be an ideal study with few false positive results. Gadolinium-enhanced MRU would be useful for those with contrast allergies and for the detection of small, non-deforming lesions that may require more soft-tissue delineation. Patients with renal insufficiency may still have accurate imaging with diffusion weighted static MRI which could

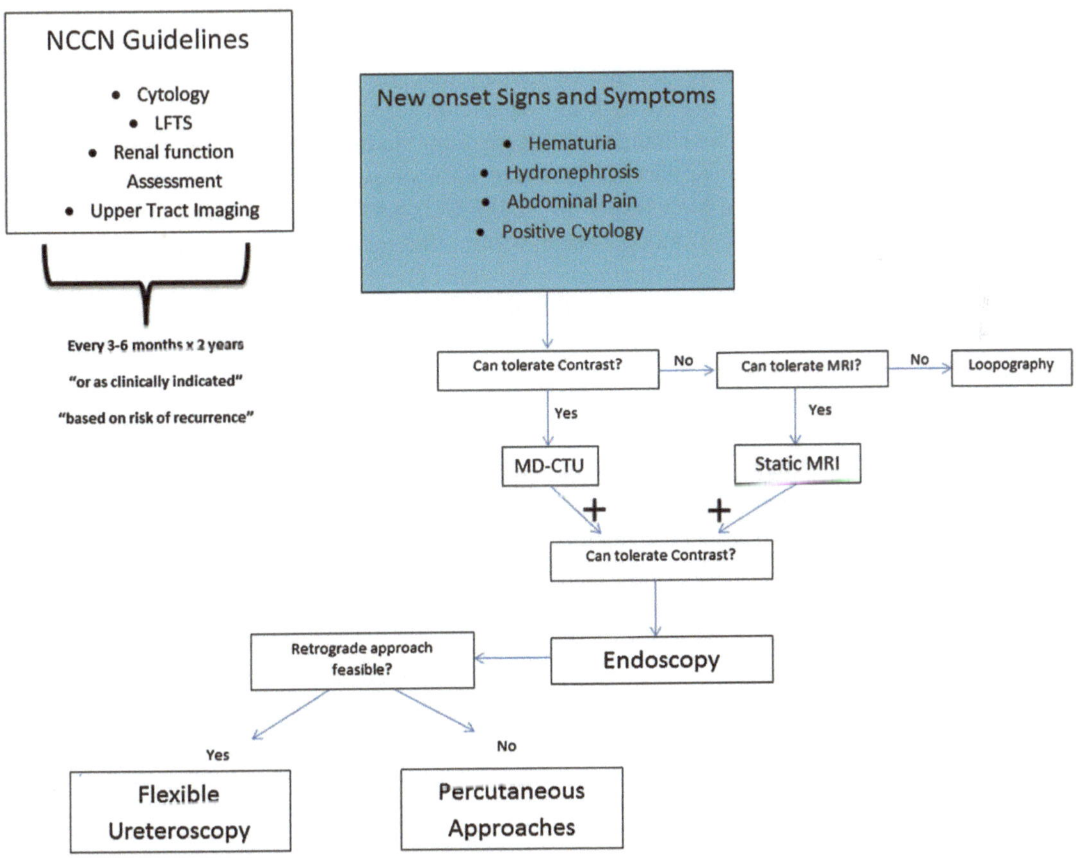

Fig. 25.3 Diagnostic approach to the upper tracts (UTs) after radical cystectomy. NCCN guidelines suggest timely UT surveillance especially in high-risk individuals. Patients who present with hematuria, a positive cytology, or lateralizing symptoms must undergo imaging and ultimately endoscopic evaluation depending on patient factors, tolerance for intervention, and feasibility

rationalize the expense and effort of ureteroscopy if a lateralizing lesion is suspected (Fig. 25.3). Loopography can be reserved for patients with bilaterally refluxing urinary diversions who cannot tolerate intravenous contrast agents and yet may require an upper tract opacification study to help with the lateralization of ureteroscopy. Contrast ultrasound is an emerging technology that may ultimately play a role in the assessment of the renal pelvis but which will likely never be applicable for ureteral relapses of UUT-UC.

Urinary Biomarkers Cytology

The use of cytology is an important tool in the work up bladder and UUT UC. The sensitivity of cytology requires the presence of shed urothelial cells in the specimen and thus has low accuracy in low grade, low-stage disease. Thus, the sensitivity of cytology may be as low as 30% for Ta or low stage T1 disease, but can rise as high as 85% in patients with CIS in which cell shedding is a histologic feature [45]. After urinary diversion, cytology samples may have high levels of mucus, enteric debris, bacterial products, and inflammatory cells which make the interpretation of cytology limited and has a positive predictive value approaching 30% [16]. It follows, therefore, that other protein-based biomarkers, which have high utility in bladder cancer, may face limitations after urinary diversion. Levels of Nuclear Matrix Protein (NMP) 22 and the protein *survivin*, for example, are found to increase in patients with some forms of urinary diversion who have no evidence of disease and may be a result of the activity of the enteric epithelium [46]. Fluorescent in situ hybridization (FISH) allows the cytologist to remove any blood cells, debris, and in many cases bacteria, to prepare a slide with host interphase nuclei. These are then stained with markers for the centromeres of chromosomes 3, 7, and 17, and a marker for the 9p21 band, all four of which are the most accurate in detecting urothelial carcinoma. The performance of FISH is higher than cytology especially in its sensitivity which is typically >94% while maintaining a high specificity of 94–98% [47]. After urinary diversion, therefore, FISH becomes particularly useful. In one study, the performance profile for cytology in detected UUT recurrences after RC showed a sensitivity, specificity, and a positive predictive value (PPV) of 80.0, 85.6, 10.7%, respectively, compared to a sensitivity, specificity, and PPV for FISH of 85.7, 86.5, and 23.1%, respectively [48]. FISH is, however, costly, and its use and a routine adjunct to the surveillance of patients after RC may be impractical. A rational use would be to combine cytology and imaging for patients at low risk of recurrence utilizing FISH for atypical cytologies, persistent microscopic or episodes of gross hematuria, or who may have developed signs of UUT relapse on upper tract imaging.

Endoscopy

Many patients who present with a high index of suspicion for UUT-UC, require endoscopic confirmation. Studies have suggested that between 50 and 75% of patients who present with primary UUT-UC do so with a dominant, enhancing mass within the renal medulla or pelvis on cross-sectional imaging [49]. Such patients will undergo nephrectomy but may require endoscopy to confirm the urothelial origin of the tumor and therefore the management of the ipsilateral ureter. The remaining patients may have either UUT-UC that is not readily imaged on cross-sectional studies or who have ureteral tumors which may be small and may cause hydronephrosis only when invasive. Endoscopy in these patients therefore becomes critical not only for tissue-typing but for lateralization and diagnosis. Still, ureteroscopy may miss occult or in situ lesions, lesions within calyceal diverticuli, or sessile lesions within inflamed hematuric pelves all of which contribute to endoscopic accuracy rates approaching 50% [50]. For patients who have an intact bladder, the task of ureteroscopy tends to be somewhat straightforward. For those patients status post urinary diversion, the ureteroscopic evaluation of the ureter is among endoscopy's most challenging tasks. Even in patients with orthotopic urinary diversions to the urethra, the location of the ureteral orifices is not reliably predictable, often 'buried' or regressed within a 'uro-scape' of redundant intestinal epithelium, and does not correlate easily with preoperative contrast-based imaging studies. Ureteral-intestinal 'neo-ureteral orifices' (NUOs) in a pouch may not always be as conveniently close to the trigone as native UOs. NUOs in a W-pouch may lie along the posterior wall, in an Indiana Pouch must be accessed through a long, surgically narrowed afferent limb, and in a Studer, may lie in the most cephalad portion of an afferent limb at or above the levels of the iliac brim of the pelvis. Patients who require upper tract evaluation, have lateralizing findings on imaging studies, and who cannot be endoscopically accessed in a retrograde manner, may require percutaneous access for an antegrade approach or for placement of an antegrade catheter that would facilitate a more traditional retrograde access technique. The basis of endoscopic techniques for UUT-UC management was derived from concepts learned in the management of nephrolithiasis. Similarly, access to the upper tracts after urinary diversion for cancer evolved from similar challenges facing patients who developed stone disease or strictures after urinary diversion [51–55]. Approximately half of patients with orthotopic diversions can be accessed de novo from a retrograde approach with failures secondary to inability to identify the afferent limb or ureteral orifice (20%), tortuosity of afferent limbs (40%), angulation (20%), and length of the afferent limb (20%) [52]. Access to an ileal conduit in several ways is more straightforward and access can be achieved in nearly 75% of cases in a retrograde fashion [56]. An antegrade percutaneous approaches is indicated if, as in large stone burdens, the urologic volume may preclude the use of the 1.9–3 Fr fulgration or biopsy devices used in flexible ureteroscopy [53].

For ileal conduit 'looposcopy', the patient is positioned supine on a fluoroscopy table, a craniotomy drape is applied to the urostomy, and flexible cystoscopy is used to perform the initial evaluation of the pouch under intravenous sedation. Peristaltic waves may intermittently diminish loop distension and it would be important that the height of the NaCl isotonic irrigant is not kept any higher than 20–30 cm above the bed. The flexible cystoscope is advanced following the central axis of the conduit, keeping the folds of enteric mucosa, which can be easily abraded and undermined, well away via irrigant dilation. Fluoroscopically following the cystoscope, the dependent end of the loop is typically reached after 15 cm. The location of the ureteral orifices may sometimes be obvious as the identification of everted ureteral mucosa or hypertrophied margins of enteric mucosa around the anastomosis. Real-time loopography can identify reflux which may help align the tip of the cystoscope with both the depth and angularity of where the anastomosis may be found. The fluoroscopic image should be rotated to keep the lumbar spine horizontal. The administration of indigo carmine or methylene blue is surprisingly ineffective in assisting the access technique. Patients may have a variable delay in their excretion of the agent and the 'jet' or blue dye seen effluxing from a native UO may not be appreciated within an ileal conduit. A Sensorwire™ is passed through the suspected ureteral orifice under fluoroscopic guidance. Any resistance without known hydronephrosis should suggest a false lumen or passage. In an ileal conduit, a wire will need to flex demonstrably immediately after the anastomosis to be reflected up the ipsilateral side or guided to traverse across the midline via the retrosigmoid mesenteric window. In either case, a 0.035 hydrophilic guidewire may be required to access the upper ureter to place a 5 French open-ended catheter through which a retrograde can be obtained or placement of a stiffer Sensor type wire. A 'super stiff' Bensten wire is probably not helpful and may be injurious via this type of diversion because the force tolerance of the anastomosis and the conduit itself may be less than native intramural ureters and bladders. A Nottingham dilator should then be used to dilate to 8 or 10 French and then exchanged for a dual lumen 8/10 coaxial dilator because the tip of the Nottingham is more flexible and forgiving on the non-dilated ureteral mucosa. The dual lumen catheter should be used to place a second 'safety' wire once a retrograde of the entire ureter has been obtained defining both the anatomy of the ureter as well as the location of the anastomosis compared to the lumbar spine and bony structures. A flexible 8 French ureteroscope can then be passed over the working wire down the conduit, across the anastomosis, and into the upper urinary tract. Resistance at the anastomosis may indicate that a lip of the ureteroscope is offset on the guiding wire and encountering the margin of the anastomosis. Rotating the scope 180 degrees often facilitates passage at this point. Once the upper urinary tract has been accessed, the user will find that ureteroscopy is far more tortuous than in the native ureter. Gentle irrigation via a handheld 60 cc syringe, dynamic rotation to maintain constant visualization of the lumen, and steady pressure of the sheath at the level of the stoma will assist in advancing the instrument. When additional stabilization is needed, placement of a nephrostomy sheath over the wire to the anastomosis will allow straighter access to the ureter and decrease forces on the walls of the conduit. Inspection of the ureter should be performed after reaching the upper pole calyx. Once access to the upper urinary tract is obtained and secured, endoscopy proceeds as if a patient has a native system and includes determination of tumor volume and extent, multifocality, evidence of invasion, involvement of the ureter, and the presence of potential skip lesions of CIS.

Conservative Management of the Upper Urinary Tract After Radical Cystectomy

Most nephroureterectomy specimens after radical cystectomy for relapsing UC reveal that a significant proportion of cancers are <T2. As urinary diversion patients are at risk for renal insufficiency, alternatives to nephrouretectomy for low risk, low-stage disease may need to be considered. On the other hand, the accuracy of ureteroscopic biopsy is notoriously poor in accurately predicting pathologic stages and choosing which patients are candidates for CT [24, 50]. The criteria for low versus high risk are derived from retrospective and smaller prospective studies of patients with primary UUT-UC. It would seem reasonable to apply these criteria to those with UUT-UC that develops after radical cystectomy. European Urologic Association guidelines suggest that low-risk patients are those with unifocal tumors that are <1 cm, are low grade, and with no evidence of infiltrative lesion on CT urography [26]. Higher risk tumors may be those that present with ipsilateral hydronephrosis, or with high-grade cells on biopsy or cytology, any tumor >1 cm, or the presence of multifocal disease. Guidelines also suggest that high-risk UUT-UC also includes any patient who recurs after radical cystectomy. The last recommendation is based on the finding that nearly a third of such patients present with advanced disease but may unnecessarily subject patients to nephroureterectomy who have biologically lower risk disease that may represent a more favorable phenotype [57]. The endoscopic management of low-risk disease, therefore, requires intense follow up and repeat ureteroscopic evaluation and treatment, all the more challenging in the surgically diverted urinary state. Most prospective studies of CT for UUT-UC display low level evidence of clinical efficacy though several studies point to equivalent overall and cancer-specific survival comparing patients with NU versus endoscopic management of low-risk disease [57, 58]. Multi-institutional studies have demonstrated no significant adverse effect of an attempt at endoscopic or regional therapy for low risk, single relapses of disease in the UUT but immediate NU must be advocated early for any patient who demonstrates progression or who is unable to undergo timely and adequate upper tract endoscopic evaluation [59]. Endoscopic management of UUT-UC would include fulguration and percutaneous approaches in which a resectoscope can be used to treat tumors too large for flexible endoscopic ablation [60]. Upper tract instillation of chemotherapeutics and BCG have long been applied to UUT-UC expecting that the same tissue responses observed in the bladder can be expected in the upper tract. Unfortunately, shorter dwell times and urothelial cell exposure to such agents, via nephrostomies or retrograde stents, has contributed to the variable efficacy of mitomycin-C and BCG therapies [61]. However, in patients with CIS only, especially bilateral disease, in whom focal or segmental nephron-sparing surgery is not feasible, BCG therapy via nephrostomy and Foley catheter drainage may play a role. In a study of 16 patients over a median follow up of 30 months with an original diagnosis of CIS UUT-UC, 10 of 16 obtained long-term durable cytology and upper tract imaging negative results [62].

Neoadjuvant platinum-based chemotherapy is becoming more popular in the management of UUT-UC prior to NU based on the favorable results of such approaches in the management if muscle-invasive bladder cancer and on the renal insufficiency after NU that precludes the use of platinum chemotherapy in the adjuvant setting [63, 64]. Staging of UUT-UC, and the rarity of the tumor, however, have greatly limited a wide availability of studies to determine the utility of this approach in primary or relapsing UUT-UC [26]. Retrospective studies focus on patients who underwent NAC versus immediate nephroureterectomy. A caveat of such an approach would be in a selection bias for those patients with high-risk disease who require early surgery versus those who may be managed on a more elective basis and can afford the 6–12 week delay to surgery required by NAC. In addition, pathologic staging after immediate NU may be either biologically different than after NAC or be different because of stage reduction by NAC. Indeed, in a retrospective study of 29 patients who underwent NAC, 65% of patients had invasive disease compared to 83% who required immediate NU [65]. Still, overall and cancer-specific survival may be better in those patients who are candidates for NAC and may thus play a role in conservation of the upper tract in patients who relapse there after radical cystectomy or who have bilateral disease.

Nephrouretectomy or Segmental Ureterectomy for UUT-UC

Patients who have high-risk disease, who elect to undergo NU, or who have completed NAC, will require open or laparoscopic NU. The goal of NU in the native kidney and ureter is to achieve the anatomic requirements of a radical nephrectomy including the entirety of the ureter and the cuff of bladder containing the intramural ureter and UVJ. After urinary diversion, the extreme distal ureter is now included in the anastomosis with bowel. For most urinary diversions, one of the ureters will be crossing the midline, usually in a retrosigmoidal window, to reach the urinary diversion or pouch. It becomes critical, therefore, to identify the ureter of the affected side, resect the distal ureter with its anastomotic tissue, and deliver the distal ureter with the proximal ureter and renal unit *in toto* without harming the contralateral urinary tract or bowel anastomosis. Most patients who require NU after urinary diversion are candidates for laparoscopic NU followed by open extraction of the specimen through a midline incision. The approach would allow open inspection of the distal ureters to ensure that the ipsilateral segment is identified. Robotic-assisted repairs of ileal ureteral strictures appears feasible with a docking of the patient side cart (PSC) similar to robotic cystectomy although with the ports more cephalad and without a reliance on extreme Trendelenberg positioning [66, 67]. Such approaches are applicable to radical nephroureterectomy whereby the nephrectomy is achieved through traditional 5 mm ports and straight laparoscopic techniques and then the patient is positioned in Trendelenberg for the robotic-assisted identification and delivery of the distal ureteral portion and repair of the defect in the ileal conduit.

Segmental ureterectomy may be useful in the management of primary UUT-UC where patients have isolated, low-grade lesions of the ureter without skip CIS who are amenable to uretero-ureterostomy repairs without tension [60]. Although relapse rates are high, reaching 50% by at a median of 4 years follow up, recurrence free survival and renal preservation appear equivalent and in some cases higher than compared NU in patients with clinical staged low-risk disease isolated to the ureter [68, 69]. After radical cystectomy, the blood supply from the superior vesicle pedicle and the iliac vessels is lost and ureteral integrity is largely maintained by collateral blood flow derived from the renal artery (although some aortic twigs to the mid-ureter may remain). Segmental resection and uretero-ureterostomy after radical cystectomy, therefore, may subject the distal ureter to ischemia and early stricture formation. As such, segmental resection may be applicable only to distal ureteral recurrences where primary ureterointestinal anastomoses can be performed under tension-free conditions.

Summary

Patients who undergo radical cystectomy (RC) for urothelial carcinoma (UC), are at life-long risk for the development of upper urinary tract (UUT) UC. Surveillance must include urinary cytology (and FISH when cytology is atypical or inadequate) and annual cross-sectional imaging. Endoscopy after urinary diversion is challenging but feasible via retrograde approaches. Antegrade access, either to allow endoscopy, or to pass a stent to allow retrograde access, is an important step to adequately diagnose patients with UUT relapses and to evaluate a patient's candidacy for CT and nephron-sparing approaches. The overall survival of UUT-UC after radical cystectomy appears related, predominately to the survival from the original bladder cancer. However, more patients with UUT-UC after radical cystectomy present with advanced disease compared to those with primary UUT-UC and they may do so despite the lack of identifiable disease on surveillance imaging. The urologist must be prepared, therefore, to act upon any signs of symptoms that could possibly be related to upper tract recurrences after radical cystectomy including microscopic or gross hematuria, flank pain or late onset hydronephrosis, or the appearance of changes on cross-sectional imaging. Patients at risk for relapse in the UUT include men who had prostatic involvement, women with urethral involvement, positive ureteral margins, and patients with persistent positive cytology after RC. With adequate surveillance, patient evaluation, and diligent follow up, early identification of UUT-UC may allow for CT and defer the sometimes debilitating effects of immediate NU.

Summary Box

- Upper urinary tract (UUT) urothelial carcinoma is a serious, sometimes fatal disease that can unnecessarily elude diagnosis in patients status post radical cystectomy and urinary diversion.
- UUT-UC after radical cystectomy presents at a more advanced stage but overall survival is related to the survival from the original bladder cancer.
- Patients at risk for relapse in the UUT include men who had prostatic involvement, women with urethral involvement, patients with positive ureteral margins, and patients with persistent positive cytology after RC.
- Ureteroscopy after urinary diversion can be accomplished in a retrograde fashion via looposcopy or facilitated by antegrade placement of a stent.

References

1. Picozzi S, Ricci C, Gaeta M, et al. Upper urinary tract recurrence following radical cystectomy for bladder cancer: a meta-analysis on 13,185 patients. J Urol. 2012;188:2046.
2. Sanderson KM, Cai J, Miranda G, et al. Upper tract urothelial recurrence following radical cystectomy for transitional cell carcinoma of the bladder: an analysis of 1,069 patients with 10-year followup. J Urol. 2007;177:2088.
3. Nison L, Roupret M, Bozzini G, et al. The oncologic impact of a delay between diagnosis and radical nephroureterectomy due to diagnostic ureteroscopy in upper urinary tract urothelial carcinomas: results from a large collaborative database. World J Urol. 2013;31:69.
4. Mitra AP, Alemozaffar M, Harris BN, et al. Outcomes after urothelial recurrence in bladder cancer patients undergoing radical cystectomy. Urology. 2014;84:1420.
5. Rink M, Adam M, Hansen J, et al. Upper tract urothelial carcinoma. An update on clinical and pathological prognostic factors. Urologe A. 2012;51:1228.
6. Rink M, Ehdaie B, Cha EK, et al. Stage-specific impact of tumor location on oncologic outcomes in patients with upper and lower tract urothelial

carcinoma following radical surgery. Eur Urol. 2012;62:677.
7. Ku JH, Moon KC, Jung JH, et al. External validation of an online nomogram in patients undergoing radical nephroureterectomy for upper urinary tract urothelial carcinoma. Br J Cancer. 2013;109:1130.
8. Elalouf V, Xylinas E, Klap J, et al. Bladder recurrence after radical nephroureterectomy: predictors and impact on oncological outcomes. Int J Urol. 2013;20:1078.
9. Ku JH, Choi WS, Kwak C, et al. Bladder cancer after nephroureterectomy in patients with urothelial carcinoma of the upper urinary tract. Urol Oncol. 2011;29:383.
10. Park J, Ha SH, Min GE, et al. The protective role of renal parenchyma as a barrier to local tumor spread of upper tract transitional cell carcinoma and its impact on patient survival. J Urol. 2009;182:894.
11. Park S, Hong B, Kim CS, et al. The impact of tumor location on prognosis of transitional cell carcinoma of the upper urinary tract. J Urol. 2004;171:621.
12. Bin X, Roy OP, Ghiraldi E, et al. Impact of tumour location and surgical approach on recurrence-free and cancer-specific survival analysis in patients with ureteric tumours. BJU Int. 2012;110:E514.
13. Milojevic B, Djokic M, Sipetic-Grujicic S, et al. Upper urinary tract transitional cell carcinoma: location is not correlated with prognosis. BJU Int. 2012;109:1037.
14. Patel N, Arya M, Muneer A, et al. Molecular aspects of upper tract urothelial carcinoma. Urol Oncol. 2014;32(28):e11.
15. Raman JD, Messer J, Sielatycki JA, et al. Incidence and survival of patients with carcinoma of the ureter and renal pelvis in the USA, 1973–2005. BJU Int. 2011;107:1059.
16. Kim SH, Yang HK, Lee JH, et al. A retrospective analysis of incidence and its associated risk factors of upper urinary tract recurrence following radical cystectomy for bladder cancer with transitional cell carcinoma: the significance of local pelvic recurrence and positive lymph node. PLoS ONE. 2014;9:e96467.
17. Haddad M, Cloutier J, Cornu JN, et al. Immediate nephroureterectomy or after attempting conservative treatment, on elective indications, for upper urinary tract urothelial carcinoma: comparison of the pathology reports on a retrospective monocentric study. J Endourol. 2015;29:969.
18. Lee JN, Kwon SY, Choi GS, et al. Impact of surgical wait time on oncologic outcomes in upper urinary tract urothelial carcinoma. J Surg Oncol. 2014;110:468.
19. Ehdaie B, Furberg H, Zabor EC, et al. Impact of smoking status at diagnosis on disease recurrence and death in upper tract urothelial carcinoma. BJU Int. 2013;111:589.
20. Solsona E, Iborra I, Dumont R, et al. Risk groups in patients with bladder cancer treated with radical cystectomy: statistical and clinical model improving homogeneity. J Urol. 2005;174:1226.
21. Kenworthy P, Tanguay S, Dinney CP. The risk of upper tract recurrence following cystectomy in patients with transitional cell carcinoma involving the distal ureter. J Urol. 1996;155:501.
22. Sved PD, Gomez P, Nieder AM, et al. Upper tract tumour after radical cystectomy for transitional cell carcinoma of the bladder: incidence and risk factors. BJU Int. 2004;94:785.
23. Yossepowitch O, Dalbagni G, Golijanin D, et al. Orthotopic urinary diversion after cystectomy for bladder cancer: implications for cancer control and patterns of disease recurrence. J Urol. 2003;169:177.
24. Wang JK, Tollefson MK, Krambeck AE, et al. High rate of pathologic upgrading at nephroureterectomy for upper tract urothelial carcinoma. Urology. 2012;79:615.
25. Stefanovic V, Polenakovic M, Toncheva D. Urothelial carcinoma associated with Balkan endemic nephropathy. A worldwide disease. Pathol Biol (Paris). 2011;59:286.
26. Roupret M, Babjuk M, Comperat E, et al. European association of urology guidelines on upper urinary tract urothelial cell carcinoma: 2015 update. Eur Urol. 2015.
27. Catto JW, Azzouzi AR, Amira N, et al. Distinct patterns of microsatellite instability are seen in tumours of the urinary tract. Oncogene. 2003;22:8699.
28. Zhang Z, Pang ST, Kasper KA, et al. FXYD3: a promising biomarker for urothelial carcinoma. Biomark Insights. 2011;6:17.
29. Zhang Z, Furge KA, Yang XJ, et al. Comparative gene expression profiling analysis of urothelial carcinoma of the renal pelvis and bladder. BMC Med Genomics. 2010;3:58.
30. Dalbagni G, Bochner BH, Cronin A, et al. A plea for a uniform surveillance schedule after radical cystectomy. J Urol. 2011;185:2091.
31. Ehdaie B, Atoria CL, Lowrance WT, et al. Adherence to surveillance guidelines after radical cystectomy: a population-based analysis. Urol Oncol. 2014;32:779.
32. Kielar AZ, Ellis JH, Cohan RH, et al. Computed tomography urography: trends in positivity rates over time. J Comput Assist Tomogr. 2008;32:46.
33. Sadow CA, Wheeler SC, Kim J, et al. Positive predictive value of CT urography in the evaluation of upper tract urothelial cancer. AJR Am J Roentgenol. 2010;195:W337.
34. Pabon-Ramos W, Caoili E, Cohan R, et al. Excretory urography: trends in clinical use and diagnostic yield. Abdom Imaging. 2010;35:607.
35. Wang LJ, Wong YC, Huang CC, et al. Multidetector computerized tomography urography is more accurate than excretory urography for diagnosing transitional cell carcinoma of the upper urinary tract in adults with hematuria. J Urol. 2010;183:48.

36. van der Molen AJ, Miclea RL, Geleijns J, et al. A survey of radiation doses in ct urography before and after implementation of iterative reconstruction. AJR Am J Roentgenol. 2015;205:572.
37. Rose TA Jr, Choi JW. Intravenous imaging contrast media complications: the basics that every clinician needs to know. Am J Med. 2015;128:943.
38. Wu GY, Lu Q, Wu LM, et al. Comparison of computed tomographic urography, magnetic resonance urography and the combination of diffusion weighted imaging in diagnosis of upper urinary tract cancer. Eur J Radiol. 2014;83:893.
39. Martingano P, Cavallaro MF, Bertolotto M, et al. Magnetic resonance urography vs computed tomography urography in the evaluation of patients with haematuria. Radiol Med. 2013;118:1184.
40. Wehrli NE, Kim MJ, Matza BW, et al. Utility of MRI features in differentiation of central renal cell carcinoma and renal pelvic urothelial carcinoma. AJR Am J Roentgenol. 2013;201:1260.
41. Schroeder J, Thacker PG, Purves TJ. Magnetic resonance urography of renal papillary necrosis. Pediatr Radiol. 2014;44:491.
42. Takahashi N, Kawashima A, Glockner JF, et al. Small (<2-cm) upper-tract urothelial carcinoma: evaluation with gadolinium-enhanced three-dimensional spoiled gradient-recalled echo MR urography. Radiology. 2008;247:451.
43. Malhi H, Grant EG, Duddalwar V. Contrast-enhanced ultrasound of the liver and kidney. Radiol Clin North Am. 2014;52:1177.
44. Noble J, Amin Z, Kessel D, et al. Recurrent upper tract urothelial tumours: the use of loopography following cystectomy for bladder cancer. Br J Radiol. 1994;67:1057.
45. Lodde M, Mayr R, Martini T, et al. Positive urine cytology and carcinoma in situ prior to second transurethral resection of the bladder correlate with positive second resection histology and the need for subsequent cystectomy. World J Urol. 2012;30:841.
46. Dong ZL, Lu ZP, Wang HZ, et al. Detection of nuclear matrix protein 22 and survivin baseline level in patients after radical cystectomy. Urol Int. 2011;87:445.
47. Phillips JL, Richardson IC. Aneuploidy in bladder cancers: the utility of fluorescent in situ hybridization in clinical practice. BJU Int. 2006;98:33.
48. Fernandez MI, Parikh S, Grossman HB, et al. The role of FISH and cytology in upper urinary tract surveillance after radical cystectomy for bladder cancer. Urol Oncol. 2012;30:821.
49. Fein AB, McClennan BL. Solitary filling defects of the ureter. Semin Roentgenol. 1986;21:201.
50. Yamany T, van Batavia J, Ahn J, et al. Ureterorenoscopy for upper tract urothelial carcinoma: how often are we missing lesions? Urology. 2015;85:311.
51. Zhong W, Yang B, He F, et al. Surgical management of urolithiasis in patients after urinary diversion. PLoS ONE. 2014;9:e111371.
52. Rivera M, Krambeck A. Retrograde ureteroscopy via a continent urinary diversion: surgical techniques and common pitfalls. J Endourol. 2014;28:763.
53. Hertzig LL, Iwaszko MR, Rangel LJ, et al. Urolithiasis after ileal conduit urinary diversion: a comparison of minimally invasive therapies. J Urol. 2013;189:2152.
54. Stuurman RE, Al-Qahtani SM, Cornu JN, et al. Antegrade percutaneous flexible endoscopic approach for the management of urinary diversion-associated complications. J Endourol. 2013;27:1330.
55. Okhunov Z, Duty B, Smith AD, et al. Management of urolithiasis in patients after urinary diversions. BJU Int. 2011;108:330.
56. Hyams ES, Winer AG, Shah O. Retrograde ureteral and renal access in patients with urinary diversion. Urology. 2009;74:47.
57. Yakoubi R, Colin P, Seisen T, et al. Radical nephroureterectomy versus endoscopic procedures for the treatment of localised upper tract urothelial carcinoma: a meta-analysis and a systematic review of current evidence from comparative studies. Eur J Surg Oncol. 2014;40:1629.
58. Seisen T, Colin P, Roupret M. Risk-adapted strategy for the kidney-sparing management of upper tract tumours. Nat Rev Urol. 2015;12:155.
59. Colin P, Neuzillet Y, Pignot G, et al. Follow-up of urothelial carcinoma: review of the Cancer Committee of the French Association of Urology. Prog Urol. 2015;25:616.
60. Lucca I, Klatte T, Roupret M, et al. Kidney-sparing surgery for upper tract urothelial cancer. Curr Opin Urol. 2015;25:100.
61. Obayashi K, Miki J, Kasai K, et al. A case of percutaneous BCG perfusion therapy for CIS of upper urinary tract CIS after radical cystectomy with ileal neobladder. Hinyokika Kiyo. 2014;60:443.
62. Miyake H, Eto H, Hara S, et al. Clinical outcome of bacillus Calmette-Guerin perfusion therapy for carcinoma in situ of the upper urinary tract. Int J Urol. 2002;9:677.
63. Lin YK, Kaag M, Raman JD. Rationale and timing of perioperative chemotherapy for upper-tract urothelial carcinoma. Expert Rev Anticancer Ther. 2014;14:543.
64. Xylinas E, Rink M, Margulis V, et al. Impact of renal function on eligibility for chemotherapy and survival in patients who have undergone radical nephroureterectomy. BJU Int. 2013;112:453.
65. Porten S, Siefker-Radtke AO, Xiao L, et al. Neoadjuvant chemotherapy improves survival of patients with upper tract urothelial carcinoma. Cancer. 2014;120:1794.

66. Tobis S, Houman J, Mastrodonato K, et al. Robotic repair of post-cystectomy ureteroileal anastomotic strictures: techniques for success. J Laparoendosc Adv Surg Tech A. 2013;23:526.
67. Dangle PP, Abaza R. Robot-assisted repair of ureteroileal anastomosis strictures: initial cases and literature review. J Endourol. 2012;26:372.
68. Hung SY, Yang WC, Luo HL, et al. Segmental ureterectomy does not compromise the oncologic outcome compared with nephroureterectomy for pure ureter cancer. Int Urol Nephrol. 2014;46:921.
69. Pedrosa JA, Masterson TA, Rice KR, et al. Oncologic outcomes and prognostic impact of urothelial recurrences in patients undergoing segmental and total ureterectomy for upper tract urothelial carcinoma. Can Urol Assoc J. 2015;9:E187.

Surveillance of the Upper Tract After Conservative Treatment

26

Joel Hillelsohn and Majid Eshghi

Conservative treatment of Urothelial Cell Carcinoma as previously discussed, is considered in cases for renal preservation and elective cases for low-grade disease or palliative considerations. Following endoscopic treatment, surveillance is key in assessing for recurrence and ensuring complete treatment. However, despite advances in imaging, surveillance requires multiple invasive procedures. Unlike bladder tumor follow up, urothelial tumors in the upper tract cannot be solely performed on an outpatient basis. Selective upper tract cytology and endoscopy requires sedation, general anesthesia, and fluoroscopy depending on the original pathology and the treatments rendered.

In a general sense, once patients have elected to undergo conservative treatment, they are signing up for lifetime surveillance. Recurrences are common and can happen long after initial resection. In a recent study by Motamedinia et al. [1] they identified recurrences as long as ten years following initial resection. In a meta-analysis by Cutress et al. [2] they found the five-year recurrence rate for ureteroscopic treatment to be 52% and percutaneous resection 37%. This recurrence rate is likely underreported since patients selected for conservative treatment are often elderly with significant comorbidities and likely did not survive long enough to have a recurrence. In the studies utilized in the meta-analysis, these patients were not censored. Cutress et al. [2] estimated the true censored five-year recurrence free survival to be only 13–54%. There is also concern for downstream seeding of the bladder. In larger studies, five-year intravesical recurrence-free survival has been estimated to range from 46 to 54% [2–5]. Finally in pooled studies progression and conversion to radical nephroureterectomy occurred in 13–50% of patients [2]. These studies emphasize the need for strict lifetime surveillance and adaptable treatment protocols.

In the early stages of treatment, most patients are quite proactive and follow up on the recommended protocols, but after a period of time an element of 'PATIENT FATIGUE' develops. Recurrence of disease is often silent and it can be hard for patients to comprehend the need for further invasive, at times painful procedures, when they feel well. To combat this 'patient fatigue', a multidisciplinary approach is often necessary to achieve a minimum basic follow-up. Furthermore, this intense lifetime surveillance is a difficult task for a young individual, but in the often elderly debilitated patients diagnosed with upper tract urothelial carcinoma it is truly a

J. Hillelsohn (✉) · M. Eshghi
Department of Urology, Westchester Medical Health Network/New York Medical College, Valhalla, NY 10595, USA
e-mail: jhillelsohn@gmail.com

M. Eshghi
e-mail: majid_eshghi@nymc.edu

M. Eshghi (ed.), *Urothelial Malignancies of the Upper Urinary Tract*,
https://doi.org/10.1007/978-3-319-51263-1_26

herculean task. This chapter will discuss recommended follow-up protocols and the management of the social aspects of follow-up with the patient and family.

Physician, Patient, Family Component

As per the EUA guidelines for the treatment of upper tract urothelial carcinoma, the five factors indicating conservative treatment are uni-focal tumors, small tumors, low-grade tumors, no evidence of infiltrative lesions on MRI or CT urogram and most significantly understanding of close follow-up [6]. Once the patients are explained the risks and benefits of conservative management, a comprehensive discussion is critical in emphasizing the need for follow-up. The patient needs to clearly understand the steps that are required for close follow-up to avoid missing recurrence or progression of disease. In our opinion, discussion with the patient should involve the family members who have an input in terms of the compliance and the patient's follow-up. We therefore recommend after the initial workup has been completed to have a full discussion with all the family members. Issues to cover include: the nature of the disease, basic understanding of the pathology, pattern of recurrence, progression, and auxiliary treatments such as topical treatment using immunotherapy or chemotherapeutic agents. Unlike other surveillance protocols for urological malignancies, such as testicular tumors or prostate cancer, there is a large need for familial support to help transition and transport the patients following multiple invasive procedures.

A typical outline of the standard conversation doing the first office visit is outlined below.

1. We first outline the patient's disease in context of their medical comorbidities, with extensive review of the diagnosis, pathology and choices of treatment including radical nephroureterectomy. Our guidelines for recommending conservative treatment and its risks and benefits are outlined in another chapter.
2. We next explain to the patients and their family the need for regular and frequent follow-ups which include procedures such as imaging, surveillance ureteroscopy, and repeat biopsies depending on the disease. Emphasis should be made on the aggressive nature of the disease. The family and patient should understand that conservative therapy rarely provides a complete cure and recurrences are common. If there is a significant change in pathology the patient may be counseled on conversion to a more invasive treatment such as radical nephroureterectomy, even if it means going on dialysis. Other possible outcomes may be neoadjuvant or salvage chemotherapy. Another point that should be addressed is that, in most cases percutaneous access is obtained for resection and/or topical chemotherapy. Therefore, the patients will have an indwelling small nephrostomy tube. The tube itself is usually clamped and used only as an access for intracavitary treatment and/or endoscopic surveillance. However, the tube can be uncomfortable for patients and can within itself carry infectious risks. It is our standard practice to have a small nephrostomy tube in the office to demonstrate the abstract concept to most patients.
3. Once the family is given the information outlined above, it is the challenging task for clinicians to evaluate the family dynamic and the patient's likelihood of follow-up. If the patient is not willing to comply with the recommended follow-up and imaging studies, they obviously should be discouraged from pursuing conservative treatment. However, if the physician feels based on his evaluation and office encounter, that the patient and other family members may not be reliable or will not be compliant, he should guide the patient and family away from conservative treatment options.
4. If the patient and clinician agree on pursuing conservative treatment, it is recommended to communicate with the patient's primary care physician and other specialists such as cardiologist, pulmonologist, hematologist, and

oncologist as per patients medical history if necessary. It is critical to maintain a strong doctor–patient relationship throughout the treatment cycle. Often patients have primary care physicians with a long-term relationship who may have a better understanding of patient's family dynamics and support system. Involving the primary care physician in the decision and discussion of care early in the treatment cycle increases compliance. In addition, during the course of treatment, patients will need regular follow ups with their primary care physicians and other specialists to be medically optimized for multiple outpatient ambulatory procedures that require anesthesia or sedation. An oncology consult is recommended to coordinate patient care for possible future treatments such as systematic chemotherapy depending on the progression, grading, and staging of the disease.

5. The physician and his staff should make every effort to ensure that the patient and the family have a clear understanding of the nature of the disease, progression, and make every effort to provide adequate educational material for the patient. We also encourage the patient to do her or his own research and pursue a second opinion before making a final decision.
6. The discussion should be outlined in the office notes with details. The patient and the family should frequently be reminded that some of these treatments are not considered standardized treatment and they always have the option to have the treatment changed to other types such as a radical nephroureterectomy.

During the course of the patient's follow-up, it is important to reemphasize the course of the treatment and potential for change of course. Any family or support dynamic change, such as divorce or death should be elucidated. Social work consultation in order to provide transport for treatments and ensure compliance is a useful tool often underutilized. During office visits for topical treatments, it is important to review the potential side effects of the treatments such as BCG or Mitomycin C as reviewed in previous chapters.

The physician and all the members of the treatment team should present a realistic level of expectation to the patient. An unrealistic outlook may cloud the critical doctor–patient relationship crucial in navigating treatment options in cases of recurrence or worsening of the disease. If a follow-up exam or negative imaging study is obtained, it should not be translated into a picture of cure or 100% remission. Rather, this should be used as a promising sign and the patient should be dissuaded from believing that a close follow-up is no longer required. Some patients in spite of multiple discussions and reminders will not comply with the recommended follow-up and procedures. They often feel well and do not have any physical sign of recurrent disease. Complacency often ensues, in the context of their growing fatigue of multiple invasive procedures. It is important for the treating physician to frequently emphasize the risk of quiet progression of the disease to the patients and this can be done in forms of written letters to other treating physicians and the patient or if necessary certified letters for legal purposes.

Surveillance Protocol

1. Post initial resection, similar to bladder treatment protocols, we start the patient with a six-week course of intracavitary treatment via a nephrostomy tube. This has been detailed elsewhere in the book.
2. After completion of a six-week course of treatment, the patient will require an in-office flexible cystoscopy and urine cytology from the bladder and nephrostomy tube.
3. Imaging studies should be obtained tailored to the patient's condition and circumstances such as indwelling nephrostomy tube, double pigtail stent, renal function, allergy to contrast, and factors that circumvent MRI or CT imaging. Therefore, a variety of methods such as sonography, CT imaging, MRI, or nephrostogram may be used. At least one imaging study must be performed in the first three months after initial treatment.

4. Upper endoscopy via flexible ureteroscopy or percutaneously through existing access should be performed following the completion of intracavitary treatment and within 3 months of initial resection. Typically, we use 12 French mini nephroscope, a flexible cystoscope, rigid and flexible ureteroscopes. After complete evaluation of the collecting system, antegrade ureteroscopy is recommended to rule out recurrence in the ureter. Flexible cystoscopy should also be performed if not done earlier in the office.
5. If a recurrence is identified, it should be resected or treated similar to the initial treatment. We recommend a deep biopsy of the areas of previous tumor if there is no visible recurrence. Sometimes with topical treatment, the surveillance endoscopy and cytology may not necessarily be positive, but there may be evidence of submucosal disease invasive disease on deep biopsy.
6. As outlined in previous chapters, a solution of 40 mg of mitomycin in 40–60 cc of saline is slowly instilled via the newly placed nephrostomy tube at the completion of the surveillance nephroscopy
7. Depending on the endoscopic findings, a three-week booster treatment with mitomycin is recommended before the nephrostomy tube is removed.
8. If there is obvious recurrence after complete resection, the patient may require alternative treatment or a second course of intracavitary treatment. There is also the option of changing the chemotherapeutic agent from Mitomycin C to BCG immunotherapy. As outlined in previous chapters, it is not uncommon for the patient to develop recurrences elsewhere such as in the distal ureter or bladder especially if the patient has had previous history of bladder or ureteral tumors. Antegrade instillation will allow for treatment of the collecting system, ureter, and the bladder with one instillation.
9. In cases of disease progression or invasion based on endoscopic biopsy or imaging, the treating physician should discuss with the patient neoadjuvant chemotherapy, nephroureterectomy, or other options in consultation with an oncologist. In cases of disease progression, a PET scan is often helpful in planning next step in treatment.
10. If the first round of surveillance is negative and nephrostomy tube has been removed, the patient will need urinary cytology, flexible cystoscopy, follow-up ureteroscopy plus MR or CT Urogram within three months.
11. With improvement of CT imaging, virtual endoscopy of the upper tract will play an increased role for detection of recurrences (see the chapter on virtual ureteroscopy).
12. After the first year following initial resection flexible cystoscopy, ureteroscopy, selective cytologies should be performed every six months for one year than annular thereafter. MR or CT Urograms as well as bladder cytologies should be performed on a regular basis.

Table 26.1 Suggested follow-up protocol

Time from initial resection	Follow up
6 weeks	Weekly intracavitary chemotherapy with mitomycin C
3 months	Flexible cystoscopy, endoscopic surveillance and biopsy, upper tract and bladder cytology and imaging
3–4 months	Booster mitomycin C instillation for 3 weeks then removal of nephrostomy tube
6 months	Flexible cystoscopy, ureteroscopy, upper tract and bladder cytology and MR or CT urogram
12 months	Flexible cystoscopy, ureteroscopy, upper tract and bladder cytology and MR or CT urogram or virtual ureteroscopy
18 months	Ureteroscopy and upper tract and bladder cytology
24 months and after, modified as needed	Flexible cystoscopy, ureteroscopy, upper tract and bladder cytology and MR or CT urogram or virtual ureteroscopy

The main focus of surveillance is the emphasis on the fact that recurrence is likely and should not be considered a setback. Constant communication with the patient is critical in reiterating need for follow-up and discussion of treatment plans. Patient fatigue with treatment is a recurrent issue that can only be addressed by engaging familial support and fostering a close therapeutic relationship with the patients. With conservative management depending on the grade and stage of the disease, complete cure cannot be guaranteed and only with strict follow-up can a patient stay ahead of the recurrent disease (Table 26.1). The follow up protocol vary significantly in different institutions.

Summary Box

- Following Upper Tract Conservative Treatment recurrences are common and strict surveillance is critical
- Surveillance involves multiple invasive procedures and can lead to 'patient fatigue' and lack of compliance
- Fostering a patient–doctor therapeutic relationship and utilizing a multidisciplinary approach is key in ensuring compliance
- A realistic outlook on the treatment as a prevention rather than a catch up approach is key to ensuring successful follow-up
- We typically examine the upper and lower tract as well as image the patient in 3–6 month intervals following initial treatment for 24 months then adjusted thereafter depending on the outcome.

Acknowledgements Author acknowledges the contribution of Gerald Matthews, MD, Westchester Medical Health Network, New York Medical College, Valhalla, NY and thanks him for his helpful comments and feedback.

References

1. Motamedinia P, Keheila M, Leavitt DA, Rastinehad AR, Okeke Z, Smith AD. The expanded use of percutaneous resection for upper tract urothelial carcinoma: a 30-year comprehensive experience. J Endourol. 2016 Mar;30(3):262–7.
2. Cutress ML, Stewart GD, Zakikhani P, Phipps S, Thomas BG, Tolley DA. Ureteroscopic and percutaneous management of upper tract urothelial carcinoma (UTUC): systematic review. BJU Int. 2012;110 (5):614–28.
3. Thompson RH, Krambeck AE, Lohse CM, Elliott DS, Patterson DE, Blute ML. Endoscopic management of upper tract transitional cell carcinoma in patients with normal contralateral kidneys. Urology. 2008;71 (4):713–7.
4. Krambeck AE, Thompson RH, Lohse CM, Patterson DE, Elliott DS, Blute ML (2007) Imperative indications for conservative management of upper tract transitional cell carcinoma. J Urol 178(3 Pt 1):792–6; (discussion 6–7).
5. Thompson RH, Krambeck AE, Lohse CM, Elliott DS, Patterson DE, Blute ML. Elective endoscopic management of transitional cell carcinoma first diagnosed in the upper urinary tract. BJU Int. 2008;102(9):1107–10.
6. Rouprêt M, Babjuk M, Compérat E, Zigeuner R, Sylvester RJ, Burger M, et al. European association of urology guidelines on upper urinary tract urothelial cell carcinoma: 2015 update. Eur Urol. 2015;68(5):868–79.

27 Analysis of Conservative Treatment of Upper Tract Urothelial Carcinoma

Joel Hillelsohn, Ariel Schulman and Majid Eshghi

Urology has always been in the forefront of technological innovations that allow urologists to explore novel approaches in patient care. However, the data on the efficacy and proper utilization of these innovations by necessity lag behind. Urologists are confronted with technological innovations that lack substantive literature. The literature is usually filled with short term, small case series. The 30-year accumulative data on the conservative treatment of upper tract urothelial cell carcinoma (UTUC) is still coming of age. The Research Office of the Endourological Society (CROES) has an ongoing international database that will hopefully bring a more comprehensive view on this subject. In this chapter, we attempt to provide the summary of available literature on this subject.

A thorough analysis of the data is extremely challenging. There is no true gold standard treatment to be compared against. Just as, TURBT and intravesical treatment data cannot always be compared to cystectomy outcome; endoscopic, and conservative treatments of the UTUC cannot always be compared against radical nephroureterectomy (RNU). There is no separate literature to be compared to conservative treatment of a solitary kidney with adjuvant intracavitary treatment. An example is one of our patients in urothelial carcinoma in a solitary kidney. He was treated for four years with combination of endoscopic and topical treatment, refusing nephroureterectomy fearing complications of hemodialysis. Once the renal function began to detoriate, the patient agreed to undergo a nephroureterectomy. The pathology showed residual disease. The patient's general condition rapidly deteriorated while on dialysis and he succumbed to a myocardial infarction a few months later. Is this considered a definitive surgical cure? Was the patient better off on conservative endoscopic and topical treatment with a nonlethal residual disease?

By far the most difficult aspect of analyzing the literature on this topic is that the literature reflects the evolution of treatment. Conservative treatment of UTUC began in the 1980s. That data from the 1980s mostly reflect older patients with multiple comorbidities. They had a choice between nephrectomy and lifetime dialysis versus an attempt at conservative or palliative treatment. This was the first stage of development in conservative treatment and the literature reflects this. In the second stage (1991 to approximately 2003)

J. Hillelsohn (✉) · A. Schulman · M. Eshghi
Department of Urology, Westchester Medical Health Network/New York Medical College, 40 Sunshine Cottage Rd., Valhalla, NY 10595, USA
e-mail: jhillelsohn@gmail.com

A. Schulman
Division of Urology, Duke University School of Medicine, Durham, NC, USA
e-mail: schulmana@wcmc.com

M. Eshghi
e-mail: majid_eshghi@nymc.edu

M. Eshghi (ed.), *Urothelial Malignancies of the Upper Urinary Tract*,
https://doi.org/10.1007/978-3-319-51263-1_27

more ureteral lesions were treated, small single renal lesion were treated with curative purpose and adjuvant treatments were more widely used. Endourologists were no longer treating patients as a last resort with conservative treatment. The final stage was the improvement of existing techniques. New retrograde and antegrade resection and ablation techniques were developed and the use of topical-intracavitary treatment was expanded with standardized follow-up and surveillance protocols. The literature from the last two stages has the largest case series and most follow-up. However, even studies published during the final stage include patients from the initial stage. Therefore, almost all the studies published on the topic are plagued by heterogeneity, reflecting multiple treatment protocols, techniques and patients with variable indications for treatment. A meta-analysis is only as good as the data it analyzes. With this background, we ventured into this difficult task to show a snapshot of information available to this date.

Ureteroscopic Resection

Ureteroscopic examination is the first line approach for diagnosis and evaluation of upper tract urothelial carcinoma. Following comprehensive staging and shared decision-making about risks and benefits of alternative therapies, a primary endoscopic approach can be pursued in properly selected cases. Multiple case series have been published with promising results with long-term patient follow-up although many remain a small size, with retrospective data collection and non-uniform case selection and management strategies. Critical review of primary endoscopic therapy should consider the impact of tumor grade, staging, endoscopic surveillance strategy, use of adjunctive topical therapy, case selection, and criteria for conversion to extirpative surgery.

Studies by Schmeller et al. [1] and Gaboardi et al. [2] reporting on lasering of UTUC on 16 and 18 patients respectively; reflect the first stage of endoscopic treatment of UTUC. These studies had a follow-up of 14 and 15 months, with 19% and 50% recurrences respectively.

A study Martinez-Piñeiro et al. [3] with 39 patients reflect the largest of the studies in the first stage of treatment. All patients who were treated either had solitary kidneys or bilateral disease. Twenty-nine percent of those patients had recurrence at a mean follow-up of 30.6 months, while 28% ultimately failed the endourologic management.

The next stage is reflected in studies by Roupret et al. [4] and Lucas et al. [5]. Roupret reported on 27 patients treated with ureteroscopy (URS) some who were treated for nonempiric reasons. He found the five-year disease-specific survival rate was 82% for low-grade tumors and 47% for high grade [4] Lucas et al., reported on 39 patients treated URS almost all for low-grade disease.

The final stage is reflected in studies such as a Cutress et al. [6] and Grasso et al. [7]. These studies contained large number of patients (76 and 63 respectively), with long follow-ups 54 versus 52 month. However, despite this seemingly robust data. These studies include patients from the first stage and like studies from Gadzinski [8], Raymundo et al. [9] and Pak et al. [10] in this final stage; patients were not censored for vital status, significant for a disease that has an OS of 72–74% [6].

A further discussion on the literature on URS resection can be found in Chap. 21.

The overall pooled data is reflected in Table 27.1 involving 537 patients with a mean follow-up of 36.7 months. There are 325/537 (55%) upper tract recurrences (range 15–90%), 91/289 (31%) bladder recurrence (range 15–43%), and 110/482 (22%) endoscopic failure (11–47%).

Analysis

Given the heterogeneity of the studies as stated above, it would be bad form to accept these pooled numbers at face value. Careful analysis of the studies shows that with longer follow-up periods upper tract recurrence rates were higher than 55%. In studies with a minimal follow-up of 40 months, recurrence rates were between

Table 27.1 Studies examining Ureteroscopic Resection for UTUC

Study	N	Follow up (mo)	UTCC recurrence (%)	Bladder recurrence N (%)	Failed endoscopic management ± (%)
Schmeller et al. 1989 [1]	16	14	3 (19)	ND	2 (13)
Gaboardi et al. 1994 [2]	18	15	8 (50)	ND	1 (6)
Engelmyer et al. 1996 [11]	10	43	7 (70)	ND	0
Martinez-Piñeiro et al. 1996 [3]	39	31	8 (29)	ND	11 (28)
Daneshmand et al. 2003 [12]	30	40	27 (90)	7 (23)	14 (47)
Johnson et al. 2005 [13]	35	32	24 (68)	ND	1 (3)
Roupret et al. 2006 [4]	27	52	4 (15)	6 (22)	7 (25.9)
Krambeck et al. 2007 [14]	37	32	23 (62)	13 (37)	11 (30)
Lucas et al. 2008 [5]	39	33	17 (46)	ND	11 (28)
Pak et al. 2009 [10]	57	53	51 (90)	ND	11 (19)
Cornu et al. 2010 [15]	35	24	21 (60)	14 (40)	4 (11)
Gadzinski et al. 2010 [16]	34	58	27 (84)	ND	ND
Raymundo et al. 2011 [9]	21	18	4 (31)	2 (15)	ND
Cutress et al. 2012 [17]	73	54	50 (69)	31 (43)	22 (30)
Grasso et al. 2012 [7]	66	52	51 (66)	18 (27)	15 (23)
Total	537	36.7	325/537 (55)	91/289 (31)	110/482 (22)

±Endourologic failure defined by pathologic progression, undergoing a RNU, or disease-specific mortality

66–90%. Furthermore in larger studies by Krambeck et al. [14] and Thompson et al. [18] tumors were treated as UTUC by visual inspection alone (~50%) in cases where pathological specimens were unable to be processed [18]. Other studies have revealed that visual presumed UTUC may actually be benign in 13–16% of cases [19–21]. This data shows that recurrences are to be expected and ought to be expressed to the patient prior to initiating treatment.

Bladder recurrence although reported in many studies, is likely cofounded by a previous history of bladder urothelial cell carcinoma. The 31% recurrence rate is likely underestimated. It was only reported in 7/15 studies and the true recurrence rate in studies with longer follow-up will likely be higher [6]. Endoscopic failure was reported at 22%, yet is likely an underestimate. There was no true way to distinguish between low-grade- and high-grade failure and in most studies did not censor for vital status. Quite simply many patients did not live long enough to fail endoscopically (Table 27.1).

Another general concern is in the area of recurrence with progression. The majority of ureteral lesions have been managed with flexible ureteroscope. This approach is typically a small biopsy with available forceps or basket removal of lesions which does not provide adequate information about the base of tumor, lamina propria, or muscle invasion. Most of these lesions are fulgrated or ablated without documented follow-up biopsy of the tumor site. It is quite plausible that some of these lesions are initially understaged with recurrences of undertreated lesions at a higher grade reported as progression. One can therefore question the accuracy of data on recurrences with progression at higher stage and consider them as initial understaging at the time of initial resection.

Percutaneous Resection

The percutaneous approach can be used second-line when complete tumor treatment or adequate staging cannot be performed in retrograde fashion. A large tumor burden, lower pole location and altered lower tract anatomy may be more favorably approached percutaneously [22, 23]. The literature for percutaneous resection (PCN) are similar or included in the ones examined for ureteroscopic resection. Therefore, they are also divided into the same three stages.

A more comprehensive discussion on the percutaneous resection can be found in Chap. 22.

Table 27.2 shows the pooled data for PCN resection. Three hundred and forty patients were reported being treated by PCN resection with a mean follow-up of 39 months. Recurrence rates was 126/340, 37% (range 13–65%), bladder recurrence 19/80 24% (range 10–42%), progression to RNU 69/340, 20% (range 6–50%).

These recurrence rates are likely the underestimates of true recurrence as outlined for the URS studies. Most studies were limited by short follow-up time, did not censor for vital status and had small retrospective cohorts consisting of many patients with low-grade and low-volume disease.

The complication rate for PCN resection though is higher than URS resection. The pooled complication rate was 64/236 or 27%. The most common complication was blood transfusion at 17%. A rare but serious concern when performing PCN resection is the possibility of tract seeding, tract seeding was seen in only 1/236 cases. This complication rate is in sharp contrast to URS studies which had a 14% complication rate, most common being ureteral strictures.

Topical Therapy

As discussed in the topical therapy chapter, there is considerable interest in utilizing topical agents in a neoadjuvant or primary therapeutic setting for UTUC. BCG is the most common agent studied for UTUC, reflecting an inherent bias in utilizing an agent that is so efficacious in urothelial carcinoma in the bladder. However, the efficacy of the topical therapy differs markedly from what is seen in the lower tract. This difference in efficacy lies in the difficulty of accessing the ureter and pelvicalyceal system. Furthermore, complete resection is difficult to assess or achieve in the upper tract. BCG is most efficacious with a completely resected tumor. Finally, despite the various methodologies of infusing the agent in an antegrade or retrograde fashion, contact with the urothelium is limited by ureteral and renal pelvis washout.

BCG has been studied in two settings; one as a primary treatment for CIS and the other as an adjuvant therapeutic agent following endoscopic resection.

BCG for Cis of the Upper Tract

BCG being used primarily UTUC was first reported on a paper by Herr in 1985 [34]. Since then its use has grown in popularity in select patients. There are many case series on its use, but there is extreme heterogeneity in patient selection, follow-up, and BCG course.

Nonomura et al. [35] had strict selection criteria for patients treated with BCG. Patients in that series had to have positive cytologies, negative multiple random biopsies of the bladder and prostatic urethra, negative upper tract radiologic findings as well as two positive cytologies from the pyeloureteral system involved. This criteria was also utilized by Okubo et al. [36], Miyake [37], Hayashida et al. [38] and Kojima et al. [39]. However other series such as Giannarini et al. [40] utilized either a positive cytology or a biopsy. Other studies such as Sharpe et al. [41], Yokogi et al. [42], Nishino et al. [43] and Irie et al. [44], simply selected patients based on a positive cytology and negative radiologic imaging. Furthermore, the response to treatment was

Table 27.2 Pooled data for PCN resection

Study	N	Follow up (mo)	Upper tract recurrence N (%)	Bladder recurrence N (%)	RNU n (%)	Complications N (%)
Tasca et al. 1992 [24]	10	19	5 (50)	ND	3 (30)	ND
Fuglsig et al. 1995 [21]	26	21	8 (31)	ND	9 (35)	2 (8) transfusion 1 (4) tumor seeding
Plancke et al. 1995 [25]	10	28	1 (10)	1 (10)	1 (10)	0/10
Patel et al. 1996 [26]	26	45	9 (35)	11 (42)	5 (19)	7 (27) overall, 3 (12) transfusion
Martinez-Piñerio et al. 1996 [27]	18	31	2 (11)	ND	1 (6)	7 (33) overall
Clarke et al. 1999 [28]	17	24	6 (33)	ND	2 (12)	2 (12) transfusion 1 (6) UTI
Goel et al. 2003 [29]	20	64	13 (65)	3 (15)	10 (50)	4 (20)
Suh et al. 2003 [30]	14	21	14 (100)	ND	5 (14)	ND
Palou et al. 2004 [31]	34	51	15 (44)	ND	9 (26)	2 (6)
Roupret et al. [32]	24	62	3 (13)	4 (17)	5 (21)	7 (29) overall, 3 (13) transfusion
Motamedinia et al. 2015 [33]	141	66	50 (35)	ND	19 (13)	ND
Overall	340	39.27	126/340 (37)	19/80 (24)	69/340 (20)	64/236 (27) overall 37/218 (17) transfusion 5/256 (2) Renal failure 1/236 (seeding of tract)

classified as simple conversion to a negative cytology not necessarily a definitive measure of response.

Table 27.3 is the pooled data for BCG for CIS. Overall 154 renal units (RU) were examined and response rate was 70% (range 50–100%), recurrence was 32% (range 10–53.9%). However, as stated above response rate was simply based on negative cytology. The recurrence rate is also likely higher, in studies with follow-up great than 40 months, the recurrence rate was 40%.

The reliance on negative cytology as evidence of efficacy of the treatment and the heterogeneity of the studies in terms of follow-up and instillation techniques, limits any set conclusion from the studies. However, it seems clear that BCG instillation for CIS of the upper tract is potentially effective.

BCG as Adjuvant After Endoscopic Resection

BCG in the adjuvant setting after endoscopic resection was first reported by Schoenberg et al. in 1991 [46]. He reported on nine patients with solitary kidneys given BCG following endoscopic resection.

This was followed by studies by Jarrett et al. [47] who reported on 17 patients (19 RU), Patel et al. [26] who reported on 13 patients (17 RU) with stage Ta disease and Clark et al. [28] who reported on 17 patients treated with BCG. These early papers showed promising disease-free rates for patients treated with adjuvant BCG ranging between 56 and 88% (Table 27.4).

Table 27.3 BCG for CIS of the upper tract

Study (year)	Patients (# of RU)	BCG scheme (weeks)	Route of administration	Response after one treatment (%)	Median follow-up (months)	Total renal unit recurrences (%)
Studer et al. (1989) [45]	8 (10)	6	PCN	4 patients (50)	23	1 (10)
Sharpe et al. (1993) [41]	11 (17)	6	Retrograde via ureteral catheterization	8 patients (73)	49	3 (17.64)
Yokogi et al. (1996) [42]	5 (8)	6	PCN (5), retrograde via ureteral catheterization (3)	5 RU (63)	28	3 (37.5)
Nishino et al. (2000) [43]	6 (8)	4–8	Retrograde via stent or ureteral catheterization	8 RU (100)	22	1 (12.5)
Nonomura et al. (2000) [35]	11 (11)	6	Retrograde ureteral stent	7 patients (64)	19.6	3 (27.3)
Okubo et al. (2001) [36]	11 (14)	6	Retrograde via ureteral catheterization (12) PCN (2)	9 RU (64%)	49.4	6 (43)
Irie et al. (2002) [44]	9 (13)	6	Retrograde via ureteral stent	13 RU (100)	36	3 (23)
Miyake et al. (2002) [37]	16 (17)	6	PCN (5), Retrograde via ureteral catheterization (11)	13 patients (81%)	30	4 (23.5)
Hayashida et al. (2004) [38]	10 (11)	6	PCN (4), Retrograde via ureteral stent (3) ureteral catheterization (1)	10 patients (100)	50.9	5 (45.5)
Kojima et al. (2006) [39]	11 (13)	8	Retrograde via stent (10), PCN (1)	9 patients (82%)	57.3	7 (53.9)
Giannarini et al. (2011) [40]	42 RU	6	PCN	25 RU (60)	42	17 (40.5)
Total	154 RU			70%		32.1%

Table 27.4 BCG as adjuvant therapy following endoscopic resection

Study (year)	Patients (RU)	Antegrade (AG)/ retrograde (RG)	Tumor stage/grade	Median follow-up (mo)	Disease free %
Schoenberg et al. (1991) [46]	9 (9)	AG/RG	7 Tx grade 1–2 2 Tx grade 3	24	56% (5/9) disease free
Jarrett et al. (1995) [47]	17 (19)	AG	4 Ta grade 1 7 Tx grade 2 6 Tx grade 3	55	67%
Patel et al. (1998) [48]	13 (17)	RG	8 Ta grade 1 5 Ta grade 2	14.6	88% (55 RU)
Clark et al. (1999) [28]	17 (18)	AG	15 Ta 2 T1 1 T2 14 grade 1–2 4 grade 3	20.5	65% (11 pts)
Rastinehad et al. (2009) [49]	50 RU	AG	27 low grade 23 high grade	61	67.3% (42 RU)
Giannarini et al. (2011) [40]	22 RU	AG	Ta or T1 70% high grade	22	41% (9 RU)
Total	135 RU				64%

Giannarini et al. [40] treated 22 RU after resection with BCG, however unlike the previous studies his recurrence rate was 59% (13 units). This marked difference, was attributed to a higher risk population with high-grade disease and a previous history of UCC of the bladder or upper tract. Rastinehad's et al. series compared 50 patients who received adjuvant BCG versus 39 patients who received no adjuvant treatment. They did not demonstrate any difference between the treated and untreated groups even when sub-selecting by grade [49]. However, this was a single center, retrospective study and despite being controlled for grade it is unclear if any other cofounding conditions led to the surgeons decision to give BCG or not.

The pooled data on Table 27.4, shows in a 135 renal units (RU) the disease-free rate after adjuvant BCG was 64% (range 41–88). The true question is would these patients have been disease free without BCG treatment. Rastinehad's single center study appears to tell us that there is no utility, however it is hard to rely on a single center, retrospective, nonrandomized study to base a standard of care. A careful analysis of the literature shows that low-grade tumors seem to have a greater response to BCG, however the true utility of BCG would likely be in patients with high-grade disease trying to avoid an RNU. In those patients, in the absence of a multicenter or randomized study, we are limited in fully evaluating the role of BCG as an adjuvant agent following endoscopic resection.

Mitomycin

Mitomycin C (MMC) has been reported as an adjuvant treatment, but the literature largely consists of small cohorts with mixed treatment. Elliot et al. reported 44 patients following endoscopic resection with 18 receiving adjuvant treatment: five receiving MMC, four thiotepa, and nine BCG [50]. Martinez-Piñero reported on 28 patients treated after resection 9 with BCG, 14 with MMC, five with thiotepa, and two with interferon [27]. In both studies lower recurrence rates were seen with MMC, but were not significant. In contrast, Keeley et al. reported on 19 patients treated with MMC following resection. Recurrence rates were higher in the group treated with MMC, which the authors contributed to a higher risk population [51]. Similarly, Palou et al. reported on 19 patients treated with BCG and MMC in the adjuvant setting. Higher recurrence rates were seen in the treated group (60% vs. 27%), which again was contributed to higher risk population [31]. Goel et al. administered MMC or epirubicin to 17 patients following PCN resection, 11 had low-grade disease and six had high grade. After a mean follow-up of 64 months, 60% of low grade cases were disease free; the other 40% had RNU. All except one of the patients with high grade died of their disease [29].

As seen above, the literature for MMC treatment is not clear, with no study showing a clear benefit, yet as for BCG the lack of any prospective trials limits the conclusions one can draw from the literature.

Other Agents

The literature on other agents such as Adriamycin, BCG and Interferon, Thiotepa, and Gemcitabine and their uses are limited to small case series without useable data, and therefore would not contribute significantly and not included in the summary [52–55].

Overview

The literature on conservative treatment for UTUC is still lacking and leaves a lot to be desired. For URS resection and PCN resections, the recurrence rates are likely an underestimate of the true recurrence. However, it is clear that recurrence is grade dependent and similar recurrence rates are seen for either technique. The main difference is the higher complication rate seen with PCN resection. For both techniques it is clear that recurrences are common and are to be expected. In terms of adjuvant therapy, the data for BCG for primary CIS is promising, but there is lacking biopsy proven data showing its efficacy. BCG for adjuvant therapy, there is conflicting data regarding its utility, but baring a true prospective trial in patients needing to avoid a RNU it may be helpful. There is even less data regarding MMC efficacy as an adjuvant agent, with some studies showing a nonsignificant response. There is likely going to be a large role in the future for biological agents such as Mitogel that will allow the upper tract prolonged contact time with MMC. Nano-particles containing chemo- and immunotherapeutic agents in near future will allow longer surface contact time which is of great value in upper tract overcoming the problem of fast transit time of these agents through the collecting system.

The endourological and conservative treatment of UTUC has reached the 30 year benchmark, we are unfortunately left with few true Grade A evidence to guide our practice. Yet the role for conservative treatment is expanding. As the technological innovations continue to improve, allowing us to better assess the upper tract with better staging; we may be on our way to treating the upper tract as the lower tract.

The next best step would be a prospective multicenter randomized study with several arms addressing all aspects, grades, stages of upper tract urothelial carcinoma with initial standardized resection and biopsies. This should be followed by intracavitary treatment that will include possibly more particulars to allow maximum contact time of the agents with urothelium.

Summary Box

- Majority of series do not allow for definitive analysis of true outcome.
- There are no standardized approaches followed by all institutions.
- There are no established definitions for disease and recurrence.
- In some cases the UTUTC is described as positive cytology.
- Most series are small and not follow a fixed template.

- Follow-up protocols are very varied.
- Definition of success, disease free, and progression are not unanimously agreed on.
- Intracavitary chemo- and immunotherapy appear to be beneficial.
- Patient's commitment is an essential part of successful outcome.
- Meticulous follow-up surveillance is essential for this highly recurrent tumor.

References

1. Schmeller NT, Hofstetter AG. Laser treatment of ureteral tumors. J Urol. 1989;141:840.
2. Gaboardi F, Bozzola A, Dotti E, et al. Conservative treatment of upper urinary tract tumors with Nd:YAG laser. J Endourol. 1994;8:37.
3. Martinez-Piñeiro JA, Garcia Matres MJ, Martinez-Piñeiro L. Endourological treatment of upper tract urothelial carcinomas: analysis of a series of 59 tumors. J Urol. 1996;156:377.
4. Roupret M, Hupertan V, Traxer O, et al. Comparison of open nephroureterectomy and ureteroscopic and percutaneous management of upper urinary tract transitional cell carcinoma. Urology. 2006;67:1181.
5. Lucas SM, Svatek RS, Olgin G, et al. Conservative management in selected patients with upper tract urothelial carcinoma compares favourably with early radical surgery. BJU Int. 2008;102:172.
6. Cutress ML, Stewart GD, Zakikhani P, et al. Ureteroscopic and percutaneous management of upper tract urothelial carcinoma (UTUC): systematic review. BJU Int. 2012;110:614.
7. Grasso M, Fishman AI, Cohen J, et al. Ureteroscopic and extirpative treatment of upper urinary tract urothelial carcinoma: a 15-year comprehensive review of 160 consecutive patients. BJU Int. 2012;110:1618.
8. Gadzinski AJ, Roberts WW, Faerber GJ, et al. Long-term outcomes of immediate versus delayed nephroureterectomy for upper tract urothelial carcinoma. J Endourol. 2012;26:566.
9. Raymundo EM, Lipkin ME, Bañez LB, et al. Third prize: the role of endoscopic nephron-sparing surgery in the management of upper tract urothelial carcinoma. J Endourol. 2011;25:377.
10. Pak RW, Moskowitz EJ, Bagley DH. What is the cost of maintaining a kidney in upper-tract transitional-cell carcinoma? An objective analysis of cost and survival. J Endourol. 2009;23:341.
11. Engelmyer EI, Belis JA. Long-term ureteroscopic management of low-grade transitional cell carcinoma of the upper urinary tract. Tech Urol. 1996;2:113.
12. Daneshmand S, Quek ML, Huffman JL. Endoscopic management of upper urinary tract transitional cell carcinoma: long-term experience. Cancer. 2003;98:55.
13. Johnson GB, Fraiman M, Grasso M. Broadening experience with the retrograde endoscopic management of upper urinary tract urothelial malignancies. BJU Int. 2005;95(Suppl. 2):110.
14. Krambeck AE, Thompson RH, Lohse CM, et al. Endoscopic management of upper tract urothelial carcinoma in patients with a history of bladder urothelial carcinoma. J Urol. 2007;177:1721.
15. Cornu JN, Rouprêt M, Carpentier X, et al. Oncologic control obtained after exclusive flexible ureteroscopic management of upper urinary tract urothelial cell carcinoma. World J Urol. 2010;28:151.
16. Gadzinski AJ, Roberts WW, Faerber GJ, et al. Long-term outcomes of nephroureterectomy versus endoscopic management for upper tract urothelial carcinoma. J Urol. 2010;183:2148.
17. Cutress ML, Stewart GD, Tudor EC, et al. Endoscopic versus laparoscopic management of noninvasive upper tract urothelial carcinoma: 20-year single center experience. J Urol. 2013;189:2054.
18. Thompson RH, Krambeck AE, Lohse CM, et al. Endoscopic management of upper tract transitional cell carcinoma in patients with normal contralateral kidneys. Urology. 2008;71:713.
19. Deligne E, Colombel M, Badet L, et al. Conservative management of upper urinary tract tumors. Eur Urol. 2002;42:43.
20. Lee BR, Jabbour ME, Marshall FF, et al. 13-year survival comparison of percutaneous and open nephroureterectomy approaches for management of transitional cell carcinoma of renal collecting system: equivalent outcomes. J Endourol. 1999;13:289.
21. Fuglsig S, Krarup T. Percutaneous nephroscopic resection of renal pelvic tumors. Scand J Urol Nephrol Suppl. 1995;172:15.
22. Jabbour ME, Smith AD. Primary percutaneous approach to upper urinary tract transitional cell carcinoma. Urol Clin North Am. 2000;27:739.
23. Irwin BH, Berger AK, Brandina R, et al. Complex percutaneous resections for upper-tract urothelial carcinoma. J Endourol. 2010;24:367.
24. Tasca A, Zattoni F. The case for a percutaneous approach to transitional cell carcinoma of the renal pelvis. J Urol. 1990;143:902.
25. Plancke HR, Strijbos WE, Delaere KP. Percutaneous endoscopic treatment of urothelial tumours of the renal pelvis. Br J Urol. 1995;75:736.
26. Patel A, Soonawalla P, Shepherd SF, et al. Long-term outcome after percutaneous treatment of transitional cell carcinoma of the renal pelvis. J Urol. 1996;155:868.

27. Martínez-Piñeiro JA, García Matres MJ, Martínez--Piñeiro L. Endourological treatment of upper tract urothelial carcinomas: analysis of a series of 59 tumors. J Urol. 1996;156:377.
28. Clark PE, Streem SB, Geisinger MA. 13-year experience with percutaneous management of upper tract transitional cell carcinoma. J Urol. 1999;161:772.
29. Goel MC, Mahendra V, Roberts JG. Percutaneous management of renal pelvic urothelial tumors: long-term followup. J Urol. 2003;169:925.
30. Suh RS, Faerber GJ, Wolf JS. Predictive factors for applicability and success with endoscopic treatment of upper tract urothelial carcinoma. J Urol. 2003;170:2209.
31. Palou J, Piovesan LF, Huguet J, et al. Percutaneous nephroscopic management of upper urinary tract transitional cell carcinoma: recurrence and long-term followup. J Urol. 2004;172:66.
32. Rouprêt M, Traxer O, Tligui M, et al. Upper urinary tract transitional cell carcinoma: recurrence rate after percutaneous endoscopic resection. Eur Urol. 2007;51:709.
33. Motamedinia P, Keheila M, Leavitt DA, et al. The expanded use of percutaneous resection for upper tract urothelial carcinoma: a 30-year comprehensive experience. J Endourol. 2015;30:262–7.
34. Herr HW. Durable response of a carcinoma in situ of the renal pelvis to topical bacillus Calmette-Guerin. J Urol. 1985;134:531.
35. Nonomura N, Ono Y, Nozawa M, et al. Bacillus Calmette-Guérin perfusion therapy for the treatment of transitional cell carcinoma in situ of the upper urinary tract. Eur Urol. 2000;38:701.
36. Okubo K, Ichioka K, Terada N, et al. Intrarenal bacillus Calmette-Guérin therapy for carcinoma in situ of the upper urinary tract: long-term follow-up and natural course in cases of failure. BJU Int. 2001;88:343.
37. Miyake H, Eto H, Hara S, et al. Clinical outcome of bacillus Calmette-Guérin perfusion therapy for carcinoma in situ of the upper urinary tract. Int J Urol. 2002;9:677.
38. Hayashida Y, Nomata K, Noguchi M, et al. Long-term effects of bacille Calmette-Guérin perfusion therapy for treatment of transitional cell carcinoma in situ of upper urinary tract. Urology. 2004;63:1084.
39. Kojima Y, Tozawa K, Kawai N, et al. Long-term outcome of upper urinary tract carcinoma in situ: effectiveness of nephroureterectomy versus bacillus Calmette-Guérin therapy. Int J Urol. 2006;13:340.
40. Giannarini G, Kessler TM, Birkhauser FD, et al. Antegrade perfusion with bacillus Calmette-Guerin in patients with non-muscle-invasive urothelial carcinoma of the upper urinary tract: who may benefit? Eur Urol. 2011;60:955.
41. Sharpe JR, Duffy G, Chin JL. Intrarenal bacillus Calmette-Guerin therapy for upper urinary tract carcinoma in situ. J Urol. 1993;149:457.
42. Yokogi H, Wada Y, Mizutani M, et al. Bacillus Calmette-Guérin perfusion therapy for carcinoma in situ of the upper urinary tract. Br J Urol. 1996;77:676.
43. Nishino Y, Yamamoto N, Komeda H, et al. Bacillus Calmette-Guérin instillation treatment for carcinoma in situ of the upper urinary tract. BJU Int. 2000;85:799.
44. Irie A, Iwamura M, Kadowaki K, et al. Intravesical instillation of bacille Calmette-Guérin for carcinoma in situ of the urothelium involving the upper urinary tract using vesicoureteral reflux created by a double-pigtail catheter. Urology. 2002;59:53.
45. Studer UE, Casanova G, Kraft R, et al. Percutaneous BCG perfusion of the upper urinary tract for carcinoma in situ. Prog Clin Biol Res. 1989;310:207.
46. Schoenberg MP, Van Arsdalen KN, Wein AJ. The management of transitional cell carcinoma in solitary renal units. J Urol. 1991;146:700.
47. Jarrett TW, Sweetser PM, Weiss GH, et al. Percutaneous management of transitional cell carcinoma of the renal collecting system: 9-year experience. J Urol. 1995;154:1629.
48. Patel A, Fuchs GJ. New techniques for the administration of topical adjuvant therapy after endoscopic ablation of upper urinary tract transitional cell carcinoma. J Urol. 1998;159:71.
49. Rastinehad AR, Ost MC, Vanderbrink BA, et al. A 20-year experience with percutaneous resection of upper tract transitional carcinoma: is there an oncologic benefit with adjuvant bacillus Calmette Guérin therapy? Urology. 2009;73:27.
50. Elliott DS, Blute ML, Patterson DE, et al. Long-term follow-up of endoscopically treated upper urinary tract transitional cell carcinoma. Urology. 1996;47:819.
51. Keeley FX, Bagley DH. Adjuvant mitomycin C following endoscopic treatment of upper tract transitional cell carcinoma. J Urol. 1997;158:2074.
52. See WA. Continuous antegrade infusion of adriamycin as adjuvant therapy for upper tract urothelial malignancies. Urology. 2000;56:216.
53. Burns JA, Williams RD, Hedican SP, O'Donnell MA: The treatment of upper tract transitional cell carcinoma with BCG plus interferon-alpha. In: American urological association annual meeting, 2001.
54. Katz MH, Lee MW, Gupta M. Setting a new standard for topical therapy of upper-tract transitional-cell carcinoma: BCG and interferon-alpha2B. J Endourol. 2007;21:374.
55. Eshghi M. Upper Tract Urothelial Carcinoma. Presentation of NY-AUA Meeting 2007.

Part IV

Ancillary Treatment

Intracavitary Topical Chemo and Immune Therapy of the Upper Tract

28

Joel Hillelsohn, Majid Eshghi and Arthur D. Smith

Abbreviations

Radical Nephroureterectomy	RNU
Upper Tract Urothelial Carcinoma	UTUC
Mitomycin C	MMC
Bacillus Calmette–Guérin	BCG
Percutaneous nephrostomy	PCN
Carcinoma in situ	CIS
Trans Urethral Resection Bladder Tumor	TURBT
Renal Units	RU
Interferon	IFN

Introduction

In general upper urinary tract urothelial carcinoma (UTUC) is traditionally treated with a radical nephroureterectomy (RNU). However, in select group of patients with a solitary kidney, chronic kidney disease, or bilateral UTUC, the benefits of oncologic control are superseded by the risks of dialysis and loss of renal function. Thus it has become standard of care to offer endourologic management of UTUC especially in low-grade disease.

As UTUC represents similar disease as in the lower urinary tract, there has been considerable interest in using adjuvant therapy such as Bacillus Calmette–Guérin (BCG) and Mitomycin C (MMC). The goal of these adjuvant therapies would be to both reduce ipsilateral recurrence and progression of disease following resection. BCG has also been used as a primary therapy for carcinoma in situ (CIS) of upper tract. However, to date no consensus has been reached regarding the clinical utility and efficacy of any chemotherapeutic or immunomodulatory agents [1]. In our practice (ME), an immediate post-op instillation of Mitomycin C (MMC) is usually performed in the operating room, similar to the procedure performed post-transurethral resection of bladder tumor (TURBT).

Differential Effectiveness of Intracavitary Therapy

The use of intravesical therapy is standard of care for most non-muscle-invasive bladder cancers [2]. However, as stated above, there remains no clear consensus or guidelines for intracavitary therapy

J. Hillelsohn (✉) · M. Eshghi
Department of Urology, Westchester Medical Health Network/New York Medical College, Valhalla, NY 10595, USA
e-mail: jhillelsohn@gmail.com

M. Eshghi
e-mail: majid_eshghi@nymc.edu

A. D. Smith
Department of Urology, Northwell Health and Hofstra University, New Hyde Park, Lake Success, NY 11040, USA
e-mail: asmith1@northwell.edu

M. Eshghi (ed.), *Urothelial Malignancies of the Upper Urinary Tract*,
https://doi.org/10.1007/978-3-319-51263-1_28

after endoscopic or percutaneous resection of UCC or in lieu of endoscopic treatment [2]. The efficacy for treating carcinoma in situ (40% recurrence, 5% progression) in the upper urinary tract without resection, according to a recent study by Giannarini et al., may be similar to the response seen in the bladder. However, their response rate was based on negative cytology on follow-up, which is specific but not sensitive, likely underestimating true recurrence. The group did not find similarly encouraging results for Ta/T1 lesions when BCG was used as an adjuvant agent [3]. A paper by Rastinehad et al. reinforced that conclusion examining 50 renal units (RU) receiving adjuvant BCG or MMC following resection versus a unmatched cohort receiving only resection and showed no difference in recurrence and progression of disease [4]. Recently an update to that series examining 141 patients reinforced that conclusion [5]. However, that series was limited, by its retrospective nature and it is not known why patients were selected for resection alone versus intracavitary treatment.

As shown above, although UTUC and lower tract urothelial carcinoma are similar histologically, agents given intravesically are more effective than given intracavitary. The reason for this is likely multifactorial. The bladder is simple to access, while accessing the ureter and pelvicalyceal system is complex. This affects our ability to surgically stage, resect, and administer topical agents to the upper tract. In regard to staging, even though advances in endoscopic instrumentation have led to improved visualization and access to the upper tracts, adequate staging remains elusive. In a recent study by Smith et al., up staging and/or upgrading from low-grade noninvasive UTUC to high-grade or invasive UTUC occurred in 43% of patients at repeat biopsy or at time of RNU [6]. Furthermore, it has been shown in studies involving intravesical BCG that its efficacy is diminished with incomplete resection, a far more likely occurrence in the upper tract. The risk of incomplete resection is also increased when utilizing the ureteroscopic approach. Therefore, when dealing with a large volume of tumor we prefer the percutaneous approach despite any increased morbidity. Finally, delivery of the agent is far more complex in the upper tract, leading to various methods of delivery summarized in Table 28.1.

Table 28.1 Mode of delivery

Antegrade via percutaneous nephrostomy tube (PCN)
Retrograde via ureteral catheter
Allowing vesicoureteral reflux via a double J pigtail stent

Delivery

As stated above a key difference in treating UTUC versus disease of the bladder is the lack of an easily accessible natural office in which to instill and monitor the agents. There is also an increased risk of systemic absorption and possible sepsis. Various methodologies have been proposed to instill the agents centering on either an antegrade or retrograde approach. Regardless of the technique chosen, it is critical to maintain a low pressure system to avoid systemic absorption through pyelovenous and pyelolymphatic backflow. It is also important the patient does not have an active infection to avoid sepsis through the same mechanism. The typical capacity of the renal parenchyma is no more than 10–15 cc. However, one must consider that continuous infusion risks inadequate exposure of the entirety of the collecting system to the agent in question and overfilling with the agent increases the risk of pyelolymphatic and pyelovenous backflow. This quagmire overfill versus inadequate exposure likely plays a role in the lower observed clinical response in UTUC versus lower urinary tract urothelial carcinoma [7].

Antegrade

The first methodology often utilized especially when administering BCG is antegrade perfusion through nephrostomy tube. This methodology first reported by Jarrett et al. consisted of a 6-week course of BCG following endoscopic resection/fulguration of tumor [8]. Patients were admitted overnight to the hospital given intravenous antibiotics and one vial of BCG was given through the nephrostomy tube for 1 h at a height of 25 cm from the kidney.

Retrograde

The standard retrograde technique revolves around instillation of a ureteral catheter or double J stent. In the case of a double J stent a cystogram is performed to ensure adequate reflux and the agent is infused either transvesically or via the ureteral catheter [9, 10]. If reflux is not seen, it is possible to resect intramural orifice to facilitate reflux, and the exact technique is discussed in the chapter on ureteroscopic tumor resection. The reflux technique however in our experience does not achieve adequate bathing of the upper tract and in our practice is limited to distal ureteral tumors with adequate resection of intramural or distal ureter.

An alternative technique was described by Patel et al. [11]: ureteral access was obtained using a rigid cystoscope and a wire is placed in the renal pelvis. Under direct vision a spinal needle was used to make a bladder puncture. A second wire was advanced through the spinal needle and advanced into the ureteral orifice. A 5-French single J stent was placed with the proximal portion at the suprapubic site and the distal end at the upper pole calyx. This access was utilized for intravesical therapy for the duration of the treatment regimen.

Our Technique (ME)

Following initial percutaneous resection of a lesion, we place a small nephrostomy tube at the PCN site. The variety of nephrostomy tubes used is discussed in Chap. 22 on percutaneous resection. A solution of 40 mg of MMC in 40–60 cc of saline is gently and slowly instilled in the collecting system utilizing a 60 cc syringe over a period of 10–15 min (Fig. 28.1). The nephrostomy tube is then capped. The patient is then sent to the recovery room with clamped foley catheter which is unclamped one-hour post infusion as done after TURBT. Nephrostomy tube is left open to a leg bag.

In order to reduce patient discomfort, we later use a small heparin lock instead of a 3-way stopcock (Fig. 28.2). This has an auto-seal mechanism, which allows for easy insertion of a syringe or IV tubing with automatic sealing when removed. The capped nephrostomy then can be buried inside gauze with a tegaderm over it. This allows the patient to bathe and better adjust to the tube (Fig. 28.3).

Around 1–2 weeks postoperatively, if a second procedure is not required for complete resection, a nephrostogram is performed to

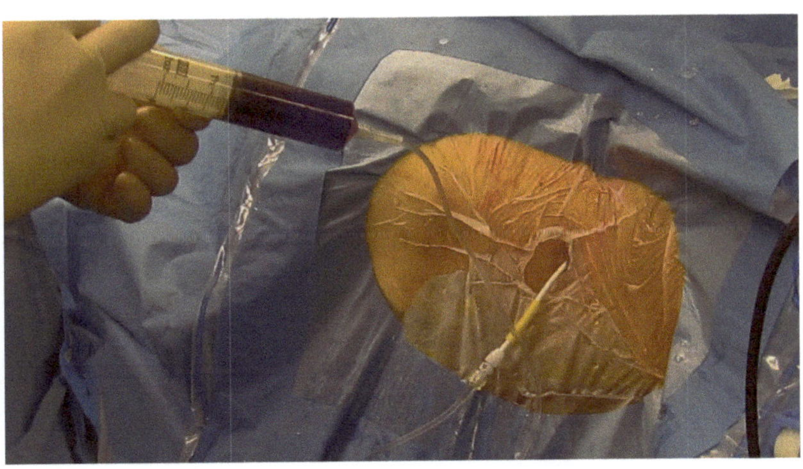

Fig. 28.1 MMC instillation after percutaneous resection, skin contact is protected to avoid contact with MMC

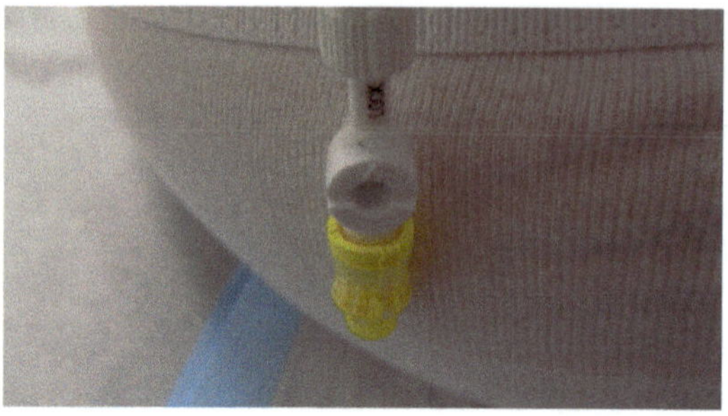

Fig. 28.2 Autoseal Heparin lock on small nephrostomy tube

confirm the placement of the nephrostomy tube and the drainage of the collecting system. The patient is also instructed to open the nephrostomy tube several times and chart the residual in order to assess the drainage of the system. Once proper location and drainage is confirmed, we then perform intracavitary treatment over a period of 6 weeks in an outpatient setting.

Office Treatment

The following is a typical description of an office intracavitary treatment:

1. Upon arrival, the patient signs consent. It is important to review with the patient the progress of care and side effects of the intracavitary therapy.
2. The patient is then asked about any clinical signs of infection, such as fever chills, dysuria, and back pain, secondary to the indwelling nephrostomy tube. Urine analysis and culture is also routinely obtained. Instillation of chemotherapeutic agents or immunotherapeutic agents in an infected system can lead to sepsis. There is no published standard prophylactic regiment, but it is our practice (ME) to give patients prophylactic antibiotics during the course of treatment, such as nitrofurantoin or sulfamethoxazole/trimethoprim.
3. It is also advisable to periodically check for fungal infections. Patients with indwelling tubes for a period of time may develop a fungal infection. If the patient has positive fungal culture, the patients are treated with standard regimen of antifungal medications such as flucanazole.
4. Before the start of the treatment, the patient is directed to void and urine culture is obtained.
5. Time out is then performed.
6. The nephrostomy tube site is then checked and cleaned. It is also gently irrigated with 10 cc of normal saline and gentamycin 80 mg. If the voided urine or the nephrostomy egress appears purulent, treatment will be postponed and a urine culture sent followed by proper treatment.
7. The patient lays in a supine position for the treatment (Fig. 28.4).

Fig. 28.3 Dressing of nephrostomy tube site

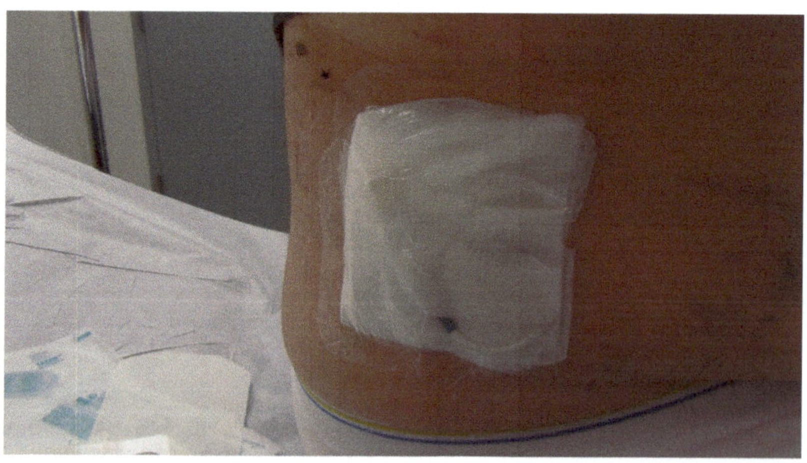

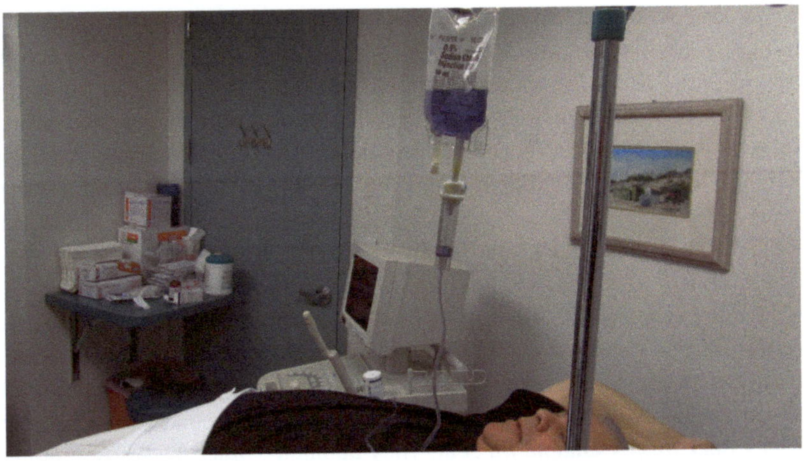

Fig. 28.4 Office intracavitary treatment with MMC (Note the solution bag should not be higher than 2–3 ft)

8. We utilize MMC as our first-line treatment (BCG is substituted if primary CIS and if refractive to MMC) and 40 mg of MMC diluted in 50–60 cc of normal saline is connected to the nephrostomy tube via an extension IV tubing and the drainage bag is hung on an IV pole delivered over a period of 40–45 min (Fig. 28.4). A simplified formula ia 4–4–4: 40 mg in 40 cc over 40 min.
9. It is important not to have the IV pole too high. It should not typically be more than 2–3 ft above the kidney level to avoid high pressure and rapid infusion of the medication into the collecting system (Fig. 28.4). The goal is to have the medication slowly dripped through the nephrostomy tube to allow for adequate intrapelvic bathing of the collecting system without over distending the renal pelvis. Overdistension could lead to systemic absorption of the agent. It is also important to allow it to slowly advance down the ureter and bladder, thereby preventing distal recurrences. At the completion of the procedure, the nephrostomy tube is typically flushed with 2–3 cc of normal saline or a solution of saline and gentamicin to avoid buildup of bacteria.
10. Sterile dressing is applied after the site of the catheter is cleaned and the patient is instructed not to void for at least an hour. In cases where MMC is used, the patients are given instructions to avoid contact of MMC with the skin since it can cause significant irritation and contact dermatitis. This needs to be emphasized several times to the patient. During the treatment, the physician and the nursing staff should be aware of this factor to avoid spilling of the medication around the skin site.
11. When giving BCG treatment the same protocol outlined above is utilized. Exact protocols that are used in intravesical treatment are followed.
12. The urine at the end of treatment is sanitarily disposed and clorox is sprayed.

Cycle of the Treatment

The cycle of the treatment as indicated earlier is 6 weeks and prior to the procedure patients are typically given six appointments usually in the morning to allow for patient monitoring during the day. If the treatment is interrupted due to a significant urinary tract infection, once the urine has cleared up and there is no evidence of significant infection, treatment is resumed to completion.

Choice of Agent

BCG

BCG is the most common agent studied for UTUC, reflecting an inherent bias in utilizing an agent that is so efficacious in urothelial carcinoma in the bladder. BCG has been studied in two settings; one as a primary treatment for CIS and the other as an adjuvant therapeutic agent following endoscopic resection. The evidence for its utility in these two settings remarkably differs.

BCG for CIS of the Upper Tract

The use of BCG for UTUC was first reported on a paper by Herr in 1985, describing the long-term remission of a patient with CIS of the renal pelvis treated with topical BCG [12]. In the most recent series examining BCG therapy for CIS of the upper tract was by Giannarini et al. They updated a series reported by Studer et al. in 1989, where eight patients with positive cytologies were treated with BCG via a percutaneous tube. Four of those patients converted into a negative cytology after 28 weeks [13]. Giannarini et al. reported on 64 renal units (RU), 55 patients, treated with topical BCG, with 42 of the units being treated for CIS. They were all diagnosed via positive cytology and/or biopsy of the upper tract. They were administered a 6-week treatment of BCG via a 10-French nephrostomy tube. Out of the 42 units treated, 17 (40%) developed recurrence and 10/17 were retreated. Of those ten who were retreated, they received either one (eight patients) or two (two patients) additional courses of BCG. Disease progression and need for RNU was seen in only 2/42 patients. The projected 5-year survival was 57% and kidney preservation was achieved in 89% of cases [3].

Sharpe et al. in a similar vein reported on 17 RU (11 patients) treated for a positive cytology of the upper tracts and no radiological evidence of UTUC. Treatment was a 6-week course of BCG administered via retrograde ureteral catheterization with an instillation time of 1 h. After one treatment course eight patients (73%) had negative cytologies after 36 months [14]. Yokogi et al. studied the benefits of BCG in eight RU (5 patients) with CIS diagnosed via positive cytology and with normal retrograde pyelography. Out of the eight units, five (63%) became and remained cytologically negative at 46 months [15]. Nishino et al. reported on six patients with cytologically proven CIS and normal retrograde pyelography. Patients were treated with BCG retrograde for 4–8 weeks. After a mean follow-up of 22 months all patients normalized their urine cytology [9].

Nonomura et al. reported on 11 patients with CIS of the upper tract treated via retrograde infusion of BCG with a stent. Of the 11 patients, seven had normal cytology after a single course and remained recurrence free for a mean period of 19 months [10]. Patients in that series had to meet strict diagnostic criteria, including positive cytologies, negative multiple random biopsies of the bladder and prostatic urethra, negative upper tract radiologic findings, and two positive cytologies from the pyeloureteral system involved.

Okubo et al. in 2001 and Miyake in 2002 both utilized diagnostic criteria similar to Nonomura et al. Okubo reported outcomes of BCG administered via retrograde ureteral catheterization for 6 weeks in 14 RU. Nine of the fourteen became negative after one course, seven remained negative for a median of 60 months [16]. Miyake evaluated 16 patients treated with BCG, 5 via a percutaneous nephrostomy tube (PCN) and 11 via retrograde ureteral catheter [10, 17]. After 30 months, 81% (13) patients had negative cytology and three had recurrence, two requiring RNU and one another course of BCG [17].

Irie et al. evaluated BCG via retrograde administration. The diagnosis was made with positive selective cytology at least two times. There were 13 units evaluated with resolution of positive cytology in all 13 units. On follow-up of 36 months, three recurrences were identified (23%) [18].

Hayashida et al. examined 11 RU (10 patients) utilizing similar diagnostic criteria as Okubo, Miyake, and Nonomura. BCG was administered either antegrade or retrograde for 6 weeks. Although initially all patients had a complete response, after a median 50.9 months, five patients recurred and died of metastatic disease (1 RNU, 1 cystectomy, 3 chemotherapy) [19].

Kojima et al. conducted a comparative study selecting patients with similar criteria as outlined in Nonomura's series, six patients were treated with RNU, and 11 patients (13 units) were treated with BCG for 8 weeks [10]. With a median follow-up of 57.3 months, the RNU group had two contralateral recurrences. In the BCG group nine patients (82%) normalized their cytology after initial treatments and of those nine only two recurred [20].

In a review by Bachir et al. they analyzed the cumulative impact of these studies (summarized on Table 28.2), and identified a cumulative 154 units treated with a minimum of 6-week therapy with BCG. Of those 154 units, 108 of them (70%) had negative urine cytology after a single course, which the author noted was similar to the response seen for BCG for bladder CIS [21]. However, it is important to note that none of these trials were randomized and all contained a small number of patients. Most of these studies selected these patients for treatment based on only a positive cytology. The reliance on negative cytology as evidence of efficacy of the treatment and the heterogeneity of the studies in terms of follow-up and instillation techniques limits any conclusion from the studies. However, it seems clear that BCG instillation for CIS of the upper tract is potentially effective.

BCG as Adjuvant After Endoscopic Resection

BCG in the adjuvant setting after endoscopic resection was first reported by Schoenberg et al. in 1991. He reported on nine patients with solitary kidneys given BCG following endoscopic resection. After a mean follow-up of 24 months, five out of nine were disease free [22]. Jarrett et al. reported on 17 patients (19 RU) who received adjuvant BCG if a second look nephroscopy and biopsy was negative. Of those 17 patients, four (23%) had grade 1, seven (41%) had grade 2, and six (35%) had grade 3. They were given BCG for 6 weeks and a third look nephroscopy was performed. Overall, after a median 55-month follow-up recurrence rate was 33% with grade 3 tumors having a recurrence rate of 50% versus 18% for low-grade [8].

Patel et al. reported on 13 patients (17 RU) with stage Ta disease (62% low grade), who received BCG after resection. After a 15-month follow-up, 88% (15 RU) remained disease free, the two recurrences both occurred in grade 2 lesions [11]. Clarke et al. reported on 17 patients treated with BCG after a negative second look nephroscopy. After a mean follow-up of 20.5 months, 11 patients were disease free. Of the six recurrences, four had grade 2 or 3 disease at diagnosis [23].

Giannarini et al. treated 22 RU after resection with BCG. After a median follow-up of 42 months, there was a recurrence rate of 59% (13 units). However, their population mainly consisted of high-risk disease, 70% had high-grade tumors and all had previous history of UCC of the bladder or upper tract [3].

Rastinehad's series of 89 RU was recently updated to include 114 RU. Of those 50 were identified that received BCG through a PCN for 6 weeks and 39 received no adjuvant treatment. Following treatment post-therapy recurrence was assessed at 3 months after resection with a third look nephroscopy. They did not demonstrate any difference between the treated and untreated groups even when sub selecting by grade [4]. However, the study is limited by lack of randomization, retrospective nature, and small sample size.

Unlike in BCG for CIS, studies overall do not support the use of adjuvant BCG. However, as noted by Bachir et al., a careful review of the studies (summarized in Table 28.3) shows that most patients in the studies had high-risk disease that tends to respond poorly to endoscopic treatment with or without BCG [21]. The series with favorable results largely consist of patient's with low-grade disease. Additionally, as noted earlier, the limitations of endoscopic treatment in ensuring complete resection of disease prior to treatment may bias the results. However, in the absence of a large sample size and a randomized study, we are limited in fully evaluating the role of BCG as an adjuvant agent following endoscopic resection.

Other Topical Therapies Used in the Adjuvant Setting

Mitomycin C

Mitomycin C has been well studied for UTUC and is the preferred initial agent in our institution (ME) following resection. Elliot et al. reported on

Table 28.2 BCG for CIS of the upper tract

Study (year)	Patients (# of RU)	BCG Cycle Length (weeks)	Route of administration	Response after one treatment (%)	Median follow-up (months)	Total renal unit recurrences (%)
Studer et al. (1989) [13]	8 (10)	6	PCN	4 patients (50)	23	1 (10)
Sharpe et al. (1993) [14]	11 (17)	6	Retrograde via ureteral catheterization	8 patients (73)	49	3 (17.64)
Yokogi et al. (1996) [15]	5 (8)	6	PCN (5), retrograde via ureteral catheterization (3)	5 RU (63)	28	3 (37.5)
Nishino et al. (2000) [9]	6 (8)	4–8	Retrograde via stent or ureteral catheterization	8 RU (100)	22	1 (12.5)
Nonomura et al. (2000) [10]	11 (11)	6	Retrograde ureteral stent	7 patients (64)	19.6	3 (27.3)
Okubo et al. (2001) [16]	11 (14)	6	Retrograde via ureteral catheterization (12) PCN (2)	9 RU (64%)	49.4	6 (43)
Irie et al. (2002) [18]	9 (13)	6	Retrograde via ureteral stent	13 RU (100)	36	3 (23)
Miyake et al. (2002) [17]	16 (17)	6	PCN (5), Retrograde via ureteral catheterization (11)	13 patients (81%)	30	4 (23.5)
Hayashida et al. (2004) [19]	10 (11)	6	PCN (4), Retrograde via ureteral stent (3) ureteral catheterization (1)	10 patients (100)	50.9	5 (45.5)
Kojima et al. (2006) [20]	11 (13)	8	Retrograde via stent (10), PCN (1)	9 patients (82%)	57.3	7 (53.9)
Giannarini et al. (2011) [3]	42 RU	6	PCN	25 RU (60)	42	17 (40.5)
Total	154 RU			70%		32.1%

44 patients following endoscopic resection with 18 receiving adjuvant treatment: 5 receiving MMC, 4 thiotepa, and 9 BCG. They found that the treated group had a smaller but not significant recurrence rate (44 vs. 65%) [24]. In a larger series with 28 patients treated after resection 9 with BCG, 14 with MMC, 5 with thiotepa, and 2 with interferon, again lower recurrence rates

Table 28.3 BCG as adjuvant therapy following endoscopic resection

Study (year)	Patients (RU)	Antegrade (AG)/ Retrograde (RG)	Tumor stage/grade	Median follow-up (mo)	Disease free %
Schoenberg et al. (1991) [22]	9 (9)	AG/RG	7 Tx grade 1–2 2 Tx grade 3	24	56% (5/9) disease free
Jarrett et al. (1995) [8]	17 (19)	AG	4 Ta grade 1 7 Tx grade 2 6 Tx grade 3	55	67%
Patel et al. (1998) [11]	13 (17)	RG	8 Ta grade 1 5 Ta grade 2	14.6	88% (55 RU)
Clark et al. (1999) [23]	17 (18)	AG	15 Ta 2 T1 1 T2 14 grade 1–2 4 grade 3	20.5	65% (11 pts)
Rastinehad et al. (2009) [4]	50 RU	AG	27 low grade 23 high grade	61	67.3% (42 RU)
Giannarini et al. (2011) [3]	22 RU	AG	Ta or T1 70% high grade	22	41% (9 RU)
Total	135 RU				64%

were seen with MMC (14.2%) and BCG (12.5%), but the sample size was too small to reach statistical significance [25].

Keeley et al. reported on 19 patients treated with MMC following resection. They received three treatments via a ureteral catheter with it clamped for 30 min. Complete response was seen in 35% of patients and partial response in 27% (reduction in tumor size by 50%) [26]. However, recurrence rate was higher in the MMC group, which the authors contributed to a higher risk population receiving MMC treatment.

Goel et al. administered MMC or epirubicin to 17 patients following PCN resection, 11 had low-grade disease and 6 had high-grade disease. After a mean follow-up of 64 months, 60% of low-grade cases were disease free; the other 40% had RNU. All except one of the patients with high-grade died of their disease [27]. Palou et al. reported on 19 patients treated with BCG and MMC in the adjuvant setting, 15 patients were treated with resection alone. Higher recurrence rates were seen in the treated group (60% vs. 27%) but the treated group consisted of patients with more high-risk disease [28].

Adriamycin

Adriamycin was investigated in a study by See, with 12 patients whom had UTUC or CIS. Each cycle had 40 mg/500 ml through a PCN for 8 h per day for 5 days. Two patients died of unrelated causes, five of the seven UTUC patients remained disease free after 21 months. Only one of the three patients who had CIS remained disease free [29].

BCG and Interferon (IFN)

Burns et al. treated 15 patients, 23 RU with BCG and IFN. Nineteen of the RU had CIS and four had papillary tumor. Response rate was 70% with the highest seen with CIS 74% [30]. Another study by Katz et al. evaluated 10 patients with BCG and infused after endoscopic resection. After a median follow-up of 24 months, eight patients had complete response and two had partial response [31].

Thiotepa

Thiotepa was the original agent used for intravesical therapy of the bladder. It was one of the only agents FDA approved for intravesical treatment of the bladder. In the early 1980s, thiotepa was the only medication available for intracavitary treatment. However, due to its low molecular weight that facilitates systemic absorption and side effects such as myelosuppression it is rarely used and has been replaced by MMC and BCG [24].

Gemcitabine

The use of gemcitabine as an adjuvant topical agent following resection stems from its use in intravenous chemotherapy for urothelial malignancies. In our experience (ME) we used intracavitary gemcitabine in two patients who had developed recurrence in spite of MMC and BCG treatment. Gemcitabine was tolerated well, and patient had mild posttreatment generalized symptoms such as body aches and mild gastrointestinal symptoms. Both of these patients eventually succumbed to cardiopulmonary complications, unrelated to the urothelial malignancy. The details of these two cases are outlined in Table 28.4.

Complications of Intracavitary Topical Therapy

Side effects of BCG treatment are similar to as seen when used transvesically. The key as in all topical intracavitary treatments is to maintain low intracavitary pressure as to avoid systemic absorption of the agent. One of the most common side effects of BCG is fever, with an occurrence rate of 67% in percutaneous series. However, fevers in that setting usually responded to broad spectrum antibiotics and did not require anti-tubercular therapy [32]. Other common complications seen in Studer and Miyake's series included irritative urinary symptoms and transient hematuria [13, 17]. Four total patients in all series reviewed and developed severe septicemia, requiring cessation of all treatment and a total of two patients developed fatal BCG septicemia [8, 13, 17]. Other complications included E. coli septicemia in two patients and three candida infections that were treated via a ureteral stent [3, 11]. Five patients progressed to end-stage renal disease and required hemodialysis [8]. There is additionally one report of aplastic anemia and death following extravasation of MMC from the upper tract [25]. However, it is worth noting that MMC is routinely used intravenously in higher doses; the minimal amount systemically absorbed following resection is unlikely to cause significant side effects. However, we always perform a nephrostogram prior to instillation of an intracavitary agent post resection. All patients undergoing intracavitary BCG immunotherapy need to be closely monitored and infectious disease consult may be necessary if patients manifest systemic signs and symptoms such as coughing, hemoptysis, chronic chills, or fever. Acute systemic manifestations may require treatment with INH. A positive PPD test in patients who were vaccinated against tuberculosis is not reliable. BCG treatment in immunosuppressed patients ALS requires special scrutiny and should be undertaken as a multidisciplinary approach in consultation with infectious disease and transplant team.

Table 28.4 Patients who received salvage gemcitabine

Age	Sex	Side	Approach	Tumor
86	Male	Left	Ureteroscopic/Nephroscopic	T3 UTCC
58	Male	Right	Ureteroscopic/Nephroscopic	T3 UTCC

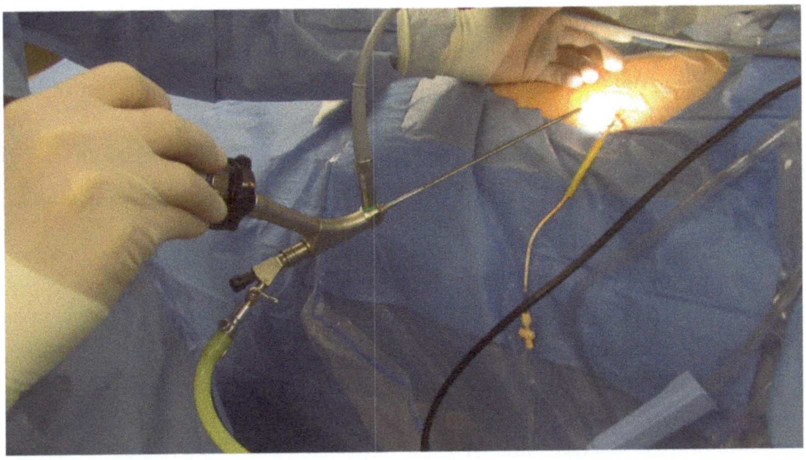

Fig. 28.5 12-F mini nephroscope

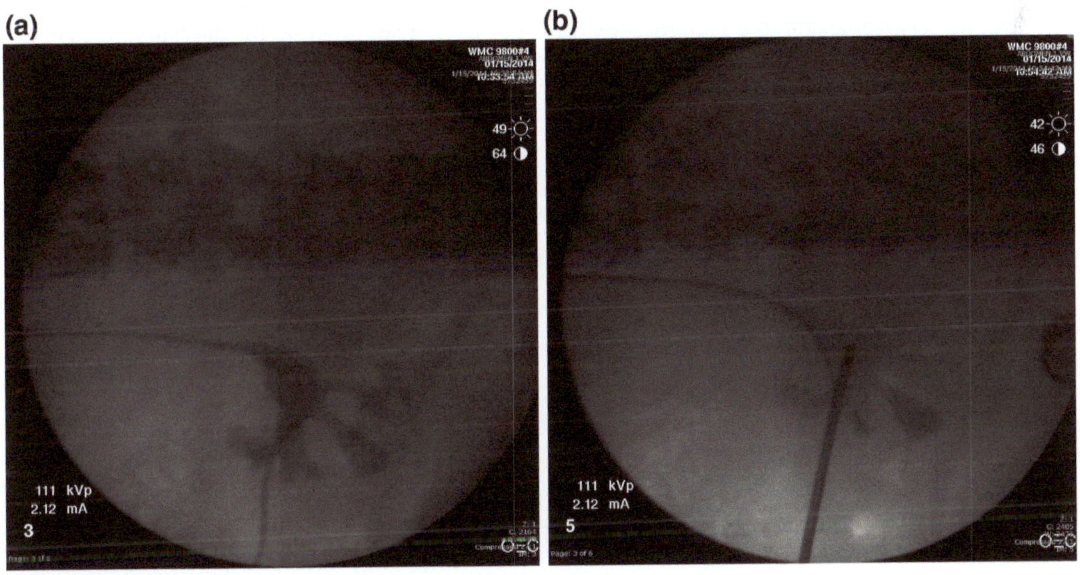

Fig. 28.6 Surveillance nephrostomy with 12-F mini nephroscope

New Advances

A potential new therapeutic option for UTUC is currently being developed by UroGen Pharmaceutical [33]. MitoGel is polymer gel infused with MMC that is liquid at cold temperature but solidifies at body temperature. It is instilled retrograde via an open-ended catheter and solidifies in the upper tract slowing down the depletion of chemotherapy which occurs during continues flow. It maintains high concentration of MMC in the upper tract for several hours as opposed to a few minutes during standard instillation. It has been designated as an orphan drug by the FDA animal trials have been successful, and clinical trials on humans are already underway [34].

Expert Commentary

As outlined above our typical treatment protocol consists of 6 weeks of therapy followed by a surveillance nephroscopy. Our choice of agent is patient specific. A patient in our institution is considered to have primary CIS, if there is multiple positive cytologies of the pelvicalyceal system, negative imaging (retrograde and/or CT Urogram/MR Urogram), negative random biopsies of the bladder, positive biopsies of the upper tract mucosa (technique is outlined in Chaps. 21, 22), and no visible lesion on ureteroscopy or nephroscopy. In those selected cases we utilize a primary 6-week treatment of BCG via a PCN. In cases of visible lesions that are endoscopically treated, our first-line treatment is MMC infused after the procedure via a PCN.

If the patient is refractive to both MMC and BCG treatments, it is our practice to attempt a course of gemcitabine, providing renal preservation is critically necessary. Our treatment protocol follows the one recommended for intravesical treatment [35]. The only difference is we advocate treatment two times a week with a week of rest in between, in order to dilute the systemic side effects often associated with treatment [35].

End Point of Treatment

The treatment using MMC or BCG is usually treatment course of 6 weeks followed by a surveillance nephroscopy. Usually for the surveillance nephroscopy, there is no need to use dilatation or large instruments and a mini-scope which is #12 French in diameter or a flexible ureteroscope can easily be introduced through the tract for inspection and biopsy (Figs. 28.5 and 28.6). We usually reassess the area of resection, re-biopsy the area, collect urine for FISH, and/or cytology for testing and in some cases administer a booster treatment of MMC. At that point depending on the pathology and any recurrent disease, the patient is counseled whether to proceed to an RNU, another intracavitary treatment course or observation. It is our practice in the absence of any recurrent disease to advice the patient to receive three more treatments of MMC or BCG, following that the nephrostomy tube is removed. However, there is often patient "fatigue" and reluctance to undergo further treatments and to continue with the PCN treatments. The methods of dealing with patient fatigue are summarized in Chap. 26 on surveillance. Following the conclusion of all treatment, the patient will follow a tight surveillance protocol for an initial evaluation in 3 months with imaging studies and ureteroscopy and this protocol will continue similar to the follow-up protocols for bladder. The process of the surveillance and follow-up is detailed in Chap. 26.

Summary Box

- Intracavitary therapy is utilized to improve response to endurologic therapy
- The best evidence exists for BCG as a primary therapy for CIS
- The literature is mixed for MMC and BCG as adjuvant agents
- There is a clear need for a prospective study on the topic
- We utilize MMC for a 6-week cycle following resection
- BCG immunotherapy in immunosuppressed patients must be done cautiously
- The future of adjuvant treatment likely lies in products such as MitoGel©.

References

1. Roupret M, Zigeuner R, Palou J, et al. European guidelines for the diagnosis and management of upper urinary tract urothelial cell carcinomas: 2011 update. Eur Urol. 2011;59:584.

2. Green DA, Rink M, Xylinas E, et al. Urothelial carcinoma of the bladder and the upper tract: disparate twins. J Urol. 2013;189:1214.
3. Giannarini G, Kessler TM, Birkhauser FD, et al. Antegrade perfusion with bacillus Calmette-Guérin in patients with non-muscle-invasive urothelial carcinoma of the upper urinary tract: who may benefit? Eur Urol. 2011;60:955.
4. Rastinehad AR, Ost MC, Vanderbrink BA, et al. A 20-year experience with percutaneous resection of upper tract transitional carcinoma: is there an oncologic benefit with adjuvant bacillus Calmette Guérin therapy? Urology. 2009;73:27.
5. Motamedinia P, Keheila M, Leavitt DA, et al. The expanded use of percutaneous resection for upper tract urothelial carcinoma: a 30-year comprehensive experience. J Endourol. 2015;30:262–7.
6. Smith AK, Stephenson AJ, Lane BR, et al. Inadequacy of biopsy for diagnosis of upper tract urothelial carcinoma: implications for conservative management. Urology. 2011;78:82.
7. Wein AJ, Kavoussi LR, Campbell MF. Campbell-Walsh urology/editor-in-chief, Alan J. Wein; [editors, Louis R. Kavoussi … et al.]. 10th ed. Philadelphia, PA: Elsevier Saunders; 2012.
8. Jarrett TW, Sweetser PM, Weiss GH, et al. Percutaneous management of transitional cell carcinoma of the renal collecting system: 9-year experience. J Urol. 1995;154:1629.
9. Nishino Y, Yamamoto N, Komeda H, et al. Bacillus Calmette-Guérin instillation treatment for carcinoma in situ of the upper urinary tract. BJU Int. 2000;85:799.
10. Nonomura N, Ono Y, Nozawa M, et al. Bacillus Calmette-Guérin perfusion therapy for the treatment of transitional cell carcinoma in situ of the upper urinary tract. Eur Urol. 2000;38:701.
11. Patel A, Fuchs GJ. New techniques for the administration of topical adjuvant therapy after endoscopic ablation of upper urinary tract transitional cell carcinoma. J Urol. 1998;159:71.
12. Herr HW. Durable response of a carcinoma in situ of the renal pelvis to topical bacillus Calmette-Guérin. J Urol. 1985;134:531.
13. Studer UE, Casanova G, Kraft R, et al. Percutaneous BCG perfusion of the upper urinary tract for carcinoma in situ. Prog Clin Biol Res. 1989;310:207.
14. Sharpe JR, Duffy G, Chin JL. Intrarenal bacillus Calmette-Guérin therapy for upper urinary tract carcinoma in situ. J Urol. 1993;149:457.
15. Yokogi H, Wada Y, Mizutani M, et al. Bacillus Calmette-Guérin perfusion therapy for carcinoma in situ of the upper urinary tract. Br J Urol. 1996;77:676.
16. Okubo K, Ichioka K, Terada N, et al. Intrarenal bacillus Calmette-Guérin therapy for carcinoma in situ of the upper urinary tract: long-term follow-up and natural course in cases of failure. BJU Int. 2001;88:343.
17. Miyake H, Eto H, Hara S, et al. Clinical outcome of bacillus Calmette-Guérin perfusion therapy for carcinoma in situ of the upper urinary tract. Int J Urol. 2002;9:677.
18. Irie A, Iwamura M, Kadowaki K, et al. Intravesical instillation of bacille Calmette-Guérin for carcinoma in situ of the urothelium involving the upper urinary tract using vesicoureteral reflux created by a double-pigtail catheter. Urology. 2002;59:53.
19. Hayashida Y, Nomata K, Noguchi M, et al. Long-term effects of bacille Calmette-Guérin perfusion therapy for treatment of transitional cell carcinoma in situ of upper urinary tract. Urology. 2004;63:1084.
20. Kojima Y, Tozawa K, Kawai N, et al. Long-term outcome of upper urinary tract carcinoma in situ: effectiveness of nephroureterectomy versus bacillus Calmette-Guérin therapy. Int J Urol. 2006;13:340.
21. Bachir BG, Kassouf W. Efficacy of instillations with chemotherapy or immunotherapy following endoscopic resection for upper tract urothelial carcinoma. Expert Rev Anticancer Ther. 2012;12:63.
22. Schoenberg MP, Van Arsdalen KN, Wein AJ. The management of transitional cell carcinoma in solitary renal units. J Urol. 1991;146:700.
23. Clark PE, Streem SB, Geisinger MA. 13-year experience with percutaneous management of upper tract transitional cell carcinoma. J Urol. 1999;161:772.
24. Elliott DS, Blute ML, Patterson DE, et al. Long-term follow-up of endoscopically treated upper urinary tract transitional cell carcinoma. Urology. 1996;47:819.
25. Martínez-Piñeiro JA, García Matres MJ, Martínez--Piñeiro L. Endourological treatment of upper tract urothelial carcinomas: analysis of a series of 59 tumors. J Urol. 1996;156:377.
26. Keeley FX, Bagley DH. Adjuvant mitomycin C following endoscopic treatment of upper tract transitional cell carcinoma. J Urol. 1997;158:2074.
27. Goel MC, Mahendra V, Roberts JG. Percutaneous management of renal pelvic urothelial tumors: long-term followup. J Urol. 2003;169:925.
28. Palou J, Piovesan LF, Huguet J, et al. Percutaneous nephroscopic management of upper urinary tract transitional cell carcinoma: recurrence and long-term followup. J Urol. 2004;172:66.
29. See WA. Continuous antegrade infusion of adriamycin as adjuvant therapy for upper tract urothelial malignancies. Urology. 2000;56:216.
30. Burns JA, WR, Hedican SP, O'Donnell MA. The treatment of upper tract transitional cell carcinoma with BCG plus interferon-alpha. In: American urological association annual meeting, 2001.
31. Katz MH, Lee MW, Gupta M. Setting a new standard for topical therapy of upper-tract transitional-cell carcinoma: BCG and interferon-alpha2B. J Endourol. 2007;21:374.

32. Liatsikos EN, Dinlenc CZ, Kapoor R, et al. Transitional-cell carcinoma of the renal pelvis: ureteroscopic and percutaneous approach. J Endourol. 2001;15:377.
33. Donin, NicholasStrauss-Ayali, DalitPantuck, Allan et al. PD13–10 Preclinical trial of serial mitogel® instillations into the pelvicalyceal system of the yorkshire swine. J Urology. 195(4):e301
34. Mitogel OLYMPUS Trial, vol. 2016 http://www.urogen.com/pipeline/utuc/.
35. Dalbagni G, Russo P, Bochner B, et al. Phase II trial of intravesical gemcitabine in bacille Calmette-Guérin-refractory transitional cell carcinoma of the bladder. J Clin Oncol. 2006;24:2729.

Systemic Chemotherapy for Upper Tract Urothelial Cancer

29

Surena F. Matin

Introduction

Upper tract urothelial cancer (UTUC) can be an aggressive disease with significant mortality [1]. Clinical predictors include biopsy grade and tumor architecture, while pathologic stage, grade, and nodal status are strongly prognostic for survival. Despite advances in imaging, endoscopy, and availability of effective chemotherapy regimens, there has not been any improvement in the survival of patients with UTUC [2, 3], suggesting that the paradigm of monotherapy by radical nephroureterectomy (RNU) needs to be reconsidered. As the median age at presentation is around 70 years [4–6] and renal insufficiency at baseline is common [7], there is additional significant loss of renal function after RNU, significantly impacting the ability of patients to receive perioperative chemotherapy and warranting a careful consideration of the use and timing of multimodality management.

S. F. Matin (✉)
Department of Urology, University of Texas MD Anderson Cancer Center, 1515 Holcombe Blvd, Unit 1373, Houston, TX 77030, USA
e-mail: surmatin@mdanderson.org

Risk Stratification

A concern arises as to who should be selected for chemotherapy, and if neoadjuvant chemotherapy (NAC) is to be considered, how can patients who are likely to benefit be appropriately selected? Appreciating that clinical staging is very poor for this disease [8], the concept of risk stratification thus becomes more important. Several studies have shown that biopsy grade [5, 6, 9], tumor architecture [10, 11], and presence of hydronephrosis [12–15] have important roles in predicting pathologic stage. Tumor grade on endoscopic biopsy is one of the strongest predictors of pathologic stage [16, 17]. While low grade on biopsy correlates with 90% accuracy low stage disease, high grade on biopsy predicts pT2 or greater stage in only 66, 67% of the patients [8, 16, 18] and predicts ≥ pT3 stage in 42% of patients [18].

Two studies have evaluated preoperative risk stratification, one which includes imaging findings [19, 20]. The study by Margulis et al. [19] provides an easy-to-use nomogram that helps identify high-risk patients, in short, patients with biopsy high grade and a sessile tumor architecture have a >80% chance of having invasive disease. In the study by Favaretto et al. [20], imaging findings portend a strong predictor for more advanced disease; however, it should be noted that falsely negative findings are often a concern for this disease resulting in a risk for under-classification.

M. Eshghi (ed.), *Urothelial Malignancies of the Upper Urinary Tract*,
https://doi.org/10.1007/978-3-319-51263-1_29

Given the inadequacy of surgical monotherapy in patients with high-risk disease, multimodality therapy has been of increasing interest. Randomized clinical trials and meta-analyses have shown a survival advantage with neoadjuvant cisplatin-based chemotherapy in bladder cancer [21, 22], providing additional impetus for considering the same for UTUC. Thus with the ability to risk-stratify patients either preoperatively or postoperatively, multimodality therapy with systemic chemotherapy can be considered.

Systemic Chemotherapy for UTUC

In early trials of chemotherapy for bladder cancer, patients with advanced UTUC were often included but did not have data reported separately [23–28]. In those reports that did describe outcomes in UTUC separately, platinum-based chemotherapy elicited response rates of 35–54% suggesting activity of chemotherapy in UTUC. Of 14 UTUC patients included in a trial of MVAC (methotrexate, vinblastine, doxorubicin, and cisplatin) in 92 patients with advanced urothelial cancer [25], two achieved pathologic complete remission (CR) and four more had clinical CR. In another phase III trial comparing MVAC with single agent cisplatin in advanced urothelial cancer, the overall response rate was 35% with a median overall survival of 11.3 months, quite similar to patients with bladder urothelial cancer [26]. In the next sections, the neoadjuvant and adjuvant chemotherapy approaches are considered.

Neoadjuvant Chemotherapy

The impetus for a neoadjuvant approach stems from 2 lines of evidence. Given the lack of improvement in survival with this disease over several decades [2, 3], some groups have argued for a paradigm shift in how this disease is managed, with consideration of NAC in all patients deemed to have clinical high-risk disease [3], given the apparent inefficacy of adjuvant chemotherapy. Since use of cisplatin-based chemotherapy is complicated by decreased renal function in the majority of patients with UTUC, and worsens post RNU [7, 29], NAC has been proposed as the primary consideration for multimodality management. With maximal renal function, full dose cisplatin-based chemotherapy can be delivered more confidently. Imaging and sometimes endoscopic assessment can be used to monitor response to chemotherapy, which can act as a possible surrogate for prognosis by itself [30]. Pathological downstaging [6, 31, 32] treatment of micrometastaes, and improved survival are obvious goals of this approach.

NAC has rarely been applied until recent studies by the MD Anderson Cancer Center provided critical data showing not only significant downstaging [31], but as well improved 5-year cancer specific and overall survival [33]. In fact, the rarity of its use is evident in a 12 center retrospective international UTUC collaboration of 1363 patients, in which only 41 patients (3%) received NAC, 5 (<1%) of whom were pT0N0 [6]. In one of the first reports of NAC for UTUC preceding the MD Anderson reports, 15 patients with locally advanced UTUC were treated with cisplatin-based combination chemotherapy consisting of MVAC 33%; methotrexate, etoposide, and cisplatin 27%; and methotrexate, vinblastine, epirubicin, and cisplatin 40%; for a mean of 2.1 cycles prior to surgery [32]. Two patients (13%) achieved a CR (pT0), which appeared durable beyond 3 years, and eight (53%) who had downstaging to $\leq$pT1N0 appeared to have better survival.

In the first report from the group at MD Anderson, 43 consecutive high-risk (defined as high grade on biopsy, sessile architecture or measurable mass on imaging) UTUC patients treated with NAC in 2004–2008 were compared to historical controls (1993–2004) with high-risk disease from the same institution [31]. Patients had similar clinical and demographic parameters except for sessile architecture being more frequent in the NAC group. Chemotherapy administered was cisplatin based in 77% (MVAC 44%; cisplatin gemcitabine ifosfamide 21%; gemcitabine, paclitaxel, and doxorubicin 14%; gemcitabine and cisplatin 12%), given for a median of

4 cycles. NAC resulted in pathologic downstaging to pT0N0 in 14% compared to 0 in the control group, similar to other studies published since [6, 32], and a significant finding since pT0 disease with initial surgery is a rare event. Pathological downstaging was significant with use of NAC ($\geq$pT2, 47% vs. 65%; $\geq$pT3/N+, 28% vs. 48%).

In another study, a prospective phase 2 bladder urothelial NAC strategy, five patients with UTUC were included and were treated with sequential chemotherapy [ifosfamide, doxorubicin, and gemcitabine (IAG), followed by cisplatin, gemcitabine and ifosfamide (CGI)], with three being found to have $\leq$pT1N0 disease at surgery [34].

In a follow-up study by the MD Anderson group, Porten et al. showed significantly improved overall and cancer-specific survival with the addition of NAC [33]. Patients who received NAC had not only improved overall survival with a 5-year OS rate of 80.2% versus 57.6% for those who underwent initial surgery ($P = 0.0015$), but also improved disease-specific survival with a 5-year DSS rate of 90.1% versus 57.6% for those who underwent initial surgery ($P = 0.0204$). In multivariate analyses, the NAC group had a lower risk of mortality (OS: hazard ratio, 0.42 [$P = 0.035$]; DSS: hazard ratio, 0.19 [$P = 0.006$]). These studies provided the first data supporting the systematic application of NAC for high-risk UTUC patients, and putatively validate the prognostic implications of downstaging for UTUC, which has previously been observed in bladder urothelial cancer [22, 35–37] but which until now had not been evaluated in UTUC.

A disadvantage of NAC is the potential for overtreatment in some patients, due to the aforementioned limitations of clinical staging and risk stratification. Given the high risk of mortality with disease recurrence, overtreatment is a reasonable risk for the well-informed patient who wishes a curative approach. The concern for progression during NAC has not been observed in these early studies, and complications from NAC precluding surgery likewise have not been realized, although a proportion of patients will only tolerate a portion of the full 4 cycles [31]. In a retrospective review of 82 patients undergoing laparoscopic RNU and lymph node dissection which included 26 receiving NAC, no increase in perioperative complication rates was evident with NAC [38]. A greater than 3-month interval between diagnosis and surgery, in the setting of NAC was also not associated with survival differences [39]. Based on the findings of these initial studies, an intergroup prospective phase 2, 2-arm study has been developed and as of early 2016 was recruiting patients with high-risk UTUC (https://clinicaltrials.gov/ct2/show/NCT02412670, accessed 3/5/2016). The study will stratify between those with adequate renal function (eGFR $\geq$ 50) to receive MVAC, and those who are renally insufficient ($30 \leq$ eGFR < 50) will receive carboplatin–gemcitabine. The primary outcome measure is pathologic complete response and the study is expected to complete in February 2020.

Adjuvant Chemotherapy

Results of adjuvant chemotherapy in UTUC are from retrospective analyses of either single centers or multi-institutional studies. A recent meta-analysis evaluated nine retrospective studies with a total of 482 patients receiving adjuvant chemotherapy [40]. In three of the studies using cisplatin, the pooled hazard ratio for overall survival was 0.43 (95% CI, 0.24–0.99, $p = 0.048$), while no benefit was seen for non cisplatin regimens [40]. However, it should be noted that in two of the three adjuvant cisplatin studies, the results were equivocal (the HR crossed 1.0), and all 3 originated from Asian countries where the renal function is likely significantly different than in the Western population. Additionally, no difference in disease-free or disease-specific survival was seen, bringing into question the applicability of this data to UTUC patients and particularly in non-Asian populations. A large reason for these inconsistent findings may be that all these studies suffered from unaddressed inherent biases of retrospective analyses. In a multicenter series, Hellenthal et al. [41] evaluated adjuvant chemotherapy in 542 patients with pT3–4 or pN+ UTUC who underwent RNU. Of the 542 patients, 121 (22%) with more advanced disease received adjuvant chemotherapy, primarily cisplatin based (MVAC or GC). Median overall survival in those receiving adjuvant chemotherapy was 24 months versus 26 months in those not receiving chemotherapy, and there were no significant differences in 5-year survival (overall 38%, cancer-specific 45%). Clearly the findings from this study were confounded by the retrospective nature of analysis, a noncomparable comparison group, and selection factors. In another multi-institutional retrospective series of 627 patients with $\geq$pT3–4, or pN+, or M + UTUC after RNU, [42] again no benefit of adjuvant chemotherapy was seen. However one has to consider that a substantial proportion (22%) in the adjuvant chemotherapy received salvage chemotherapy, not true adjuvant chemotherapy.

In the only prospective adjuvant chemotherapy study for UTUC, carboplatin and paclitaxel were given for 4 cycles in 36 patients with $\geq$pT3 or pN+ UTUC [43]. After a median follow-up of 41 months, 5 year OS was 52% and 5 year DFS was 40%, which does not appear to be different than studies evaluating surgery alone [9]. Common adverse events were related to neutropenia. In general, carboplatin-containing regimens are considered inferior to cisplatin combinations with respect to survival based on data of treatment of metastatic urothelial bladder cancer [44–47], but it is unknown if the same holds true in the adjuvant setting.

In reality, most patients are not candidates for cisplatin-based chemotherapy due to preexistent renal dysfunction which worsens after RNU [7, 29]. In a study by Kaag et al., only 49% of patients preoperatively and 19% of patients post RNU had an eGFR > 60 ml/min/1.73 mg/m^2 as measured by the Modification of Diet in Renal Disease (MDRD) formula [7]. This finding was validated by another report by Lane et al. [29].

One advantage of adjuvant systemic chemotherapy, however, may be a reduced risk of intravesical recurrence of urothelial cancer [48–50]. Whether this holds true with the application of NAC is currently unknown. The POUT trial, a phase 3 randomized trial of adjuvant chemotherapy versus surveillance in UTUC, is a European multicenter randomized controlled trial of 345 patients after RNU with pT2–pT4 pN0–3 or pT1 pN1–3 disease. Those who are fit for adjuvant chemotherapy will be randomized to 4 cycles of adjuvant platinum-based chemotherapy (experimental group) or surveillance (control group). The study was opened in May 2012, is currently enrolling and will have a primary endpoint of disease-free survival, with anticipated completion in May 2020 (available at https://clinicaltrials.gov/ct2/show/NCT01993979, accessed 3/5/2016).

In summary, the use of adjuvant systemic chemotherapy has not shown dramatic or consistent beneficial outcomes. Until results of the POUT trial become available, adjuvant chemotherapy can be individually considered for well-informed patients who are at high risk of relapse, such as those with $\geq$pT3 or pN+ UTUC with adequate renal function to tolerate a cisplatin-based regimen. For pT2N0 tumors, the presence of other adverse prognostic features such as lymphovascular invasion may direct use of adjuvant chemotherapy [51].

Conclusions

NAC for UTUC has become standard in recent years based on strong retrospective data, and a prospective trial currently underway will validate this for the community at large. The POUT trial will inform whether adjuvant chemotherapy is an effective approach for locally advanced and node-metastatic UTUC. Until these data are available to provide stronger guidance, patients need to be counseled as to the options available as well as be informed of the limited data available so they can act as partners in their care and in particular to help the care team prioritize the trade-off in risks of either approach.

Summary Box

- Patients with UTUC frequently have baseline renal dysfunction, and there is additional significant loss of renal function after nephroureterectomy, precluding many patients from being able to receive adjuvant chemotherapy. This historical approach has yet to improve survival for this disease.

- Neoadjuvant chemotherapy (NAC) takes advantage of a patient's maximal renal function, allowing optimal delivery of cisplatin-based regimens, which are the most effective against urothelial cancer.
- Candidates for NAC are those found to have biopsy high-grade disease, sessile tumors, and imaging findings of local invasion. Typically 4 cycles of ddMVAC, MVAC, or GC are given.
- It should be noted that patients with clinically node positive disease are a different disease group. These patients should receive chemotherapy as their primary treatment. If a radiographic CR is seen after 6 cycles, consolidative surgery can be considered.
- NAC does not appear to preclude the ability to proceed to surgery. Some patients may only tolerate a portion of the 4 cycles in which case NAC is discontinued and surgery performed after 4 weeks of recover.

Acknowledgements The author would like to recognize the Monteleone Family Professorship for Research in Kidney and Bladder Cancer and the Eleanor and Scott Petty Fund for UTUC Research for their support.

References

1. Konety BR, Joyce GF, Wise M. Bladder and upper tract urothelial cancer. J Urol. 2007;177(5):1636–45.
2. Adibi M, Youssef R, Shariat SF, Lotan Y, Wood CG, Sagalowsky AI, et al. Oncological outcomes after radical nephroureterectomy for upper tract urothelial carcinoma: comparison over the three decades. Int J Urol. 2012;19(12):1060–6.
3. Brown GA, Busby JE, Wood CG, Pisters LL, Dinney CP, Swanson DA, et al. Nephroureterectomy for treating upper urinary tract transitional cell carcinoma: time to change the treatment paradigm? BJU Int. 2006;98(6):1176–80.
4. Munoz JJ, Ellison LM. Upper tract urothelial neoplasms: incidence and survival during the last 2 decades. J Urol. 2000;164(5):1523–5.
5. Lughezzani G, Jeldres C, Isbarn H, Sun M, Shariat SF, Alasker A, et al. Nephroureterectomy and segmental ureterectomy in the treatment of invasive upper tract urothelial carcinoma: a population-based study of 2299 patients. Eur J Cancer. 2009;45(18):3291–7.
6. Margulis V, Shariat SF, Matin SF, Kamat AM, Zigeuner R, Kikuchi E, et al. Outcomes of radical nephroureterectomy: a series from the upper tract urothelial carcinoma collaboration. Cancer. 2009; 115(6):1224–33.
7. Kaag MG, O'Malley RL, O'Malley P, Godoy G, Chen M, Smaldone MC, et al. Changes in renal function following nephroureterectomy may affect the use of perioperative chemotherapy. Eur Urol. 2010;58(4):581–7.
8. Skolarikos A, Griffiths TR, Powell PH, Thomas DJ, Neal DE, Kelly JD. Cytologic analysis of ureteral washings is informative in patients with grade 2 upper tract TCC considering endoscopic treatment. Urology. 2003;61(6):1146–50.
9. Hall MC, Womack S, Sagalowsky AI, Carmody T, Erickstad MD, Roehrborn CG. Prognostic factors, recurrence, and survival in transitional cell carcinoma of the upper urinary tract: a 30-year experience in 252 patients. Urology. 1998;52(4):594–601.
10. Fritsche HM, Novara G, Burger M, Gupta A, Matsumoto K, Kassouf W, et al. Macroscopic sessile tumor architecture is a pathologic feature of biologically aggressive upper tract urothelial carcinoma. Urol Oncol. 2010.
11. Remzi M, Haitel A, Margulis V, Karakiewicz P, Montorsi F, Kikuchi E, et al. Tumour architecture is an independent predictor of outcomes after nephroureterectomy: a multi-institutional analysis of 1363 patients. BJU Int. 2009;103(3):307–11.
12. Brien JC, Shariat SF, Herman MP, Ng CK, Scherr DS, Scoll B, et al. Preoperative hydronephrosis, ureteroscopic biopsy grade and urinary cytology can improve prediction of advanced upper tract urothelial carcinoma. J Urol. 2010;184(1):69–73.
13. Cho KS, Hong SJ, Cho NH, Choi YD. Grade of hydronephrosis and tumor diameter as preoperative prognostic factors in ureteral transitional cell carcinoma. Urology. 2007;70(4):662–6.
14. Ito Y, Kikuchi E, Tanaka N, Miyajima A, Mikami S, Jinzaki M, et al. Preoperative hydronephrosis grade independently predicts worse pathological outcomes in patients undergoing nephroureterectomy for upper tract urothelial carcinoma. J Urol. 2011;185(5):1621–6.
15. Ng CK, Shariat SF, Lucas SM, Bagrodia A, Lotan Y, Scherr DS, et al. Does the presence of hydronephrosis on preoperative axial CT imaging predict worse outcomes for patients undergoing nephroureterectomy for upper-tract urothelial carcinoma? Urol Oncol. 2011;29(1):27–32.

16. Keeley FX, Kulp DA, Bibbo M, McCue PA, Bagley DH. Diagnostic accuracy of ureteroscopic biopsy in upper tract transitional cell carcinoma. J Urol. 1997;157(1):33–7.
17. Williams SK, Denton KJ, Minervini A, Oxley J, Khastigir J, Timoney AG, et al. Correlation of upper-tract cytology, retrograde pyelography, ureteroscopic appearance, and ureteroscopic biopsy with histologic examination of upper-tract transitional cell carcinoma. J Endourol. 2008;22(1):71–6.
18. Brown GA, Matin SF, Busby JE, Dinney CP, Grossman HB, Pettaway CA, et al. Ability of clinical grade to predict final pathologic stage in upper urinary tract transitional cell carcinoma: implications for therapy. Urology. 2007;70(2):252–6.
19. Margulis V, Youssef RF, Karakiewicz PI, Lotan Y, Wood CG, Zigeuner R, et al. Preoperative multivariable prognostic model for prediction of nonorgan confined urothelial carcinoma of the upper urinary tract. J Urol. 2010;184(2):453–8.
20. Favaretto RL, Shariat SF, Savage C, Godoy G, Chade DC, Kaag M, et al. Combining imaging and ureteroscopy variables in a preoperative multivariable model for prediction of muscle-invasive and non-organ confined disease in patients with upper tract urothelial carcinoma. BJU Int. 2012;109(1):77–82.
21. Ribic CM, Sargent DJ, Moore MJ, Thibodeau SN, French AJ, Goldberg RM, et al. Tumor microsatellite-instability status as a predictor of benefit from fluorouracil-based adjuvant chemotherapy for colon cancer. N Engl J Med. 2003;349 (3):247–57.
22. Grossman HB, Natale RB, Tangen CM, Speights VO, Vogelzang NJ, Trump DL, et al. Neoadjuvant chemotherapy plus cystectomy compared with cystectomy alone for locally advanced bladder cancer. N Engl J Med. 2003;349(9):859–66.
23. Tannock I, Gospodarowicz M, Connolly J, Jewett M. M-VAC (methotrexate, vinblastine, doxorubicin and cisplatin) chemotherapy for transitional cell carcinoma: the Princess Margaret Hospital experience. J Urol. 1989;142(2 Pt 1):289–92.
24. Lerner SE, Blute ML, Richardson RL, Zincke H. Platinum-based chemotherapy for advanced transitional cell carcinoma of the upper urinary tract. Mayo Clin Proc. 1996;71(10):945–50.
25. Sternberg CN, Yagoda A, Scher HI, Watson RC, Herr HW, Morse MJ, et al. M-VAC (methotrexate, vinblastine, doxorubicin and cisplatin) for advanced transitional cell carcinoma of the urothelium. J Urol. 1988;139(3):461–9.
26. Loehrer PJ Sr, Einhorn LH, Elson PJ, Crawford ED, Kuebler P, Tannock I, et al. A randomized comparison of cisplatin alone or in combination with methotrexate, vinblastine, and doxorubicin in patients with metastatic urothelial carcinoma: a cooperative group study. J Clin Oncol Off J Am Soc Clin Oncol. 1992;10(7):1066–73.
27. Bamias A, Aravantinos G, Deliveliotis C, Bafaloukos D, Kalofonos C, Xiros N, et al. Docetaxel and cisplatin with granulocyte colony-stimulating factor (G-CSF) versus MVAC with G-CSF in advanced urothelial carcinoma: a multicenter, randomized, phase III study from the Hellenic Cooperative Oncology Group. J Clin Oncol Off J Am Soc Clin Oncol. 2004;22(2):220–8.
28. Kaufman DS, Carducci MA, Kuzel TM, Todd MB, Oh WK, Smith MR, et al. A multi-institutional phase II trial of gemcitabine plus paclitaxel in patients with locally advanced or metastatic urothelial cancer. Urol Oncol. 2004;22(5):393–7.
29. Lane BR, Smith AK, Larson BT, Gong MC, Campbell SC, Raghavan D, et al. Chronic kidney disease after nephroureterectomy for upper tract urothelial carcinoma and implications for the administration of perioperative chemotherapy. Cancer. 2010;116 (12):2967–73.
30. Splinter TA, Denis L, Scher HI, Schroder FH, Dalesio O. Neoadjuvant chemotherapy of invasive bladder cancer. The prognostic value of local tumor response. Prog Clin Biol Res. 1989;303:541–7.
31. Matin SF, Margulis V, Kamat A, Wood CG, Grossman HB, Brown GA, et al. Incidence of downstaging and complete remission after neoadjuvant chemotherapy for high-risk upper tract transitional cell carcinoma. Cancer. 2010;116(13):3127–34.
32. Igawa M, Urakami S, Shiina H, Kishi H, Himeno Y, Ishibe T, et al. Neoadjuvant chemotherapy for locally advanced urothelial cancer of the upper urinary tract. Urol Int. 1995;55(2):74–7.
33. Porten S, Siefker-Radtke AO, Xiao L, Margulis V, Kamat AM, Wood CG, et al. Neoadjuvant chemotherapy improves survival of patients with upper tract urothelial carcinoma. Cancer. 2014;120 (12):1794–9.
34. Siefker-Radtke A, Millikan RE, Kamat A, Shen Y, Williams D, Grossman H, Dinney C, A phase II trial of sequential neoadjuvant chemotherapy with ifosfamide, doxorubicin, and gemcitabine (IAG), followed by cisplatin, gemcitabine and ifosfamide (CGI) in locally advanced urothelial cancer (UC): final results from the M.D. Anderson Cancer Center. J Clin Oncol. 2008; 26 (May 20 suppl; abstr 5079).
35. Palapattu GS, Shariat SF, Karakiewicz PI, Bastian PJ, Rogers CG, Amiel G, et al. Cancer specific outcomes in patients with pT0 disease following radical cystectomy. J Urol. 2006;175(5):1645–9; discussion 9.
36. Tilki D, Svatek RS, Novara G, Seitz M, Godoy G, Karakiewicz PI, et al. Stage pT0 at radical cystectomy confers improved survival: an international study of 4,430 patients. J Urol. 2010;184(3):888–94.
37. Stein JP, Lieskovsky G, Cote R, Groshen S, Feng AC, Boyd S, et al. Radical cystectomy in the treatment of invasive bladder cancer: long-term results in 1,054 patients. J Clin Oncol Off J Am Soc Clin Oncol. 2001;19(3):666–75.
38. Rajput MZ, Kamat AM, Clavell-Hernandez J, Siefker-Radtke AO, Grossman HB, Dinney CP, et al. Perioperative outcomes of laparoscopic radical

nephroureterectomy and regional lymphadenectomy in patients with upper urinary tract urothelial carcinoma after neoadjuvant chemotherapy. Urology. 2011.
39. Sundi D, Svatek RS, Margulis V, Wood CG, Matin SF, Dinney CP, et al. Upper tract urothelial carcinoma: impact of time to surgery. Urol Oncol. 2010.
40. Leow JJ, Martin-Doyle W, Fay AP, Choueiri TK, Chang SL, Bellmunt J. A systematic review and meta-analysis of adjuvant and neoadjuvant chemotherapy for upper tract urothelial carcinoma. Eur Urol. 2014;66(3):529–41.
41. Hellenthal NJ, Shariat SF, Margulis V, Karakiewicz PI, Roscigno M, Bolenz C, et al. Adjuvant chemotherapy for high risk upper tract urothelial carcinoma: results from the upper tract urothelial carcinoma collaboration. J Urol. 2009; 182(3):900–6.
42. Vassilakopoulou M, de la Motte Rouge T, Colin P, Ouzzane A, Khayat D, Dimopoulos MA, et al. Outcomes after adjuvant chemotherapy in the treatment of high-risk urothelial carcinoma of the upper urinary tract (UUT-UC): results from a large multicenter collaborative study. Cancer. 2011.
43. Bamias A, Deliveliotis C, Fountzilas G, Gika D, Anagnostopoulos A, Zorzou MP, et al. Adjuvant chemotherapy with paclitaxel and carboplatin in patients with advanced carcinoma of the upper urinary tract: a study by the Hellenic Cooperative Oncology Group. J Clin Oncol Off J Am Soc Clin Oncol. 2004;22(11):2150–4.
44. Bellmunt J, Ribas A, Eres N, Albanell J, Almanza C, Bermejo B, et al. Carboplatin-based versus cisplatin-based chemotherapy in the treatment of surgically incurable advanced bladder carcinoma. Cancer. 1997;80(10):1966–72.
45. Dreicer R, Manola J, Roth BJ, See WA, Kuross S, Edelman MJ, et al. Phase III trial of methotrexate, vinblastine, doxorubicin, and cisplatin versus carboplatin and paclitaxel in patients with advanced carcinoma of the urothelium. Cancer. 2004;100 (8):1639–45.
46. Petrioli R, Frediani B, Manganelli A, Barbanti G, De Capua B, De Lauretis A, et al. Comparison between a cisplatin-containing regimen and a carboplatin-containing regimen for recurrent or metastatic bladder cancer patients. A randomized phase II study. Cancer. 1996;77(2):344–51.
47. Dogliotti L, Carteni G, Siena S, Bertetto O, Martoni A, Bono A, et al. Gemcitabine plus cisplatin versus gemcitabine plus carboplatin as first-line chemotherapy in advanced transitional cell carcinoma of the urothelium: results of a randomized phase 2 trial. Eur Urol. 2007;52(1):134–41.
48. Soga N, Arima K, Sugimura Y. Adjuvant methotrexate, vinblastine, adriamycin, and cisplatin chemotherapy has potential to prevent recurrence of bladder tumors after surgical removal of upper urinary tract transitional cell carcinoma. Int J Urol. 2008;15 (9):800–3.
49. Ku JH, Choi WS, Kwak C, Kim HH. Bladder cancer after nephroureterectomy in patients with urothelial carcinoma of the upper urinary tract. Urol Oncol. 2009.
50. Kwak C, Lee SE, Jeong IG, Ku JH. Adjuvant systemic chemotherapy in the treatment of patients with invasive transitional cell carcinoma of the upper urinary tract. Urology. 2006;68(1):53–7.
51. Lee KS, Kim KH, Yoon YE, Choi KH, Yang SC, Han WK. Impact of adjuvant chemotherapy in patients with upper tract urothelial carcinoma and lymphovascular invasion after radical nephroureterectomy. Korean J Urol. 2015;56(1):41–7.

The Role of Radiation Therapy for Upper Urinary Tract Malignancies

30

Alfredo I. Urdaneta and Mitchell S. Anscher

Principle

Radiation therapy can be defined as the clinical modality that deals with the use of ionizing radiation in the treatment of malignant, and to a lesser degree, benign processes. The goal of treatment with radiation is to deliver a specific tumoricidal dose to the target while limiting the dose to the surrounding organs at risk (OAR) of developing acute and late side effects from radiation. In theory, one could eradicate any tumor if one could deliver enough radiation dose to all malignant cells. In practice this may not be possible, due to the detrimental impact on normal organs through which the beam must traverse in order to reach the target, thus limiting the total dose that can be safely administered. This conundrum brings up an important concept in radiation biology, i.e., the therapeutic ratio, which can be defined as the probability of tumor response or control that can be achieved with a given risk of dose limiting normal tissue damage, supporting a risk–benefit approach to designing a radiation treatment plan (Fig. 30.1) [1]. Using this concept, the goal is to reach the maximum potential for tumor control that does not create an unacceptable risk of normal tissue damage. In the case of upper urinary tract malignancies, the OAR for radiation damage include: small and large bowel, bladder, liver, stomach, spinal cord as well as the remaining kidney. One can control, to a great extent, how much dose these structures will receive by changing the treatment technique, such as intensity modulated radiation therapy (IMRT), stereotactic radiation therapy (SBRT), and the delivery of ionizing radiation in the operating room at the time of resection (IORT). Additionally, the use of charged particles, such as protons, may have an advantage in some situations by permitting the delivery of a higher dose to small targets while reducing the exposure to surrounding tissues [2].

A complete description of all of the physical, biological, and chemical aspects of radiation and its interaction with matter are beyond the scope of this chapter, but a basic understanding of this process is required to better appreciate the therapeutic principles of this treatment modality. Radiation can be categorized as either indirectly or directly producing DNA damage, which is the predominant mechanism through which radiation exerts its effects on cells (Fig. 30.2). Particles that carry a neutral electric charge, such as photons produced by linear accelerators, generally create DNA damage indirectly in that they first transfer their energy through absorption in tissue

A. I. Urdaneta · M. S. Anscher (✉)
Department of Radiation Oncology, Virginia Commonwealth University School of Medicine, 401 College Street, PO Box 980058, Richmond, VA 23298, USA
e-mail: mitchell.anscher@vcuhealth.org

A. I. Urdaneta
e-mail: alfredo.urdaneta@vcuhealth.org

M. Eshghi (ed.), *Urothelial Malignancies of the Upper Urinary Tract*, https://doi.org/10.1007/978-3-319-51263-1_30

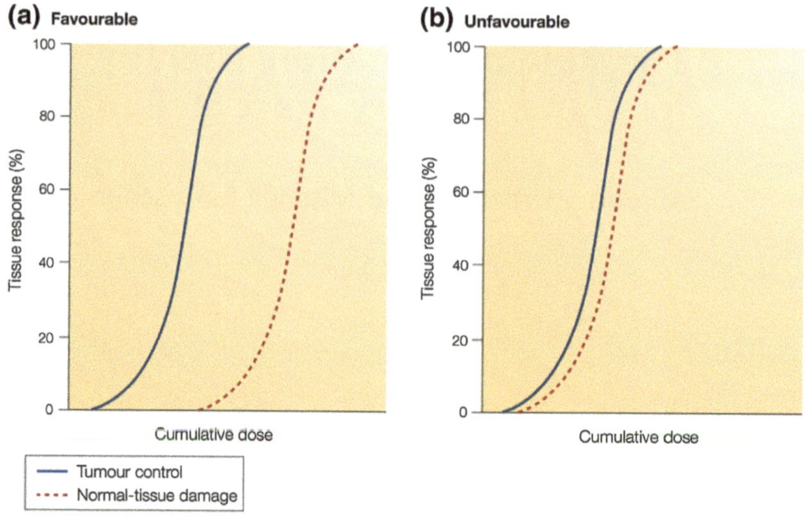

Fig. 30.1 Graphical representation of the therapeutic index in relation to cumulative dose. **a** A favorable therapeutic ratio indicates that the probability of tumor control is much greater than the probability of normal tissue injury and complications at any given dose, i.e., the therapeutic index is large. **b** An unfavorable therapeutic ratio indicates that the probability of tumor control and complications are similar at any given dose, i.e., the therapeutic index is small. From Bernier et al. [1]; used with permission

to create charged particles (secondary electrons), which in turn will interact with water molecules to generate free radicals. Conversely, charged particles, such as heavy ions like carbon or protons, are more likely to interact with tissue to release a secondary electron that interacts directly with the DNA to produce damage without the generation of free radicals (Fig. 30.2).

Photon interaction in tissue at therapeutic energies is dominated by a process called Compton scattering, in which the incidental photon interacts with an electron causing the electron to be dislodged from its orbital shell (Fig. 30.2). In this process, the photon transfers part of its energy to the electron (i.e., making it recoil), and as shown in Fig. 30.2, it is the resultant recoil electron that creates the damage, either by directly interacting with DNA, or creating free radicals that go on to damage DNA. This photon–electron interaction results in a new photon of less energy traveling in a different direction from the original, and an electron traveling through tissue (Fig. 30.2), such that the overall momentum of the two is conserved, analogous to the interaction between two billiard balls on a pool table. If the new photon retains enough energy, this photon–electron interaction will be repeated until the photon either exits the body or loses all of its energy. These interactions result in a gradual energy deposition "scattered" along the path of the beam (Fig. 30.3), with the greatest energy deposition occurring within 1–2 cm of the entry point of the beam into tissue and gradually decreasing with depth. Thus, if a tumor is located deep within the body, the dose from a single photon beam will be higher in the tissues in front of the tumor than in the tumor itself, which, in part accounts for the limitations of photon therapy to deliver high tumoricidal doses to a target while maintaining the nearby OAR below tolerated dose thresholds. Owing to their sparsely ionizing nature, however, photon beams will travel a long distance in tissue (Fig. 30.3), and by using multiple beams entering from different directions, one can create an energy deposition profile in which the highest dose is delivered within the region of overlap of the various beams, ideally surrounding the tumor, with significantly lower doses being delivered to tissues in regions outside of the overlap zone.

Compared to photons, charged particles such as protons, deliver their energy to tissue through many more interactions for a given distance traversed, causing atomic excitation and ionization

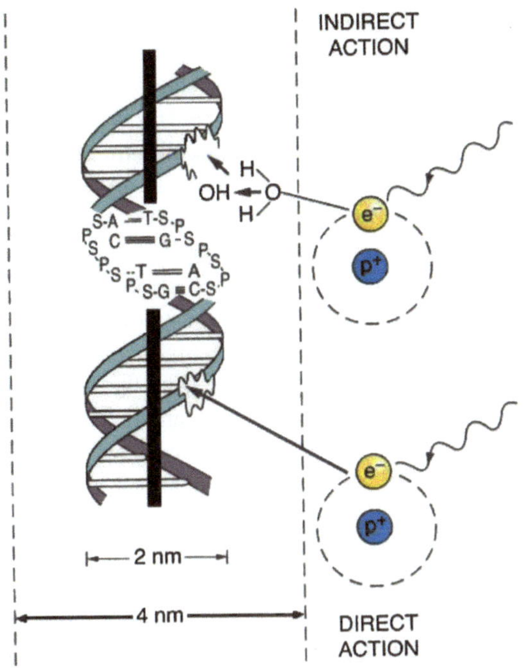

Fig. 30.2 Direct and indirect actions of radiation. The structure of DNA is shown schematically. In direct action, a secondary electron resulting from the absorption of an X-ray or heavy particle interacts with the DNA to produce an effect. In indirect action, the secondary electron interacts with, for example, a water molecule to produce a hydroxyl radical (OH^-); which in turn produces the damage to the DNA. From Pham et al. [5]; used with permission

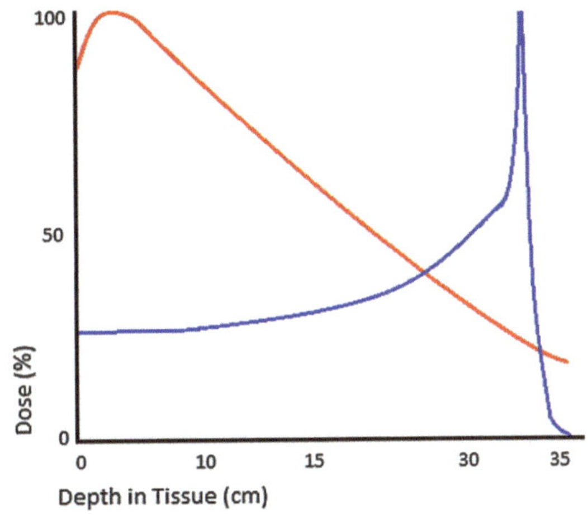

Fig. 30.3 Schematic graph showing the difference in the distribution of radiation dose as a function of depth in tissue for a 6 MV photon (*red curve*) and a 225 meV proton beam (*blue curve*). Notice that the photon has its maximum depth dose distribution at about 1.5 cm with a gradual decrease along the path of the beam. In contrast to the photon, the proton beam has very low depth dose distribution as it enters the tissue with its highest dose being delivered at around 30 cm (Bragg peak) with no exit dose

that leads to biological damage. Heavy charged particles including protons and heavy ions have straighter ionization tracks compared to photons, due to the fact that they are not as easily scattered as electrons, which have less mass and are considered light charged particles. The amount of energy that is transferred by an ionizing particle to the traversed material per unit distance is referred to as linear energy transfer. Thus, heavy charged particles have a high linear energy transfer, compared to photons. This property of heavy charged particles, combined with several other factors unique to the energy and speed of the particle, will result in most of the energy being deposited at the end of its track, creating a spike in the profile of absorbed energy called the Bragg peak, with no further energy deposition beyond that point. Thus, in contrast to photon beams, particle beams have a lower entrance dose and no exit dose. This property can be very useful as the energy of the particles can be adjusted to preferentially deliver dose at greater depths where a tumor might be located and at the same time keep the absorbed energy in superficial structures low, but most importantly the energy deposition beyond that peak will be essentially zero (Fig. 30.3). In practice, the enormous cost of particle accelerators, and uncertainties in the exact profile of beam deposition in different tissues and tissue interfaces have limited the implementation of this technology into the clinic until very recently [3].

Radiation Technique and Modalities

The delivery of ionizing radiation in the treatment of malignant tumors can be divided into two very distinct and different techniques: external beam radiation therapy (EBRT) and brachytherapy. In the case of malignant tumors arising in the upper urinary tract, external beam radiation and its different treatment planning modalities have been used with conflicting results, largely due to the fact that the only prospective studies that looked at neoadjuvant or adjuvant radiation therapy in malignancies arising in the kidney used planning techniques that would now be considered obsolete (i.e., two dimensional treatment planning). Modern approaches, such as three-dimensional conformal (3DCRT), and intensity modulated radiation therapy (IMRT), that allow for a better conformation of the high dose regions to the target, have not been prospectively studied. More advanced modalities, such as stereotactic radiation therapy (SBRT), intraoperative radiation therapy (IORT), and the use of charged particles such as protons are currently being investigated. The use of brachytherapy, in which a radioactive source is placed inside an organ (interstitial) or in a space next to the area of interest (intracavitary, intraluminal or intravascular) has not been evaluated, probably due to the difficulty in the placement, planning, and delivery of such therapy in tumors of the upper urinary tract.

Three-Dimensional and Intensity Modulated Radiation Therapy

Before the advent of high quality imaging such as computerized tomography (CT) and magnetic resonance imaging (MRI), radiation planning was based on crude estimates of the height and width of the tumor (two dimensional), often without determination of thickness, which necessitated big treatment fields that included larger volumes of normal tissue, limiting the total dose that could be delivered safely. With higher quality imaging and more sophisticated planning systems that integrate volumetric imaging and even organ motion, treatment plans more conformal to the target could be created allowing the radiation oncologist to deliver higher doses while better excluding normal tissue from the high dose region. These treatment plans are built using a large number of beams of various sizes and shapes as well as different orientations to create a dose distribution that conforms to the target. Delivery techniques vary between institutions but mainly involve either the use of thick lead alloy beam blocks custom made for each patient or, more commonly now, a built-in electronic beam blocking system called a multileaf collimator to help modulate the intensity of the radiation beam in order to better conform it to the target. One of the main differences between three-dimensional and intensity modulated radiation therapy, besides the delivery technique, is the number of treatment fields used to deliver each. A 3DCRT plan usually involves the use of three or four fields. In IMRT, the modulation of the beam allows the use of more than four fields (often 6 or more), providing better conformality of the high

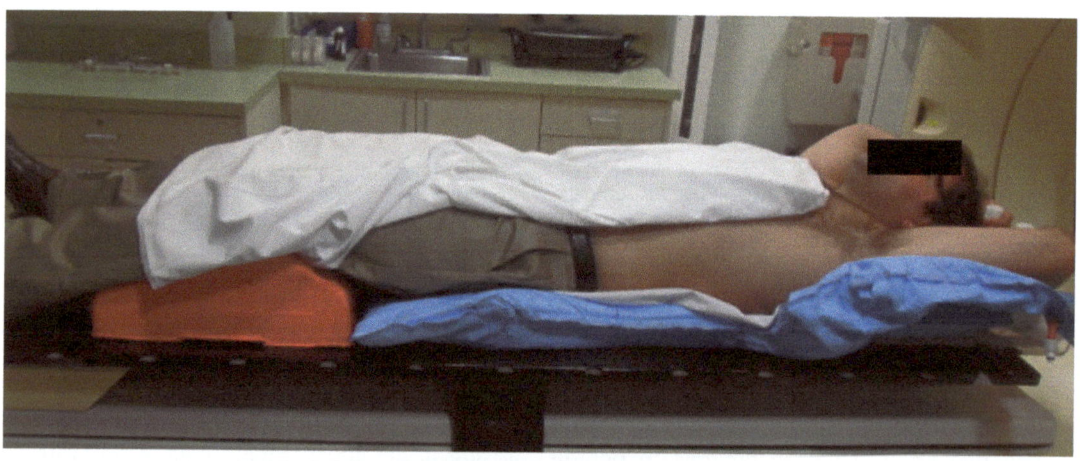

Fig. 30.4 Custom immobilization device used for daily setup reproducibility

dose region, but at the expense of larger volumes of normal tissue being exposed to low doses of radiation. In addition, the use of individually constructed patient immobilization devices improves daily reproducibility of the treatment setup. An example of a patient immobilization device is shown in Fig. 30.4. Also, the integration of megavoltage and/or kilovoltage diagnostic imaging capabilities into linear accelerators now allows the radiation oncologist to better exploit image-based patient positioning verification in combination with 3DCRT or IMRT treatment delivery techniques, which is referred to as image-guided radiation therapy (IGRT) Fig. 30.5 shows a Varian linear accelerator with onboard cone beam imager for IGRT used at our institution. These newer approaches are crucial to guarantee the accuracy and safety of these complex treatment delivery plans. These modern treatment techniques have not been explored in recent treatment protocols.

Stereotactic Radiation Therapy

The ability to better identify a potential target, thanks to higher quality imaging such as MRI and positron emitted tomography (PET), combined with the technological advances in treatment delivery described earlier, have led to the use of stereotactic techniques in the delivery of radiation therapy, not only in the setting of metastatic disease to the brain (stereotactic radiosurgery, or SRS) but also outside the brain for metastatic disease to the lungs and liver and more recently as an alternative to treatment of unresectable primary tumors (stereotactic ablative radiation therapy, or SABR). This allows the delivery of a very high dose of radiation to the target, with a very small (less than 10 mm) margin, in a single session or a few fractions (≤ 5) that could potentially overcome the historical belief that these tumors are resistant to standard dose fractionation schedules. Treatment planning techniques vary

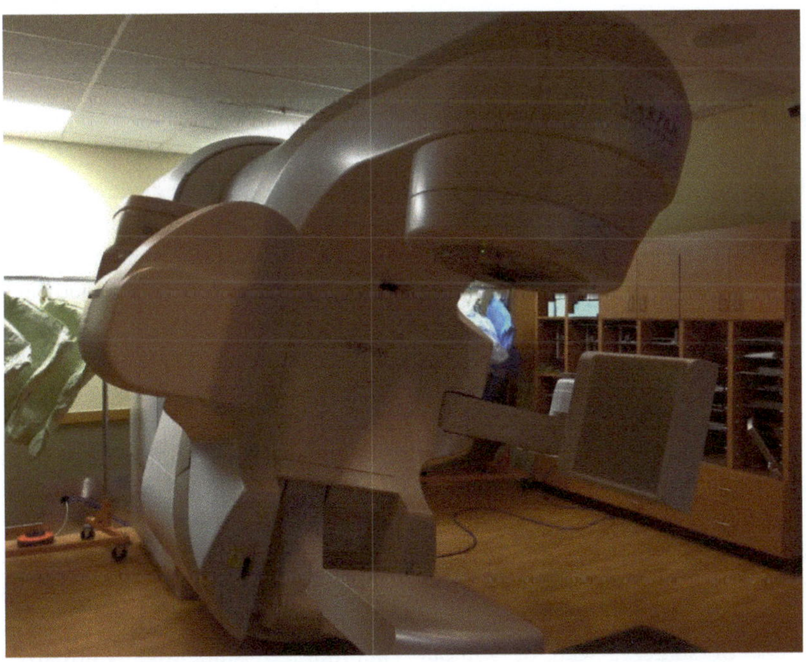

Fig. 30.5 Varian linac accelerator with both, megavoltage and kilovoltage imaging, capable of registering real-time cone beam computerized tomography for image-guided radiation therapy. The treatment beam emerges from the head of the machine at the *top* of the picture. The retractable imaging components of the machine are deployed in this picture and are located on the *right* and *left side* of the linear accelerator. Both treatment and imaging can be accomplished quickly and without the need to move the patient

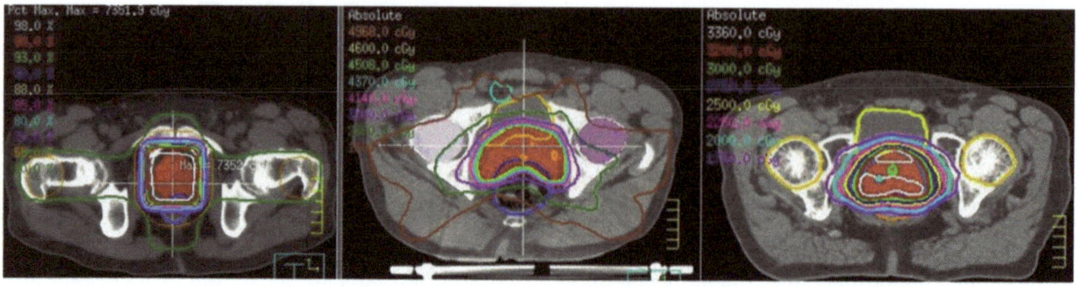

Fig. 30.6 Comparison of dose distributions for definitive treatment of prostate cancer. From *left* to *right*; 3D conformal radiation therapy, intensity modulated radiation therapy and stereotactic radiation therapy. The techniques of IMRT and SBRT permit a more conformal distribution of dose to the target, in this case the prostate plus a small margin, shown in *red*. While the high dose region is smaller using IMRT versus 3D, the volume of tissue exposed to low doses often is greater. The SBRT approach provides very rapid falloff of dose with distance from the target

by institution but more commonly involve techniques similar to those used in IMRT. Due to the high doses given per fraction, accurate target definition, and sophisticated treatment planning and delivery (using IGRT) are essential for such an approach. In the setting of the primary treatment of upper urinary tract malignancies, this is still considered an experimental technique, since few patients have been followed long term, and its use outside research protocols should be discouraged. This technique is well established in the treatment of limited metastatic disease to the brain, lung, and liver and currently is being investigated in the treatment of limited disease to the bone. Comparison between a 3DCRT, IMRT, and SBRT treatment plan, in this case for prostate cancer, is shown in Fig. 30.6.

Intraoperative Radiation Therapy (IORT)

As clinical advances in radiation therapy continue to pursue the goal of delivering higher doses of radiation to the tumor or tumor bed, while limiting the dose to the surrounding normal tissues, the strategy of directly irradiating these areas at the time of surgery, with or without additional external beam radiation therapy delivered in the preoperative or postoperative setting, has been the subject of investigation for many years. The major advantage of IORT is that critical normal structures, such as the small bowel, can be manually moved out of the path of the radiation beam. Other structures that are not mobile can be directly visualized and taken care to minimize the dose to which they are exposed. Initially this technique was quite cumbersome, since patients had to be transported under anesthesia to the radiation oncology department, where they underwent treatment with a non-dedicated linear accelerator. In the last 20 years, the development of operating rooms that are appropriately shielded for either a dedicated intraoperative electron beam accelerator or a high dose rate brachytherapy unit, have made this technique more popular in Europe, Asia, and in a few centers in the United States. Treatment planning and dose delivery relays largely on the surgeon's ability to resect the gross disease, and without the definitive pathological analysis of the specimen, treatment dosages can be at times arbitrary. This technique has been used in the treatment of retroperitoneal sarcomas, breast and rectal malignancies and as adjuvant treatment for ureteric malignancies in Asia. One of the biggest limitations of this therapy is the expense that is required to fit an operating room with the appropriate shielding. Currently the use of mobile self-shielded low energy linear accelerators is making this approach available at a larger number of sites across Europe and Asia.

The group at the University of Heidelberg reported the use of intraoperative radiation therapy in patients with primary or recurrent renal cell carcinoma. A total of 11 patients were analyzed. Macroscopic disease was left behind in seven patients with only one being able to undergo a complete resection. Treatment was delivered using a 6–10 meV beam to deliver a single dose of 15–20 Gy to the renal bed and paraaortic nodes. Three weeks later, patients started a course of adjuvant external beam radiation therapy to a total dose of 40 Gy in 20 fractions. Mean follow-up was 24.3 months with a mean disease-free survival and overall survival of 6.4 and 11.5 months, respectively. Local tumor control was 100%. Grade 1–2 small bowel toxicity was reported in three patients and no grade 3–4 toxicities were seen [4].

Another technique used to deliver radiation therapy at the time of surgery involves the use of an absorbable, flexible, mesh with multiple small (nonabsorbable) radioactive seeds attached to it, (iodine-125, palladium-103 or cesium-131). The clinical target volume is defined at the time of surgery, intraoperatively, after reviewing frozen section slides from the surgical specimen to identify areas of positive or close margins. The number of seeds will depend on the size of the area to be treated and is usually decided at the time of surgery. This mesh is sutured in place, assuring that it encompasses the tumor bed and regions with close or positive margins, and that the mesh remains in full contact with the predetermined treatment region. This technique is usually used to achieve a high dose to the areas at greatest risk of tumor recurrence, where external beam radiation dosing is limited due to the proximity of organs at risk for radiation toxicity.

Recently, the group at Brigham and Women's Hospital reported the safety and efficacy of delivering radiation therapy to deep cavity sarcomas using an iodine-125 (I-125) brachytherapy mesh implant. They reviewed their experience in 46 patients with primary or recurrent deep cavity sarcomas who had a macroscopically complete oncological resection and placement of an I-125 mesh to areas of positive or close margins. The plan was to deliver 20 Gy (as a form of boost in association with 45 Gy of externally delivered radiation therapy either pre or postoperatively) or 60 Gy (as a definitive dose) in cases of local recurrence following an initial course of EBRT and surgical resection. Median follow-up was 34.8 months, and the most common indication for mesh placement was microscopically positive margin. Postoperative complications were seen in 48% of the patients including 77% that had preoperative EBRT. Grade III/IV complications were seen in 11 patients including eight that had pre-operative radiation therapy, most commonly in the form of wound infection. No grade V toxicity was seen. The 5-year crude cumulative incidence of infield, regional, and distant recurrence was 26.3, 54.2, and 54.1%, respectively [5].

Patient Considerations and Technical Aspects

After proper evaluation, the patients began the process of having their treatment set up and planned, which is referred to as simulation. As part of this process, a device is constructed in which the patient lies during treatment, the purpose of which is to ensure accurate reproducibility of the setup and comfort during treatment to minimize patient motion (Fig. 30.4). This is usually accomplished by having the patient lay supine in a vacuum bag or similar device that is custom molded to the individual patient's external anatomy, with additional support at the level of the ankles, knees, and arms, making sure that the position of the arms will not interfere with the path of the beam. Once the immobilization device is ready, the patients undergo a planning CT scan in the treatment position. Once the image acquisition is complete, the scans are loaded into a computer-based 3D planning system and, if desired, fused with other imaging modalities, such as MRI and PET, to delineate the grossly visible tumor volume (GTV) and the known areas of potential spread. The OAR's (bladder, small and large bowel, liver, stomach, etc.) are contoured and subsequently a plan is created respecting normal tissue dose limitations established by the treatment protocols, while achieving the prescribed dose per fraction and total dose to the tumor and areas at risk for spread of disease. These steps are followed for three-dimensional, IMRT and SBRT. Patients undergoing IORT will undergo dose delivery at the time of surgery, often either followed or preceded by external beam radiation therapy.

Outcome Data

The role of radiation therapy as an adjuvant treatment after surgery is unclear for primary tumors of the upper urinary tract. Current treatment guidelines do not advocate for the use of radiation as part of a definitive approach. Prospective studies either in the neoadjuvant or adjuvant setting using what would now be considered archaic techniques showed no benefit in primary malignancies of the kidney. More recently single institution reviews looking at newer techniques in either setting have revitalized the interest in such approaches, as well as in the definitive setting for patients that cannot undergo a surgical resection. For tumors arising from the renal pelvis and ureter, where local failures are slightly more common than in the kidney, some benefit may be obtained in specific cases, such as those with positive surgical margins. The role of radiation therapy in the setting of metastatic disease whether for long or short-term palliation is well established.

Renal Cell Carcinoma

Adjuvant Therapy

The results of retrospective series in the 1950s and 1960s regarding the use of adjuvant radiation therapy for primary renal cell carcinoma were conflicting. An initial report by Flocks et al. in 1958 of over 300 patients with primary renal cell carcinoma, suggested a 10-year overall survival benefit of 9% [6]. Contrary to these findings, Peeling et al. in 1969 reported on 348 patients from the London Hospital treated between 1940 and 1965, showing that the addition of radiation therapy to nephrectomy conferred a significant detriment to overall survival, with a 5-year overall survival of 25% in those receiving radiation versus 52% in those treated with surgery alone [7].

The first prospective randomized trial evaluating nephrectomy with or without radiation therapy was published in 1973 by Finney et al. The radiation treatment consisted of 5500 rad given in 27 fractions using an anteroposterior (AP) oriented field plus a posterior angled beam, from the 11th thoracic vertebral body (VB) to the 3rd lumbar VB, including the paraaortic lymphatic chain. A total of 52 patients were treated with radiation and 48 without. Local control was 86 and 87% for nephrectomy with or without radiation, respectively. Overall survival at 5 years was 47% for patients without radiation compared to 36% with the addition of adjuvant therapy. It is important to note that four out of the 52 patients treated with adjuvant therapy with right-sided tumors died of liver toxicity [8]. In 1987, the Copenhagen Renal Cancer Study Group reported on the results of 72 patients who had undergone nephrectomy for stage II–III renal adenocarcinoma. Patients were randomized to observation or adjuvant radiation therapy consisting of a total dose of 50 gray (Gy) to the kidney bed, ipsilateral and contralateral paraaortic lymph nodes, given at 2.5 Gy per fraction 4 times per week. Median follow-up was 4 years. An analysis was performed on 60 eligible patients, 27 with adjuvant radiation and 33 without. Local control was 53% for the nephrectomy arm and 57% for adjuvant radiation therapy with a median time to relapse of 10.2 months. Median survival for the radiated group was 26 months and had not been reached for the surgery alone group. Of note 44% of patients in the radiation group had severe toxicity, including duodenal stenosis and ulceration [9].

As new techniques became available, the use of stereotactic radiation as an alternative to surgery in medical inoperable patients or patients refusing surgery was explored. Beitler et al., reported the outcome of nine patients with primary renal cell carcinoma that had refused surgery or that were medically inoperable who underwent treatment with SBRT to a total dose of 40 Gy given in 5 fractions over 3 weeks using 4–6 field arrangement only to the primary tumor. Target volumes ranged from 4.14 to 742.9 cc. Two patients had bilateral disease. With a median follow-up of 26.7 months, four out of the nine patients were alive with one of the patients developing a new lesion outside the radiated field. Median follow-up for the surviving patients is 57.8 months. Two patients developed nausea and vomiting during the treatment with one of them experiencing a 30 lbs. weight loss in 30 days following treatment for bilateral kidney disease [10]. The group at Karolinska Institute published the results of eight patients treated on a prospective protocol for inoperable primary or recurrent renal cell carcinoma. Patients were treated with a regimen consisting of 8 Gy times 5 fractions for a total dose of 40 Gy. One patient failed at 15 months at a distant site and the other seven patients were locally controlled with a median survival >58 months [11]. Svedman et al. summarized their experience with SBRT for patients with metastatic renal cell carcinoma to the contralateral kidney after a previous nephrectomy. Treatment varied from a total dose of 30–40 Gy given in 3–4 fractions depending on tumor size and location. With a median follow-up of 39 months, six out of the seven patients evaluated had local control. There were no grade ≥ 3 toxicities and five patients had no change in their kidney function [12].

More recently Pham et al., published the interim analysis of a phase 1 trial looking at SBRT for medically inoperable primary renal cell carcinomas. Patients with tumor volume <5 cm had a single dose of 26 Gy. For patients with tumor volumes ≥ 5 cm, the total dose was 42 Gy in 3 fractions. Planning required a minimum of 8 fields. Twenty patients were enrolled with a follow-up of at least 1 year. Sixty percent had grade 2 or less toxicity with no grade 3 or higher toxicity reported. The report includes a summary table of the dose constraints established for the target as well as the OAR compared to the achieved median dose for single and three fraction regimens. Table 30.1 summarizes the dose constraints on target volumes and organs at risk utilized by the authors [13]. Staehler et al. reported the outcomes of 40 patients with inoperable primary renal tumors (29 renal cell carcinoma and 11 transitional cell carcinoma [TCC]) treated with single fraction SBRT to a total dose of 25 Gy. With a median follow-up of 28.1 months, local tumor control at 9 months was close to 97% with complete remission in 19 patients including all TCC histologies. Median progression-free and overall survival had not been reached at the time of analysis. There were five grade 1 toxicities with no grade 2 or higher toxicities reported. Renal function remained stable on all patients [14]. The results of treatment using SBRT for renal cell carcinoma are summarized in Table 30.2.

Other modalities, such as, the use of charged particles has also been explored. A report from the National Institute of Radiological Sciences in Japan; which, at the time of the report, had the only heavy ion accelerator for medical use in the world and analyzed the outcome of 10 patients with primary renal cell carcinoma treated with carbon ion radiotherapy to a median total dose of 72 (62–80) Gray equivalent (GyE) delivered in

Table 30.1 Dose constraints used for planning both single and fractionated stereotactic radiation therapy

Organ	26 Gy in 1 fraction	42 Gy in 3 fractions
PTV	D99 = 26 Gy	D99 = 42 Gy
Spinal canal	12 Gy point dose	18 Gy point dose
Skin (5 mm s.c.)	18 Gy (max dose)	24 Gy (max dose)
Small bowel	30 cm^3 < 12.5 Gy	D0.035 cm^3 < 30 Gy
Stomach	–	<30 Gy
Liver	700 cm^3 $\leq$ 15 Gy	700 cm^3 $\leq$ 15 Gy
Large bowel	No constraint	No constraint

From: Hall and Giaccia [2]; used with permission

Table 30.2 Summary of recent published trials of SBRT for renal cell carcinoma (treatment delivered to the primary site)

Study (reference)	Study design	N	Total dose (Gy)/ #fractions	Median FU (months)	Outcome	Adverse events grade ≥3
Beitler et al. [10]	Retrospective	9	40/5	26.7	4/9 patients alive at 72 months	1/9 (GI)
Wersäll et al. [11]	Prospective	8	40/5	37	>58 months median survival	None
Ponsky et al. [20]	Prospective	3	16/4 Followed by partial nephrectomy at 8 weeks	14	one patient had pathologic complete response. NED at 1 year	None
Svedman et al. [12]	Retrospective	7	30–40/3–4	39.2	Local control 6/7 patients	
Staehler et al. [14]	Prospective	40	25/1	28.1	Local control at 9 months was 98%	None
Pham et al. [13]	Prospective (phase 1)	20	26/1 (<5 cm) 42/3 (≥5 cm)	NR	Grade ≤2 toxicity 60% (nausea, chest wall pain and fatigue)	None

16 fractions. The 5-year local control, cause-specific survival and progression-free survival were 100% for all end points. There were no acute toxicities higher than grade 1 and only one patient, with a T4 muscle invasive tumor, developed a late skin ulcer [15].

Neoadjuvant Therapy

In 1954 Sir Eric Riches described the use of preoperative radiation therapy in a patient that had been deemed inoperable and subsequently underwent a complete resection [16]. There had been other reports on the feasibility and potential benefit of preoperative radiation, and in 1973 results from the Rotterdam carcinoma of the kidney trial were published. A total of 141 patients were randomized to 3000 Gy of preoperative radiation therapy given in 3 weeks followed by immediate nephrectomy or nephrectomy alone. Patients were stratified according to primary tumor stage (T1–T3). There was no difference in overall survival or cause-specific survival, although gross complete resection for T3 tumors was improved from 27 to 50% for preoperative radiation [17]. After the preliminary analysis, the study continued, increasing the dose to 40 Gy, but no benefit was seen with the higher dose [18]. The group in Scandinavia conducted a prospective trial that included 88 patients with renal cell carcinoma that were treated with preoperative radiation to 3300 Gy at 2.2 Gy/fraction to the flank, followed by a nephrectomy in 3 weeks after radiotherapy or nephrectomy alone. Patients undergoing nephrectomy alone had a 5-year survival rate of 63% compared to 47% for patients that underwent neoadjuvant radiation. These studies have been criticized for the low dose used and the lack of CT-based planning [19].

An interim analysis from a phase 1 clinical trial from the Cleveland Clinic in 2007 suggested that SBRT prior to nephrectomy was safe at low doses and merited further evaluation; in it three patients underwent SBRT to a total dose of 16 Gy in 4 fractions to the tumor bed followed by a partial nephrectomy at 8 weeks. One patient had no evidence of residual disease at the time of surgery [20].

Renal Pelvis and Ureter

The role of radiation therapy in the treatment of primary malignancies of the renal pelvis and ureter is not well defined. Williams et al. showed that patients with higher grade tumors, as well as patients with muscle invasive disease, had a worse prognosis compared to those with earlier stage or lower grade disease, and these patients represent a group that might benefit from adjuvant therapy [21, 22]. To this date, there are no prospective randomized trials evaluating the value of postoperative radiotherapy in this patient population. Results of retrospective studies show ambiguous results although the combination of radiation and chemotherapy has been the subject of recent publications, as discussed below.

In 1968 Brady et al., reported on six patients who underwent radiation therapy for either unresectable disease [2], extensive regional nodal involvement at the time of surgery [2] or local recurrence [2]. Doses ranged from 2200 to 6000 rad. All patients were alive without evidence of disease at 1 year and three out of the six were alive without evidence of disease at 5 years. One patient had persistent mild radiation induced cystitis 84 months after treatment [23]. The group at M.D. Anderson summarized their experience on eight patients with documented infiltrative disease who underwent radiation therapy to the ureteral bed following nephroureterectomy. Doses planned ranged from 4000 to 6000 rad using opposed anterior and posterior fields. Persistent or recurrent disease was documented in only one patient with survival ranging from 9 to 53 months [24]. Brookland et al. described their experience in 11 out of 23 patients with high grade or invasive disease who underwent adjuvant radiation following radical surgery. Five patients in the nonirradiated and one in the radiated arm experienced a local recurrence. Median survival of the nonirradiated and irradiated patients was 26 and 35 months, respectively [25].

In the last two decades, several publications using more sophisticated radiation techniques have been published showing overall an improvement in local control with unclear benefit for overall survival. The group at the University of Kansas showed an improved actuarial local control at 5 years from 34 to 88% by adding adjuvant radiation therapy mainly to the tumor bed. In total, 26 patients with stage III–IV transitional cell carcinoma (TCC) of the renal pelvis and ureter underwent a radical resection after which nine patients had adjuvant radiation therapy. Median dose was 50 Gy with an average of three fields used in their treatment design. Absolute overall survival at 5 years was 24 and 44% in the nonradiated versus the radiated arm, respectively. On multivariate analysis, high grade and the use of adjuvant radiation therapy were significant factors influencing local recurrence [26]. Hall et al. from the University of Texas Southwestern Medical Center reported the outcome of 74 patients with stage III ($n = 49$) and stage IV ($n = 25$) TCC of the upper urinary tract treated with radical nephroureterectomy followed by observation ($n = 46$) or adjuvant therapy, including radiation therapy ($n = 28$), chemotherapy ($n = 10$) or chemo radiation ($n = 3$). Median FU was 21 months. Isolated local recurrence was seen in five patients with stage III, two followed by observation, two with adjuvant radiation alone and one with adjuvant chemo radiation, and one patient with stage IV disease treated with chemotherapy alone. The actuarial disease specific survival for patients with stage III disease was 45 and 40% for patients with adjuvant therapy and observation, respectively. For patients with stage IV disease median survival was poor at 7 month compared to 9 months for those who underwent adjuvant treatment versus no adjuvant therapy, respectively [27].

More recently Czito et al., published their experience on 31 patients with advanced TCC of the renal pelvis and ureter treated with radical nephroureterectomy followed by adjuvant radiation therapy ($n = 22$) and more recently, adjuvant chemotherapy (methotrexate, cisplatinum and vinblastine) followed by concurrent chemotherapy (cisplatinum) and radiation therapy ($n = 9$). Median radiation dose was 46.9 Gy, and treatment fields used a combination of two–four field techniques. Target included the tumor bed and regional lymph nodes. Median follow-up for all patients was 2.6 years and 8.5 years for the surviving patients. A total of 16 patients experience a relapse with seven being locoregional, all of which, except one, also had distant disease. No difference between the radiation alone or chemo radiation adjuvant treatment regimens was seen. The overall 5-year actuarial and disease specific survival was 39% (27% in the radiation alone and 67% in the chemo radiation arms) and 52% (41% in the radiation alone arm and 76% for the chemo radiation arm), respectively. This study concluded that the use of combined adjuvant therapy should be the subject of future studies [28]. The group from Fudan University in Shanghai summarized the outcome of 133 patients with TCC of the upper urinary tract, 67 of whom underwent adjuvant radiation therapy at the discretion of the provider; comparison of the radiated and nonirradiated groups did not show any specific indication for referral to adjuvant therapy. Radiation dose ranged from 46 to 50 Gy using multiple field arrangements, including field size reductions during treatment to decrease toxicity to surrounding organs. The clinical target volume included the ipsilateral renal fossa and/or tumor bed, the course of the ureter, the whole bladder, and the paracaval and paraaortic lymph nodes. All patients underwent adjuvant intravesical chemotherapy. Primary end point was safety and locoregional failure and overall survival. Median follow-up was 26.6 months. Overall survival at 1, 3 and 5 years for the RT group and the non-RT group were 98.8% versus 75.5%, 61.1% versus 53.6%, and 49.6% versus 44.7%, respectively. For patients with T3 and T4 tumors, median survival time was 29.9 months for the RT arm compared to 11.4 months in the non-RT group. On multivariate analysis, age <60, T1–T2 tumors, absence of synchronous lymph node metastasis and use of radiation were predictor of improved overall survival. There were no tumor bed recurrences in the RT group and 4 in the non-RT group. Regional nodal relapse as a primary site of failure was seen 9.5% compared to 24.6% in the RT group and the non-RT group, respectively. Only two patients developed grade 3 gastrointestinal toxicity and five developed grade 3 thrombocytopenia [29].

A group out of the University of Yamanashi in Japan recently reported the use of SBRT in three patients over the age of 80 with TCC of the ureter who were deemed not surgical candidates or refused surgery. Treatment volumes encompassed the gross disease with an unspecified margin. Doses ranged from 50 to 60 Gy delivered in 10 fractions. All three patients showed tumor regression at 3 months with no evidence of tumor regrowth at 12 months. One patient died of comorbidities at 13 months, one patient died 33 months posttreatment without evidence of disease, and one patient suffered a tumor recurrence in the bladder at 22 months and passed away after 38 months from the time of initial treatment. No acute or chronic toxicity was reported [30].

Summary Box

- Historically, radiation therapy has not played a major role in the primary management of upper urinary tract malignancies.
- Newer approaches to radiation therapy, such as intensity modulated radiation therapy, stereotactic radiotherapy, and particle therapy (e.g., protons) may permit the delivery of higher doses to deep seated tumors with improved sparing of surrounding normal tissues, thereby overcoming the limitations faced in older series.
- Thus, for locally advanced malignancies of the kidney, ureter and renal pelvis, adjuvant radiotherapy may help prevent locoregional recurrence and subsequently improve survival.

- For medically inoperable patients, or for those who refuse surgery, radiotherapy as primary treatment may provide prolonged local control and even cure in selected patients.
- Radiotherapy continues to play an important role in the management patients with metastatic cancers of the upper urinary tract, and may provide an opportunity for prolonged survival in selected patients with oligometastatic disease.

References

1. Bernier J, Hall EJ, Giaccia A. Radiation oncology: a century of achievements. Nat Rev Cancer. (Historical Article Review). 2004;4(9):737–47.
2. Hall EJ, Giaccia AJ. Radiobiology for the radiologist. 7th ed. Philadelphia: Lippincott Williams & Wilkins; 2011.
3. Khan FM. The physics of radiation therapy. 4th ed. Philadelphia: Lippincott Williams & Wilkins; 2010.
4. Eble MJ, Lehnert T, Herfarth C, Wannenmacher M. Intraoperative radiotherapy as adjuvant treatment for stage II/III rectal carcinoma. Recent Results Cancer Res. (Clinical Trial Controlled Clinical Trial). 1998;146:152–60.
5. Fairweather M, Wang J, Devlin PM, Hansen J, Baldini EH, Ready JE, et al. Safety and efficacy of radiation dose delivered via iodine-125 brachytherapy mesh implantation for deep cavity sarcomas. Ann Surg Oncol. 2015;22(5):1455–63.
6. Flocks RH, Kadesky MC. Malignant neoplasms of the kidney; an analysis of 353 patients followed five years or more. J Urol. 1958;79(2):196–201.
7. Peeling WB, Mantell BS, Shepheard BG. Post-operative irradiation in the treatment of renal cell carcinoma. Br J Urol. 1969;41(1):23–31.
8. Finney R. An evaluation of postoperative radiotherapy in hypernephroma treatment—a clinical trial. Cancer. 1973;32(6):1332–40.
9. Kjaer M, Iversen P, Hvidt V, Bruun E, Skaarup P, Bech Hansen J, et al. A randomized trial of postoperative radiotherapy versus observation in stage II and III renal adenocarcinoma. A study by the Copenhagen Renal Cancer Study Group. Scand J Urol Nephrol. (Clinical Trial Comparative Study Randomized Controlled Trial). 1987;21(4):285–9.
10. Beitler JJ, Makara D, Silverman P, Lederman G. Definitive, high-dose-per-fraction, conformal, stereotactic external radiation for renal cell carcinoma. Am J Clin Oncol. 2004;27(6):646–8.
11. Wersall PJ, Blomgren H, Lax I, Kalkner KM, Linder C, Lundell G, et al. Extracranial stereotactic radiotherapy for primary and metastatic renal cell carcinoma. Radiother Oncol. (Clinical Trial Research Support, Non-U.S. Gov't). 2005;77(1):88–95.
12. Svedman C, Karlsson K, Rutkowska E, Sandstrom P, Blomgren H, Lax I, et al. Stereotactic body radiotherapy of primary and metastatic renal lesions for patients with only one functioning kidney. Acta Oncol. (Research Support, Non-U.S. Gov't). 2008; 47(8):1578–83.
13. Pham D, Thompson A, Kron T, Foroudi F, Kolsky MS, Devereux T, et al. Stereotactic ablative body radiation therapy for primary kidney cancer: a 3-dimensional conformal technique associated with low rates of early toxicity. Int J Radiat Oncol Biol Phys. (Clinical Trial, Phase I Research Support, Non-U.S. Gov't). 2014;90(5):1061–8.
14. Staehler M, Bader M, Schlenker B, Casuscelli J, Karl A, Roosen A, et al. Single fraction radiosurgery for the treatment of renal tumors. J Urol. (Evaluation Studies). 2015;193(3):771–5.
15. Nomiya T, Tsuji H, Hirasawa N, Kato H, Kamada T, Mizoe J, et al. Carbon ion radiation therapy for primary renal cell carcinoma: initial clinical experience. Int J Radiat Oncol Biol Phys. 2008;72(3): 828–33.
16. Riches EW. Irradiation therapy in urology: the kidney. Br J Urol. 1954;26(4):319–25.
17. van der Werf-Messing B. Proceedings: carcinoma of the bladder treated by preoperative irradiation followed by cystectomy. The second report. Cancer. 1973;32(5):1084–8.
18. van der Werf-Messing B, van der Heul RO, Ledeboer RC. [Renal adenocarcinoma; a prospective therapy study in Rotterdam]. Ned Tijdschr Geneeskd. 1980;124(31):1298–303.
19. Juusela H, Malmio K, Alfthan O, Oravisto KJ. Preoperative irradiation in the treatment of renal adenocarcinoma. Scand J Urol Nephrol. (Clinical Trial Randomized Controlled Trial). 1977;11(3):277–81.
20. Ponsky LE, Mahadevan A, Gill IS, Djemil T, Novick AC. Renal radiosurgery: initial clinical experience with histological evaluation. Surg Innov. 2007;14(4):265–9.
21. Williams CB, Mitchell JP. Carcinoma of the renal pelvis: a review of 43 cases. Br J Urol. 1973; 45(4):370–6.
22. Williams CB, Mitchell JP. Carcinoma of the ureter—a review of 54 cases. Br J Urol. 1973;45(4):377–87.
23. Brady LW, Gislason GJ, Faust DS, Kazem I, Antoniades J, Davis JA. Radiation therapy. A valuable adjunct in the management of carcinoma of the ureter. JAMA. 1968;206(13):2871–4.
24. Babaian RJ, Johnson DE, Chan RC. Combination nephroureterectomy and postoperative radiotherapy

for infiltrative ureteral carcinoma. Int J Radiat Oncol Biol Phys. 1980;6(9):1229–32.
25. Brookland RK, Richter MP. The postoperative irradiation of transitional cell carcinoma of the renal pelvis and ureter. J Urol. 1985;133(6):952–5.
26. Cozad SC, Smalley SR, Austenfeld M, Noble M, Jennings S, Reymond R. Adjuvant radiotherapy in high stage transitional cell carcinoma of the renal pelvis and ureter. Int J Radiat Oncol Biol Phys. 1992;24(4):743–5.
27. Hall MC, Womack JS, Roehrborn CG, Carmody T, Sagalowsky AI. Advanced transitional cell carcinoma of the upper urinary tract: patterns of failure, survival and impact of postoperative adjuvant radiotherapy. J Urol. 1998;160(3 Pt 1):703–6.
28. Czito B, Zietman A, Kaufman D, Skowronski U, Shipley W. Adjuvant radiotherapy with and without concurrent chemotherapy for locally advanced transitional cell carcinoma of the renal pelvis and ureter. J Urol. (Comparative Study). 2004;172(4 Pt 1): 1271–5.
29. Chen B, Zeng ZC, Wang GM, Zhang L, Lin ZM, Sun LA, et al. Radiotherapy may improve overall survival of patients with T3/T4 transitional cell carcinoma of the renal pelvis or ureter and delay bladder tumour relapse. BMC Cancer. 2011;11:297.
30. Maehata Y, Kuriyama K, Aoki S, Araya M, Marino K, Onishi H. Stereotactic body radiotherapy for localized ureter transitional cell carcinoma: three case reports. Case Rep Urol. 2015;2015:519897.

Epilogue

During the trailblazing years of endourology in the early 1980s, any unusual or challenging case provided an opportunity to envision, develop, and try new approaches within this field.

Between 1983 and 1984, one such clinical scenario was an elderly female patient with poor renal function and transitional cell carcinoma of the renal pelvis who had refused nephrectomy to avoid hemodialysis, which she resented more than the thought of living fighting potential recurrence of cancer. This was the circumstance for the first planned percutaneous renal pelvic tumor resection, which was followed by intracavitary instillation of thio-TEPA, a commonly used topical agent then, to decrease the recurrence of the bladder tumors. The protocol used was similar to the one used in treatment of bladder cancers. We reported this case in video format with my colleagues, Dr. Arthur Smith and Dr. Gopal Badlani in AUA meeting in 1985 [1]. To my knowledge, this was the first reported elective systemic endoscopic resection combined with intracavitary treatment in management of the upper tract urothelial tumors. The conservative management of UTUC has evolved significantly since then with a lot more to be accomplished as outlined in the pages of this book.

It is often difficult or unrealistic to format the treatment of all patients into preconceived or algorithmic models especially in cases of UTUC. This group of patients has often multiple factors that will not allow every patient to fall in or follow one of the arms of the algorithm. Instead in this portion of the textbook, I have outlined fifteen actual clinical cases from an approximate period of three decades. These sample cases of different aspects and stages of upper tract urothelial carcinoma will illustrate a timeline with changes reflecting better, newer technology as well as a retrospective review of these not run-of-the-mill cases. The study of these actual clinical scenarios will allow for a brief recapitulation of all the modalities that have been described in the previous chapters in a variety of forms. We are practically seeing the applications of all the modalities that have been described in the pages of this textbook. In some cases, multiple modalities have been used, as is the case usually in the management of these patients as they transition through different phases from diagnosis to the endpoint of treatment. These case reviews demonstrate ***success as well as failure*** and as was mentioned earlier, not all of these cases can be compared to radical nephroureterectomy or segmental resection as alternative options. Two such examples: case 1 of 58-year-old male patient with a small renal pelvic tumor managed endoscopically when standard treatment of the time was nephroureterectomy and the second case 8 of an 80-year-old female with solitary kidney presented with anuria secondary to large lesion causing complete obstruction and was resected percutaneously

M. Eshghi (ed.), *Urothelial Malignancies of the Upper Urinary Tract*,
https://doi.org/10.1007/978-3-319-51263-1

without recurrence while she went on to undergo additional unrelated cancer surgeries. They should also serve as a constant reminder of the need for diligent and unrelenting continuous follow-up surveillance of patients with upper tract urothelial carcinoma … ***a disease with high potentials for recurrence and progression*** and nephroureterectomy considered ***only if and when necessary***.

Majid Eshghi, MD, FACS, MBA
Valhalla, New York
January 2018

Reference

1. Smith A, Eshghi M, Badlani G: Percutaneous renal surgery, parts 1–2, AUA 2015, Abstract Book.

Case Studies: A Spectrum of Upper Tract Urothelial Carcinoma

Neel Patel, Cristina Fox and Majid Eshghi

Corresponding author:
Majid Eshghi, MD, FACS, MBA
Chief Section of Endourology and Minimally Invasive Urology, Westchester Medical Health Network/New York Medical College, Department of Urology, Valhalla, NY, United States

Case Study 1

A 58-year-old male with one episode of hematuria underwent a complete urological workup that was negative except for the intravenous pyelogram showing a small filling defect in the right renal pelvis. A flexible ureteroscopy revealed a small papillary lesion and the rest of the collecting system was free of any pathology. Considering that 25 years ago, we did not have proper ureteroscopic equipment to adequately biopsy and ablate this lesion, patient underwent a percutaneous approach and the lesion was completely removed using a cold cup and the base was fulgurated. A similar case is demonstrated in Chap. 14, Video 14.1 and Video 14.2. He was followed closely for 15 years before he retired and moved to another state and reported negative follow up studies. He was given recommendation of close urological follow-up (Fig. C.1).

Comment

Today this patient will be managed completely in a retrograde fashion: biopsy, urinary cytology, cell block and laser ablation. This would be similar to the procedure shown in Video 14.1. It also highlights that low-grade urothelial carcinoma of the upper tract can be managed successfully with complete resection and proper surveillance.

Case Study 2

Patient is a 73-year-old non-smoker female with a history of renal stones who was found to have significant left hydronephrosis on her follow-up ultrasound. Her previous imaging studies 2 years earlier were negative. The patient was completely asymptomatic and denied flank pain fever, urinary tract infection, or hematuria. CT scan imaging revealed a filling defect in the left distal ureter associated with left hydroureteronephrosis. No stone was identified in the distal ureter. Office cystoscopy was negative and urine cytology showed some atypical cells.

A left ureteroscopy was performed showing a papillary lesion that was resected using a rigid ureteroesectoscope. Evaluation of the rest of the

M. Eshghi (ed.), *Urothelial Malignancies of the Upper Urinary Tract*,
https://doi.org/10.1007/978-3-319-51263-1

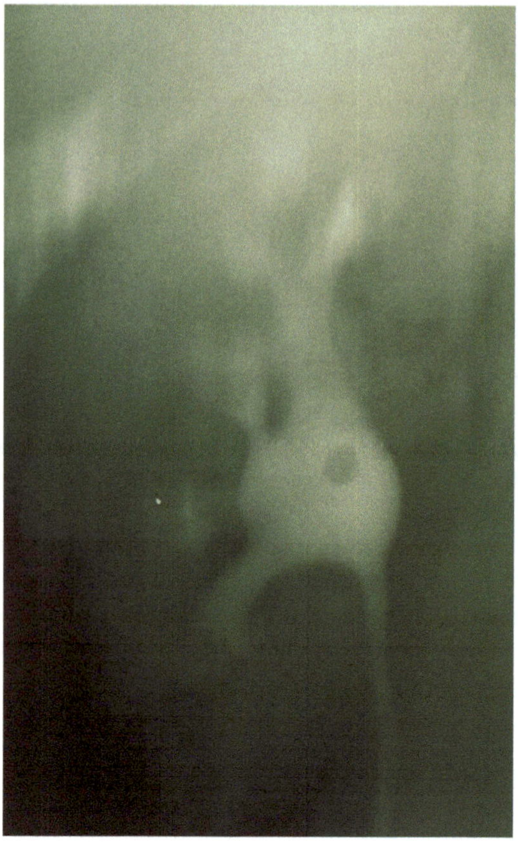

Fig. C.1 Intravenous pyelogram prior to percutaneous nephrostomy, which shows a small filling defect in the renal pelvis

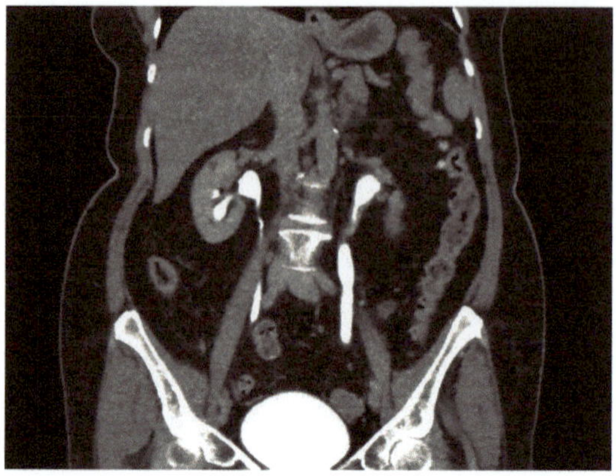

Fig. C.2 CT showing L hydroureter from distal ureteral lesion

collecting system was negative. The left orifice and intramural ureter were resected to allow for free reflux into the distal segment. Double pigtail stent was placed and mitomycin was instilled into the renal pelvis with an open-ended catheter placed next to the stent. A Foley was placed and clamped while the open-ended catheter was removed. The Foley was unclamped after one hour. Pathology was consistent with papillary urothelial carcinoma with no muscle invasion.

Patient underwent a 6 week course of intravesical mitomycin and was instructed to lie on her left side for at least one hour. Follow-up ureteroscopy revealed no residual tumor. She underwent another instillation of mitomycin at the end of the procedure, it was felt although the lesion was low-grade mitomycin C would provide additional benefit. Urine cytology has remained negative. She has been placed on a surveillance protocol with periodic imaging and endoscopy. At 9 months, surveillance endoscopy showed completely normal bladder and ureter with multiple negative cytologies. Office ureteroscopy and cystoscopy repeated 18 months later is negative. Figures C.2, C.3, C.4 and C.5; Video C.1 and Video C.2.

Comment

This case illustrates aggressive endoscopic resection of low-grade bulky tumor of distal ureter using rigid ureteroresectoscope followed with topical chemotherapy via intentionally created vesicoureteral reflux. Complete, deep resection of tumor and wide resection of the orifice and intramural ureter are essential for a successful outcome. Resection of ureteral orifice allows for office ureteroscopy without anesthesia.

Case Study 3

Patient is a 78-year-old male who was referred from nephrologist after a routine evaluation for chronic kidney disease. In 2014, renal and bladder ultrasound revealed severe left hydronephrosis. Due to elevated creatinine, diabetes, and an aortic aneurysm, a contrast study had not been done. The patient had several additional comorbidities. He underwent a cystoscopy and retrograde pyelogram revealing a

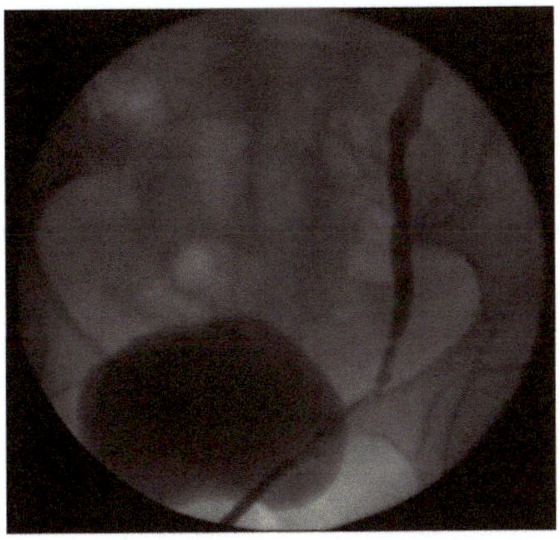

Fig. C.3 Left retrograde pyelogram showing distal ureteral filling defect

three-centimeter-long filling defect suggesting urothelial carcinoma in the left distal ureter nearing the ureterovesical junction. The patient underwent incision of a narrow distal ureter and ureteroscopic resection of this lesion using the 11.5 French rigid ureteroresectoscope. Pathologic analysis of the specimen revealed noninvasive, low-grade papillary urothelial carcinoma.

One month subsequent to this original resection, the patient underwent repeat cystoscopy, retrograde pyelography, and ureteroscopic biopsy of the distal ureter demonstrating mucosa negative for tumor, only characteristic of fibrous soft tissue. Three months subsequent to the initial resection, the patient developed recurrent hydronephrosis and flank pain secondary to a distal ureteral stricture, requiring ureteral balloon dilation and stenting. Surveillance pyelography, ureteroscopy with biopsy, and stent exchange were subsequently performed at 6-month intervals in addition to serial urine cytology, all of which were negative for malignant cells.

The patient underwent CT, albeit without contrast secondary to his chronic kidney disease with a creatinine of approximately 2.4. In late 2015, CT demonstrated hydronephrosis and thickening the distal ureter, and in early 2016 surveillance cystoscopy revealed a few superficial bladder tumors that were fulgurated.

Additionally, ureteroscopy revealed some narrowing of the left distal ureter. Post dilation, retrograde pyelography revealed a filling defect of the mid ureter. Ureteroscopy revealed 3 small mid ureteral tumors which were ablated with a combination of Holmium and Nd–Yag lasers. The lesions were pathologically classified as low grade, noninvasive papillary urothelial carcinoma with no invasion to lamina propria. The patient will continue with endoscopic surveillance. CT

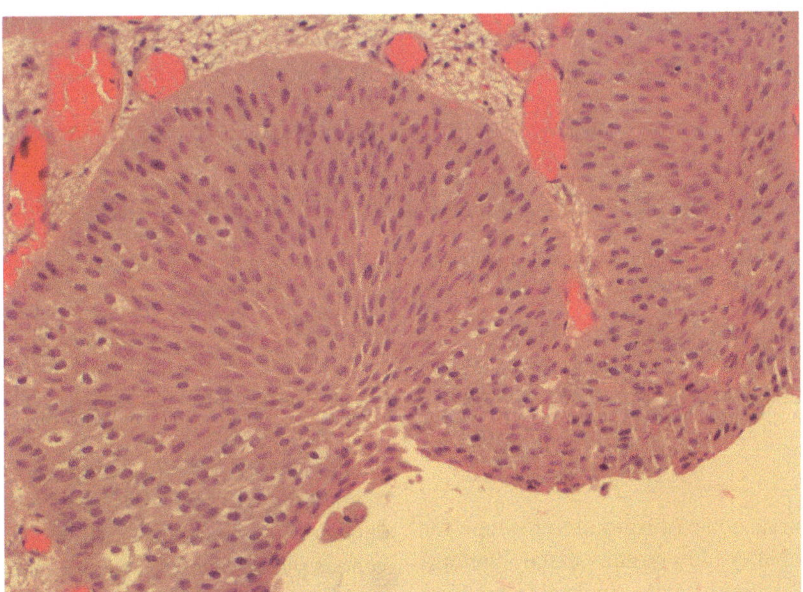

Fig. C.4 Left distal ureter biopsy showing low-grade urothelial carcinoma with no lamina propria or muscle invasion

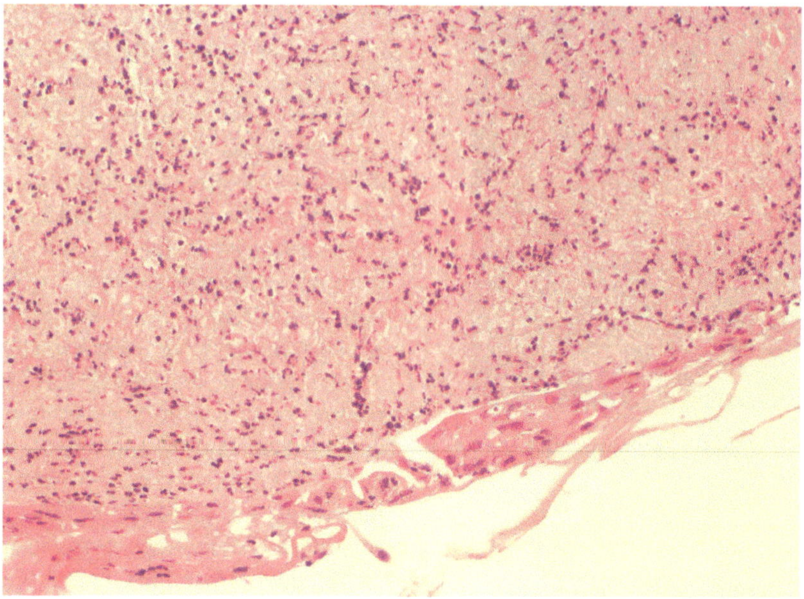

Fig. C.5 Distal ureteral biopsy showing urothelium lined with acute inflammation and necrosis/infarction, negative for dysplasia or malignancy; V-1; this segment shows ureteroresectoscopic resection of the tumor; V-2; follow-up endoscopy showing no residual tumor

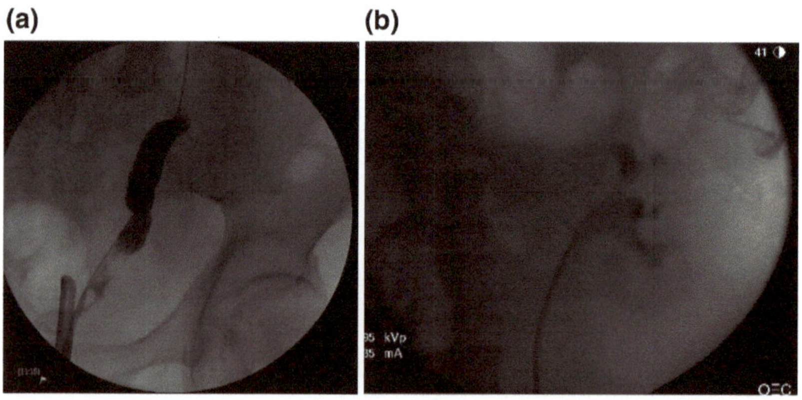

Fig. C.6 **a**, **b** 2014 retrograde pyelogram during a ureteroscopic resection of distal ureteral tumor demonstrating 2–3 cm filling defect in distal ureter as well as torturous ureter and hydronephrosis

scan of the abdomen did not show any evidence of metastatic disease (Figs. C.6, C.7 and C.8).

Comment

This case illustrates: use of rigid ureteroscope for resection of bulky low-grade distal ureteral tumor in a patient with multiple medical comorbidities.

Case Study 4

Patient is a 68-year-old male with a strong history of smoking and uric acid stones presented with an episode of gross hematuria 30 years ago. Intravenous pyelogram showed a slight filling defect of the left upper pole calyx. One of the first generation flexible ureteroscope with active deflection was

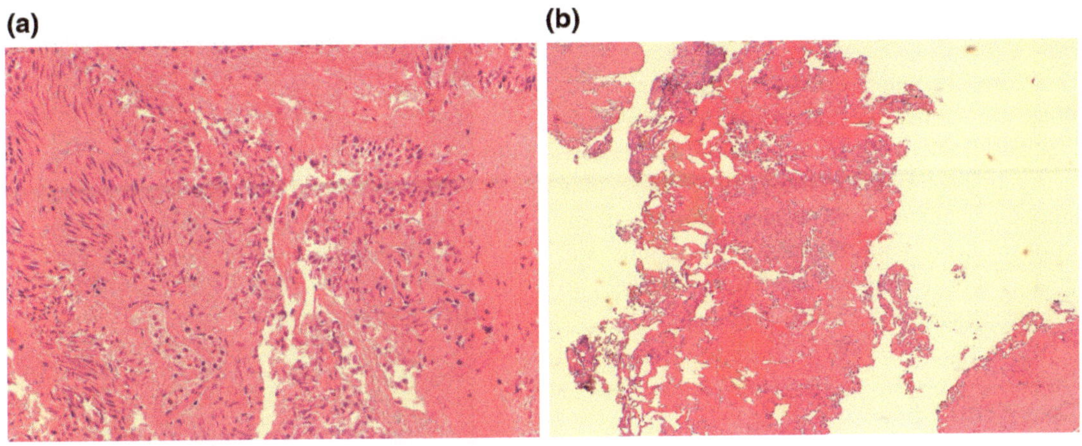

Fig. C.7 Pathologic slide from 2014 ureteroscopic resection of distal left ureteral tumor consistent with low grade, papillary urothelial carcinoma. Muscle bundles are free of tumor

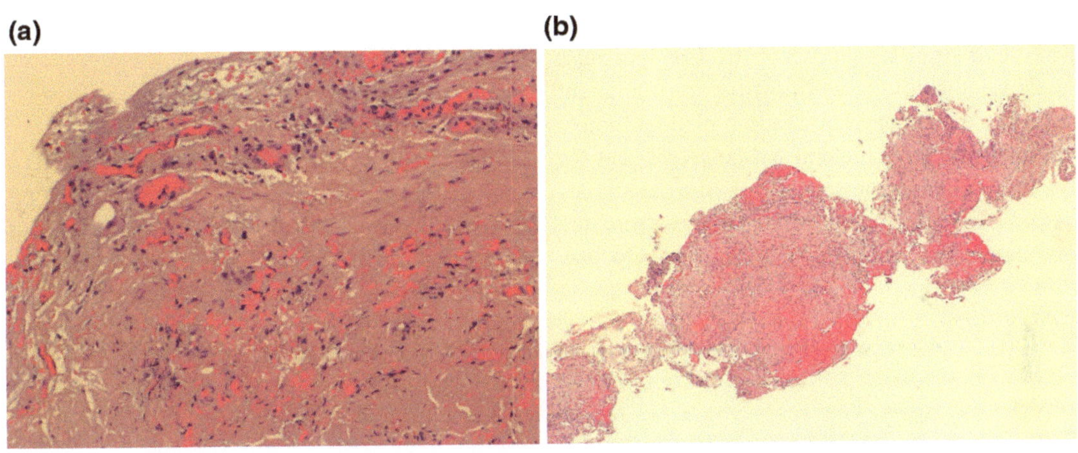

Fig. C.8 Pathologic slide from 2014 repeat surveillance biopsy of distal ureter performed 6 months post resection demonstrating fibrocollagenous tissue and areas of hemorrhage with no evidence of malignant cells

used to perform a biopsy of the upper calyx, which showed high-grade urothelial carcinoma. The patient underwent a left nephroureterectomy. Serial surveillance of the patient has been done by in office cystoscopy, annual urine cytology, as well as CT urogram and renal/bladder ultrasound. The patient has documented presence of multiple simple right renal cysts measuring approximately 6×6 cm in the upper pole, approximately 1.3×1.4 cm in the midpole cortex, and 1.0×0.7 cm in the midpole parenchyma. These lesions have been stable in size over the many years of surveillance. In the first few years of follow–up, the patient had one episode of superficial bladder cancer which was resected without recurrence.

Several years post nephrouterectomy, the patient developed one episode of obstructive uropathy, necessitating ureteroscopy. However, currently, the stones have been successfully managed medically without recurrence. The long-term sequela of the remote neoplasm experienced by this patient has been the gradual development of chronic kidney disease. The patient's creatinine has slightly increased to 1.1, he is post one MI and on multiple medications for hypertension. He has had no recurrence to this date (Figs. C.9, C.10 and C.11).

Comment

This case illustrates: early diagnostic and sampling using flexible ureteroscopes providing adequate tissue diagnosis of high-grade disease justifying nephroureterectomy, in the face of a suboptimal contralateral kidney, partially compromised with stone disease. Prior to this era, most nephroureterectomies were based on imaging studies and clinical findings.

Case Study 5

This is a 71-year-old female with findings of microscopic hematuria. Her initial workup demonstrated a cystoscopy and CT Urogram at the time were within normal limits; however the urine cytology was equivocal. The patient's repeat urine cytology was positive for malignant cells. She then underwent random bladder biopsy and intra-operative ureteral washes were sent for cytology. The biopsies consisting of five samples were all negative, while the cytology from the left ureter was negative A urine cytology was again obtained in the office which revealed high-grade urothelial cell carcinoma.

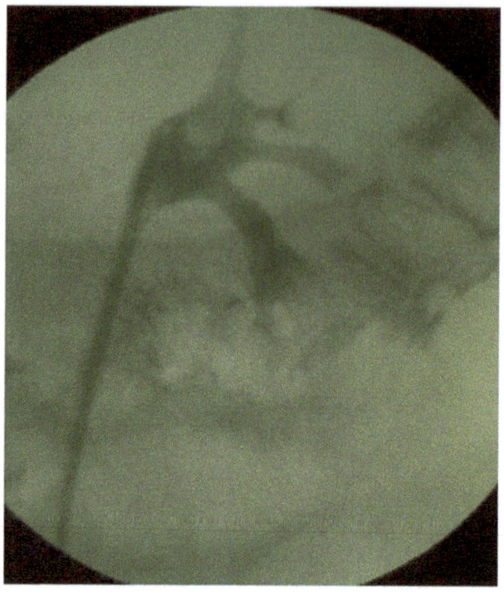

Fig. C.9 Retrograde pyelogram prior to ureteroscopic biopsy of upper calyceal area 30 years ago

The patient underwent a second round of random bladder biopsies as well as bilateral retrograde pyelogram and cytology. No abnormalities or filling defects were seen with the

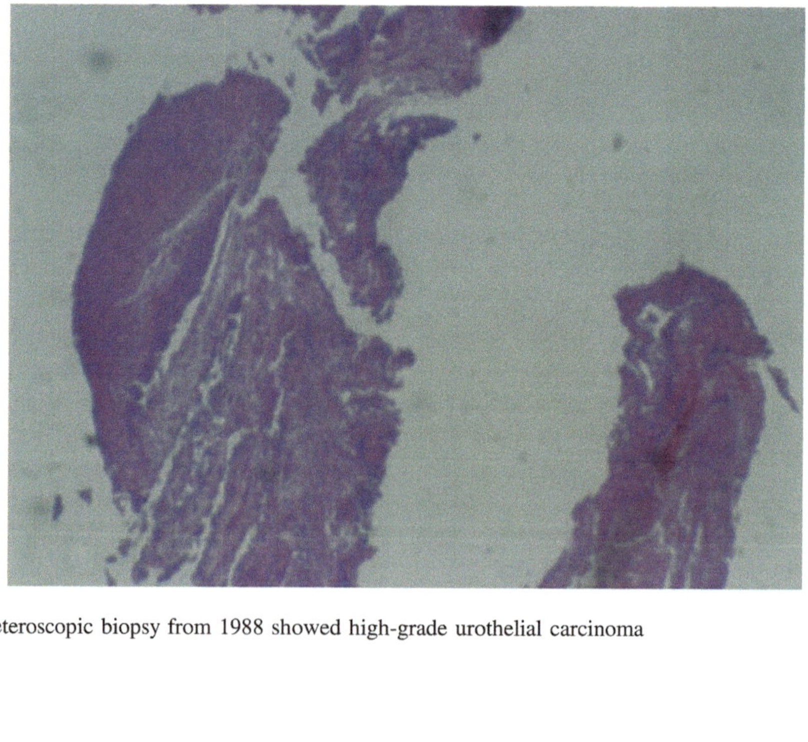

Fig. C.10 Ureteroscopic biopsy from 1988 showed high-grade urothelial carcinoma

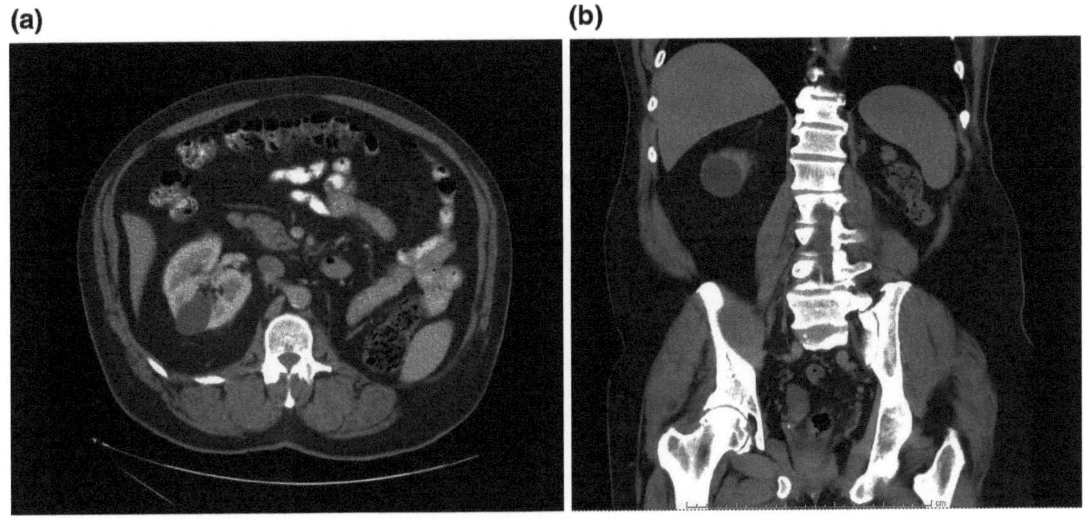

Fig. C.11 CT scan of abdomen and pelvis demonstrating simple renal cysts in right kidney several years post left nephroureterectomy

retrograde pyelogram, while the bladder biopsies were again negative with muscularis propria present in each specimen. The intra-operative cytology showed high-grade urothelial cell carcinoma from the bladder and positive malignant cells from the left ureteral washing. Left ureteroscopy with biopsy and cytology were performed which showed left renal pelvis lesion with urothelial atypia and left ureteral wash with positive malignant cells. The patient underwent a repeat left ureteroscopy and biopsy of a left upper pole lesion, which revealed atypical urothelial cells and fibrous connective tissue.

A thorough discussion was held with the patient regarding her history of multiple urine cytologies with various findings ranging from benign to atypical to malignant, as well as multiple bladder biopsies showing no malignancy, and a finding of a left renal pelvic lesion that revealed atypical urothelial cells. Patient was given all treatment options: surveillance, endoscopic management, and neoadjuvant chemotherapy followed by left nephroureterectomy. The patient opted for a course of neoadjuvant chemotherapy followed by left nephroureterectomy. Final pathology showed no detectable residual disease (Figs. C.12, C.13 and C.14).

Comment

This case illustrates high-grade lesion with CIS and positive cytology responding to neoadjuvant chemotherapy. Obtaining a definitive biopsy can

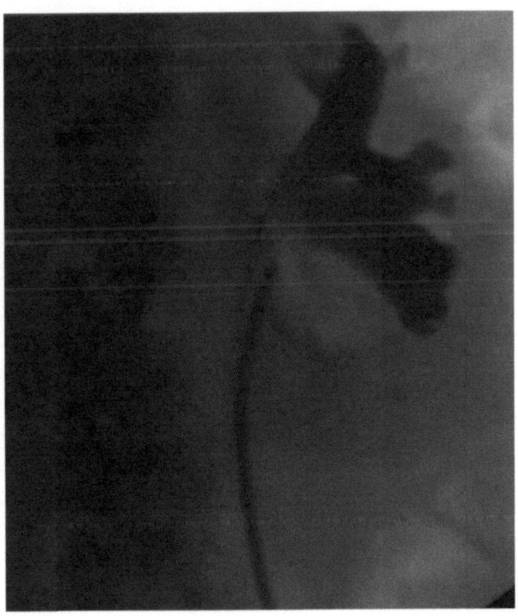

Fig. C.12 Retrograde pyelogram showing no filling defects

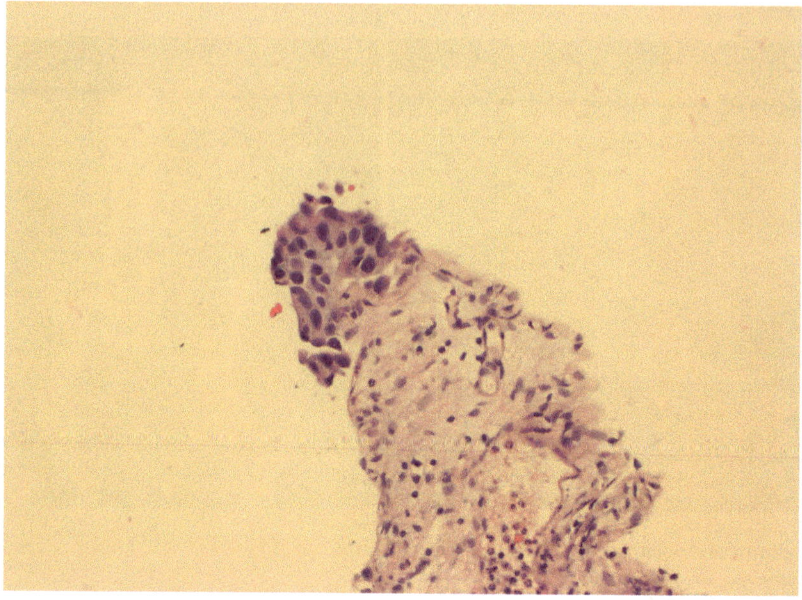

Fig. C.13 Left renal pelvis biopsy showing focal marked urothelial atypia—fibrous connective tissue with chronic inflammation

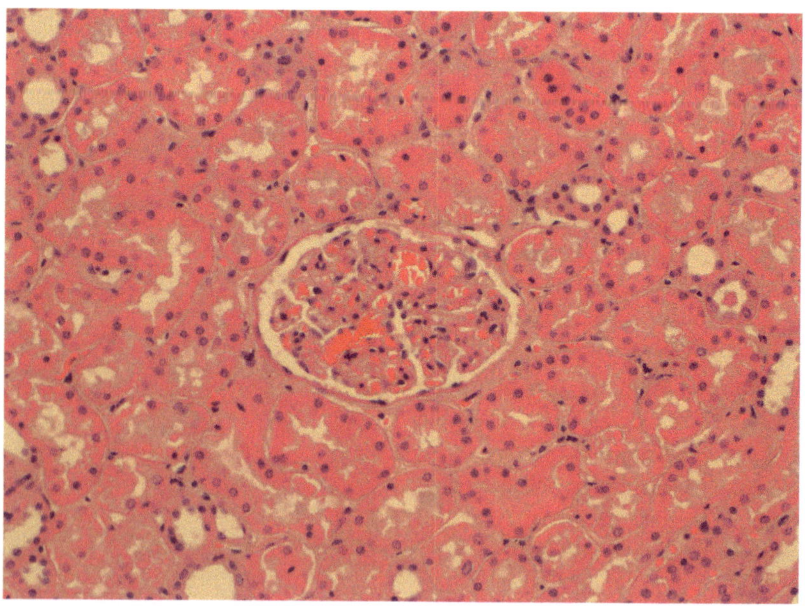

Fig. C.14 Nephroureterectomy specimen showing benign unremarkable renal parenchyma and renal pelvis with no residual tumor seen

be challenging in some of these cases. It is hard to assess long-term complete response without nephroureterectomy.

Case Study 6

A 77–year-old man with a strong history of smoking was evaluated for gross painless hematuria. Initial CT and Cystoscopy were found to be negative. Despite initial negative findings, the patient continued to have intermittent gross hematuria. Due to high index of suspicion because of strong history of smoking a follow-up, CT Urogram that was performed later that showed mild to moderate right hydronephrosis with tapering of the right distal ureter.

The patient underwent right ureteroscopy and was found to have a right distal ureteral stricture and dilated ureter proximal to this area. Multiple cold cup biopsies were taken after the initial dilation of the intramural ureter. Endoscopy of the rest of the ureter and collecting system did not show additional pathology. Pathology was positive for a diagnosis of high-grade urothelial carcinoma involving the lamina propria, but the muscularis propria free of tumor.

The patient underwent a robotic assisted laparoscopic partial cystectomy with right distal ureterectomy and ureteral reimplantation. His final pathology showed high-grade urothelial carcinoma within the right distal ureteral segment measuring 0.6 × 0.3 cm with involvement into the muscle, negative proximal and distal margins as well as lack of lymphovascular invasion. This was classified as pT2pNxMx. The patient was placed on a surveillance protocol involving imaging, cystoscopy, and urine cytology. The importance of surveillance protocol was emphasized to the patient and he agreed to be compliant (Figs. C.15, C.16, C.17 and C.18).

Comment

This case illustrates a non-papillary infiltrating tumor causing obstruction. Endoscopic management is not a good option for such cases. A similar pattern of infiltrative disease is sometimes seen in renal pelvis and upper ureter as well without obvious papillary or sessile tumor. Ureteral wall thickening, ureteral obstruction, and abnormal cytology are telltale signs.

Case Study 7

A 58-year-old female was evaluated with a 10-month history of intermittent gross hematuria and right flank pain. Computed tomography revealed mild hydronephrosis and thickening of upper ureter. Previous ureteroscopy and biopsies at another institution were not diagnostic. She underwent repeat ureteroscopy which only revealed firm ureteral wall with slightly abnormal looking mucosa. Deep biopsies of renal pelvis and very proximal ureter revealed high-grade urothelial carcinoma.

She was recommended to undergo radical nephroureterectomy due to changes of ureteral wall, UPJ area and high-grade carcinoma. Final pathology revealed infiltrative high-grade urothelial carcinoma (Fig. C.19).

Comment

The significance of this case is infiltrative submucosal disease without any papillary or elevated mucosal lesions. These lesions are like ***fire under the ash*** requiring aggressive treatment before they completely penetrate through the wall and as was described in case study number 6 with the difference that in distal ureter the patient could have the option of distal ureterectomy and reimplantation.

Case Study 8

An 80-year-old female with a left solitary kidney was evaluated for anuria and serum creatinine of 3.9. Her past cancer history included a Rt nephrectomy for renal cell carcinoma, hysterectomy, colectomy, breast lumpectomy, resections

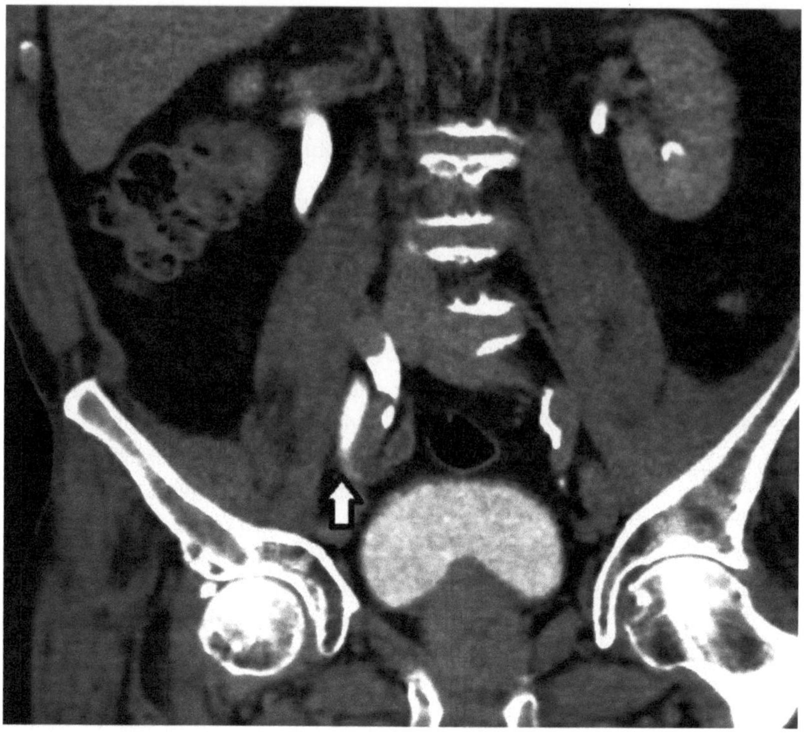

Fig. C.15 CT showing right hydroureter with distal tapering of ureter

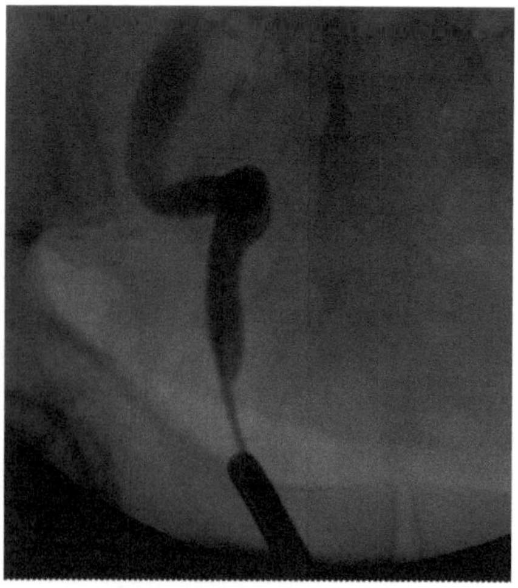

Fig. C.16 Right retrograde pyelogram showing distal filling defect with proximal dilated ureter

of melanoma and basal cell carcinoma. She also had history of open heart and aortic surgery.

Imaging studies revealed a large filling defect in the renal pelvis and associated hydronephrosis. Considering her strong history of malignancies and multiple comorbidities she decided to undergo organ preserving endoscopic treatment.

She underwent percutaneous resection of a large broad based papillary renal pelvic tumor that had caused UPJ obstruction. Pathological diagnosis was low-grade papillary urothelial carcinoma (Video C.3).

She underwent a 6-week course of intracavitary mitomycin C. Follow-up nephroscopy and biopsies were negative. She received a second booster intracavitary treatment before the removal of the nephrostomy tube.

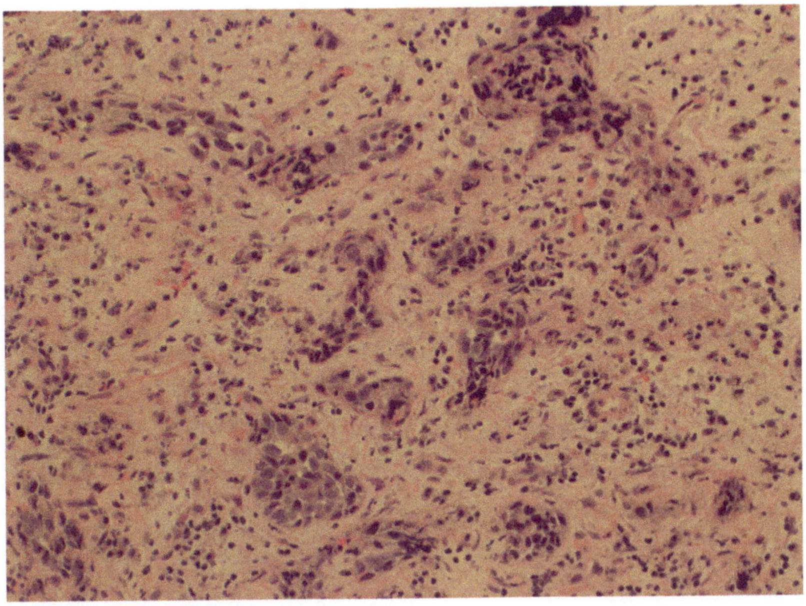

Fig. C.17 Right ureter biopsy showing high-grade urothelial carcinoma involving lamina propria, muscle is free of invasion

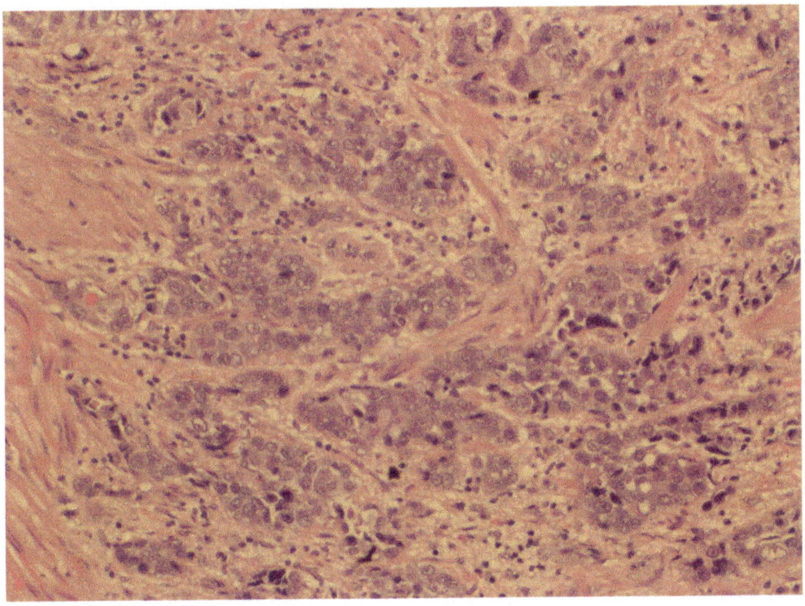

Fig. C.18 Right ureter s/p ureterectomy showing high-grade urothelial carcinoma with muscle invasion

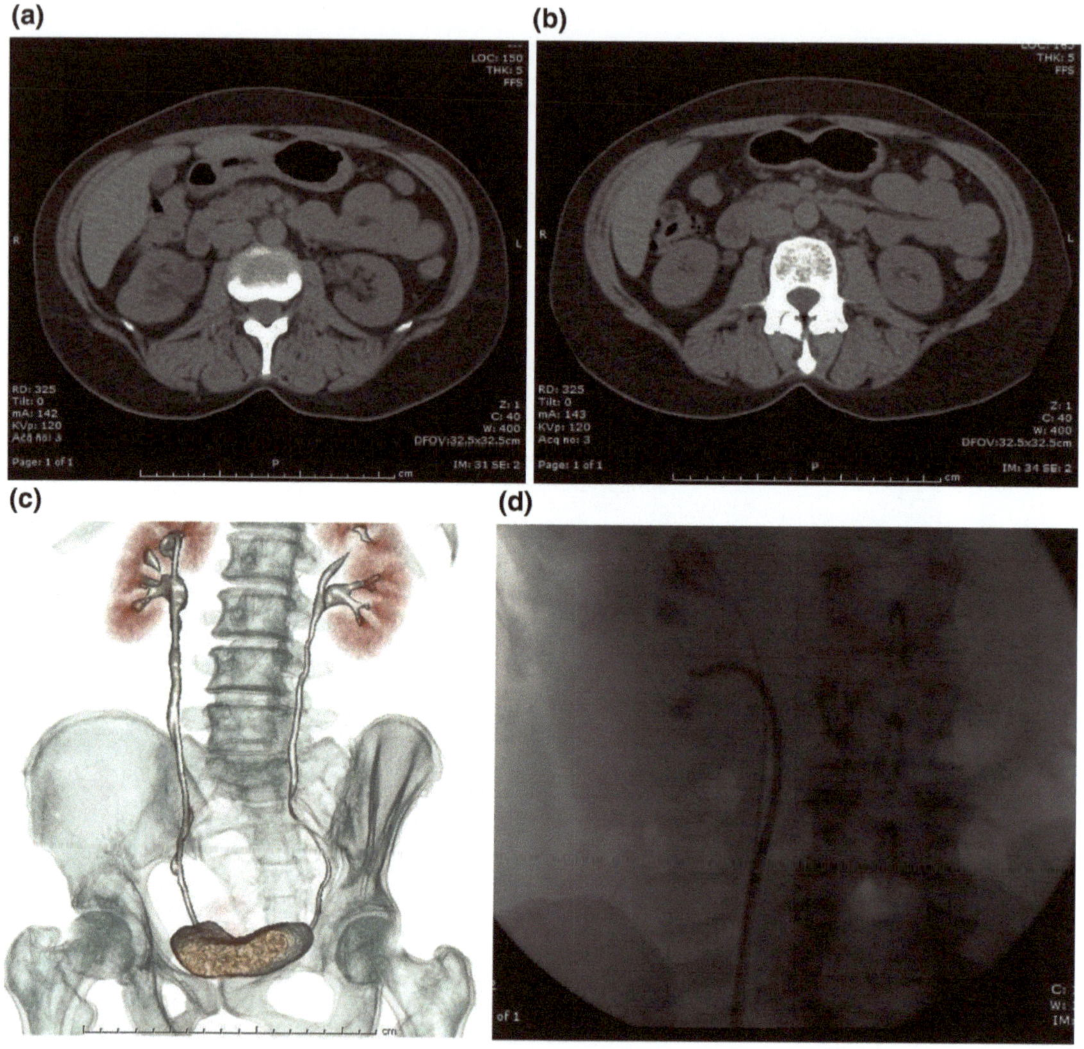

Fig. C.19 **a** Cross-sectional CT image of the UPJ area shows thickening of the wall; **b** additional section lower down shows thickening of the upper ureteral wall without any intraluminal filling defect; **c** CT urogram reconstruction of the collecting system showing irregularity and thickening of RT upper ureter and renal pelvis without any intraluminal filling defect. There is an indwelling double pigtail stent in place; **d** ureteroscopic DEEP biopsy renal pelvis; **e** ureteroscopic renal pelvis biopsy showing high-grade urothelial carcinoma; **f** low-power section of nephroureterectomy specimen showing high-grade disease; **g** high-power view shows high-grade urothelial carcinoma

A retrograde pyelogram and ureteroscopy after 6 months showed no evidence of recurrence with negative urine cytology.

She developed another colon cancer a year later requiring resection and was in coma in ICU setting for a month before complete recovery.

Three years after her original renal tumor resection she slowly developed deterioration of renal function without evidence of any recurrence (Fig. C.20).

Comment

This is a perfect example of an ***absolute imperative case***, due to multiple comorbidities and

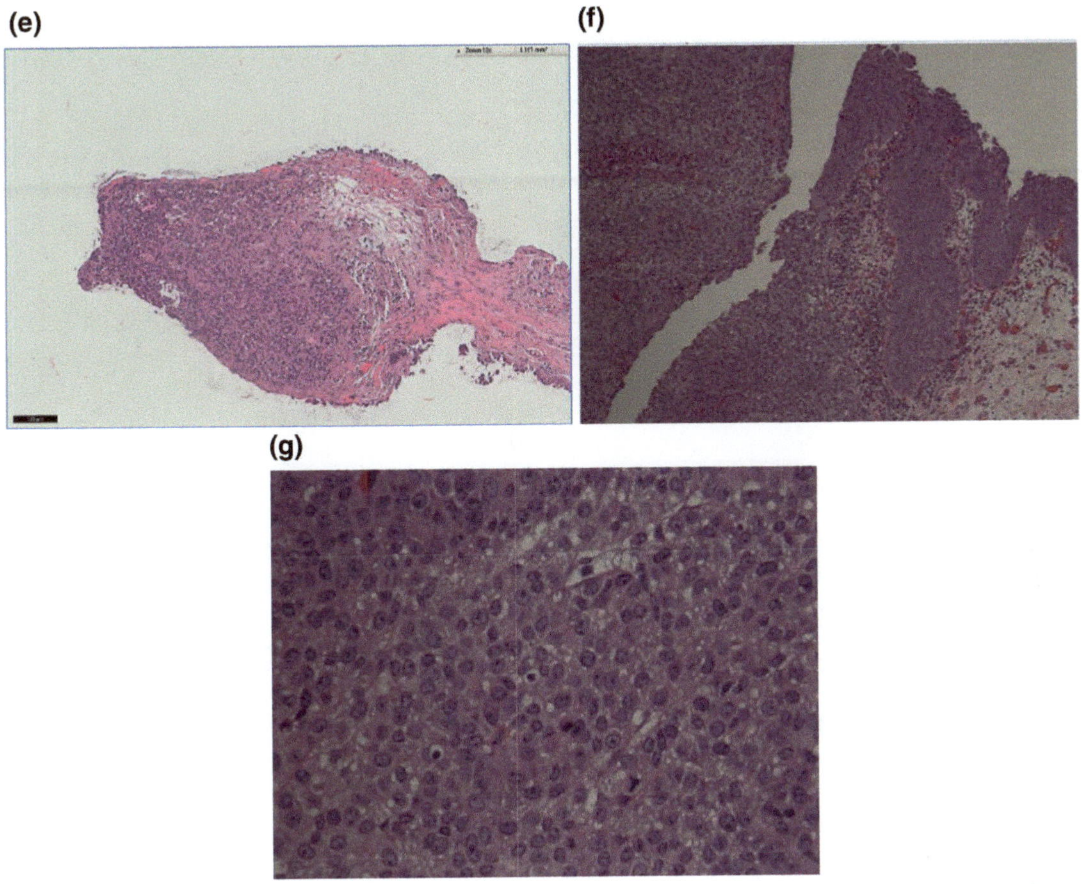

Fig. C.19 (continued)

strong history of several malignancies, with an excellent outcome. Patient and family's compliance with follow-up protocol played an important role towards this outcome.

Case Study 9

This patient is a 69-year-old male with history of colorectal cancer one and half years ago who was found to have a filling defect in the upper pole of the left kidney on subsequent imaging. The patient underwent chemotherapy for colon cancer and on interval imaging the filling defect was not seen on CT images. The patient was quite frail with multiple comorbidities and slight elevation of creatinine. Due to possibility of cancer recurrence, patient and his oncologist were concerned about renal function in case he would need further chemotherapy. Approximately a year later, during follow-up imaging he was found to have recurrence of the filling defect and he underwent left ureteroscopy and biopsy which was not quite adequate but suggesting low-grade urothelial carcinoma.

We evaluated patient at this time and he underwent ureteroscopy of the left kidney for repeat biopsy. Tumor was present and located in a highly superior calyx which was bulky making ureteroscopic management inadequate. Pathology at that time was consistent with low-grade urothelial carcinoma. Patient then underwent a percutaneous nephroscopic complete resection of the upper calyceal tumor. Percutaneous access was obtained by urology into the upper pole calyx allowing us to perform complete resection

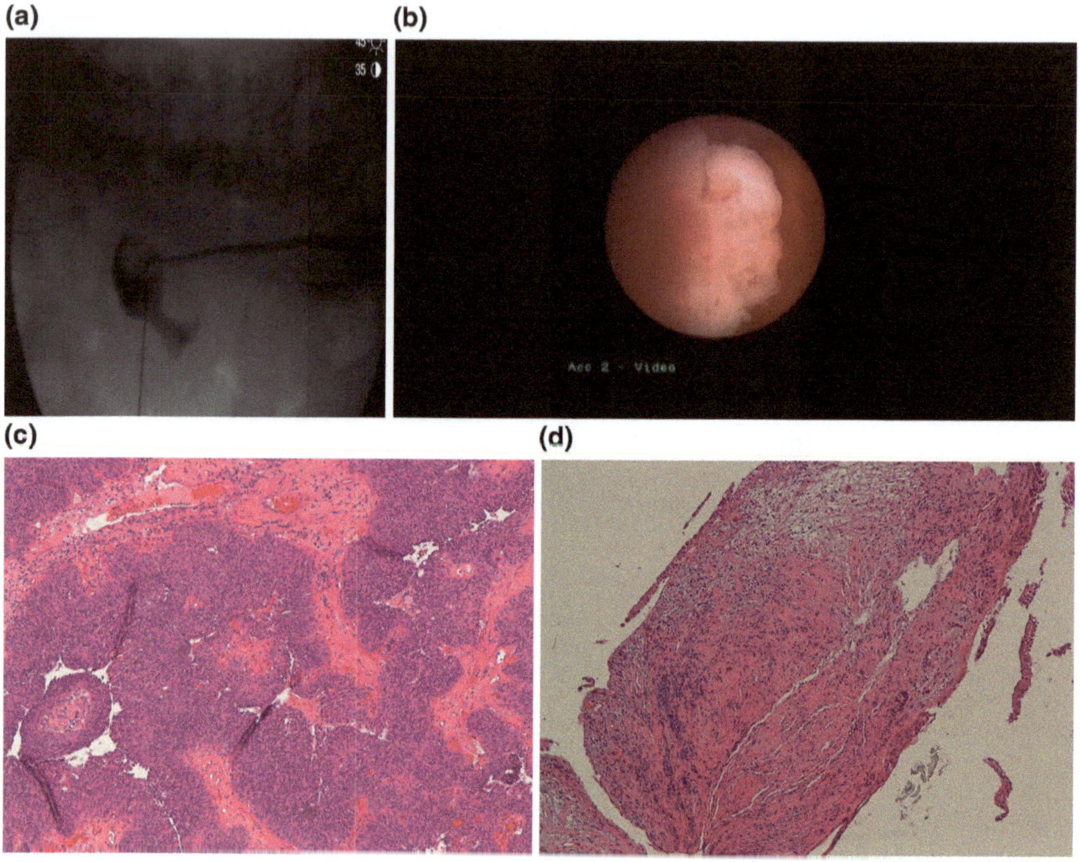

Fig. C.20 **a** A retrograde pyelogram at the time percutaneous resection. Note the large filling defect in the renal pelvis; **b** endoscopic view of renal pelvis tumor showing a large papillary tumor; **c** low-power view of tumor described as low-grade papillary carcinoma; **d** follow-up biopsy of renal pelvis after resection and mitamycin C intracavitary treatment shows no obvious recurrence; **e** retrograde pyelogram 6 months later; **f** radiographic and endoscopic images of ureteroscopy after six months showed no residual or recurrence

and ablation of all tumor burden within the calyx using a urethroresectoscope. Pathology from this procedure with complete resection revealed high-grade urothelial carcinoma.

As a result of the upstaging of the disease, treatment options were discussed including Left nephroureterectomy, which the patient refused due to fear of impaired renal function. Additional treatment options were discussed at this time and patient agreed to intracavitary instillation of mitomycin C through a nephrostomy tube.

Surveillance nephroscopy revealed no new areas of tumor recurrence in the left calyx, renal pelvis, and proximal ureter. With thorough inspection of the left upper pole calyx, sites of prior resection showed fibrosis and sloughing of tissue. Multiple biopsies were taken of these areas which showed urothelial denudation, submucosal fibrosis, fat necrosis and no evidence of malignancy. A nephrostomy was placed and patient underwent maintenance instillation of mitomycin C before the removal of nephrostomy. Patient undergoes imaging, cytology, and endoscopic surveillance (Figs. C.21, C.22, C.23, C.24 and C.25).

Comment

This case illustrates bulky lesion in the calyceal area, which cannot be adequately managed in a retrograde fashion. Additionally, the percutaneous resection

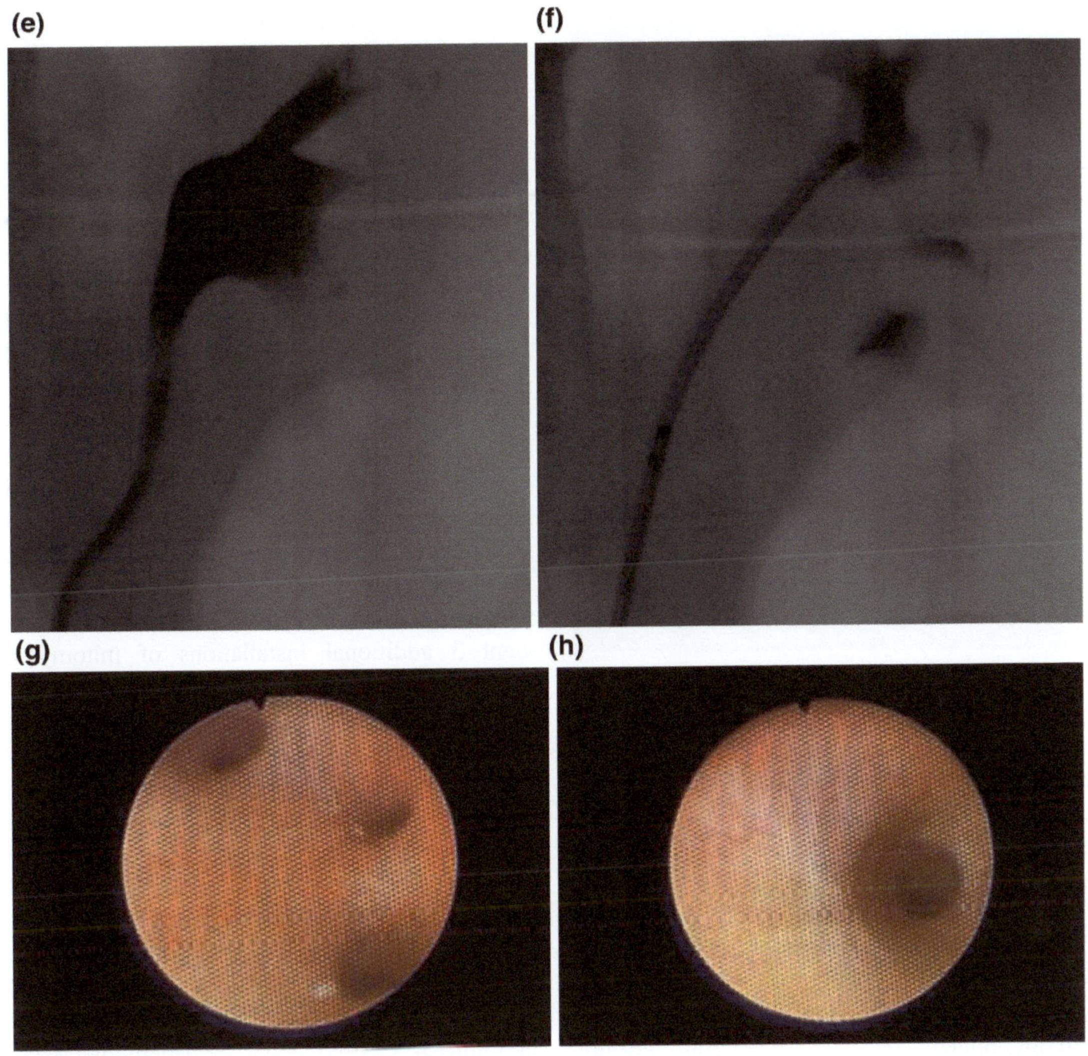

Fig. C.20 (continued)

showed upstaging to high-grade disease indicating inadequacy of retrograde tumor management in some cases. We recommend percutaneous resection for all bulky renal pelvis and large deep calyceal tumor to avoid understaging. A 19–22 Fr slender urethroresectoscope is ideal for such resections.

Case Study 10

This patient is an 81-year-old diabetic male patient with an initial diagnosis of transitional cell carcinoma of the bladder with concomitant carcinoma in situ in 2001. At that time, the patient was treated with a transurethral resection of the tumor burden followed by intravesical BCG and interferon for 6 weeks. After completion of the induction course, the patient was maintained on maintenance BCG, with completion in 2003. The patient was then monitored with surveillance cystoscopy and imaging. In 2006, the patient demonstrated a distal right ureteral tumor and underwent a distal ureterectomy with pathologic diagnosis of high-grade T1 transitional cell carcinoma. He remained disease free until 2009 when he developed recurrence of

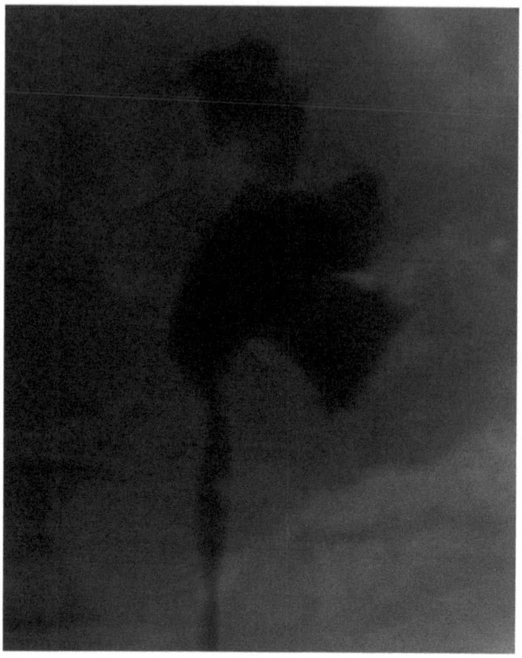

Fig. C.21 Left retrograde pyelogram showing upper calyx filling defect

bladder CIS and underwent an additional 6-week course of BCG. Subsequent to this, the patient experienced continued hematuria and persistently positive urine FISH.

In 2010, an interval surveillance CT urogram revealed a subtle left upper pole lesion, which was not present in an MR urogram earlier that same year. Consequently, the patient underwent a cystoscopy, bilateral retrograde pyelogram, left ureteroscopy, and biopsy of the left upper pole lesion. Intraoperatively, the patient was found to have a normal bladder mucosa, normal retrograde pyelography of the collecting systems bilaterally, except for a questionable lesion within the left upper pole calyx, from which biopsy was taken, and selective cytology was also obtained. Cytology and pathologic analysis confirmed urothelial cells consistent with transitional cell carcinoma. Given the location and volume of the lesion, the patient underwent percutaneous resection of the calyceal lesion using a 24 FR urethroresctoscope as per his choice. The lesion was resected deeply and into the neck of the calyceal infundibulum and a nephrostomy tube was placed for installation of mitomycin. The patient refused a nephroureterectomy. He underwent a 6-week course of intracavitary treatment using mitomycin. Follow-up surveillance endoscopy using a 12 French mini nephroscope revealed no additional lesions and several deep biopsies of the previous tumor bed were performed, which showed fibrotic tissue without evidence of disease. The patient underwent 3 additional installations of mitomycin before the nephrostomy was removed.

Given the extensive comorbidity index of this patient including hypertension, diabetes, morbid obesity, coronary artery disease necessitating coronary stenting, as well as a 2011 diagnosis of Gleason 6 adenocarcinoma of the prostate, treated with radiation therapy; when a surveillance MRI revealed a suspicious left upper pole lesion, a percutaneous renal biopsy was performed revealing high-grade infiltrating transitional cell carcinoma in a milieu of chronic inflammation and fibrosis. Consequently, the patient underwent laparascopic nephroureterectomy. Pathologically, the specimen was high-grade transitional cell carcinoma with infiltration to the renal medulla and cortex, involving the upper part of the right

(a) (b)

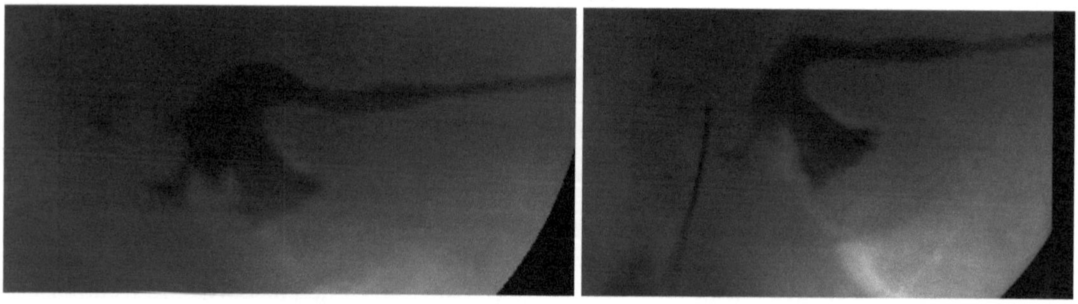

Fig. C.22 **a**, **b** percutaneous nephrostomy performed to gain access to *left upper* pole calyx for tumor resection

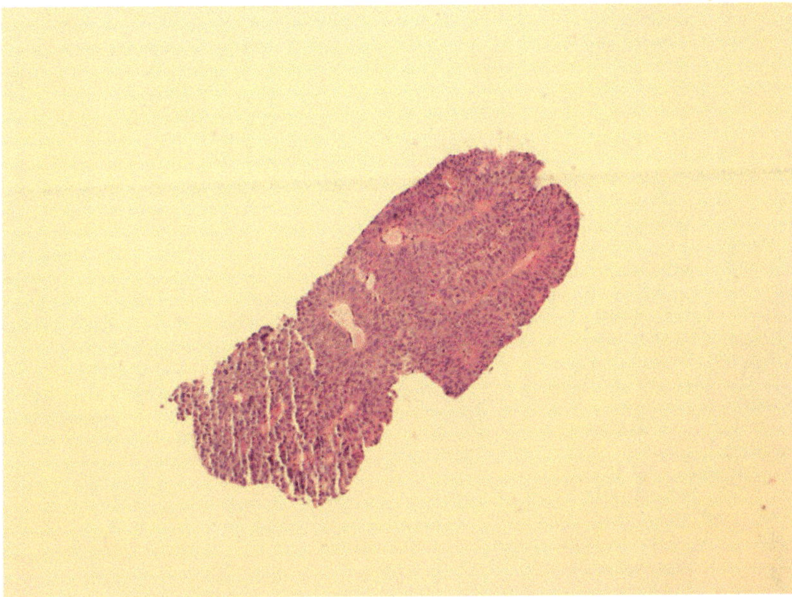

Fig. C.23 Left kidney upper calyx biopsy showing low-grade papillary urothelial carcinoma

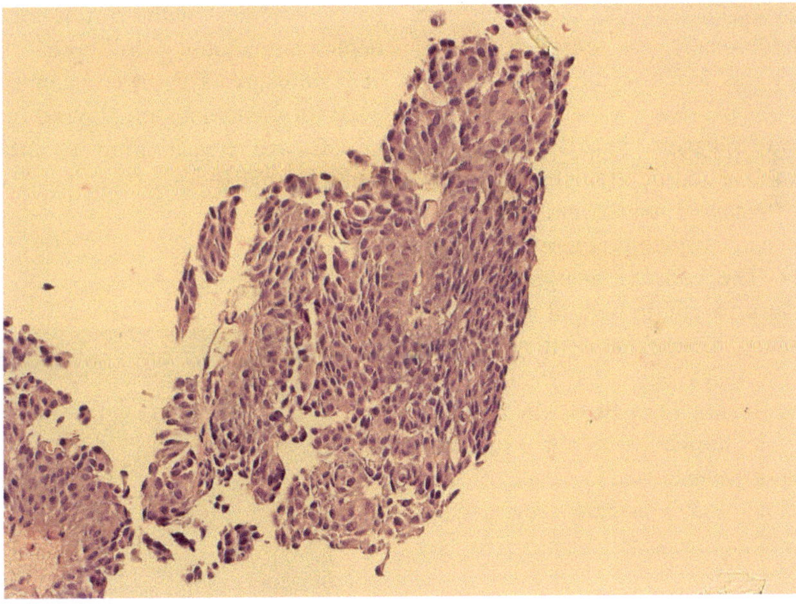

Fig. C.24 Left percutaneous renal calyx biopsy showing high-grade urothelial carcinoma

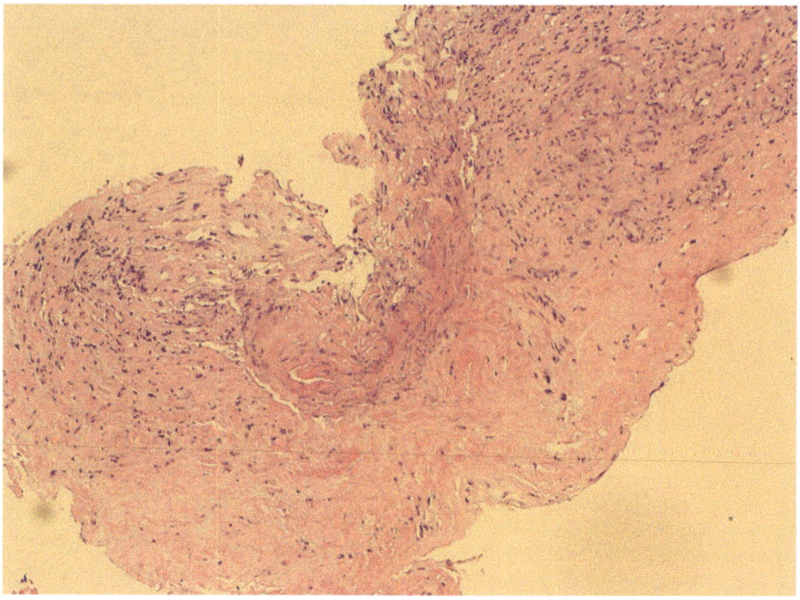

Fig. C.25 Left kidney previous tumor site biopsy showing urothelial denudation with submucosal fibrosis and fat necrosis, no evidence of malignancy

kidney, but sparing the renal capsule, pelvis, and sinus fat. Additionally, a small focus of high-grade CIS was found at the ureterovesical junction.

At the time of diagnosis in 2012, MRI confirmed 1.5 cm para-aortic lymphadenopathy; hence, the patient underwent adjuvant chemotherapy and maintains close follow-up with oncology. The patient undergoes regular surveillance MR urogram, in light of a diagnosis of chronic kidney disease, as well as regular surveillance cystoscopy and urine cytology. At the present time, he has a low PSA, MR urogram and PET CT are normal, with no suspicious lesions or filling defects and absence of any lymphadenopathy, and a negative cystoscopy (Figs. C.26, C.27, C.28, C.29, C.30, C.31 and C.32).

Comment

This cases illustrates: initial conservative treatment as per patient's resistance due to multiple co morbidities with recurrence necessitating nephrouretrectomy followed by adjuvant chemotherapy. This case again emphasizes the need for continuous monitoring of patients with UTUC and transitioning to other modalities when one fails.

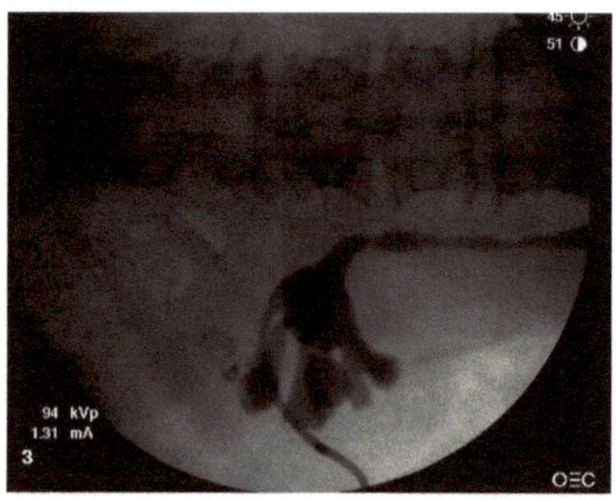

Fig. C.26 2010 antegrade nephrostogram intraoperatively demonstrating *left upper* pole filling defect consistent with calyceal mass. This finding was treated endoscopically

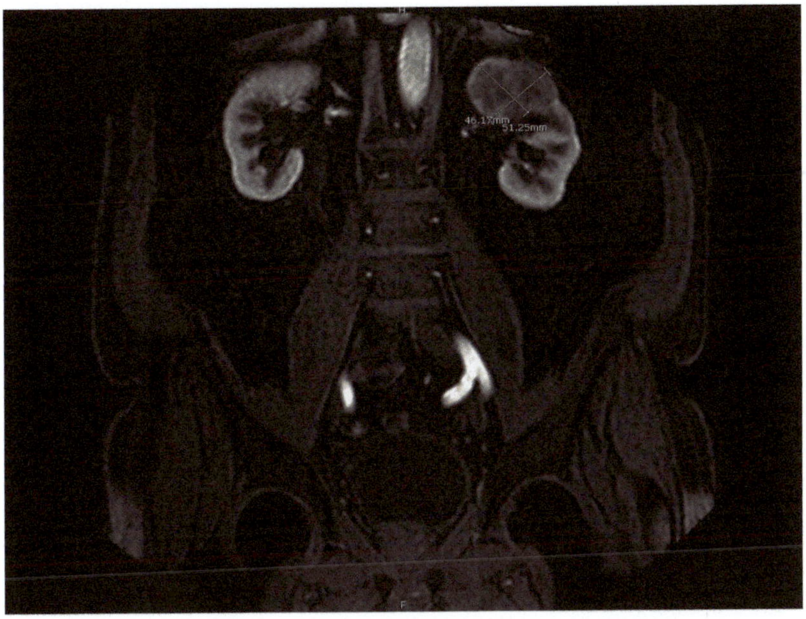

Fig. C.27 2012 MRI of the abdomen and pelvis demonstrating *left upper* pole heterogeneous, enhancing mass measuring 4.6 × 5.1 × 4.6 cm. This mass was treated with nephroureterectomy and neoadjuvant chemotherapy due to hilhar lymphadenopathy

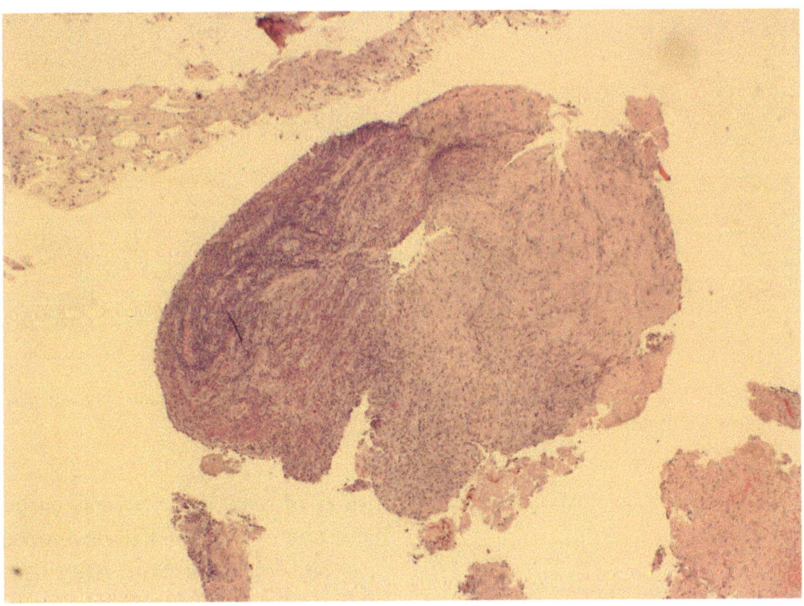

Fig. C.28 Pathology slide from 2011 ureteroscopic biopsy of *left upper* pole calyx consistent with fibro-connective and granulation tissue with focal areas of necrosis

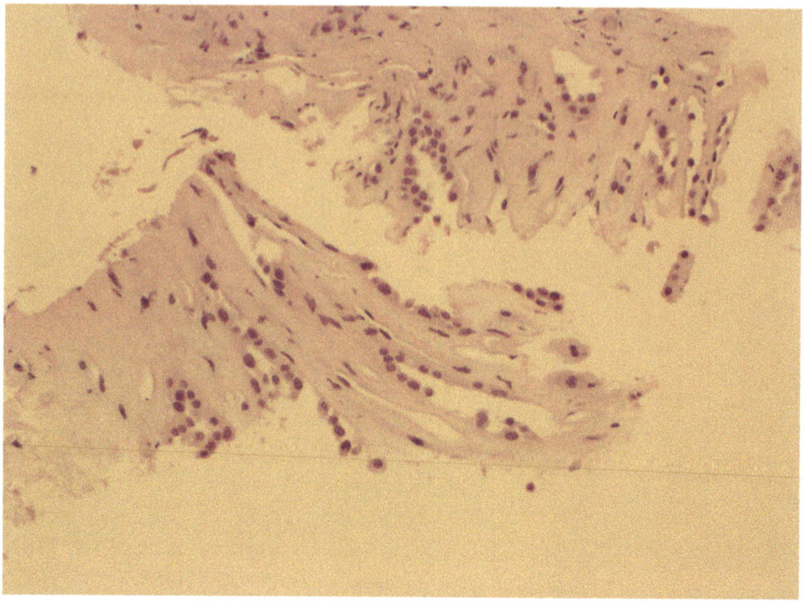

Fig. C.29 Pathology slide from 2011 ureteroscopic biopsy of *left upper* poly calyx demonstrated scattered atypical cells, suspicious for urothelial neoplasm but not fully characterized

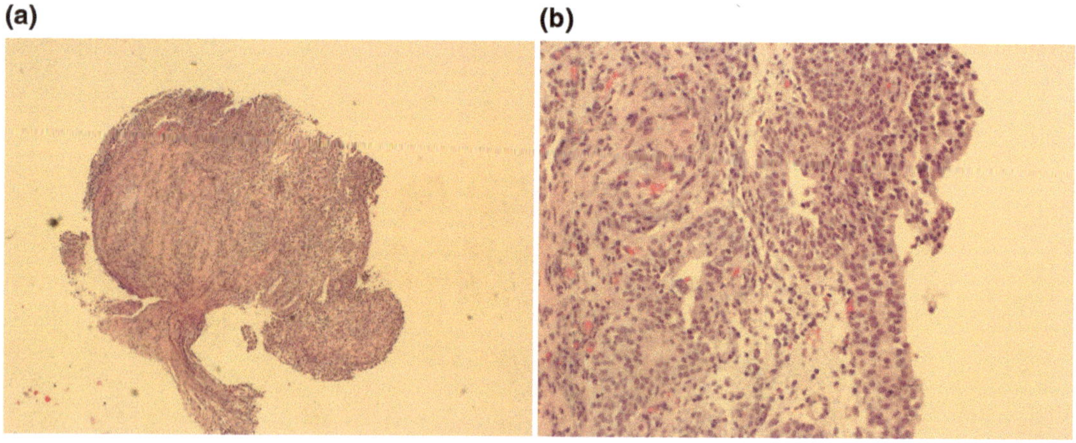

Fig. C.30 **a**, **b** Pathologic slide from repeat 2011 ureteroscopic biopsy of left upper pole calyceal mass demonstrating urothelium with dysplasia in a milieu of chronic inflammation

Case Study 11

A 50-year-old female with strong history of smoking developed gross hematuria and several bladder tumors were resected endoscopically. Her past medical history included a Rt pyeloplasty, that had failed and was successfully managed with ureteroscopic cold knife endopyelotomy, history of renal stone 5 years earlier. In between these two events she had developed gross hematuria and left flank pain. After ureteroscopy and biopsy revealed high-grade left ureteral tumor she underwent Lt radical nephroureterectomy.

During her followup after the bladder tumor resection her urine cytology was intermittently positive or showed atypical cells in spite of negative imaging studies and thorough RT

(a) (b)

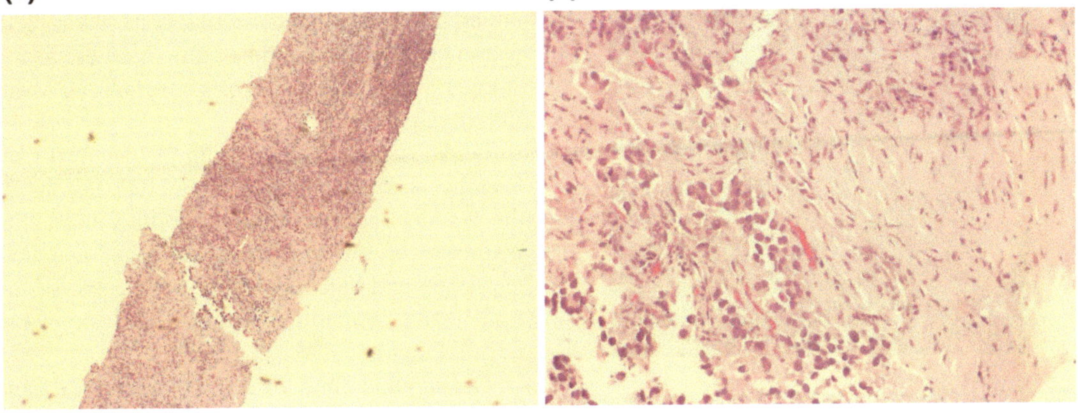

Fig. C.31 **a**, **b** 2012 CT scan guided renal biopsy of *left upper* pole mass consistent with infiltrative high-grade urothelial carcinomas

(a) (b)

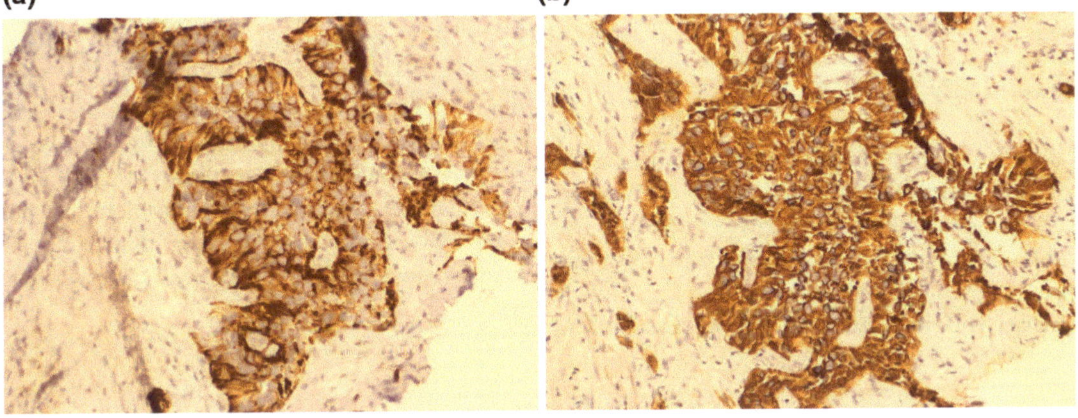

Fig. C.32 **a**, **b** Pathology slides from 2012 renal biopsy preparation demonstrating positivity for CD20 (**a**, *left*) and Cytokeratin AE1 (**b**, *right*)

ureterorpyeloscopy. She underwent random biopsies of ureter and renal pelvis that were also negative. Approximately two years later, she developed visible mucosal lesions in the upper calyces that were managed endoscopically. Because of positive cytology. She underwent placement of a nephrostomy resection of recurrent tumor and intracavitary treatment with mitomycin C and BCG. After approximately one year she had a small lesion in the collecting system with suspicious cytology. She refused the recommendation of nephroureterectomy.

After placement of a small pigtail nephrostomy tube, she underwent a course of intracavitary treatment using gemcitabine with remission.

She succumbed to cardiopulmonary complications secondary to her strong history of smoking. Two years later, there was no evidence of active urothelial carcinoma at the time of her death (Figs. C.33, C.34, C.35, C.36 and C.37).

Comment

This case depicts a continuum of urothelial carcinoma metachronously affecting all different segments of the urinary tract and the need for vigilant follow-up of these patients. In 2010 she had intracavitary salvage treatment with gemcitabine. It was also the first case to our

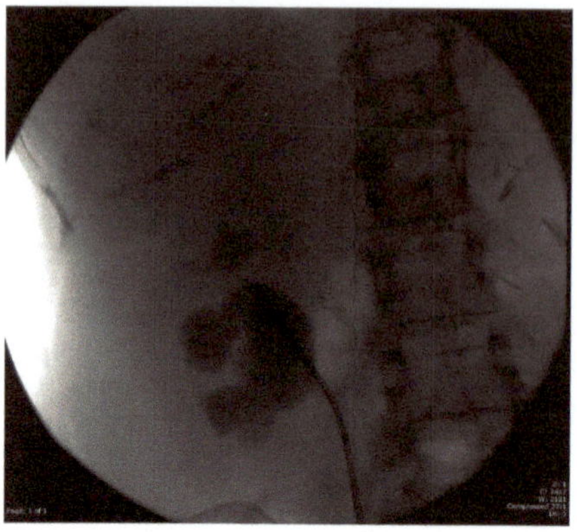

Fig. C.33 Ureteroscopic biopsy of renal lesion showing urothelial carcinoma

knowledge where salvage intracavitary gemcitabine treatment was successfully used.

Case Study 12

Patient is a 65-year-old female with history of gross hematuria presenting originally in 2009. Workup at that time including a CT showed fullness of the right collecting system with trace enhancement and filling defect of the proximal ureter. Patient underwent rigid ureteroresctoscopic resection of low-grade urothelial lesion of the proximal right ureter. The rest of the collecting system was clear of tumor. She has multiple comorbidities: heavy smoker, multiple sclerosis, achalasia, and fibromyalgia.

On subsequent follow-up in 2010 repeat cystoscopy showed papillary frond like lesions in the bladder (consistent with papillary urothelial neoplasm of low malignant potential) and ureteroscopy and barbotage were performed for the right ureter, which demonstrated no lesions and negative cytology.

During this time patient continued to have stable findings in the bladder with no recurrence of disease seen in the right collecting system. In 2012, when right-sided ureteroscopy was performed it revealed tumor in the upper and lower pole calyx, after biopsies were taken laser ablation was performed. Pathology revealed low-grade papillary urothelial carcinoma. Random bladder biopsies performed at that time were negative for malignancy. After placement of a percutaneous nephrostomy Mitomycin C was instilled in an antegrade fashion into the right collecting system draining down into the bladder treating both upper and lower urinary tract.

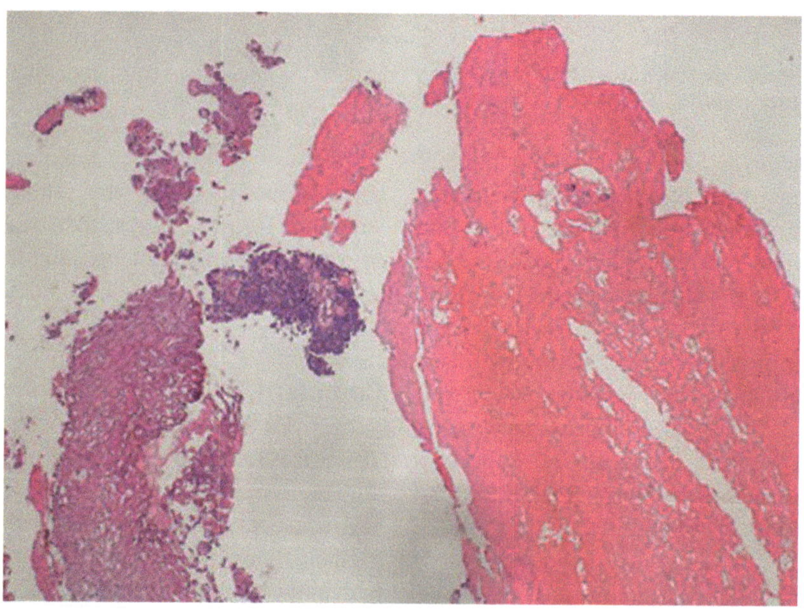

Fig. C.34 Whole mount of the biopsy sample showing urothelial carcinoma

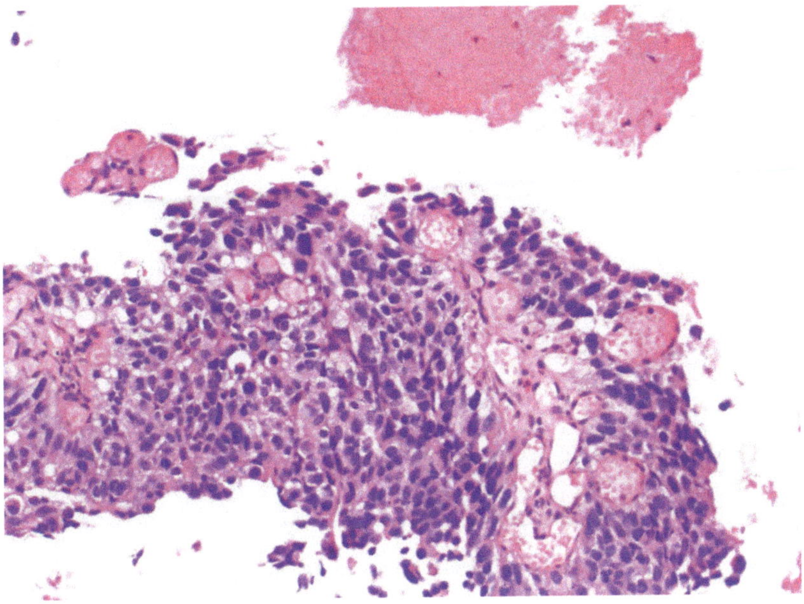

Fig. C.35 High-power view of biopsy which shows superficial papillary carcinoma

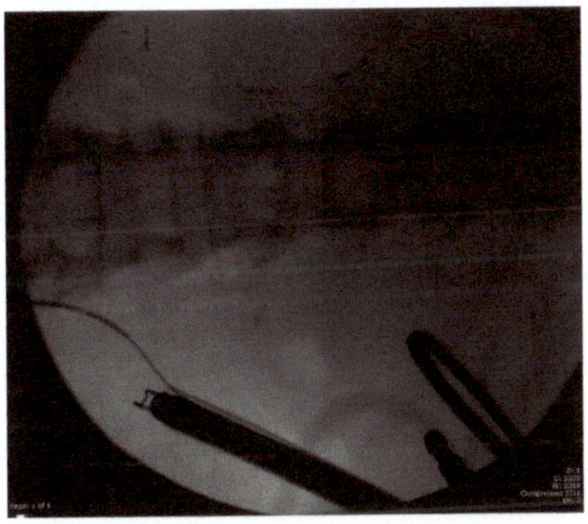

Fig. C.36 Percutaneous resection of tumor

Since 2013–2017, patient has been managed with surveillance protocol consisting of urine cytology and imaging every 6 months. Patient has undergone multiple repeat cystoscopies in the office with plan for biopsy and investigation of the upper tracts when tumor has been seen. Multiple ureteroscopies and bladder biopsies at various times each year have periodically revealed bladder tumors that have been consistent with papillary urothelial neoplasm of low malignant potential. She has had good control of

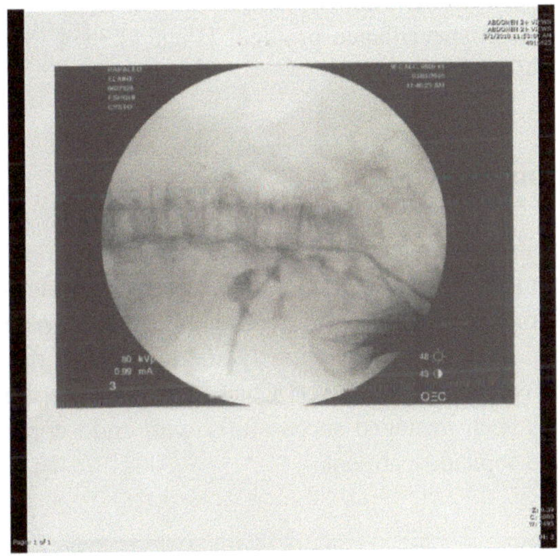

Fig. C.37 Nephrostogram after tumor resection

her disease with no progression. The patient was offered nephroureterectomy several times which she refused.

On recent evaluation there was evidence of recurrence in the right collecting system which was biopsied and ablated using a combination of holmium and neodymium YAG laser. Pathology

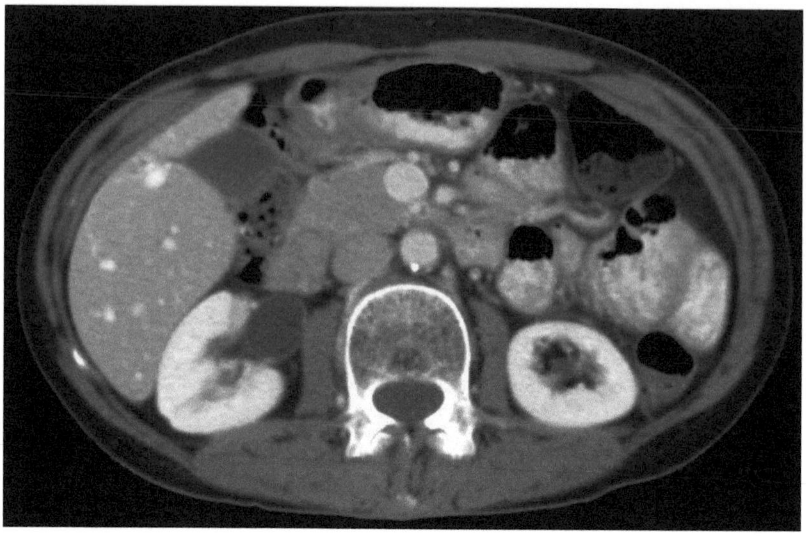

Fig. C.38 CT showing fullness of right proximal ureter with wall enhancement

revealed papillary urothelial carcinoma. She completed a course of antegrade intracavitary BCG treatment and is clear of active disease or CIS on surveillance protocol (Figs. C.38, C.39, C.40 and C.41).

Comment

This case illustrates a frail patient with multiple comorbidities with recurrence of tumor in bladder and progression from PUNLMP to low grade and areas of CIS. Obviously she has a high risk of recurrence, but over a period of 9 years she has been managed successfully with endoscopic and topical treatment.

Case Study 13

A 72-year-old male patient with history of neurogenic bladder on clean intermittent catheterization and poorly functioning left kidney was managed with TURBT and BCG immunotherapy after he developed bladder cancer. During follow-up, bladder evaluations were negative and right upper tract cytology was positive. We evaluated the patient for upper tract workup and treatment. Random biopsies were negative. After percutaneous nephrostomy for deep biopsy of pelvis which was negative, urine showed positive cytologies. He underwent antegrade intracavitary BCG immunotherapy with the presumptive diagnosis of upper tract CIS. Post treatment, several urine cytology samples from nephrostomy and bladder were negative. This patient is being monitored closely with endoscopy, imaging and urinary cytologies (Figs. C.42 and C.43).

Comment

This case illustrates the fact that in absence of bladder pathology a positive urine cytology with no visible tumor most probably reflects upper tract CIS. Before initiating intracavitary chemo- or immunotherapy of upper tract, one must perform a thorough investigation of the bladder and the contralateral kidney to exclude them as the source for positive cytology. Conversion of nephrostomy urine cytology from positive to negative is considered a positive response to intracavitary immunotherapy with BCG.

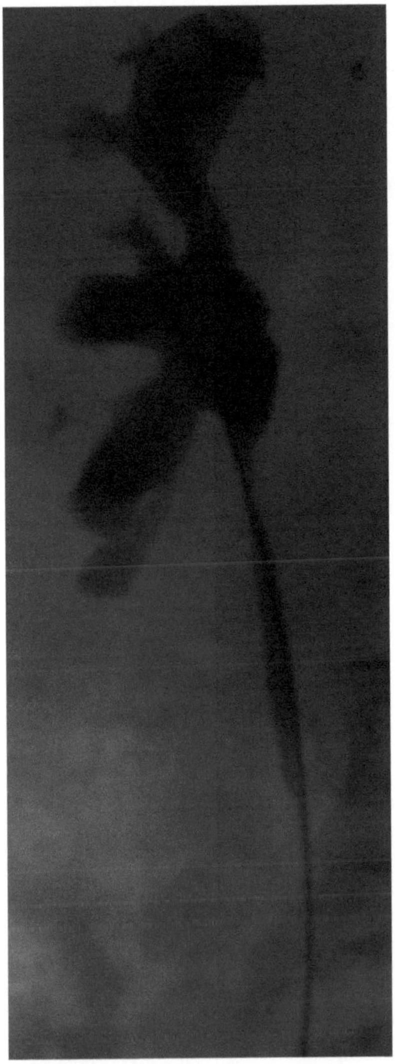

Fig. C.39 Right retrograde pyelogram showing lower pole filling defect

Case Study 14

A 69-year-old male who had donated his left kidney to his brother 14 years earlier was diagnosed with NMI bladder cancer 7 years ago. After transurethral resection of the tumor he underwent intravesical BCG immunotherapy. Over a period of 3 years he had two courses of BCG treatment with maintenance. Four years ago his urinary cytology became positive. Cystoscopy bladder biopsies, retrograde pyelogram and ureteroscopy were all negative. Selective cytology of right collecting system was suspicious. We evaluated this patient for assessment of possible urothelial carcinoma or CIS of his right solitary kidney. Biopsies of ureter and collecting system did not reveal any obvious pathology. With the assumption of positive cytology in absence of bladder pathology suggesting CIS of upper tract he underwent percutaneous intracavitary topical treatment following which nephrostomy and voided urine cytologies were negative or atypical over a period of two months and nephrostomy tube was removed. Follow-up urine cytology was strongly positive with grossly negative CT scan. At the time of cystoscopy a slight mucosal irregularity was noted at the site of left ureteral orifice, a retrograde pyelogram and ureteroscopy showed bulky intraluminal urothelial carcinoma. Distal ureterectomy with excision of bladder cuff was carried out with evidence high grade invasive urothelial carcinoma with periureteral disease. He underwent adjuvant chemotherapy. The patient's brother was under the care of a nephrologist who was informed to have the patient go through diagnostic workup or a nephrectomy since the transplanted kidney had failed by then and he was on hemodialysis (Figs. C.44, C.45, C.46 and C.47). Figs. C.48 and C.49 are examples of transplant kidney.

Comment

This case illustrates the significance of complete nephroureterectomy in patients with upper tract urothelial carcinoma. Obviously donor nephrectomy screening rules out pre-existing malignancies and the nephrectomy is a considered a benign procedure and the distal ureter is never removed. The critical point in this type of case is periodic assessment of the ureteral stump when urothelial malignancies have developed later either in the donor or recipient.

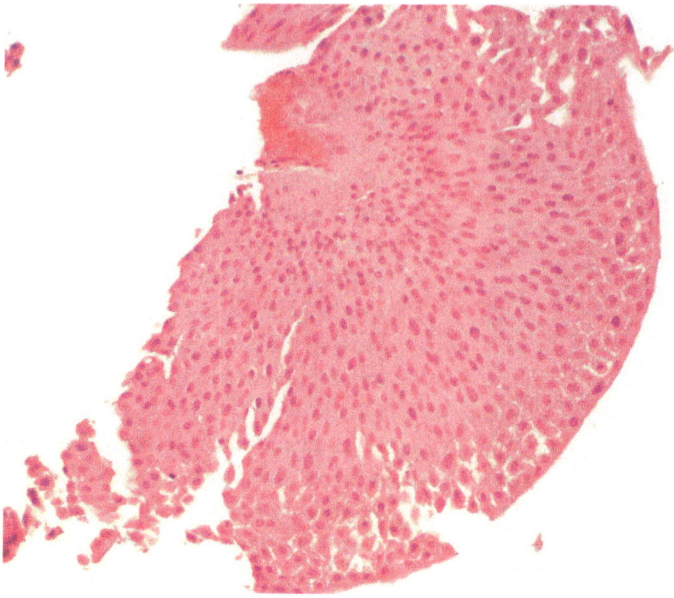

Fig. C.40 Bladder biopsy showing papillary urothelial neoplasm of low malignant potential

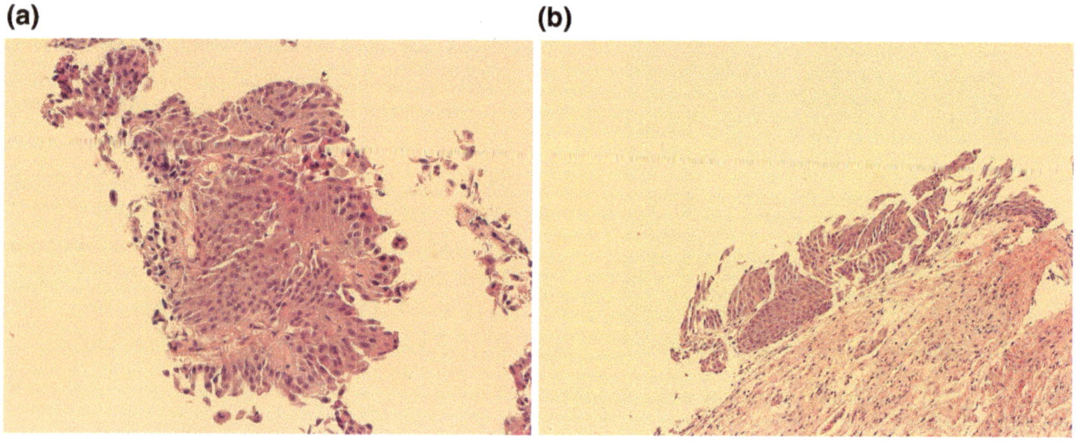

Fig. C.41 **a** Right calyx biopsy showing low-grade papillary urothelial neoplasm; **b** bladder biopsy showing low-grade papillary urothelial carcinoma

Case Study 15

The patient is a 42-year-old female with a history of smoking, diagnosed with multiple bilateral large cystine stones secondary to congenital cystinuria at the time of diagnosis in 2013. She had been experiencing several months of constitutional symptoms, flank pain, and a thirty-pound unexplained weight loss. This was the very first time that she was diagnosed with renal stones and had no prior history of any intervention or medical treatment. The patient was also found to have an exophytic, contrast enhancing right upper pole mass on CT. Renal biopsy confirmed pathologic diagnosis of high-grade urothelial carcinoma. Preoperative renal scan revealed equal differential function

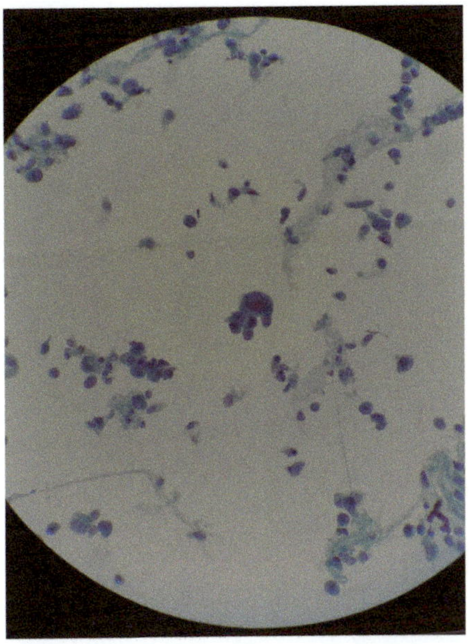

Fig. C.42 Urine cytology from the right kidney showing malignant cell

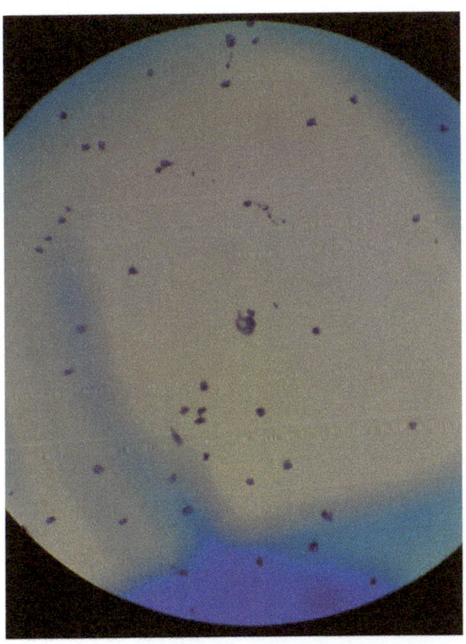

Fig. C.43 Urine cytology prepped slide from the right kidney after antegrade intracavitary BCG treatment showing no malignant cells

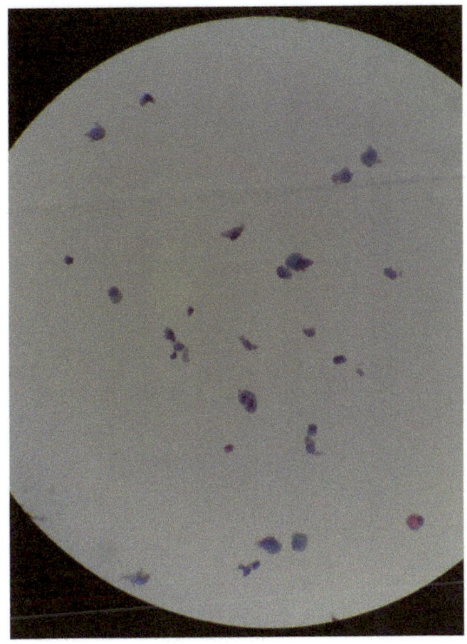

Fig. C.44 Urine cytology showing malignant cells

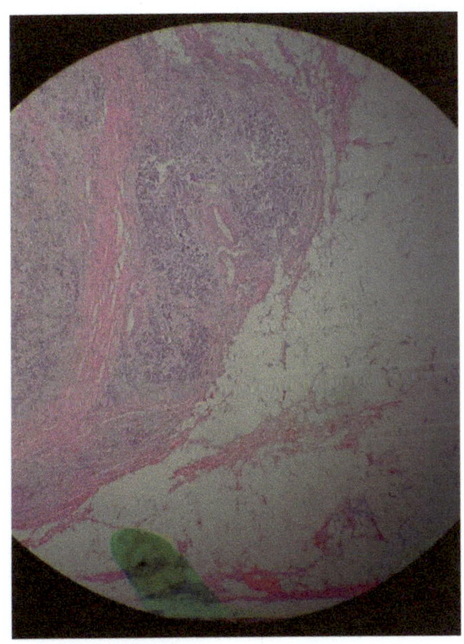

Fig. C.45 Low-power view of distal ureteral stump showing high-grade invasive urothelial carcinoma

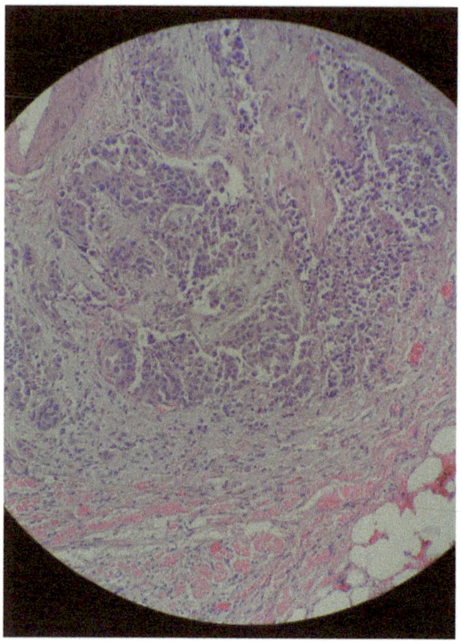

Fig. C.46 High-power view shows high-grade invasive urothelial carcinoma

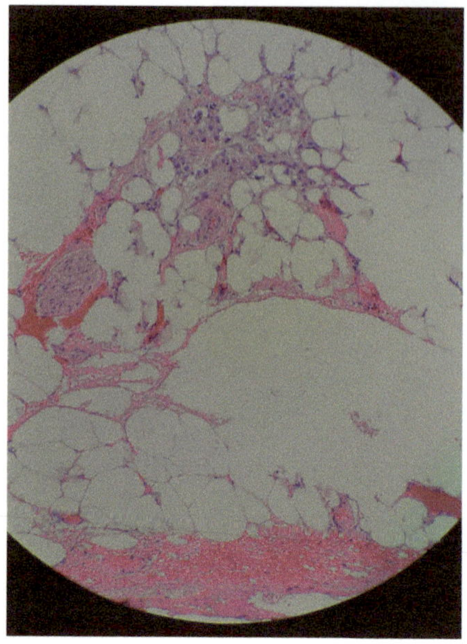

Fig. C.47 Para ureteral tissue shows clusters of high-grade urothelial carcinoma

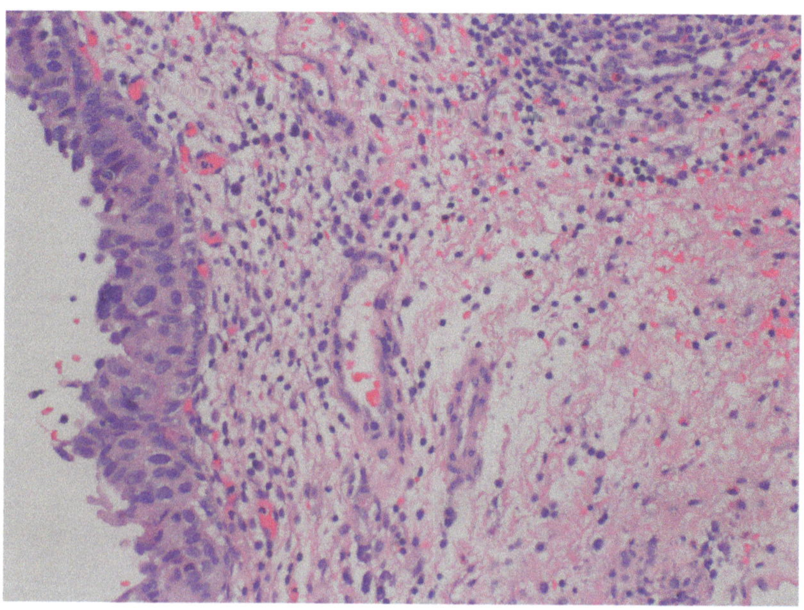

Fig. C.48 Section of a transplant ureter shows high-grade urothelial in situ carcinoma

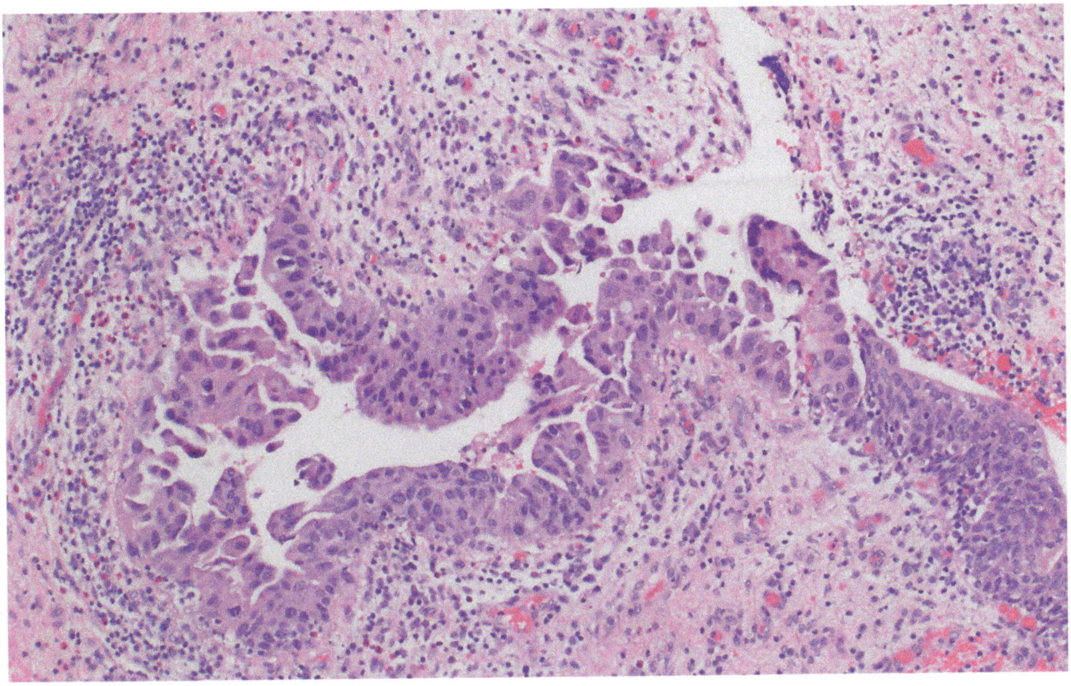

Fig. C.49 Section through the transplant renal pelvis in the same patient shows similar findings

and serum creatinine was 1.1 at baseline. Given the aggressive nature of the disease, the patient underwent a right nephroureterectomy and right retroperitoneal lymph node dissection. The specimen was 7 cm, with negative margins pathologically consistent with biopsy and five of the six nodes were negative for metastasis with the remaining node positive for urothelial carcinoma; staging the patient as T2N2.

Post nephrectomy, given the abundant stone burden, the patient underwent multiple left percutaneous nephrolithotomies and ureteroscopic procedures. She was also managed medically to defray additional stone formation. On routine surveillance MRI, the patient was found to have a mass in the nephrectomy bed, measuring 3.4 × 3.6 × 3.5 cm and adjacent lesion in the liver. The patient underwent extensive laparoscopic lysis of adhesions, resection of the retroperitoneal mass, partial hepatectomy, and partial omentectomy. The boundaries of disease were marked by metallic clips. Pathologic analysis revealed recurrence of high-grade urothelial carcinoma with metastasis of the omentum and extensive necrosis of the liver parenchyma. The patient underwent adjuvant chemotherapy and radiation to the marked area. She tolerated both interventions well, undergoes regular surveillance CT and /MRI and PET scans and urine cytology.

The stone burden continues to be significant; therefore, she periodically requires ureteroscopy, stone removal or laser lithotripsy, and stent exchange. Recent surveillance CT shows mild hydronephrosis with stable nephrocalcinosis, and no evidence of soft tissue mass or lymphadenopathy. The patient impressively maintains completely normal functional status and her current creatinine is 1.60 (Figs. C.50, C.51, C.52, C.53, C.54, C.55, C.56, C.57, C.58, C.59, C.60 and C.61).

Comment

This case illustrates a multidisciplinary approach of nephroureterectomy, lymph node dissection, resection of recurrent mass at the tumor bed, liver, and omentum. This was followed by adjuvant chemotherapy and radiation to the site of the recurrence identified by metal clips. Most of the modalities described in this book have been used in management of this patient reflecting transitioning through several phases of treatment. This young patient elected to undergo an aggressive approach and has been free of obvious recurrence for 5 years.

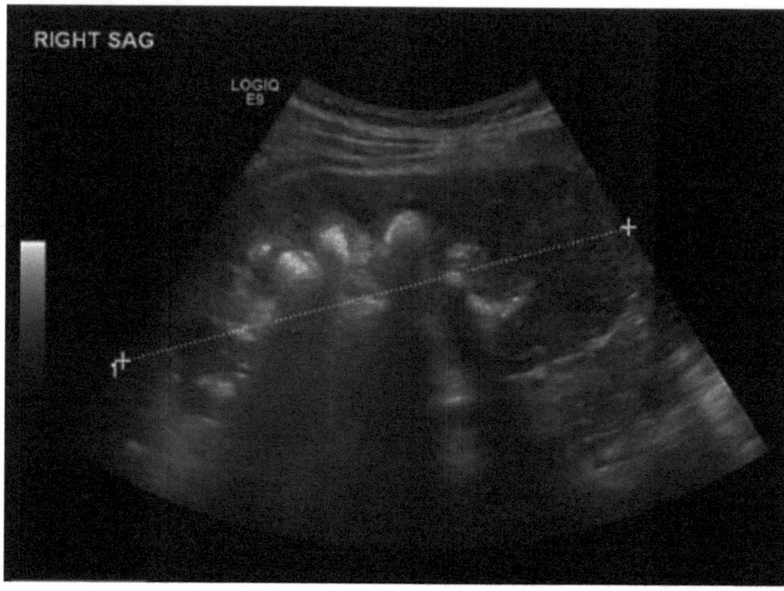

Fig. C.50 2013 renal ultrasound of left kidney demonstrating large staghorn calculi obscuring the renal pelvis

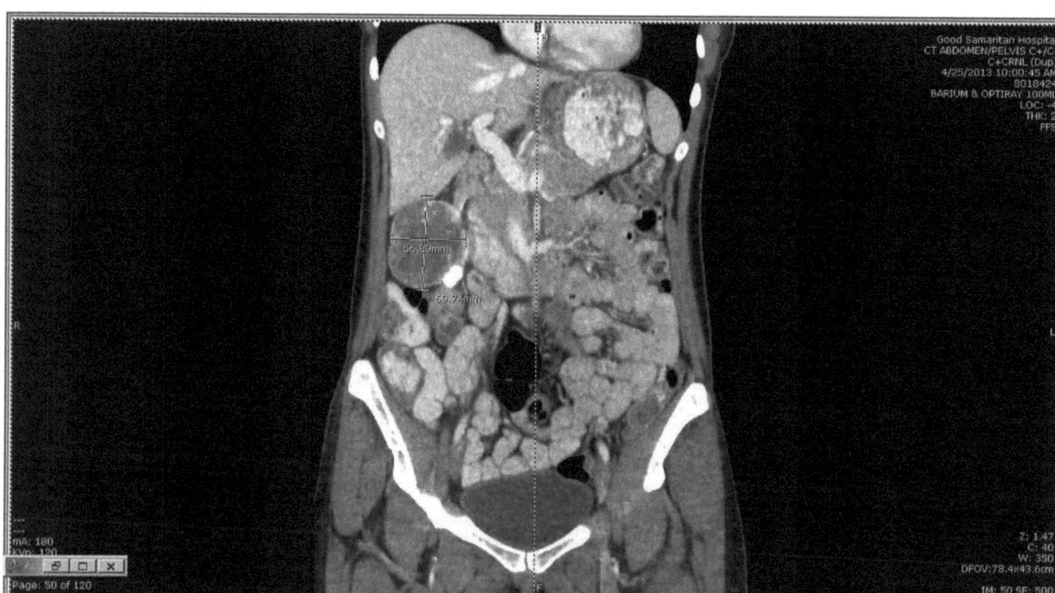

Fig. C.51 2013 CT scan of abdomen and pelvis, renal mass protocol demonstrating a 5.6 × 7 cm exophytic, enhancing, heterogeneous, right renal mass

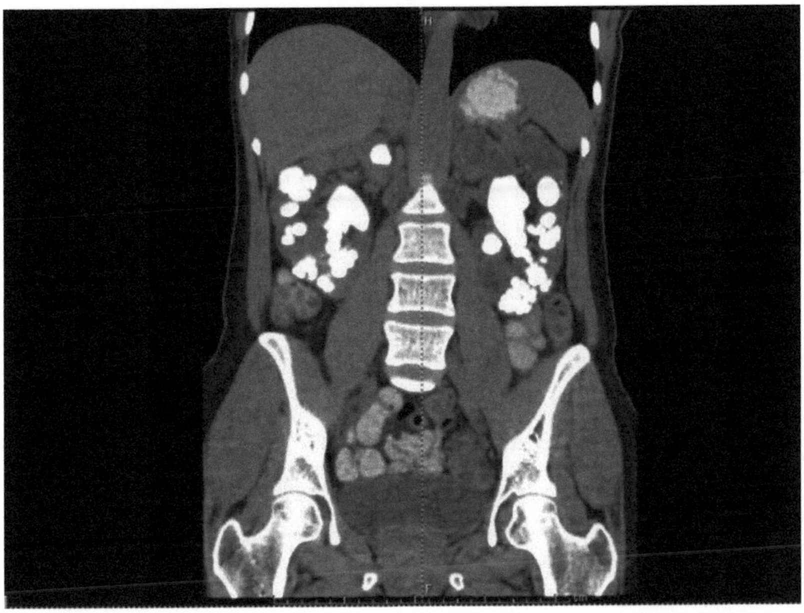

Fig. C.52 2013 CT scan of abdomen and pelvis demonstrating bilateral renal stone burden prior to nephroureterectomy

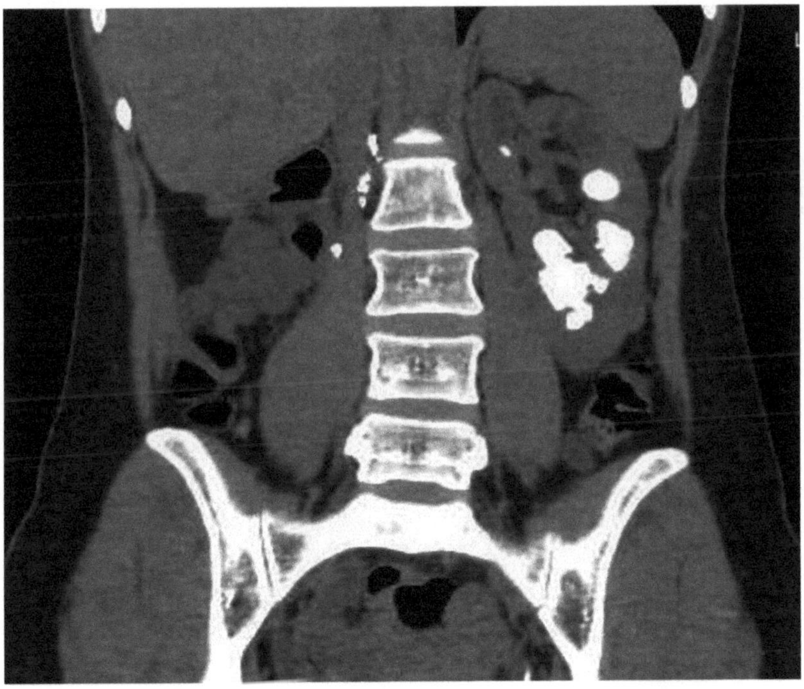

Fig. C.53 2015 CT scan of abdomen and pelvis demonstrating persistent residual renal stone burden in left kidney after nephroureterectomy of right kidney for urothelial carcinoma

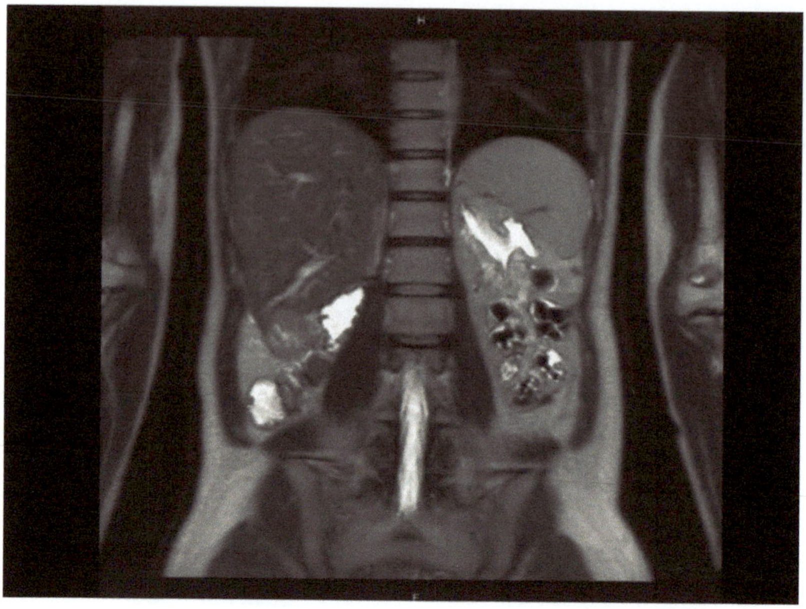

Fig. C.54 2014 MRI of the abdomen demonstrating the ~3.5 cm mass representing recurrence of urothelial carcinoma of the right retroperitoneal renal fossa

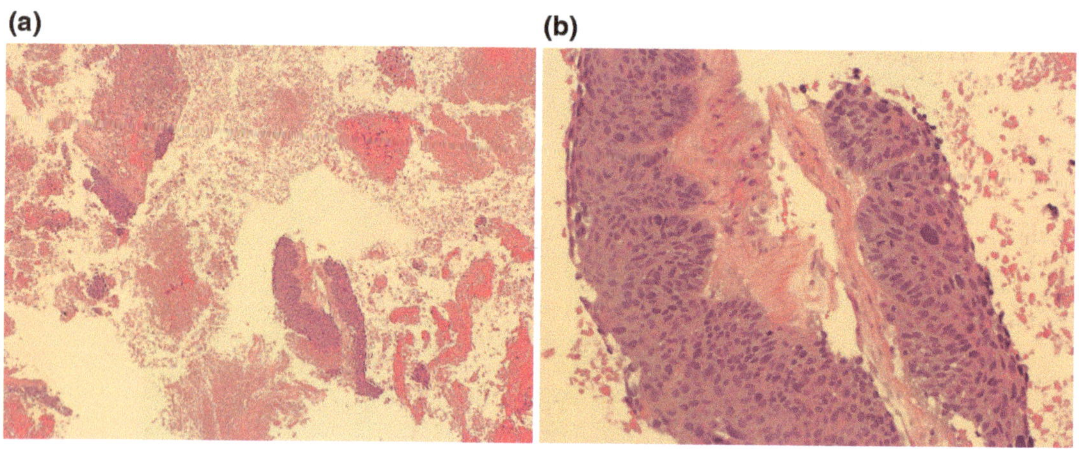

Fig. C.55 a, b Pathology slide from 2013 CT guided renal biopsy of right renal mass consistent with high-grade invasive urothelial carcinoma with elements of necrosis

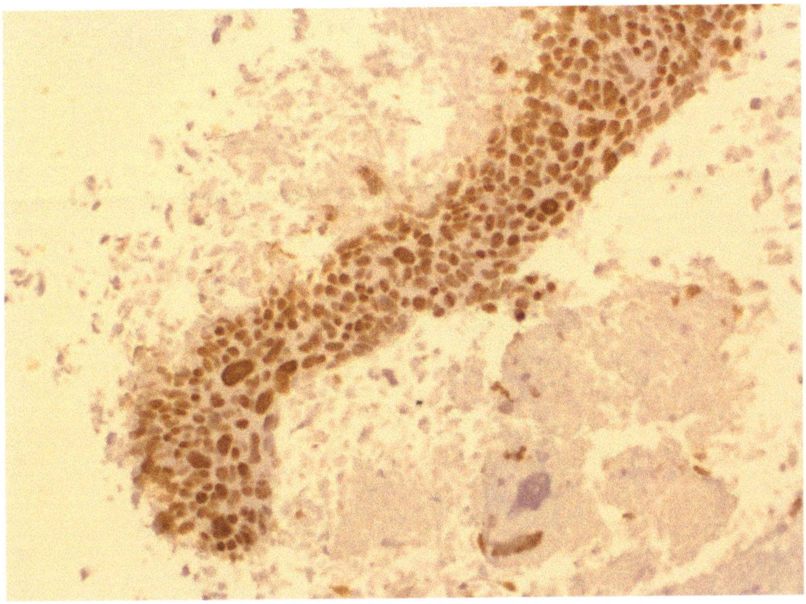

Fig. C.56 Pathology slide from 2013 renal biopsy demonstrating positive P63 staining which is consistent with urothelial carcinoma

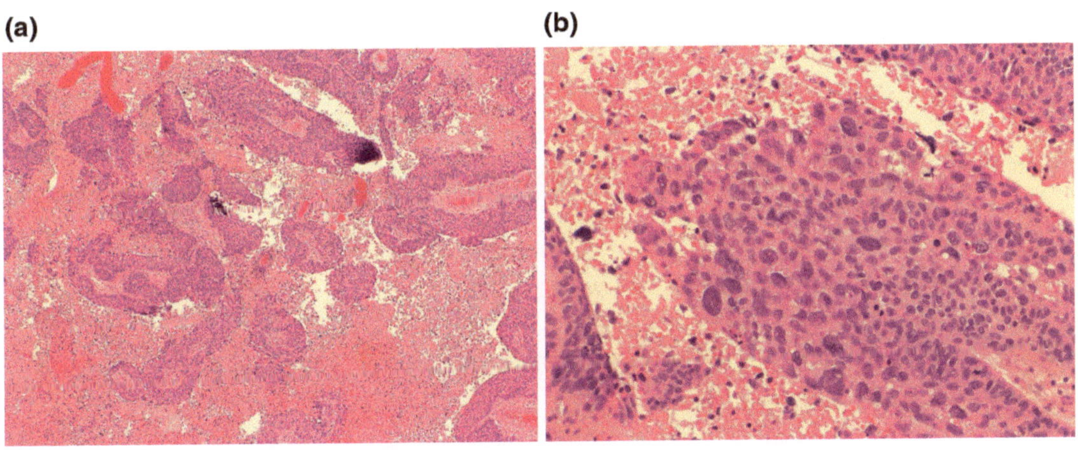

Fig. C.57 **a**, **b** Pathology slides of right kidney specimen from 2013 nephroureterectomy demonstrating high-grade papillary urothelial carcinoma. Analysis of kidney demonstrated negative resection margin with no lymphovascular invasion

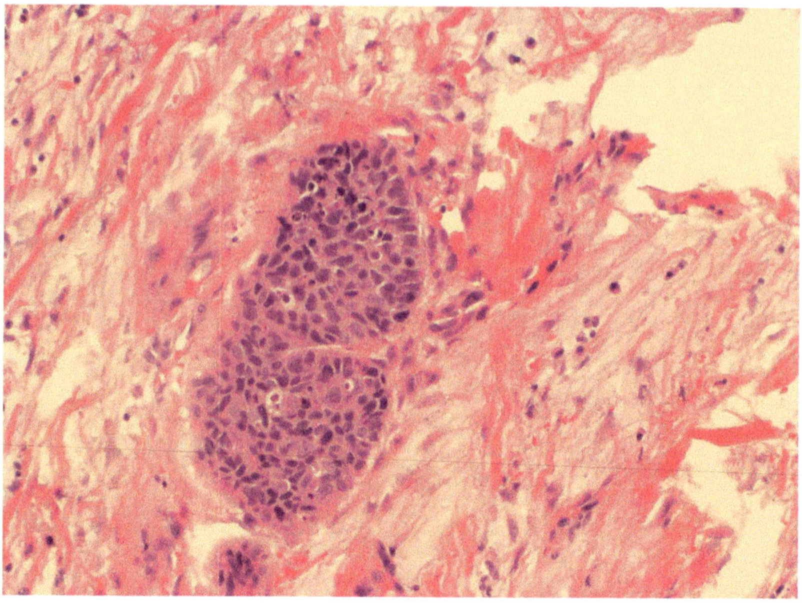

Fig. C.58 Pathology slide of right ureter from 2013 nephroureterectomy demonstrating high-grade papillary urothelial carcinoma

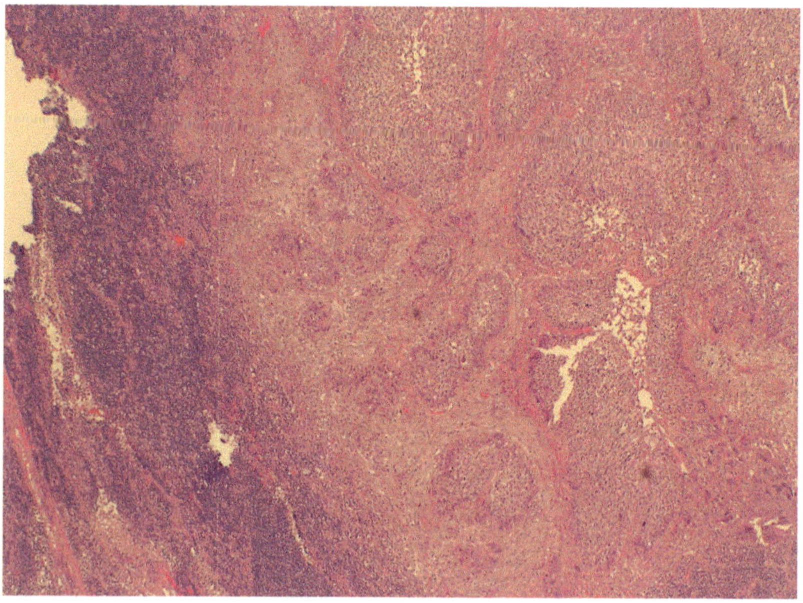

Fig. C.59 Pathology slide of precaval right lymph node at time of 2013 nephroureterectomy demonstrating presence of metastatic urothelial carcinoma

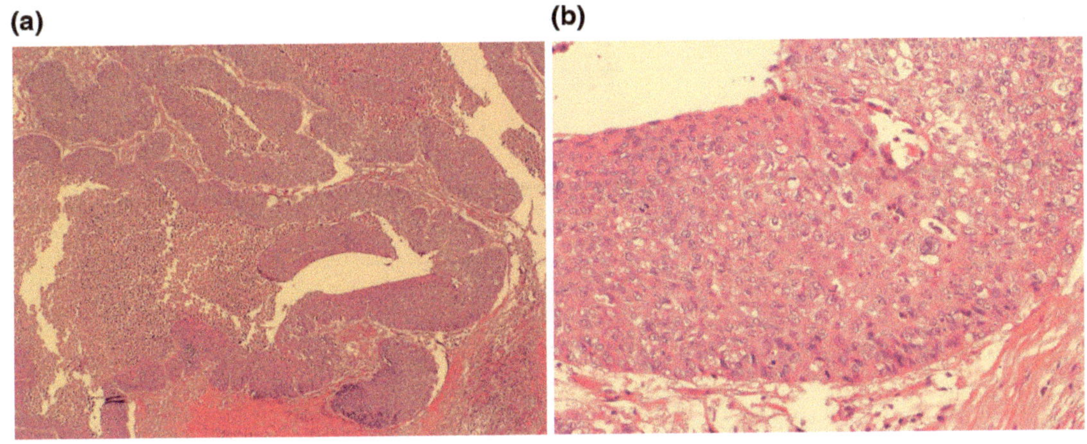

Fig. C.60 **a**, **b** Pathology slide of retroperitoneal mass from 2014 resection consistent with urothelial carcinoma involving fibroadipose tissue and liver parenchyma with extensive necrosis

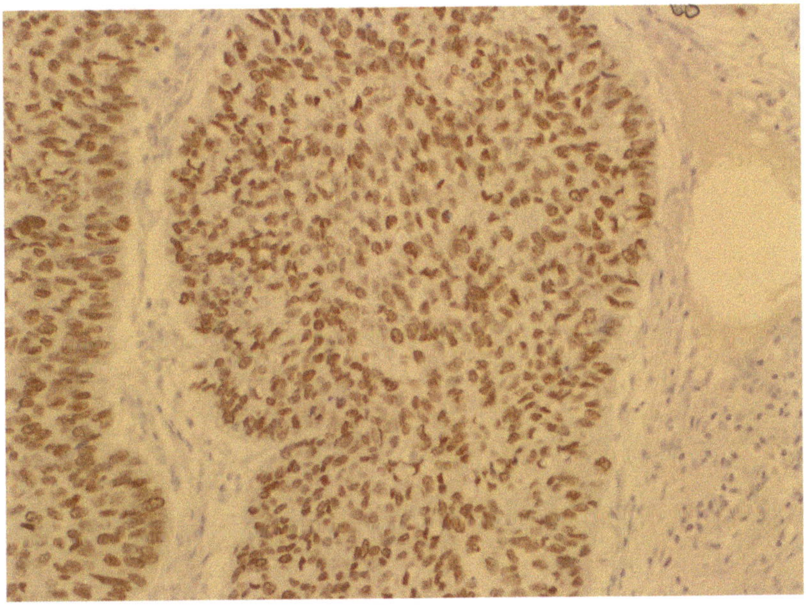

Fig. C.61 Additional pathology slide preparation from 2014 retroperitoneal resection stained positive diffusely for P63

In My Mind's Eye[1]

Majid Eshghi

Hamlet, who had the most vivid imagination of all Shakespeare's characters, spoke those words over 400 years ago (1599–1602). Chares H. Duell, the commissioner of the United States Post Office in 1899, uttered: "Everything that can be invented has been invented." The reality is that regardless of myriad inventions and novelties it is impossible to prevent the inquisitive human mind from bursting with new ideas and envisioning newer methods and more efficient tools. It is amazing what the human mind can foresee! Such has been the case in medicine and especially so in the field of urology: to improve treatments we sometimes need to go beyond standard boundaries to look for novel ideas at the edge. Thirty years ago, I envisioned the art on these two pages as a reminder that, with the rapid development of upper tract endoscopy, the sky would be the limit for what we would be able to achieve in the ensuing years. I usually used them as closing slides during lectures to remind the audience to never stop imagining and keep searching to reach the unreachable for better and easier ways to serve our patients and in the words of Cervantes: "Para llegar a las estrellas inalcanzables (ref 2)."

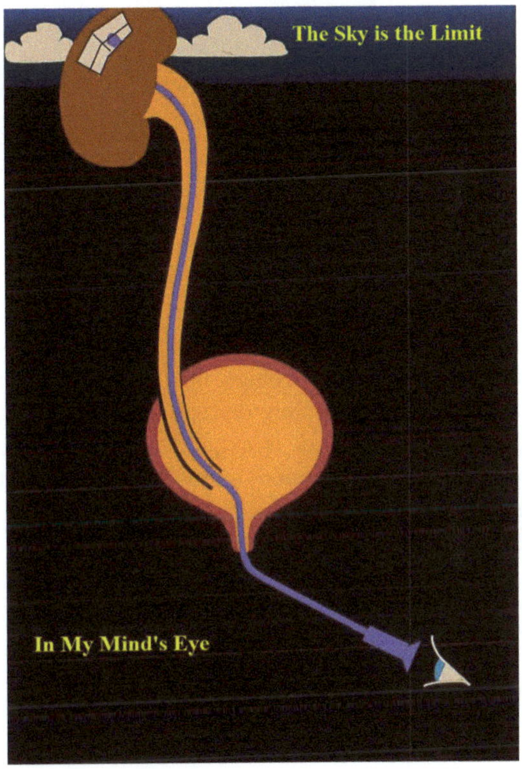

M. Eshghi (ed.), *Urothelial Malignancies of the Upper Urinary Tract*,
https://doi.org/10.1007/978-3-319-51263-1

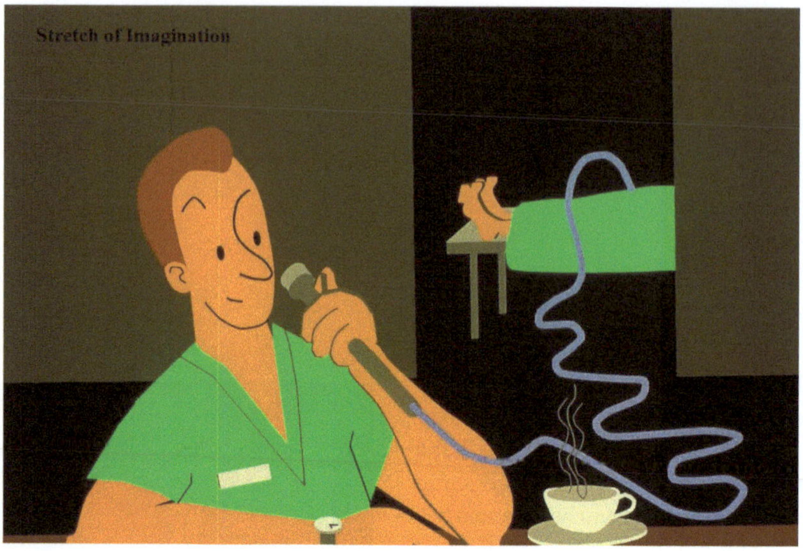

TELEMEDICINE

By the time this publication is completed, there will already be numerous new methods, treatment protocols and innovations being introduced into clinical urology that have not been addressed or adequately discussed in this book, for now this subject is exhausted (ref 3). The purpose of this section is to provide a brief description or snapshot of only some of what we know that is on the horizon.

References

1. Hamlet, The Prince of Denmark; 1599–1602, William Shakespeare
2. Don Quixote, published 1615, Miguel de Cervantes
3. Bernard Shaw; dramatic opinions and essays, volume 2; this subject is exhausted, so am I.

Review of Future Developments

Ali Fathollahi and Majid Eshghi

Laboratory

Serum Tumor Marker

In a research published in March 2016, researchers in China investigated potential association of increased plasma fibrinogen level and UTUC. The results of the study showed increased plasma fibrinogen was an independent prognostic risk factor for poor outcomes in UTUC. This may serve as an effective biomarker in the future.

UGT1A

UGT1A is a major phase II drug metabolism enzyme. It is known to play an important role in preventing bladder cancer initiation by detoxifying carcinogenic compounds. A significant decrease in the expression of UGT1A in UUTUC was seen suggesting its preventive role. Loss of UGT1A expression was also found to correlate with tumor progression and a predictor of poor prognosis.

Imaging

PET Scan

There is an emerging role for wider use of PET scan with a variety of agents for early diagnosis and assessment of the tumor stage. PET had traditionally been thought not to be much applicable in detecting tumors of the urinary tract system, because of its excretion throughout the urinary tract and resulting in obscured images. However, a few studies have shown that different hydration protocols might help bypass this limitation and detect UTUC. PET scan has also been shown to be superior in detecting metastatic disease that might be otherwise missed by CT. Researchers in Tokyo Medical and Dental University investigated the diagnostic accuracy of FDG PET/CT for detecting metastasis and its impact on patient management with UTUC. They performed 18F-FDG PET/CT after CT for initial staging ($n = 47$) and for restaging at recurrence ($n = 9$) on patients with UTUC. In the lesion-based analysis, 142 lesions were diagnosed as metastases. The sensitivity of PET/CT was significantly better than that of CT (85 vs. 50%, $p = 0.0001$). In the patient-based analysis, 22 patients were diagnosed as having metastases. The sensitivity/specificity/accuracy of PET/CT tended to be superior to those of CT, but these values were not significantly different (95, 91, and 93% vs. 82, 85, and 84%; $p = 0.25$, 0.50, and 0.063, respectively). The clinicians changed their assessments of disease extent and management plans in 18 (32%) and 11 (20%) patients, respectively, based on the PET/CT results.

MRI

High-power MRI imaging and diffusion studies are showing promising results in predicting grade and invasiveness of renal pelvic tumors. Hydration of patient prior to MRI along with diuresis will allow filling of collecting system without the use of contrast agents. Yoshida et al. demonstrated applicability of diffusion-weighted MRI

M. Eshghi (ed.), *Urothelial Malignancies of the Upper Urinary Tract*,
https://doi.org/10.1007/978-3-319-51263-1

(DW MRI) for a series of UTUC. DW MRI imaging was carried out in 10 consecutive patients with suspected UTUC. While conventional imaging, detected seven renal pelvic tumors definitely, on DW MRI, all nine tumors showed hyperintensity with negligible urinary intensity. A case of benign stenosis had negative DW MRI. In another study in France, Roy et al. assessed the value of DW MRI in detecting malignant UTUC, and showed that adding another parameter, called apparent diffusion coefficient (ADC) is useful in differentiating malignant lesions (78.3 and 95.5% sensitivity and specificity, respectively). Of note, they did not find ADC different in differentiating low-grade versus high-grade tumors. Yoshida et al., however, found that ADC value can serve as an indicator of tumor grade in UTUC. They showed that high-grade tumors had lower ADC value and that ADC can be used as an independent preoperative indicator of shorter cancer specific survival.Virtual Ureteroscopy

Image processing becomes more efficient, intuitive and computerized to make it less laborious. As these imaging techniques show more sensitivity there will be less need for more invasive endoscopic surveillance.Elastography-Contrast Enhanced Ultrasound

Have shown encouraging results in some areas of urology imaging. They have not yet shown a specific role in collecting system imaging.

Endoscopy

The utilization of O-Arm in combination with ureteroscopy may allow instant CT imaging assessment of depth of treated areas with laser and possibly in the future with microwave fibers placed through the working channels of ureteroscopes it may be possible to treat small parenchymal endophytic lesions. Additionally HIFU can potentially be delivered via an ultrasound probe similar to the principles used in intraluminal ultrasound. Prototypes of small fiber scopes (3Fr) are being tested for clinical which may allow for office ureteroscopy in uncomplicated cases.

NBI-Blue Light-Spectra

The endoscopic imaging has significantly evolved in the last decade with new digital video endoscopes with camera chips at the tip of the scopes providing superb high definition intraluminal images with true colors and impressive surface details. **Narrow Band Imaging and Blue Light** are already in clinical use in the United States and the Spectra (Karl Storz Endoscoy America, Secondo, CA) system is in its early stages of use in Europe. NBI and Blue Light have been discussed earlier. Spectra system and Clara are based on principles similar to NBI and utilization of red green and blue (RGB) bands (Figs. B.1, B.2 and B.3).

Prototype versions of miniature fiberscopes measuring about 3 Fr have been tested which may eventually allow for office ureteroscopy for surveillance. Once this technology is perfected it could potentially decrease the need for operating room procedures.

Optical Coherence Tomography

Optical Coherence Tomography (OCT) is a high-resolution imaging technology that can be applied during URS and is analogous to ultrasound. It uses backscattered light instead of back

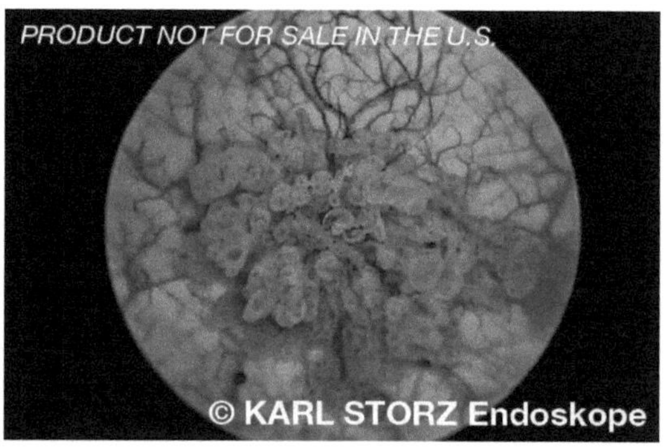

Fig. B.1 Spectra system and Clara

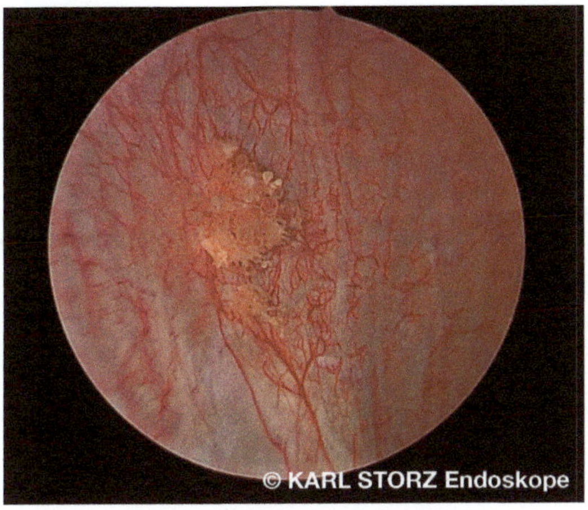

Fig. B.2 Spectra system and Clara

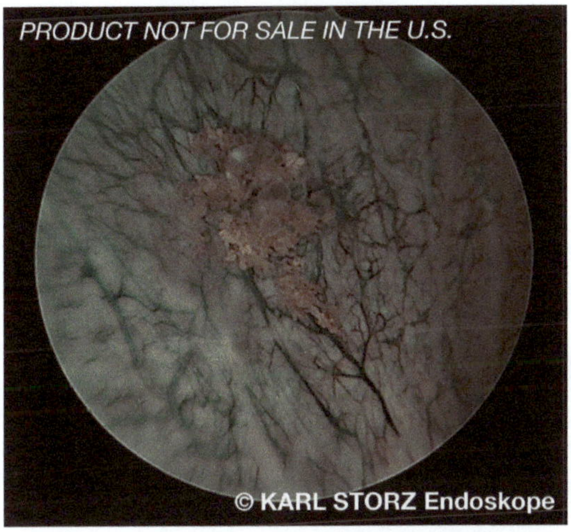

Fig. B.3 Spectra system and Clara

reflected sound waves to produce cross-sectional images and has the potential to provide real-time information on grade and stage in UTUC [1]. Bus et al. did a study on 26 patients who underwent diagnostic URS including biopsies and OCT imaging, followed by nephroureterectomy or segmental ureteral resection. They found that in 83% of the specimen staging of lesions were in accordance with final histopathology. Interpretation of OCT findings should be cautious with large lesions filling ureteral lumen and inflammation, which may also lead to a false-positive result.

Magnetic Tracking

It is conceivable that in near future, as was demonstrated in laboratory research, computer models of radiologic images showing certain pathologies can be accessed with a more precise accuracy using magnetic tracking devices.

Confocal Laser Endomicroscopy (CLE)

Recent advances in fiber-optics technology have enabled packaging of a confocal microscope into a small probe format compatible with standard endoscopes. A 488 nm low-power laser scans a targeted tissue below the surface. The tissue is nonspecifically stained with intravenous fluorescein. Under excitation, the fluorescein emits light that is filtered through a pinhole so that only in-focus light is measured by a photodetector while the out-of-focus light is rejected, resulting in optical sectioning of the regions of interest with micron-scale resolution comparable to histology. Nuclear features are not routinely visualized, since fluorescein highlights the extracellular matrix and does not cross intact cell membranes. CLE images are acquired as video sequences at a rate of 12 frames per second via direct contact of the probe with tissues of interest. This technique has more value when combined with other technologies.

Bui et al. implemented this technique in imaging of UTUC. It showed characteristic features of tumors, including papillary structure, pleomorphic cells, and fibro vascular stalks.

Diagnostic accuracy of bladder cancer using white light source together with CLE, as clinically relevant, has been reported as having 89% sensitivity and 88% specificity (Fig. B.4).

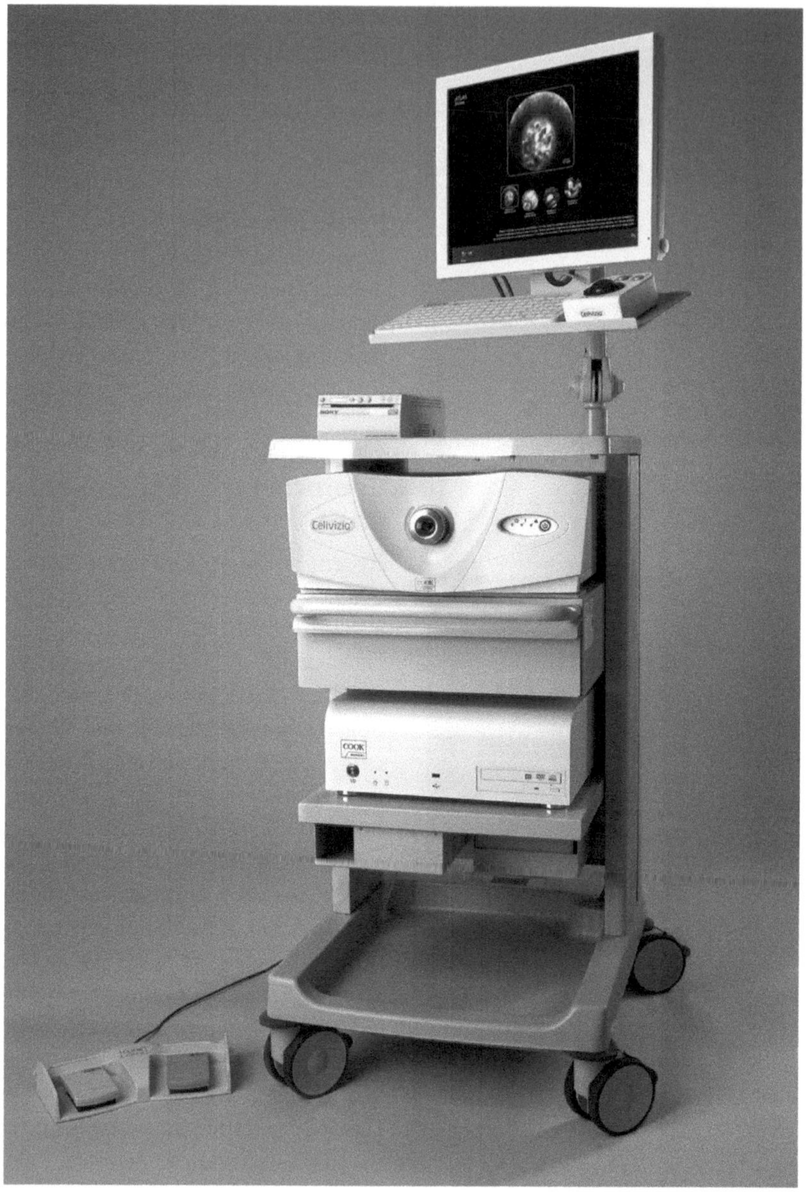

Fig. B.4 Cellvizio_DS27996 *Source* Permission is Dr. Eshghi's chapter, Future Technology, in Urothelial Malignancies of the Upper Tract to be published by Springer in 2017

Chemo- and Immunotherapy: Novel Treatment in Gemcitabine-Resistant Disease

Yeh et al. in Taiwan studied patients with gemcitabine-resistant advanced urothelial cancer. They demonstrated that increased TG-interacting factor (TGIF) in specimens is associated with worse prognosis in patients with UTUC. Their results showed that increased TGIF is significantly associated with chemo-resistance, poor progression-free survival, and higher cancer-related deaths from UTUC. In addition, histone deacetylases inhibitor trichostatin A (TSA) inhibited TGIF, p-AKTSer473 expression and migration ability. Synergistic effects of gemcitabine and TSA on NGR cells were also demonstrated.

The Nanoparticles appear to be very promising in delivery of immuno therapy as the next line of treatment of the upper tract urothelial carcinoma.

Mitogel (UroGen): Early laboratory and clinical trials with gels containing chemotherapeutic agent mitomycin C shows promising results with the goal of increasing contact time of urothelium with the treating agent. In general nanoparticle delivery may become the treatment of choice for urothelial carcinoma.

An interim report on clinical use of Mitogel showed in 34 patients for low grade disease showed 58.8% initial response, 22 patients has compassionate use with 44% response.

Suggested Readings

Asai S, Fukumoto T, Tanji N, et al. Fluorodeoxyglucose positron emission tomography/computed tomography for diagnosis of upper urinary tract urothelial carcinoma. Int J Clin Oncol. 2015; 20(5):1042–7.

Bui D, Mach KE, Lopez A, Liu JJ, Chang T, Lavelle J, Leppert JT, Liao JC. Optical biopsy of upper tract urothelial carcinoma with confocal laser endomicroscopy. Eur. Urol. 2014; 13:e630.

Bus MT, de Bruin DM, Faber DJ, et al. Optical coherence tomography as a tool for in vivo staging and grading of upper urinary tract urothelial carcinoma: a study for diagnostic accuracy. J Urol. 2016;27 S0022–5347(16) 30924s7

Bus MT, Muller BG, de Bruin DM et al. Volumetric in vivo visualization of upper urinary tract tumors using optical coherence tomography: a pilot study. J Urol. 2013;190:2236–2242.

Ceriani L, Suriano S, Ruberto T et al. Could different hydration protocols affect the quality of 18F-FDG PET/CT images? J Nucl Med Technol. 2011;39:77–82

Chang TC, et al. Interobserver agreement of confocal laser endomicroscopy for bladder cancer. J. Endourol. Endourol. Soc. 2013; 27:598–603. This paper describes the interobserver agreement of confocal laser endomicroscopy of bladder lesions and provides updated optical diagnostic criteria.

Goh AC, Tresser NJ, Shen SS, Lerner SP. Optical coherence tomography as an adjunct to white light cystoscopy for intravesical real-time imaging and staging of bladder cancer. Urology 2008;72:133–137.

Koji Izumi, Satoshi Inoue, Hiroki Ide, et al. MP27-01. UDP-glucuronosyltransferase 1A (UGT1A) immunohistochemistry in urothelial carcinoma of the upper urinary tract as a strong prognosticator, Abstract, AUA Meeting 2016.

Lerner, Seth, Non Surgical Management of low grade upper tract urothelial cancer: An interim analysis of the international multicenter Olympus trial, Plenary, AUA Meeting 2018 (LBA-25).

Neumann H, Kiesslich R, Wallace MB, Neurath MF. Confocal laser endomicroscopy: technical advances and clinical applications. Gastroenterology. 2010;139:388–392. 392. e1–392.e2.

Pan, Chong-Xian. State of the Art Lecture predicting chemo sensitivity in urothelial malignancy: Nanotech and precision medicine. Plenary, AUA 2018.

Roy C, Labani A, Alemann G, et al. DWI in the etiologic diagnosis of excretory upper urinary tract lesions: can it help in differentiating benign from malignant tumors? A retrospective study of 98 patients. AJR Am J Roentgenol. 2016;207 (1):106–13. doi:10.2214/AJR.15.15652.Epub 2016 Apr 11.

Sonn GA, et al. Optical biopsy of human bladder neoplasia with in vivo confocal laser endomicroscopy. J. Urol. 2009;182:1299–1305. [PubMed: 19683270] This paper was the initial feasibility study of in vivo confocal laser endomicroscopy in the urinary tract

Stephanie P, Chen and Joseph C. Liao. Confocal laser endomicroscopy of bladder and upper tract urothelial carcinoma: a new era of optical diagnosis? Curr Urol Rep. 2014;15(9): 437.

Tanaka H, Yoshida S, Komai Y, et al. Clinical value of 18f-fluorodeoxyglucose positron emission tomography/computed tomography in upper tract urothelial carcinoma: impact on detection of metastases and patient management. Urol Int. 2016;96(1):65–6.

Wu K, et al. Dynamic real-time microscopy of the urinary tract using confocal laser endomicroscopy. Urology. 2011;78:225–231. [PubMed: 21601243] This paper describes the suggested optical diagnostic criteria for normal urothelium, benign inflammatory urothelium, low-grade urothelial carcinoma, and high-grade urothelial carcinoma.

Yeh BW, Li WM, Li CC, et al. Histone deacetylase inhibitor trichostatin A resensitizes gemcitabine-resistant urothelial carcinoma cells via suppression of TG-interacting factor. Toxicol Appl Pharmacol. 2016;290:98–106.

Yeh CL, Chen SW, Chen YK. Delayed diuretic FDG PET/CT scan facilitates detection of renal urothelial cell carcinoma. Clin Nucl Med 2009;34:829–830

Yoshida S, Masuda H, Ishii C, Saito K, et al. Initial experience of functional imaging of upper urinary tract neoplasm by diffusion-weighted magnetic resonance imaging. Int J Urol. 2008;15 (2):140–3. doi:10.1111/j.1442–2042.2007.01950.x.

Yoshida S, Uchida Y, Kobayashi S, et al. MP27-07: Apparent diffusion coefficient as a prognostic biomarker of upper urinary tract cancer. AUA abstract, May 7, 2016

Zhang B, Song Y, Jin J, et al. Preoperative plasma fibrinogen level represents an independent prognostic factor in a Chinese cohort of patients with upper tract urothelial carcinoma. PLoS One. 2016;11(3):e0150193. doi:10.1371/journal.pone.0150193. eCollection 2016.

Appendix A: Glossary and Abbreviations

Ali Fathollahi

The wide use of Internet has opened the medical literature to the public and thus created a new genre of readers and researchers reviewing such literature. This is not a single group and the reasons are multifaceted; a simple high school report, college reports, medical students researching under a mentor, journalists, pharmaceutical marketing and patients searching medical entities to understand their medical problems better are just some examples. Not all of these varied pools of readers have an adequate knowledge of all medical terms forcing them to frequently refer to dictionaries or similar resources which at times do not provide the specific information as presented in the texts. The purpose of this section is to provide accurate information on some of the entities for such individuals and make the text more user friendly.

A

Ablation	the surgical removal or destruction of body tissue
Adriamycin	an antineoplastic (anti-tumoral) agent
Adjuvant therapy	an addition designed to help reach the ultimate goal. Adjuvant therapy for cancer usually refers to surgery followed by chemo- or radiotherapy to help cure or decrease the risk of the cancer recurring (coming back)
Analgesia	the inability to feel pain
Anaphylactic	relating to or caused by a severe, potentially life-threatening allergic reaction

B

Bacille Calmette Guerin	also known as BCG, a weakened (attenuated) version of bacteria called *Mycobacterium bovis* which is closely related to *Mycobacterium tuberculosis*, the agent responsible for tuberculosis. Intravesical (instillation inside the bladder) BCG therapy is highly effective for managing high-risk non-muscle-invasive (not penetrating the bladder muscle) urothelial carcinoma of the bladder
Balkan nephropathy	a chronic kidney disease associated with a high frequency of urothelial atypia, occasionally culminating in tumors of the renal pelvis and urethra
BCG	see Bacille Calmette Guerin
Biomarker	a measurable substance in an organism whose presence is indicative of some phenomenon such as disease, cancer, infection, or environmental exposure
Bladder cuff	the area around ureteral orifices in the bladder which is usually resected as part of surgery to treat upper tract urothelial cancers
Bugbee	a monopolar, flexible electrode which is used in cystoscopes, resectoscopes and ureteroscopes. The Bugbee electrode is used for the ablation coagulation (desrtroying by burning)of soft tissue

M. Eshghi (ed.), *Urothelial Malignancies of the Upper Urinary Tract*,
https://doi.org/10.1007/978-3-319-51263-1

C

Calyx the first unit in the system of ducts in the kidney carrying urine from kidney to the renal pelvis and through the ureters

Carcinoma a cancer arising in the epithelial tissue of the skin or of the lining of the internal organs

Carcinoma in situ also known as in situ neoplasm (tumor) is a group of abnormal cells. While they are a form of neoplasm there is disagreement over whether CIS should be classified as cancer. These abnormal cells grow in their normal place, thus "in situ" (from Latin for "in its place")

Cardiopulmonary of or relating to the heart and the lungs

Chemotherapy the treatment of disease by the use of chemical substances, especially the treatment of cancer by cytotoxic and other drugs

Circumaortic around the aorta (main abdominal artery)

CIS see Carcinoma in situ

Cold Cup Forceps a type of forceps used to obtain biopsy material from the urinary tract

Comorbidity the simultaneous presence of two or more chronic diseases or conditions in a patient

Continent urinary diversion is an internal urinary reservoir that a surgeon creates from a section of the bowel

Corticomedullary relating to, or joining, the renal medulla (center) and cortex (outer shell)

CT urogram also CTU, an imaging exam used to evaluate urinary tract, including the kidneys, the bladder and the tubes (ureters) that carry urine from the kidneys to the bladder

Cubital of the forearm or the elbow

Cyclosporine a drug used to prevent the rejection of grafts and transplants

Cystectomy a surgical operation to remove the urinary bladder

Cystoscope a telescopic instrument inserted into the urethra (urinary channel) for examining the inside of the urinary bladder

Cystogram an imaging visually used to visualize the urinary bladder. Using a urinary catheter, radiocontrast is instilled in the bladder, and X-ray imaging is performed

D

DaVinci a robotic surgical system made by the American company Intuitive Surgical. Approved by the Food and Drug Administration (FDA) in 2000, it is designed to facilitate complex surgery using a minimally invasive approach, and is controlled by a surgeon from a console

Debulking surgical removal of as much of a malignant tumor as possible

Deflection in endoscopic instrumentation, angling or a turning aside or deviation from a straight line to allow better visualization

Desmoplasia growth of fibrous or connective tissue, usually as a result of an insult

Dorsal lithotomy position a supine position in which the hips and knees are fully flexed with the legs spread apart and raised and the feet resting in straps

Double J stent a type of ureteral stent (narrow tube)

Doxorubicin see Adrianycin

Doppler a diagnostic mode of ultrasonic beam; the ultrasound reflected from moving structures changes its frequency and thus allowing for measurement of flow and speed

E

E coli. a bacterium

Endo-GIA stapler a device for fastening together tissues, e.g., bowel inside body

Endourology a minimally invasive technique using small scopes to treat a variety of urinary tract conditions

Extravasation leakage of a fluid out of urinary tract

F

Fiberoptic the use of thin flexible fibers of glass or other transparent solids to transmit light signals, chiefly for telecommunications or for internal examination of the body

FISH a way to visualize and map the genetic material in an individual's cells, including specific genes or portions of genes

Fluconazole an antifungal medicine. It is used to treat infections caused by fungus, which can invade any part of the body

Fluorescence in situ hybridization see FISH

Fr French size is three times the diameter in millimeters. A round catheter of 3 French has an external diameter of 1 mm

Fulguration destruction of living tissue by electric sparks generated by a high-frequency current

Fungal of or caused by a fungus or fungi

Furosemide a diuretic medication used to treat fluid build-up due to heart failure, liver scarring, or kidney disease

G

Gadolinium a chemical substance used as a contrast in MRI

Gemcitabine an antineoplastic agent used in chemotherapy

Genome the complete set of genes or genetic material present in a cell or organism

Gibson incision an oblique incision made in lower lateral part of abdomen to access lower part of ureter and bladder

Gonadal Vessels Veins and arteries going to/coming from gonads (testis or ovary)

Guidewire A wire or spring used as a guide for placement of a larger device, such as a catheter or scope

H

Heparin Lock a type of intermittent intravenous device for the administration of heparin, fluids and variety of medications. It does not require a continuous flow of fluids; the intravenous fluid flow can be disconnected and the heparin lock filled with a heparin solution that maintains patency of the needle

Hematuria the presence of blood in urine

Holmium:YAG a laser whose beam is in the near infrared spectrum at 2100 nm; used for photocoagulation and photoablation

Horseshoe kidney a congenital disorder in which the patient's kidneys fuse together at the bottom to form a horseshoe-shape during development in the womb

Hounsfield unit a quantity commonly used in computed tomography (CT) scanning to express tissue density numbers in a

	standardized and convenient form
Hydronephrosis	literally "water inside the kidney"—refers to distension and dilation of the renal pelvis and calyces, usually caused by obstruction of the free flow of urine from the kidney
Hyperchromatism	the development of excess chromatin (genetic material) or of excessive nuclear staining especially as a part of a pathological process
Hyperechoic	In ultrasound, denoting a region in which the echoes are stronger (brighter in images) than normal or than surrounding structures
Hypertrophy	excessive development of an organ or part; specifically increase in bulk without multiplication of parts
Hypoechoic	In ultrasound, denoting a region in which the echoes are weaker (darker in images) than normal or than surrounding structures

I

Ileal ureter	restoration of continuity of urinary tract by replacing a part or all ureter with a segment of small bowel
IFN	see Interferon
Iliac artery	main artery in pelvis branching from aorta
Immunotherapy	the prevention or treatment of disease with substances that stimulate the immune response
Indwelling tube	left within a bodily organ or passage to maintain drainage, prevent obstruction, or provide a route for administration of food or drugs
Infundibulum	a funnel-shaped part connecting calyx to renal pelvis
Interferon	a group of signaling proteins made and released by host cells in response to the presence of several pathogens, such as viruses, bacteria, parasites, and also tumor cells. They are important for fighting viral infections and for the regulation of the immune system
Intramural	situated or done within the walls of a structure
Intravesical	inside bladder

J

Jejunum	second part of the small intestine in humans

K

KTP laser	a type of laser, in the blue-green to green (532-nm) spectrum, used for hemostasis and tissue ablation

L

Leukoplakia	a whitish patch or plaque that cannot be characterized clinically or pathologically as any other disease, and is not associated with any physical or chemical causative agent, except the use of tobacco
Lumbotomy	a type of incision to make access to kidney from back
Lumen	the cavity of a tubular organ or part
Lymphadenectomy	surgical removal of one or more groups of lymph nodes

M

Magnetic Resonance Imaging (MRI)	a technique that uses a magnetic field and radio waves to create detailed

	images of the organs and tissues within your body
Meatotomy	refers to an incision or tearing done to enlarge the urethra or ureter
Mesh	a synthetic material that is used to provide additional support to weakened or damaged tissue
Miniperc	performing percutaneous nephrostomy access with a smaller caliber tract
Mitomycin C	any of a group of antibiotics produced by the soil actinomycete *Streptomyces caespitosus* that inhibit DNA synthesis and are used against bacteria and cancerous tumor cells
Mitosis	a type of cell division that results in two daughter cells each having the same number and kind of chromosomes as the parent nucleus, typical of ordinary tissue growth
MMC	see Mitomycin C
MRI	see Magnetic Resonance Imaging
Multivariate analysis	the statistical process of simultaneously analyzing multiple independent (or predictor) variables with multiple dependent (outcome or criterion) variables
Mutagen	an agent, such as radiation or a chemical substance, that causes genetic mutation
Myelosuppression	decrease in production of cells responsible for providing immunity (leukocytes), carrying oxygen (erythrocytes), and/or those responsible for normal blood clotting (thrombocytes)

N

Nd:YAG	a laser whose beam is in the near infrared spectrum at approximately 1060 nm; used for photocoagulation and photoablation
Neodymium: yttrium–aluminum–garnet	see Nd:YAG
Nephroscopy	inspecting and passing instruments into the interior of the kidney
Nephrostogram	a radiograph of the kidney after opacification of the renal pelvis by injecting a contrast agent through a nephrostomy tube
Nephrostomy tract	an artificial opening created between the kidney and the skin which allows for the urinary diversion directly from the upper part of the urinary system (renal pelvis)
Nitrofurantoin	a synthetic compound with antibacterial properties, used to treat infections of the urinary tract

O

Opacify	on radiology studies, to make visible
Orthotopic neobladder	a bladder fashioned from intestine, placed at the site of the excised natural bladder, and draining through the intact urethra

P

Packed Red Blood Cells	red blood cells (RBC, also called erythrocytes) that have been collected, processed, and stored in bags as

blood product units available for blood transfusion

Palliative relieving pain or alleviating a problem without dealing with the underlying cause

Paraaortic near aorta (main abdominal artery)

Paracaval near inferior vena cava (main abdominal vein)

Parathormone also parathyroid hormone, a hormone that regulates calcium levels in a person's body

PCN the placement of a small, flexible rubber catheter (tube) through the skin into the kidney to drain the urine

Pelvicalyceal pertaining to the renal pelvis and calices

Percutaneous made, done, or effected through the skin

Percutaneous Nephrostomy Tube see PCN

PET scan an imaging test that uses a radioactive drug (tracer) to help reveal abnormal biologic activity in cancer patients

Pfannenstiel incision also known as Bikini incision, a type of transverse low abdominal surgical incision for cosmetic purposes that allows access to the abdomen. It is most common method for performing Caesarian sections today

Pigtail stent a type of ureteral stent

Pleomorphic variability in the size, similar to double J stent shape and staining of cells and/or their nuclei

Positron Emission Tomography scan see PET scan

PRBC see Packed Red Blood Cells

Pyelolymphatic pertaining to the renal pelvis and renal lymphatics

Pyeloureteritis inflammation of a ureter and the renal pelvis

Pyelovenous pertaining to the renal pelvis and renal veins

R

Radical nephroureterectomy (RNU) The standard treatment strategy to remove a patient's kidney, ureter, and bladder cuff for bulky, high-grade, or invasive upper tract urothelial carcinoma (UTUC)

Rads unit of absorbed radiation dose

Reflux see Vesicoureteral Reflux

Reimplantation a surgery to reattach tubes (ureters) that connect the bladder to the kidneys

Renal parenchyma functional parts of the human kidney, including the elements of the organ that create urine

Renal pelvis The area at the center of the kidney. Urine collects in the renal pelvis and is funneled into the ureter

Renal sinus a cavity within the kidney which is occupied by the renal pelvis, renal calyces, blood vessels, and fat

Retina a layer at the back of the eyeball containing cells that are sensitive to light and that trigger nerve impulses that pass via the optic nerve to the

	brain, where a visual image is formed
Retrograde pyelogram	a urologic procedure where the physician injects contrast into the ureter in order to visualize the ureter and urinary ducts inside the kidney. The flow of contrast (up from the bladder to the kidney) is opposite the usual flow of urine, hence the retrograde name
Rhabdomyolysis	the destruction of striated muscle cells
Segmental ureterectomy	excision of a segment of the ureter
Sensor Guide Wire	a guiding wire with a floppy smooth surface

S

Sepsis	the presence in tissues of harmful bacteria and their toxins, typically through infection of a wound
Septicemia	blood poisoning, especially that caused by bacteria or their toxins
Sequential compression device	used in patients who are on bed rest or immobile because of an illness, injury, or surgery to prevent developing deep vein thrombosis (DVT)
Somatic	of or relating to the body. Also, of or relating to the body wall
Spatulate	make the edge of ureter wider at the tip by incising it
Spinal needle	a needle, provided with a stylet, for entering the inside of an obstructed or normal space with a bore of at least 1 mm and 40 mm or more in length. This type of needle has a variety of applications in different interventions
Sulfamethoxazole/trimethoprim	an antibiotic used to treat a variety of bacterial infections usually called sulfa drug
Suprapubic	from the Latin "supra", meaning above, and "pubis", meaning the front bone of the pelvis

T

T1	in staging of urinary tract transitional cell cancer, tumor has spread to the subepithelial connective tissue but does not involve the bladder wall muscle (lamina propria, the tissue below the inside lining of the bladder)
T2	in staging of urinary tract transitional cell cancer, tumor has spread to the muscle of the bladder wall
T2a	in staging of urinary tract transitional cell cancer, tumor has spread to the inner half of the muscle of the bladder wall, which may be called the superficial muscle
T2b	in staging of urinary tract transitional (urothelial) cell cancer, tumor has spread to the deep muscle of the bladder (the outer half of the muscle)
T3	in staging of urinary tract transitional cell cancer, tumor has grown into the perivesical tissue (the fatty tissue that surrounds the bladder)

T3a	in staging of urinary tract transitional cell cancer, tumor has grown into the perivesical tissue, as seen through a microscope
T3b	In staging of urinary tract transitional cell cancer, tumor has grown into the perivesical tissue macroscopically, meaning that the tumor(s) is large enough to be seen during imaging tests or to be seen or felt by the surgeon
T4	in staging of urinary tract transitional cell cancer, tumor has spread to any of the following: the abdominal wall, the pelvic wall, a man's prostate or seminal vesicle (the tube(s) that carry semen), or a woman's uterus or vagina
Ta	In staging of urinary tract transitional cell cancer, refers to noninvasive papillary carcinoma
TCC	see Transitional Cell Carcinoma
Tegaderm	a transparent medical dressing manufactured by 3 M. Tegaderm transparent dressings can be used to cover and protect wounds and catheter sites
Tetraploid	(of a cell or nucleus) containing four homologous sets of chromosomes i.e. two times more than normal cells
Thio- Tepa	A sulfur-containing analog of tepa, used in the treatment of certain malignant diseases such as leukemia, lymphoma, and carcinoma
Thoracoabdominal	of, relating to, involving, or affecting the chest and the abdomen
Thromboprophylaxis	a measure taken to prevent the development of blood clot
Trabeculated	thick walled and hypertrophied muscle bundles in bladder, typically seen in instances of chronic obstruction
Transitional Cell Carcinoma (TCC)	also urothelial cell carcinoma or UCC is a type of cancer that typically occurs in the urinary system: the kidney, urinary bladder, and accessory organs. It is the most common type of bladder cancer and cancer of the ureter, urethra, and urachus
Transurethral resection of bladder tumor (TURBT)	a surgical procedure that is used both to diagnose bladder cancer and to remove cancerous tissue from the bladder
Transvesical	passing through or performed by way of the urinary bladder
Trocar	a surgical instrument with a three-sided cutting point enclosed in a tube, used for withdrawing fluid from or entry to a body cavity for surgical reasons
Tumoricidal	destroying tumor cells

U

UCC	see Transitional Cell Carcinoma
UPJ	junction between renal pelvis and the proximal ureter

Upper urinary tract urothelial carcinoma (UTUC)	Tumors of the renal calyces, renal pelvis and ureters start in the layer of tissue that lines the bladder and the upper urinary tract, called the urothelium. Cancer that starts in the urothelium is called urothelial (or transitional cell) cancer. This is the most common type of cancer found in the bladder as well
Ureter	the duct by which urine passes from the kidney to the bladder
Ureteral Catheter	a long, small gauge catheter designed for insertion directly into a ureter, either through the urethra and bladder or posteriorly via the kidney
Ureteral orifice	the opening of the ureter in the bladder situated one at each lateral angle of the trigone; wide ostium usually indicates vesicoureteral reflux
Ureteritis cystica	benign inflammatory reaction of the urothelium to infection or mechanical irritation
Ureteral stricture	a narrowing in ureteral lumen
Ureteroneocystostomy	reimplantation of the ureter into the bladder
Ureteroscope	a tube-like instrument with: a light and lens or camera chip at its tip for examining the inside of the ureter and renal pelvis
Ureteroscopy	an examination or procedure using a ureteroscope performing variety of diagnostic or curative procedures
Urethra	the duct by which urine is transported out of the body from the bladder, and which in male also transports semen
Urinary diversion	any one of several surgical procedures to reroute urine flow from its normal pathway. It may be necessary for diseased or defective ureters, bladder or urethra, either temporarily or permanently. Some diversions result in a stoma
Urine Cytology	a test to look for abnormal cancerous cells in urine
Urinoma	collection of urine outside the urinary tract
Urothelial Cell Carcinoma	see Transitional Cell Carcinoma
Urothelium	an example of "transitional epithelium". It is the type of epithelium that lines much of the urinary tract including the renal pelvis, the ureters, the bladder, and parts of the urethra
URS	see ureteroscopy
UTUC	see Upper urinary tract urothelial carcinoma

V

Vesicoureteral Reflux	the backward flow of urine from the bladder into the kidneys
Virtual Endoscopy	an imaging technique in which cross-sectional images acquired by computed

tomography or magnetic resonance imaging are processed by computer to reconstruct a three-dimensional display similar to that seen through an endoscope

Voiding urination

Voxel a value on a regular grid in three-dimensional space

VUR see Vesicoureteral Reflux

W

Weck ligaSure a multifunctional tissue sealing system, featuring an integrated cutting mechanism for use in open and endoscopic

X

Xyphoid process a small cartilaginous process (extension) of the lower part of the sternum, which is usually ossified in the adult human

Y

Yag yag laser a form of laser for tissue ablation

Z

Zygote the cell resulting from the union of an ovum (female egg) and a spermatozom (male sperm)

Appendix B: Product and Manufacturer Information

Ali Fathollahi

Throughout this book, the authors mention or refer to several medical products and manufacturers. This is by no means an endorsement or considered promoting these products, rather mere reflection of authors' preference, availability of products at their institute and their routines. The editor did not require disclosures from the authors in regards to their relations with the manufacturers and industry.

The following list, though not comprehensive, was created to help the practicing physicians, to have access to some of the products mentioned in this textbook through their manufacturers.

- **Richard Wolf Medical Instruments Corporation**
  353 Corporate Woods Parkway
  Vernon Hills, Illinois 60061
- **UROVISION GmbH**
  Medi-Globe-Str. 1–5
  83101 Achenmühle—Germany
- **COOK MEDICAL INC.**
  P.O. Box 4195
  Bloomington, IN 47402-4195
  U.S.A.
- **BOSTON SCIENTIFIC**
  300 Boston Scientific Way.
  Marlborough, MA 01752-1234
- **Coloplast US** Headquarters
  1601 West River Road North
  Minneapolis, MN 55411
- **KARL STORZ Endoscopy-America, Inc.**
  2151 E. Grand Avenue,
  EL Segundo, CA 90245-5017
- **COBRA ENGINEERING**
  23801 E. La Palma Avenue
  Yorba Linda, CA 92887
- **Olympus America Inc.**
  3500 Corporate Parkway
  P.O. Box 610
  Center Valley, PA
- **Greenwald Surgical Co., Inc.**
  2688 DeKalb Street
  Lake Station, IN 46405-1519
- DELTA MEDIX PC LOCATIONS
  503 Sunset Drive
  Dickson City, PA 18519
- **Lumenis Ltd.**
  Yokneam Industrial Park
  Hakidma 6
  P.O.B. # 240
  Yokneam 2069204
  Israel
- **Intuitive Surgical, Inc.**
  1020 Kifer Road
  Sunnyvale, CA 94086-5304
- **COVIDIEN, Medtronic**
  710 Medtronic Parkway
  Minneapolis, MN 55432-5604
- **Teleflex**
  3015 Carrington Mill Boulevard
  Morrisville, NC 27560

M. Eshghi (ed.), *Urothelial Malignancies of the Upper Urinary Tract*,
https://doi.org/10.1007/978-3-319-51263-1

- **Ethicon US, LLC.**
  Route 22 West
  Somerville, NJ 08876
  4545 Creek Road
  Cincinnati, OH 45242
- **PHOTOCURE INC**
  104 Carnegie Center
  Suite 303
  Princeton, NJ 08540
  USA

Index

Note: Page numbers followed by *f* and *t* indicate figures and tables respectively

M. Eshghi (ed.), *Urothelial Malignancies of the Upper Urinary Tract*,
https://doi.org/10.1007/978-3-319-51263-1

L

M

N

FSC
www.fsc.org
MIX
Papier | Fördert
gute Waldnutzung
FSC® C083411

Kolibri 360 GmbH
Ferdinand-Jühlke-Straße 7
99095 Erfurt, Deutschland
produktsicherheit@kolibri360.de